3D Printing of Pharmaceuticals and Drug Delivery Devices

3D Printing of Pharmaceuticals and Drug Delivery Devices

Special Issue Editor
Dimitrios A. Lamprou

MDPI • Basel • Beijing • Wuhan • Barcelona • Belgrade • Manchester • Tokyo • Cluj • Tianjin

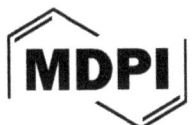

Special Issue Editor
Dimitrios A. Lamprou
Queen's University Belfast
UK

Editorial Office
MDPI
St. Alban-Anlage 66
4052 Basel, Switzerland

This is a reprint of articles from the Special Issue published online in the open access journal *Pharmaceutics* (ISSN 1999-4923) (available at: https://www.mdpi.com/journal/pharmaceutics/special_issues/3D_Printing_Pharmaceutics).

For citation purposes, cite each article independently as indicated on the article page online and as indicated below:

LastName, A.A.; LastName, B.B.; LastName, C.C. Article Title. *Journal Name* **Year**, *Article Number*, Page Range.

ISBN 978-3-03936-423-7 (Hbk)
ISBN 978-3-03936-424-4 (PDF)

Cover image courtesy of Loreto Valenzuela.

© 2020 by the authors. Articles in this book are Open Access and distributed under the Creative Commons Attribution (CC BY) license, which allows users to download, copy and build upon published articles, as long as the author and publisher are properly credited, which ensures maximum dissemination and a wider impact of our publications.

The book as a whole is distributed by MDPI under the terms and conditions of the Creative Commons license CC BY-NC-ND.

Contents

About the Special Issue Editor ix

Essyrose Mathew, Giulia Pitzanti, Eneko Larrañeta and Dimitrios A. Lamprou
3D Printing of Pharmaceuticals and Drug Delivery Devices
Reprinted from: *Pharmaceutics* 2020, 12, 266, doi:10.3390/pharmaceutics12030266 1

Sarah A. Stewart, Juan Domínguez-Robles, Victoria J. McIlorum, Elena Mancuso, Dimitrios A. Lamprou, Ryan F. Donnelly and Eneko Larrañeta
Development of a Biodegradable Subcutaneous Implant for Prolonged Drug Delivery Using 3D Printing
Reprinted from: *Pharmaceutics* 2020, 12, 105, doi:10.3390/pharmaceutics12020105 11

Bhupendra Raj Giri, Eon Soo Song, Jaewook Kwon, Ju-Hyun Lee, Jun-Bom Park and Dong Wuk Kim
Fabrication of Intragastric Floating, Controlled Release 3D Printed Theophylline Tablets Using Hot-Melt Extrusion and Fused Deposition Modeling
Reprinted from: *Pharmaceutics* 2020, 12, 77, doi:10.3390/pharmaceutics12010077 27

Shrawani Lamichhane, Jun-Bom Park, Dong Hwan Sohn and Sangkil Lee
Customized Novel Design of 3D Printed Pregabalin Tablets for Intra-Gastric Floating and Controlled Release Using Fused Deposition Modeling
Reprinted from: *Pharmaceutics* 2019, 11, 564, doi:10.3390/pharmaceutics11110564 43

Nagi Reddy Dumpa, Suresh Bandari and Michael A. Repka
Novel Gastroretentive Floating Pulsatile Drug Delivery System Produced via Hot-Melt Extrusion and Fused Deposition Modeling 3D Printing
Reprinted from: *Pharmaceutics* 2020, 12, 52, doi:10.3390/pharmaceutics12010052 57

Suet Li Chew, Laura Modica de Mohac and Bahijja Tolulope Raimi-Abraham
3D-Printed Solid Dispersion Drug Products
Reprinted from: *Pharmaceutics* 2019, 11, 672, doi:10.3390/pharmaceutics11120672 71

Petra Arany, Eszter Róka, Laurent Mollet, Anthony W. Coleman, Florent Perret, Beomjoon Kim, Renátó Kovács, Adrienn Kazsoki, Romána Zelkó, Rudolf Gesztelyi, Zoltán Ujhelyi, Pálma Fehér, Judit Váradi, Ferenc Fenyvesi, Miklós Vecsernyés and Ildikó Bácskay
Fused Deposition Modeling 3D Printing: Test Platforms for Evaluating Post-Fabrication Chemical Modifications and In-Vitro Biological Properties
Reprinted from: *Pharmaceutics* 2019, 11, 277, doi:10.3390/pharmaceutics11060277 83

Juan Domínguez-Robles, Niamh K. Martin, Mun Leon Fong, Sarah A. Stewart, Nicola J. Irwin, María Isabel Rial-Hermida, Ryan F. Donnelly and Eneko Larrañeta
Antioxidant PLA Composites Containing Lignin for 3D Printing Applications: A Potential Material for Healthcare Applications
Reprinted from: *Pharmaceutics* 2019, 11, 165, doi:10.3390/pharmaceutics11040165 107

Juan Domínguez-Robles, Caterina Mancinelli, Elena Mancuso, Inmaculada García-Romero, Brendan F. Gilmore, Luca Casettari, Eneko Larrañeta and Dimitrios A. Lamprou
3D Printing of Drug-Loaded Thermoplastic Polyurethane Meshes: A Potential Material for Soft Tissue Reinforcement in Vaginal Surgery
Reprinted from: *Pharmaceutics* 2020, 12, 63, doi:10.3390/pharmaceutics12010063 121

Marius Tidau, Arno Kwade and Jan Henrik Finke
Influence of High, Disperse API Load on Properties along the Fused-Layer Modeling Process Chain of Solid Dosage Forms
Reprinted from: *Pharmaceutics* **2019**, *11*, 194, doi:10.3390/pharmaceutics11040194 137

Muqdad Alhijjaj, Jehad Nasereddin, Peter Belton and Sheng Qi
Impact of Processing Parameters on the Quality of Pharmaceutical Solid Dosage Forms Produced by Fused Deposition Modeling (FDM)
Reprinted from: *Pharmaceutics* **2019**, *11*, 633, doi:10.3390/pharmaceutics11120633 155

Pariksha Jolene Kondiah, Pierre P. D. Kondiah, Yahya E. Choonara, Thashree Marimuthu and Viness Pillay
A 3D Bioprinted Pseudo-Bone Drug Delivery Scaffold for Bone Tissue Engineering
Reprinted from: *Pharmaceutics* **2020**, *12*, 166, doi:10.3390/pharmaceutics12020166 177

Eleftherios G. Andriotis, Georgios K. Eleftheriadis, Christina Karavasili and Dimitrios G. Fatouros
Development of Bio-Active Patches Based on Pectin for the Treatment of Ulcers and Wounds Using 3D-Bioprinting Technology
Reprinted from: *Pharmaceutics* **2020**, *12*, 56, doi:10.3390/pharmaceutics12010056 195

Andrew V. Healy, Evert Fuenmayor, Patrick Doran, Luke M. Geever, Clement L. Higginbotham and John G. Lyons
Additive Manufacturing of Personalized Pharmaceutical Dosage Forms via Stereolithography
Reprinted from: *Pharmaceutics* **2019**, *11*, 645, doi:10.3390/pharmaceutics11120645 219

Pamela Robles-Martinez, Xiaoyan Xu, Sarah J. Trenfield, Atheer Awad, Alvaro Goyanes, Richard Telford, Abdul W. Basit and Simon Gaisford
3D Printing of a Multi-Layered Polypill Containing Six Drugs Using a Novel Stereolithographic Method
Reprinted from: *Pharmaceutics* **2019**, *11*, 274, doi:10.3390/pharmaceutics11060274 239

Atheer Awad, Fabrizio Fina, Sarah J. Trenfield, Pavanesh Patel, Alvaro Goyanes, Simon Gaisford and Abdul W. Basit
3D Printed Pellets (Miniprintlets): A Novel, Multi-Drug, Controlled Release Platform Technology
Reprinted from: *Pharmaceutics* **2019**, *11*, 148, doi:10.3390/pharmaceutics11040148 255

Marijana Madzarevic, Djordje Medarevic, Aleksandra Vulovic, Tijana Sustersic, Jelena Djuris, Nenad Filipovic and Svetlana Ibric
Optimization and Prediction of Ibuprofen Release from 3D DLP Printlets Using Artificial Neural Networks
Reprinted from: *Pharmaceutics* **2019**, *11*, 544, doi:10.3390/pharmaceutics11100544 273

Henrika Wickström, Rajesh Koppolu, Ermei Mäkilä, Martti Toivakka and Niklas Sandler
Stencil Printing—A Novel Manufacturing Platform for Orodispersible Discs
Reprinted from: *Pharmaceutics* **2020**, *12*, 33, doi:10.3390/pharmaceutics12010033 289

Katarzyna Rycerz, Krzysztof Adam Stepien, Marta Czapiewska, Basel T. Arafat, Rober Habashy, Abdullah Isreb, Matthew Peak and Mohamed A. Alhnan
Embedded 3D Printing of Novel Bespoke Soft Dosage Form Concept for Pediatrics
Reprinted from: *Pharmaceutics* **2019**, *11*, 630, doi:10.3390/pharmaceutics11120630 305

Heidi Öblom, Erica Sjöholm, Maria Rautamo and Niklas Sandler
Towards Printed Pediatric Medicines in Hospital Pharmacies: Comparison of 2D and 3D-Printed Orodispersible Warfarin Films with Conventional Oral Powders in Unit Dose Sachets
Reprinted from: *Pharmaceutics* **2019**, *11*, 334, doi:10.3390/pharmaceutics11070334 . . . . **321**

Mohammad A. Azad, Deborah Olawuni, Georgia Kimbell, Abu Zayed Md Badruddoza, Md. Shahadat Hossain and Tasnim Sultana
Polymers for Extrusion-Based 3D Printing of Pharmaceuticals: A Holistic Materials–Process Perspective
Reprinted from: *Pharmaceutics* **2020**, *12*, 124, doi:10.3390/pharmaceutics12020124 . . . . **355**

Andrew Kjar and Yu Huang
Application of Micro-Scale 3D Printing in Pharmaceutics
Reprinted from: *Pharmaceutics* **2019**, *11*, 390, doi:10.3390/pharmaceutics11080390 . . . . **389**

Maisa R. P. Araújo, Livia L. Sa-Barreto, Tais Gratieri, Guilherme M. Gelfuso and Marcilio Cunha-Filho
The Digital Pharmacies Era: How 3D Printing Technology Using Fused Deposition Modeling Can Become a Reality
Reprinted from: *Pharmaceutics* **2019**, *11*, 128, doi:10.3390/pharmaceutics11030128 . . . . **411**

About the Special Issue Editor

Dimitrios A. Lamprou (Ph.D., MBA) is a Reader in Pharmaceutical Engineering and the MSc Programme Director at the School of Pharmacy of Queen's University Belfast (UK). Dimitrios has authored 80+ articles, 200+ conference abstracts and over 90 Oral/Invited presentations, and has secured over £2M of research funding. His research and academic leadership have been recognized by a range of awards, including the Royal Pharmaceutical Society (RPS) Science Award and the Scottish Universities Life Sciences Alliance (SULSA) Leaders Scheme Award. He is Chair of the United Kingdom and Ireland Controlled Release Society (UKICRS), Associate Editor for Heliyon (the Drug Delivery, Pharmaceutical Science, Pharmacology and Toxicology section) and Guest Editor of over 10 Special Issues in international refereed journals. His group is applying nano and microfabrication techniques in pharmaceutical and medical device manufacturing. The nano/microfabrication facility contains 5 microfluidic systems, 4 electrospinners (melt and solution), 12+ 3D printers covering all available types on the market, and other advanced characterization technologies.

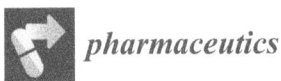

Editorial

3D Printing of Pharmaceuticals and Drug Delivery Devices

Essyrose Mathew [1], Giulia Pitzanti [1,2], Eneko Larrañeta [1] and Dimitrios A. Lamprou [1,*]

1. School of Pharmacy, Queen's University Belfast, 97 Lisburn Road, Belfast BT9 7BL, UK; emathew01@qub.ac.uk (E.M.); e.larraneta@qub.ac.uk (E.L.)
2. Department of Life and Environmental Sciences (Unit of Drug Sciences), University of Cagliari, 09124 Cagliari, Italy; giulia.pitzanti@unica.it
* Correspondence: d.lamprou@qub.ac.uk; Tel.: +44-(0)28-9097-2617

Received: 12 March 2020; Accepted: 13 March 2020; Published: 15 March 2020

Abstract: The process of 3D printing (3DP) was patented in 1986; however, the research in the field of 3DP did not become popular until the last decade. There has been an increasing research into the areas of 3DP for medical applications for fabricating prosthetics, bioprinting and pharmaceutics. This novel method allows the manufacture of dosage forms on demand, with modifications in the geometry and size resulting in changes to the release and dosage behaviour of the product. 3DP will allow wider adoption of personalised medicine due to the diversity and simplicity to change the design and dosage of the products, allowing the devices to be designed specific to the individual with the ability to alternate the drugs added to the product. Personalisation also has the potential to decrease the common side effects associated with generic dosage forms. This Special Issue Editorial outlines the current innovative research surrounding the topic of 3DP, focusing on bioprinting and various types of 3DP on applications for drug delivery as well advantages and future directions in this field of research.

Keywords: 3D printing; bioprinting; additive manufacturing; computer-aided design (CAD); drug delivery; personalized medicine; pharmaceutics

---

1. Introduction

Three-dimensional printing (3DP) has become one of the most innovative technologies in the pharmaceutical field. Within the last decade, there has been a significant expansion in the manufacture of drug delivery and medical devices. Additive manufacturing (AM) includes a variety of processes in which a layer-by-layer process is used to fabricate a solid object. The 3DP techniques, which can be used in the pharmaceutical field and are also covered under this editorial include Stereolithography (SLA), Selective Laser Sintering (SLS), inkjet-based 3DP, extrusion-based Fused Deposition Modeling (FDM) and Bioprinting. 3DP allows the potential for printing dosage forms on demand, with low cost and ease of use. AM is leading towards personalised medicine as the dosing and release characteristics of the drug delivery devices can be easily changed by altering the geometries of the 3D design using computer-aided design (CAD). The research outlined below and in this Special Issue addresses the current areas of research in bioprinting and 3D printing of drug delivery systems, focusing on the advantages and future directions in the use of AM in the pharmaceutical industry.

2. Fused Deposition Modelling (FDM)

FDM is one of the most commonly explored additive manufacturing methods due to the low cost of printers, print quality and ability to use drug-loaded filaments through hot-melt extrusion (HME). In this issue, the most common way of incorporating drug into the system was by creating drug-loaded filament created through HME with Chew et al. being the only exception, choosing to soak the polymer filaments in a drug-loaded solution. The articles within the Special Issue that used the FDM method of printing are outlined in this section.

Current implants are made with non-biodegradable polymers, which require surgical removal from the body after use. 3DP allows tailored dosage forms to be created specific to the patient and their condition, using biodegradable polymers, which can be broken down in the body into products that can be easily excreted. Dimensions of already marketed implants were used to create the hollow 3DP implants using filaments made from HME. Polylactic acid (PLA) and Poly(vinyl alcohol) (PVA) filaments were used to print hollow implants with a PVA window. Implants were loaded with a model compound by directly packing the powder inside. After in vitro testing, the implants showed the potential to adapt the dosage forms according to the material and implant designs used. Additional modification of the implant design with coatings was also explored in this paper by Stewart et al., showing the potential to extend the release profiles of the implants. The simplicity of the method outlined above allows the potential for easy set up within a clinical setting so such drug delivery devices can be printed on demand [1].

Giri et al. presented a novel approach to the fabrication of gastro-retentive floating tablets (GRFT) by using HME in order to create drug-loaded filaments that can be used on an FDM printer to create 3D printed tablets. GRFT has the ability to stay above the normal gastric content of the stomach for a prolonged period of time allowing them to overcome common issues with oral dosage forms such as unpredictable gastrointestinal transit and emptying times and metabolic degradation. Theophylline was used along with hydroxypropyl cellulose (HPC) matrix to create drug-loaded filaments using HME. Tablets with varying infill densities and shell thicknesses were created. The resulting tablets were assessed by determined the drug content, dissolution rates, physiochemical properties and floating behaviour. The developed FDM printed GRFTs possessed buoyancy for 10 h and had zero-order release kinetics. Overall, the 3DP tablets had better controlled release rates in comparison to current pharmaceutical manufactured tablets. This study highlights the potential for HME coupled with 3D printing to produce effective oral dosage forms of GRFTs providing greater versatility and a simplified manufacturing method in comparison to conventional methods [2].

Lamichhane et al. used FDM printing technology to develop floating gastro-retentive tablets with controlled release properties. The polymers used to create the pregabalin-loaded filaments were hypromellose acetate succinate (HPMCAS) and polyethylene glycol (PEG 400). FDM was used to create cylindrical tablets with varying infill densities. Differential scanning calorimetry (DSC), Fourier-transform infrared (FTIR) spectroscopy, X-ray powder diffraction (XRPD), and thermogravimetric analysis (TGA) were used to evaluate the properties of the resulting tablets, showing that extrusion and printing process does not affect drug stability and crystallinity. It was shown that the presence of a top/bottom layer determined the floating capabilities of the printed tablets. In particular, closed systems retain the buoyancy for >24 h, open systems, on the contrary, failed to float. Moreover, open systems with a low infill percentage showed a faster drug release compared to open and closed systems with a high infill ratio. Thus, they optimised the formulation designing a tablet with a closed bottom layer and a partially opened top layer. This formulation showed a zero-order drug release and retained its floating ability for 24 h. This study showed that FDM printing technology is a suitable technology for the development of floating gastro-retentive tablets [3].

HME was used to also create HPC and ethyl cellulose-based filaments, which were used as a feedstock for printing the shells using FDM. Directly compressed theophylline tablets were used as the core. Theophylline is used for the treatment of symptomatic treatment of chronic asthma. The aim was to develop a tablet with floating capabilities as well as the ability to have pulsatile release after the relative lag time to be able to improve the therapy for patients with asthma. The FDM printed shells varied in shell thickness, infill density and wall thickness. All of the geometries of printed core-shell tablets showed good floating capabilities with no lag time as well as good dissolution properties. This meant that lag time could be varied from 30 min to 6 h according to the requirement.

The proportion of EC in the formulation had a significant effect on the floating lag time. The proposed floating pulsatile system showed promise for effective delivery of drugs that require a high residence time in the stomach. This method of drug delivery minimises adverse effects and can increase patient compliance. This method of printing also allows the use of thermolabile drugs to be delivered through this system, as the inner core is not directly exposed to the high temperatures of FDM printing [4].

Chew et al. used 5-aminosalicyclic acid (5-ASA) and fluorescein sodium (FS) to create fixed dose combination solid dispersion drug products. The drugs were impregnated into PVA filament by soaking the filament in a drug solvent mixture for 24 h, the filament was then heated to achieve rapid solvent evaporation. The influence of the use of different solvents during drug loading was also studied in order to understand the optimal drug loading as well as the mechanical and physiochemical properties of the filaments prior to printing the drug using FDM 3D printing. The results showed that the drug loading could be improved up to 3 times according to the choice of solvent due to its polarity. In this paper, it was proven that methanol (MeOH) had better properties as the solvent in comparison to ethanol (EtOH) for FS and 5-ASA. The resultant 3DP product using both drugs were solid dispersion fixed dose combination with favourable release profiles and behaviours [5].

Arany et al., produced cylindrical plates to test chemical, physical, mechanical and biological properties of 3DP materials. The plates were developed through FDM 3DP technology. First, PLA plates were printed and then the PLA plates were chemically modified with the addition of positive charged groups in order to decrease their lipophilicity. The material was characterised to assess the effective surface modification and the increased hydrophilicity. The MTT assay performed in Caco-2 cells demonstrated the cytocompatibility of the material. Moreover, the 3D printed plates showed an antifungal activity against Candida albicans. This work put the basis for further studies in the chemical functionalization of 3D printed materials [6].

Domínguez-Robles et al., used HME to develop antioxidant PLA filaments containing Lignin (LIG). In addition, tetracycline (TC), which has known antibiotic and antioxidant capabilities, was combined with PLA and LIG. The addition of LIG leaded to a filament with lower resistance to fracture. Moreover, as the LIG content was increased the materials showed a reduction in their wettability properties. The 2,2-diphenyl-1-picrylhydrazyl (DPPH) assay showed the antioxidant properties of the PLA filament containing LIG. The antimicrobial properties of the material were examined through bacterial adhesion studies performed on *S. aureus*. The addition of only LIG did not confer any antimicrobial properties to the material but the further addition of TC significant redacted the bacterial adherence. PLA-LIG filament was used to develop meshes for wound healing applications. Curcumin (CUR) was selected as a model drug and applied on the top of the mesh. The permeation studies showed that the grid size of the mesh affects the release rate of CUR. Small size leaded to a slower release. The combination of the mesh with a soluble PVA film further delayed the release rate. Accordingly to this study, PLA-LIG filament can be used to print personalised meshes for wound dressing applications [7].

Pelvic Organ Prolapse (POP) and stress urinary incontinence (SI) are currently treated with surgical implantation of vaginal meshes, with these conditions affecting 30–40% of women worldwide. These mesh reinforcements are often made from poly(propylene) (PP) or polyester, which have been approved by the Food and Drug Administration (FDA) for vaginal applications. However, since their approval there has been an increased number of complications associated with vaginal meshes, some of which include chronic pain, infection and high inflammatory response. Domínguez-Robles et al., proposed the use of an alternative material for these meshes, the Thermoplastic polyurethane (TPU), which is more flexible in nature. FDM was used to print meshes using Levofloxacin (LFX) loaded TPU filaments created using HME. The printed meshes were characterised using fracture force studies, FTIR, SEM, X-ray microcomputed tomography (μCT), release studies and bacterial testing. The μCT showed the LFX was evenly distributed throughout the TPU matrix at all the concentrations of drug used. Mechanical testing also revealed that the currently used PP is more rigid in nature compared to TPU and therefore, TPU is more suitable for vaginal meshes due to its elasticity. The printed TPU meshes also showed significant bacteriostatic activity against both *Staphylococcus aureus* and *Escherichia coli* cultures meaning infection rates associated with vaginal meshes could be reduced. This study effectively showed the use of 3DP as a novel approach for producing anti-infective drug loaded vaginal meshes with better mechanical properties in comparison to the PP meshes that currently being used [8].

Tidau et al., developed high-loaded theophylline filaments using a co-rotating twin-screw extruder. The polymers selected were polyethylene oxide and hypromellose (HPMC). Afterwards, the filaments were utilised to develop tablets of three different geometries (cylinders, rings and spheres) with fused layer modeling (FLM). The size and the morphology of the particles of the raw material were investigated. The filaments and the dosage forms were characterised in terms of mechanical properties, surface morphology, mass and content uniformity. A dissolution test was performed in order to evaluate the release rate of theophylline from the different dosage forms. The results showed that for HPMC in particular the larger load of theophylline resulted in increased flexural strength; however, the accuracy of the printing process decreased resulting in defects in the microstructure. No significant effect on the dissolution profiles was observed by increasing the load of theophylline. The work highlights how the amount of API used influence the 3DP process [9].

Alhijjaj et al., highlighted the need for a greater understanding of the process parameters of AM required for the development of 3DP from a group of proof of concept studies to an advanced tool used in the manufacture of pharmaceuticals. In this study, the processing parameters of FDM printing were explored. The macroscopic and microstructural reproducibility of the FDM process was examined, showing that the prints poorly matched the target dimensions, an issue that was also highlighted by Healy et al., in the SLA printing process. Weights of the printed grids was also another area that was highlighted in this study, with the weights varying according to print speed. The temperature of the print however, showed to have little effect on the print weight. A principal component analysis showed that there is an interaction between the accuracy of the weight and/or dosing and the dimensional authenticity, indicating the need for a compromise between these quality parameters. Summed Standard Deviation (SSD) was used as measure of the goodness of printing conditions, which can produce the best overall printing reproducibility, which was calculated by adding together all the standard deviations of each measured value for every condition with the lowest SSD value showing the most reproducible prints. In this study, the processing parameters of 120 °C and 90 mm/s had the lowest SSD, indicating that these were the parameters with the most reproducible prints [10].

3. Three-Dimensional Bioprinting

Three-dimensional bioprinting, includes all the variety of 3DP modes and is been used in different pharmaceutical studies and tissue engineering. Current treatments for bone fractures and bone defects involve bone grafts or metal prosthetic implants, which can be restrictive because of the substantial loss of tissue from surgery, prolonged recovery periods and donor site morbidity. Therefore, there is a need for a novel method of treatment for bone fractures and defects. Kondiah et al., explored 3D bio-printed pseudo-bone drug delivery scaffolds that have been fabricated from polypropylene fumarate (PPF), free radical polymerised polyethylene glycol-polycaprolactone (PEG-PCL-PEG) and Pluronic (PF127). The scaffolds were optimised using MATLAB software and artificial neural networks (ANN) with the ANN optimised scaffolds showing controlled release of Simvastatin for over 20 days. Simvastatin was incorporated into the scaffold due to its abilities to promote bone healing and repair. The bio-printed scaffolds were tested on fracture-induced human clavicle bones. The matrix analysis showed that after the application of the scaffolds, the fractured bone had similar matrix hardness and matrix resilience to healthy human clavicle bones. This highlights the potential for bioprinted pseudo bone scaffolds to fill in fracture sites, resulting in great adhesion of the fractured bone and restoration to intended mechanical strength [11].

Andriotis et al. developed a 3D bioprinted wound dressing using pectin-based bio ink. The properties of the pectin bioinks were optimised by the addition of chitosan and cyclodextrin inclusion complexes with propolis extract to improve the antimicrobial and wound healing properties of the inks. The inks were able to form transparent films when dried and exhibited fast disintegration upon contact with aqueous media. The in vitro wound healing studies showed that the addition of cyclodextrin/propolis extract inclusion complexes (CCP) enhanced wound healing as well as the antimicrobial properties of the patches, with a 95% increase in antimicrobial activity of the films. Addition of CCP up to a certain point also enhanced the bio-adhesive properties of the dressing. However, in higher concentrations of CCP, the cell viability was reduced >10% w/w. This may have been due to the presence of insoluble film material in the higher concentrations of CPP, which could physically obstruct the cells. Overall, this study was able to effectively show the potential for use of biodegradable, 3D printable inks for fabrication of direct and indirect wound dressings [12].

4. Stereolithography (SLA)

Healy et al., used SLA as the AM process to create oral dosage forms of 2.5% and 5% concentration of aspirin and paracetamol. A novel photopolymerisable resin was used and drugs were printed using an SLA 3D printer. Healy et al., were able to fabricate 28 drug dosage forms in one print cycle, showing the potential for bulk manufacture of oral dosage forms through SLA. This study also highlighted the effect of addition of drug on the dimensions of the printed dosage forms, with the printed form dimensions being different to the design. This highlights an area, which requires research, in the future, on how addition of materials can affect the printed product. The results from release studies showed that there was an increased in release of active drug when drug loading was increased, this highlights the potential for patient specific drugs to be created with the ability to modulate drug release. Overall, this study effectively highlighted the potential for creating solid dosage forms using SLA printing, with the research leading towards the ability to create personalised medication and the ability to modulate drug release from printed products [13].

Robles-Martinez et al., were able to construct a novel SLA printing method that allowed the production of multi-layered tablets (polypills) that had flexible drug content and shape. The drugs chosen for the work were paracetamol, caffeine, naproxen, chloramphenicol, prednisolone and aspirin. Three different tablets shapes were printed: cylinder, ring, and ring with a soluble filler. Raman microscopy confirmed the spatial separation of the drugs but also showed the ability of certain drugs (naproxen, aspirin, and paracetamol) to diffuse between the layers due to its solid-state characteristics. Dissolution tests showed that the polypill geometry and the type of excipient affected the drug release allowing distinct release profiles for each of the six drugs. This study showed the possibility to use SLA 3DP for fabricating multi-drugs tablets to improve personalisation for patients [14].

5. Other forms of Additive Manufacture

5.1. Selective Laser Sintering (SLS)

Similarly to SLA, this method of AM works with lasers but powder materials are fused together, whereas SLA works with a resin. Awad et al., utilised SLS 3DP, for the first time, to produce small oral dosage forms with modified release properties. They fabricated single miniprintlets using paracetamol as a model drug and dual miniprintlets where paracetamol is combined with ibuprofen. For the single miniprintlets, ethyl cellulose (EC) was employed as the main polymer matrix. In the case of dual miniprintlets one layer contained EC for sustained release whereas the second layer containing Kollicoat IR (a graft copolymer comprised of PEG: PVA, 1:3) for immediate release. In order to assess the effect size has on dissolution properties, miniprintlets of two different diameters, 1 mm and 2 mm, were developed. The single miniprintlets exhibited slow paracetamol release, which was reduced when increasing the diameter. For the dual miniprintlets, the diameter does not affect the paracetamol release profile. This work demonstrates the possibility to use SLS 3D printing to combine multiple Active Pharmaceutical Ingredients (APIs) with distinct release properties in a single dosage form [15].

5.2. Digital Light Processing (DLP)

DLP is another method of 3DP, which is similar to SLA. Is a resin-based method, however, rather than using a laser-focused UV beam, DLP uses UV light from a projector to cure each layer of the 3D printed product. Madzarevic et al., prepared ibuprofen tablets through DLP 3DP technology. Eleven formulations were prepared following the D-optimal mixture design from Design Expert software. It was noticed that an increase of water content leads to an enhancement of printing time. Two artificial neural networks (STATISTICA 7.0 and MATLAB R2014b) were used in order to evaluate how the components and the printing parameters affect the ibuprofen release. The data obtained from these two software were compared with the one obtained experimentally. The drug release predicted with STATISTICA 7.0 was quite similar to the one obtained experimentally. This study described that suitable ANN allows to recognise the input–output relationship in DLP printing of pharmaceutics [16].

5.3. Stencil Printing

Wickstrom et al., propose a new method of printing that has not been used in the production of pharmaceuticals. This study aimed to evaluate the feasibility of creating drug containing polymer inks, which could be used in the manufacture of flexible dosage forms, with products having acceptable content of uniformity and mass. Haloperidol (HAL) discs were printed using a prototype stencil printer, with polyester used as the stencil material. The stencil geometry was used to define the dose, with doses being altered by changing aperture areas and stencil heights. The therapeutic HAL was successfully created for treatment of 6–17 year-old children that fulfilled both mass and content of uniformity requirements. HAL dose was achieved by using 16% hydroxypropyl methylcellulose (HPMC) and 1% of lactic acid. The results show that the drug was amorphous after printing and the pH remained above pH 4. Disintegration studies showed that the orodispersible discs printed showed disintegrations times below 30 s. Therefore, it was concluded that the novel method of batchwise stencil printing, could be used as a viable method for the production of pharmaceuticals [17].

5.4. Embedded 3D Printing (e-3DP)

Embedded 3D printing is a novel form of AM in which a viscoelastic ink is extruded into a solidifying reservoir using a deposition nozzle at a predefined path. Rycerz et al., presented one of the first examples in using e-3DP in the pharmaceutical field to fabricate chewable oral dosage forms with dual drug loading. The two drugs used were paracetamol and ibuprofen, which were suspended in locust gum solution and an embedding medium of a gelatin-based matrix material. These were printed at an elevated temperature of 70 °C and then solidify at room temperature. The dosing of the printed dosage forms were varied by specifically altering the printing patterns. The rheology, printing speed and the needle size of the embedded phase were examined. This proof of concept study showed the potential for e-3DP to be used to print oral dosage forms that could include various materials, allow personalised dosing and geometry for novel oral dosage forms in paediatrics [18].

5.5. Semisolid Extrusion Printing (EXT) and Inkjet Printing (IJP)

Öblom et al., compared the conventional manufacturing method to produce patient-tailored doses of the anticoagulant drug warfarin at Helsinki University Hospital (HUS) Pharmacy, Finland's largest hospital pharmacy, with two innovative printing techniques, named semisolid extrusion 3D printing (EXT) and inkjet printing (IJP). The printed orodispersible films (ODFs) showed a good thickness and flexibility and a better uniformity than the oral powders in unit dose sachets (OPSs). OPSs and ODFs remained stable for a period of one month and were appropriated for being given to the patients through a naso-gastric tube. In order to provide additional information about the dosage form and to reduce the errors that occur in the administration of medication a Quick Response (QR) code was printed onto the ODFs using IJP. The study demonstrated how printing technologies are promising techniques for the development of patient-specific dosage forms [19].

6. Critical Literature Reviews

This Special Issue also includes three review articles on the areas of FDM and 3DP as a whole. Azad et al., highlighted that is important to find out which polymers are appropriate for pharmaceuticals extrusion-based 3DP, focusing on FDM and pressure-assisted microsyringe (PAM). They also evaluated how the printing operations are affected by the material properties and by the comportment of the mixture of polymer and active component. They confronted 3DP with the current process of direct compression and evidenced the importance to know the rheological properties of the polymers and polymer–API mixture in order to predict their impact on the printing process and on the final dosage form. They also discussed which kind of characterisation methods are required for 3D printed structure, drug, polymer and other functional excipients. Finally, examined the challenges and opportunities related to pharmaceutical extrusion-based 3Dp [20].

The review of Kjar and Huang first described the different AM techniques and the resolution related to each technique described. They discussed the application of 3DP technology in the pharmaceutical field specific to micron sized manufacture. Finally, they highlighted the challenges and opportunities related to the use of AM in drug delivery and development with the main challenges outlined being gaining approval from regulatory authorities as well as changing from small- to large scale-manufacture of 3D printed products [21].

Araújo et al., aimed to present the possibility of turning current pharmacies into digital pharmacies with the ability to print dosage forms for patients on demand. The versatility of using FDM 3DP was explored, referring to HME as mentioned in previous papers using FDM, as an effective method for the addition of drugs allowing customizable dosage forms. Pharmaceutical companies will need to work in unison with these digital pharmacies for the large-scale production of extruded filaments, which the digital pharmacies can later use to print. The regulatory concerns surrounding 3DP were also evaluated showing that patents have hindered 3DP products from reaching the market and there should be greater cooperation between regulatory and patenting authorities to ensure that 3DP products can reach the market [22].

7. Conclusions/Future Directions

There is an increasing research using multiple types of 3DP. However, one of the main advantages common to all available types of 3DP is the ability to create personalised medicine. AM, due to its ease of use, speed and accessibility is increasingly promoting the creation of medical devices and pharmaceutical products on demand for patients within a clinical setting. The ability to change the release profile and dosing of a 3D printed tablet simply by changing the geometries using CAD and the ability to incorporate drugs into FDM printed injectable devices or mesh implants using HME, opens up a wide range of possibilities within the application of 3DP in the medical field.

However, more research does need to be conducted in the field before the production of 3D-printed products on demand can become a reality within a clinical setting, such as the effect of process parameters on the print quality and how reproducibility in 3DP can be improved. FDM is also limited to the number of drugs that can be loaded into filaments, as they need to withstand the high temperatures of the process. However, if research continues to rise in the area of 3DP, due to the versatility of 3D printed products and the number of manufacturing advantages that 3DP offers there is potential for more 3DP to leave the proof of concept stage and be developed into a widely used manufacturing tool.

The number of manuscripts published in this Special Issue focused on 3DP of oral dosage suggests an increasing interest in personalised medicine. Additionally, this Special Issue included several works describing the use of 3DP for other applications such as medical devices. Therefore, 3DP can be applied in a wide variety of fields within biomedical sciences. However, before this technology can be extensively applied for medical applications, multiple regulatory questions should be addressed. One of the main unanswered questions is the quality assurance if the dosage form/medical device is created on demand for each patient. In order to accelerate the acceptance of this technology, the US FDA published guideline documents for medical devices manufacturing using 3DP technology. Accordingly, we anticipate that more 3D printed pharmaceutical/medical products will reach to the market within the next few years.

Funding: This research received no external funding.

Conflicts of Interest: The authors declare no conflict of interest.

References

1. Stewart, S.A.; Domínguez-Robles, J.; McIlorum, V.J.; Mancuso, E.; Lamprou, D.A.; Donnelly, R.F.; Larrañeta, E. Development of a Biodegradable Subcutaneous Implant for Prolonged Drug Delivery Using 3D Printing. *Pharmaceutics* **2020**, *12*, 105. [CrossRef]
2. Giri, B.R.; Song, E.S.; Kwon, J.; Lee, J.-H.; Park, J.-B.; Kim, D.W. Fabrication of Intragastric Floating, Controlled Release 3D Printed Theophylline Tablets Using Hot-Melt Extrusion and Fused Deposition Modeling. *Pharmaceutics* **2020**, *12*, 77. [CrossRef]
3. Lamichhane, S.; Park, J.-B.; Sohn, D.H.; Lee, S. Customized Novel Design of 3D Printed Pregabalin Tablets for Intra-Gastric Floating and Controlled Release Using Fused Deposition Modeling. *Pharmaceutics* **2019**, *11*, 564. [CrossRef]
4. Reddy Dumpa, N.; Bandari, S.; A Repka, M. Novel Gastroretentive Floating Pulsatile Drug Delivery System Produced via Hot-Melt Extrusion and Fused Deposition Modeling 3D Printing. *Pharmaceutics* **2020**, *12*, 52. [CrossRef] [PubMed]
5. Chew, S.L.; Modica de Mohac, L.; Tolulope Raimi-Abraham, B. 3D-Printed Solid Dispersion Drug Products. *Pharmaceutics* **2019**, *11*, 672. [CrossRef] [PubMed]
6. Arany, P.; Róka, E.; Mollet, L.; Coleman, A.W.; Perret, F.; Kim, B.; Kovács, R.; Kazsoki, A.; Zelkó, R.; Gesztelyi, R. Fused Deposition Modeling 3D Printing: Test Platforms for Evaluating Post-Fabrication Chemical Modifications and In-Vitro Biological Properties. *Pharmaceutics* **2019**, *11*, 277. [CrossRef] [PubMed]
7. Domínguez-Robles, J.; Martin, N.K.; Fong, M.L.; Stewart, S.A.; Irwin, N.J.; Rial-Hermida, M.I.; Donnelly, R.F.; Larrañeta, E. Antioxidant PLA composites containing lignin for 3d printing applications: A potential material for healthcare applications. *Pharmaceutics* **2019**, *11*, 165.
8. Domínguez-Robles, J.; Mancinelli, C.; Mancuso, E.; García-Romero, I.; Gilmore, B.F.; Casettari, L.; Larrañeta, E.; Lamprou, D.A. 3D Printing of Drug-Loaded Thermoplastic Polyurethane Meshes: A Potential Material for Soft Tissue Reinforcement in Vaginal Surgery. *Pharmaceutics* **2020**, *12*, 63.
9. Tidau, M.; Kwade, A.; Finke, J.H. Influence of High, Disperse API Load on Properties along the Fused-Layer Modeling Process Chain of Solid Dosage Forms. *Pharmaceutics* **2019**, *11*, 194. [CrossRef]
10. Alhijjaj, M.; Nasereddin, J.; Belton, P.; Qi, S. Impact of Processing Parameters on the Quality of Pharmaceutical Solid Dosage Forms Produced by Fused Deposition Modeling (FDM). *Pharmaceutics* **2019**, *11*, 633. [CrossRef]
11. Kondiah, P.J.; Kondiah, P.P.; Choonara, Y.E.; Marimuthu, T.; Pillay, V. A 3D Bioprinted Pseudo-Bone Drug Delivery Scaffold for Bone Tissue Engineering. *Pharmaceutics* **2020**, *12*, 166. [CrossRef] [PubMed]
12. Andriotis, E.G.; Eleftheriadis, G.K.; Karavasili, C.; Fatouros, D.G. Development of Bio-Active Patches Based on Pectin for the Treatment of Ulcers and Wounds Using 3D-Bioprinting Technology. *Pharmaceutics* **2020**, *12*, 56. [CrossRef] [PubMed]
13. Healy, A.V.; Fuenmayor, E.; Doran, P.; Geever, L.M.; Higginbotham, C.L.; Lyons, J.G. Additive Manufacturing of Personalized Pharmaceutical Dosage Forms via Stereolithography. *Pharmaceutics* **2019**, *11*, 645. [CrossRef] [PubMed]
14. Robles-Martinez, P.; Xu, X.; Trenfield, S.J.; Awad, A.; Goyanes, A.; Telford, R.; Basit, A.W.; Gaisford, S. 3D printing of a multi-layered polypill containing six drugs using a novel stereolithographic method. *Pharmaceutics* **2019**, *11*, 274. [CrossRef]
15. Awad, A.; Fina, F.; Trenfield, S.J.; Patel, P.; Goyanes, A.; Gaisford, S.; Basit, A.W. 3D printed pellets (miniprintlets): A novel, multi-drug, controlled release platform technology. *Pharmaceutics* **2019**, *11*, 148. [CrossRef]
16. Madzarevic, M.; Medarevic, D.; Vulovic, A.; Sustersic, T.; Djuris, J.; Filipovic, N.; Ibric, S. Optimization and prediction of ibuprofen release from 3D DLP printlets using artificial neural networks. *Pharmaceutics* **2019**, *11*, 544. [CrossRef]

17. Wickström, H.; Koppolu, R.; Mäkilä, E.; Toivakka, M.; Sandler, N. Stencil Printing—A Novel Manufacturing Platform for Orodispersible Discs. *Pharmaceutics* **2020**, *12*, 33.
18. Rycerz, K.; Stepien, K.A.; Czapiewska, M.; Arafat, B.T.; Habashy, R.; Isreb, A.; Peak, M.; Alhnan, M.A. Embedded 3D Printing of Novel Bespoke Soft Dosage Form Concept for Pediatrics. *Pharmaceutics* **2019**, *11*, 630. [CrossRef]
19. Öblom, H.; Sjöholm, E.; Rautamo, M.; Sandler, N. Towards Printed Pediatric Medicines in Hospital Pharmacies: Comparison of 2D and 3D-Printed Orodispersible Warfarin Films with Conventional Oral Powders in Unit Dose Sachets. *Pharmaceutics* **2019**, *11*, 334.
20. Azad, M.A.; Olawuni, D.; Kimbell, G.; Badruddoza, A.Z.M.; Hossain, M.; Sultana, T. Polymers for Extrusion-Based 3D Printing of Pharmaceuticals: A Holistic Materials–Process Perspective. *Pharmaceutics* **2020**, *12*, 124. [CrossRef]
21. Kjar, A.; Huang, Y. Application of Micro-Scale 3D Printing in Pharmaceutics. *Pharmaceutics* **2019**, *11*, 390. [CrossRef] [PubMed]
22. Araújo, M.R.; Sa-Barreto, L.L.; Gratieri, T.; Gelfuso, G.M.; Cunha-Filho, M. The digital pharmacies era: How 3D printing technology using fused deposition modeling can become a reality. *Pharmaceutics* **2019**, *11*, 128.

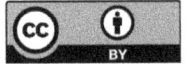

© 2020 by the authors. Licensee MDPI, Basel, Switzerland. This article is an open access article distributed under the terms and conditions of the Creative Commons Attribution (CC BY) license (http://creativecommons.org/licenses/by/4.0/).

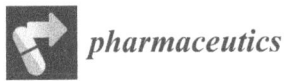

Article

Development of a Biodegradable Subcutaneous Implant for Prolonged Drug Delivery Using 3D Printing

Sarah A. Stewart [1], Juan Domínguez-Robles [1], Victoria J. McIlorum [1], Elena Mancuso [2], Dimitrios A. Lamprou [1], Ryan F. Donnelly [1] and Eneko Larrañeta [1,*]

[1] School of Pharmacy, Queen's University Belfast, 97 Lisburn Road, Belfast BT9 7BL, UK; sstewart35@qub.ac.uk (S.A.S.); j.dominguezrobles@qub.ac.uk (J.D.R.); vmcilorum01@qub.ac.uk (V.J.M.); d.lamprou@qub.ac.uk (D.A.L.); r.donnelly@qub.ac.uk (R.F.D.)

[2] Nanotechnology and Integrated Bio-Engineering Centre (NIBEC), Ulster University, Jordanstown BT37 0QB, UK; e.mancuso@ulster.ac.uk

* Correspondence: e.larraneta@qub.ac.uk

Received: 30 December 2019; Accepted: 24 January 2020; Published: 28 January 2020

Abstract: Implantable drug delivery devices offer many advantages over other routes of drug delivery. Most significantly, the delivery of lower doses of drug, thus, potentially reducing side-effects and improving patient compliance. Three dimensional (3D) printing is a flexible technique, which has been subject to increasing interest in the past few years, especially in the area of medical devices. The present work focussed on the use of 3D printing as a tool to manufacture implantable drug delivery devices to deliver a range of model compounds (methylene blue, ibuprofen sodium and ibuprofen acid) in two in vitro models. Five implant designs were produced, and the release rate varied, depending on the implant design and the drug properties. Additionally, a rate controlling membrane was produced, which further prolonged the release from the produced implants, signalling the potential use of these devices for chronic conditions.

Keywords: implantable devices; subcutaneous; biodegradable; 3D printing; prolonged drug delivery

1. Introduction

Implantable drug delivery devices are those that, when implanted into the body, release drugs at a defined rate and for a defined period. They offer advantages over other routes of drug delivery. They may achieve a therapeutic effect with lower drug concentrations [1–3] by potentially achieving higher drug concentrations at the site of interest, thus, reducing systemic drug exposure and minimising the potential for unwanted side-effects [4,5]. In addition, these devices allow personalised medicine, increased patient compliance [6] and prolonged delivery of treatment over weeks, months or years [7] in a device which may be removed if adverse effects require early termination of treatment [8,9]. Implantable delivery systems have been used for a range of clinical applications, most commonly contraception (e.g., Nexplanon® and NuvaRing®) and cancer treatment (e.g., Vantas®) [3,10]. Nexplanon® is a subcutaneous implant made from poly(ethylene vinyl acetate) which delivers etonogestrel over a period of three years before requiring removal [11,12]. Vantas® is a subcutaneous implant made from a methacrylate-based hydrogel which delivers the drug histrelin for the treatment of prostate cancer over a period of one year [13]. Implantable drug delivery devices also have the potential to be used for other conditions such as the delivery of localised anaesthetics [14] or antibiotics [15].

Currently, the majority of implantable drug delivery devices which are available are manufactured from non-biodegradable polymers [10]. Thus, these implants require surgical removal once they have achieved their purpose. The surgical removal of non-biodegradable implants can often be more traumatic than their insertion [16]. Alternatively, biodegradable polymers offer the significant advantage of not requiring removal after their use, whilst still offering the potential for early removal, if required. They are designed to degrade naturally to products that can be excreted easily by the body [17]. Commonly used biodegradable and biocompatible polymers include poly(lactic acid) (PLA), poly(glycolic acid) (PGA), poly(lactic-co-glycolic acid) (PLGA) and poly(caprolactone) (PCL). Previously, these polymers have been successfully used in nanoparticle-based drug delivery systems and solid and microparticle parenteral implants [18] such as: Zoladex® (AstraZeneca, Cambridge, UK), a solid PLGA parenteral implant for the delivery of goserelin for the treatment of prostate cancer in men or breast cancer or endometriosis in women [19]; and Profact Depot® (Sanofi-Aventis, Paris, France), which is also a solid PLGA parenteral implant, for the delivery of buserelin. Other parenteral implantable systems use polymeric microparticles as the delivery carrier including: Sandostatin LAR® (Novartis, Basel, Switzerland) to deliver octreotide; or Risperdal Consta® (Janssen, Beerse, Belgium) to deliver risperidone [20].

The potential for personalisation of an implantable drug delivery device is substantial and becomes more likely due the increasing interest in 3D printing technologies. The high degree of flexibility and controllability of 3D printing would allow the preparation of tailored dosage forms with a release profile designed to exactly match the individual patient and condition to be treated [21]. Moreover, some of the disadvantages associated with 3D printing, such as high cost and speed, are improving as the technology becomes more widely used. The 3D printing approach to research newer (implantable) drug delivery devices can usher in a new era of treatments to various diseases.

The concept of drug delivery via an implantable device is not a new one. However, an implantable device that is cheap; easily manufactured; biodegradable; biocompatible and with a release rate that may be tailored to an individual patient, drug or clinical application is a very desirable goal, but one that is, as yet unachieved.

Current research is often still focussed on the use of materials that are not biodegradable [22,23]. The aims of this study are 1) to develop 3Dprinted implantable devices for drug delivery using biocompatible/biodegradable materials and 2) to study the influence of the implant geometry on the drug release kinetics. For this purpose, we prepared different PLA and PVA implant designs using fused deposition modelling (FDM) 3D printing technology. These implants were designed containing "windows" of different sizes to allow drug release. Finally, a coating procedure using PCL was used to evaluate the possibility of obtaining a more sustained release from these implants. The resulting implants were characterised using different techniques such as X-ray micro-computed tomography and texture analysis. The last step was to evaluate the drug release kinetics from these implants by using different model molecules and two in vitro models.

2. Materials and Methods

2.1. Materials

Granulate PLA (Ingeo™ Biopolymer 4043D) was purchased from NatureWorks (Minnesota, MN, USA). Filament PVA was purchased from Ultimaker (Ultimaker, Netherlands). Methylene blue, ibuprofen sodium, poly(ethylene glycol) (PEG) (M_W = 1000 Da), agarose powder and phosphate buffered saline (PBS) tablets pH 7.4 were purchased from Sigma-Aldrich (Dorset, UK). Sodium azide was purchased from Fluorochem Ltd. (Hadfield, UK). Ibuprofen acid was purchased from PharmInnova (Waregem, Belgium). Poly(caprolactone) (PCL) 6506 (M_W = 50,000 Da) and PCL 2054 (M_W = 550 Da) were provided by Perstorp (Perstorp, Sweden).

2.2. Methods

2.2.1. Implant Designs

Hot-melt extrusion was used to produce the PLA filament, which would be used for the implant manufacture in combination with the PVA filament. PLA pellets were added to a filament extruder (3devo, Utrecht, The Netherlands) at an extrusion speed of 5 rpm and a filament fan speed of 70%. Finally, the temperature was adjusted through a control panel positioned at the side of the extruder, and it was between 170 and 190 °C, due to the existence of four heaters [24].

Hollow implants were designed using a computer-aided design (CAD) software and printed using an Ultimaker3 3D printer (Ultimaker, Geldermalsen, The Netherlands) using Cura® software. The Ultimaker3 system was equipped with two 0.4 mm extruder nozzles equipped with PLA and PVA, respectively. The print speed was 70 mm/s, the print temperature used was 205 °C, the build plate temperature was 85 °C and the layer height used was 0.2 mm. Five implant configurations were designed and produced (Figure 1A) 2.5 × 40.0 mm PVA implant (weight 0.15 ± 0.001 g); (Figure 1B) 2.5 × 40.0 mm PLA implant with one (1.0 × 38.0 mm) PVA "window" (weight 0.13 ± 0.007 g); (Figure 1C) 2.5 × 40.0 mm PLA implant with eight (1.0 × 1.0 mm) PVA "windows" (weight 0.13 ± 0.001 g); (Figure 1D) 2.5 × 40.0 mm PLA implant with two (1.0 × 1.0 mm) PVA "windows" (weight 0.14 ± 0.005 g) and (Figure 1E) 2.5 × 40.0 mm PLA implant with one (1.0 × 1.0 mm) PVA "window" (weight 0.14 ± 0.003 g). The thickness of the PVA "window" was 0.4 mm in all cases. Finally, implants were filled with a model compound by directly packing powder inside.

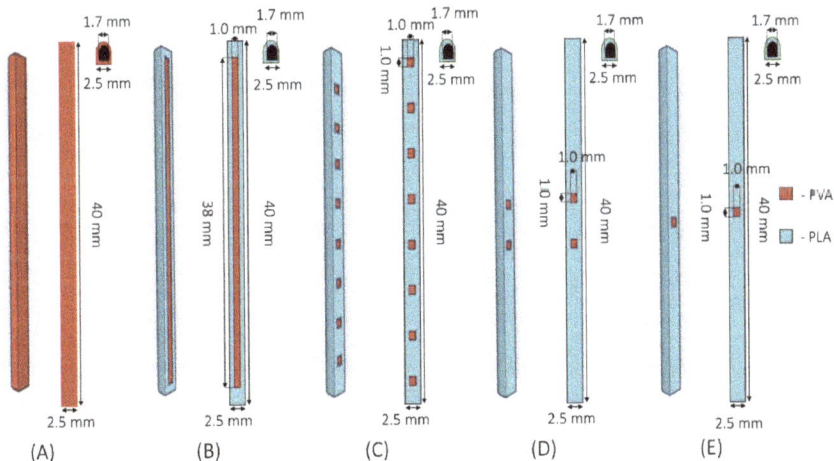

Figure 1. Schematic showing the implant designs: (**A**) 2.5 × 40.0 mm poly(vinyl alcohol) (PVA) implant; (**B**) 2.5 × 40.0 mm poly(lactic acid) (PLA) implant with one (1.0 × 38.0 mm) PVA "window"; (**C**) 2.5 × 40.0 mm PLA implant with eight (1.0 × 1.0 mm) PVA "windows"; (**D**) 2.5 × 40.0 mm PLA implant with two (1.0 × 1.0 mm) PVA "windows" and (**E**) 2.5 × 40.0 mm PLA implant with one (1.0 × 1.0 mm) PVA "window".

Finally, methylene blue (MB)-loaded implants (Figure 1B implant design) were coated with a formulation containing 50/50 PCL 6506/PCL 2054. This particular PCL composition was used because the coating of the implants with only PCL 6506 yielded implants that were not capable of releasing their MB cargo (data not shown). For this purpose, 5 g of this mixture was dissolved in 10 mL of dichloromethane (Merck, Darmstadt, Germany). Implants were coated following a dip-coating procedure using the previously prepared solution. The thickness of the resulting coating was measured using a digital calliper after pealing it from the implant. The coating showed a thickness of 0.11 ± 0.01 mm.

2.2.2. Implant Characterisation

Optical coherence tomography (OCT) using an EX1301 OCT microscope (Michelson Diagnostics, Kent, UK) enabled visualisation of the dissolving PVA "windows" and the drug within the filled implant. The morphology of the implants was evaluated using electronic and optical microscopy. A Hitachi TM3030 benchtop scanning electron microscope (SEM) (Tokyo, Japan) and a Leica EZ4 D digital microscope (Leica, Wetzlar, Germany) were used.

X-ray micro-computed tomography (μCT) scans were performed on 3D printed implants following the same methodology reported by Matthew et al. and Dominguez-Robles et al. [25,26]. Briefly, the 3D reconstruction volumes and inner structures of the implants were observed by using a Bruker SkyScan 1275 system (Bruker, Germany) with a Hamamatsu L11871 source. The microfocus of the X-ray source of the micro-CT scanner had a maximum voltage of 40 kV and maximum current of 250 μA. Samples were mounted vertically on dental wax and positioned 59.791 mm from the source, where the camera-to-source distance was 286 mm. No filter was applied for an exposure time of 49 ms. The images generated were 1944 × 1413 pixels with a resolution of 17 μm per pixel. Then the data were collected and Data Viewer as well as CT-An software were used to analyse them. Finally, CTVol software was applied to generate 3D reconstruction images.

The mechanical properties of the prepared implants were evaluated following a three-point bending test using a TA-XT2 Texture Analyser (Stable Micro Systems, Haslemere, UK). For all measurements the texture analyser was set in compression mode, with a cuboidal probe (9.5 cm in length) with a sharp end (1.1 mm thick) using a setup previously described by Donnelly et al. [27]. The probe was moved towards the implant at a speed of 0.5 mm/s. From the peak maximum of the force–distance curve, the break strength of each implant was calculated.

2.2.3. Analytical Methods

Methylene blue (MB), ibuprofen sodium (IS) and ibuprofen acid (IA) were chosen as model compounds due to their different solubilities to assess any effect this may have on the release profiles. MB was quantified using UV spectroscopy (FLUOstar Omega Microplate Reader, BMG LABTECH, Ortenberg, Germany) at a wavelength of 668 nm. IS and IA were quantified using reverse-phase high-performance liquid chromatography (RP-HPLC) (Agilent 1220 series system, Agilent Technologies UK Ltd., Stockport, UK). The column used to achieve separation was Agilent Eclipse XDB-C18 (5 μm pore size, 4.6 × 150 mm) column (Agilent Technologies UK Ltd., Stockport, UK). The mobile phase used was composed of acetonitrile and 0.1% phosphoric acid at a ratio of 70:30, with a flow rate of 1 mL/min, injection volume of 50 μL and a sample runtime of 5 min. UV detection was carried out at 220 nm. The mobile phase was degassed by sonication for 30 min prior to use. The column temperature was regulated to 25 °C.

2.2.4. In Vitro Drug Release Experiments

Implants were loaded with MB, IS or IA and placed in 500 mL of PBS (or PBS with 0.05% sodium azide for IS and IA release) at 37 °C and shaken at 40 rpm. Samples (0.5 mL) of the release medium were taken at specified time points and replaced with equal volume of PBS [28].

As well as the agitated vessel in vitro release model, an agarose gel in vitro release model was also investigated to more closely mimic in vivo conditions [29]. Agarose powder was dissolved in PBS (for MB release) or PBS containing 0.05% of sodium azide (for IS release) and heated to prepare a 0.6% agarose solution. One-third of the required agarose solution was cast into a Petri dish (10 cm in diameter) and the implant (implant design E) was placed in the centre of this and the agarose solution was allowed to solidify. Subsequently, the remaining agarose solution was cast over this initial layer and allowed to solidify [29]. The Petri dishes were then covered with Parafilm M®, to prevent water evaporation, and placed into an airtight container within a non-agitated incubator at 37 °C. Cylindrical samples (0.5 cm diameter) of agarose were removed at predefined time points (Figure 2). Samples were weighed and analysed for their drug content using an appropriate method, as described in Section 2.2.3. Due to the symmetry of the agarose gel, it was assumed that the drug concentration was constant within each zone with the same distance from the implant "window" [29].

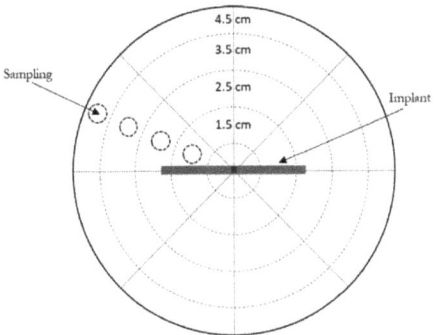

Figure 2. Schematic illustration of the in vitro experimental setup used to sample drug release into agarose gel.

2.3. Data Analysis

Release profiles from each of the implants were compared by calculating and comparing the difference (F_1) and similarity (F_2) factor. F_1 was calculated using Equation (1) that measures the percentage difference between two curves at each time point and is a measurement of the relative error between the two curves. Where, n is the number of time points, R_t is the reference dissolution value at time t, and T_t is the test dissolution value at time t [30,31].

$$F_1 = \left\{ \left[\sum_{t=1}^{n}(R_t - T_t) \right] / \left[\sum_{t=1}^{n} R_t \right] \right\} \times 100 \quad (1)$$

F_2, shown in Equation (2), is a logarithmic transformation of the sum-squared error of differences between the test and reference products over all time points, n.

$$F_2 = 50 \times \log \left\{ \left[(1/n) \sum_{t=1}^{n}(R_t - T_t) \right]^{-0.5} \times 100 \right\} \quad (2)$$

In order for two dissolution profiles to be considered similar, the F_1 value should be lower than 15 × (0–15) and F_2 value should be more than 50 × (50–100) [30,31].

Where appropriate, all data were expressed as a mean ± standard deviation (SD) and compared using one-way analysis of variance (ANOVA) with Tukey's post-hoc. In all cases, $p < 0.05$ was the minimum value considered acceptable for rejection of the null hypothesis.

3. Results and Discussion

3.1. Implant Design and Characterisation

A rod-shaped implant with a size of 2.5 × 40.0 mm was chosen because this shape and these dimensions are similar to dimensions that have already been shown to be acceptable in commercially available products and applicator devices have already been developed for an implant of these dimensions [32]. Implants were loaded with MB (68.6 ± 5.1 mg), IS (68.1 ± 3.0 mg) or IA (72.3 ± 3.2 mg).

Images of the produced implants are shown in Figure 3A–H. These images give an appreciation of the actual geometry of the 3D printed "windows" in comparison to what was designed. Figure 3C, E shows that, although the 1.0 × 1.0 mm has been printed to the correct size, they are more circular in shape than square like the design. This is because the resolution of FDM printers is not as high as that displayed by other types of 3D printing such as stereolithography [33].

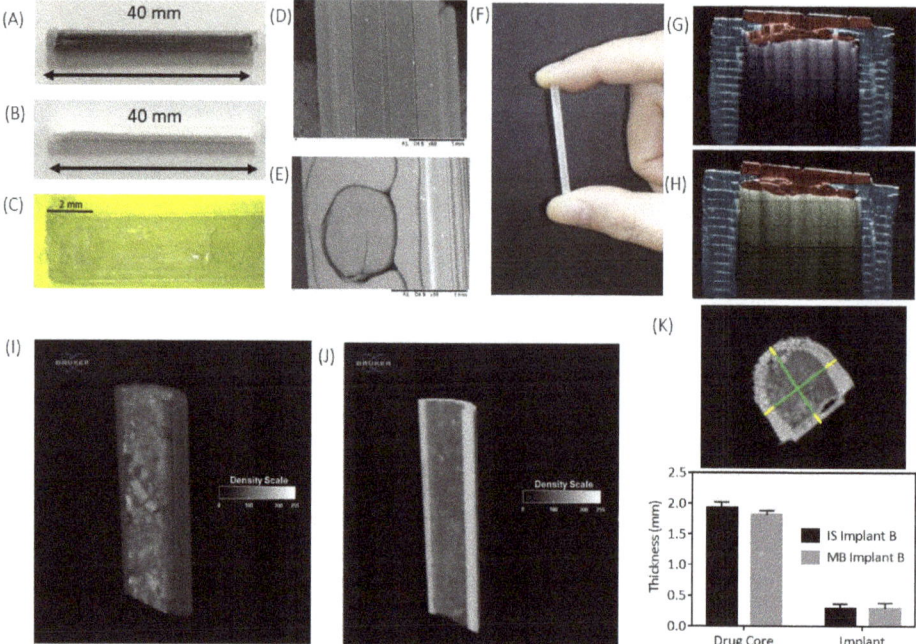

Figure 3. Images of (**A**) methylene blue-filled implant (Implant B); (**B**) ibuprofen sodium-filled implant (Implant B); (**C**) digital microscope image of a section of Implant C, (**D**) a scanning electron microscope (SEM) image of a section of a 38.0 × 1.0 mm poly(vinyl alcohol) (PVA) membrane, (**E**) SEM images of a 1.0 × 1.0 mm poly(vinyl alcohol) (PVA) membrane, (**F**) an image to show the size of the printed implant, (**G**) optical coherence tomography (OCT) image of an MB-filled implant and (**H**) OCT images of an IS-filled implant. Characterisation of implants through microCT analysis. Cross-section reconstructions in the y–z plane of the implants containing (**I**) MB and (**J**) IS. (**K**) Representative x–y cross-section of a 3D-printed implant used for quantitative analysis and dimensional measurements calculated at different locations over the implant 3D volume for the core/shell of the samples reported in (A) and (B), respectively.

Implants A–E loaded with MB, Implants B and E loaded with IS and Implant B loaded with IA were tested using the agitated vessel release model. Implant E loaded with MB or IS was tested using the agarose gel release model. IA was not included in the agarose release model because of its poor solubility and the difficulties this would present to maintain sink conditions. These molecules were used due to their differing solubility values: MB 40 mg/mL [34]; IS 100 mg/mL [35] and IA 0.021 mg/mL [36]. These three molecules cover a wide range of hydrophobicity. Therefore, they are good candidates to establish how this parameter affects drug release from the 3D printed implantable devices. The influence of the solubility on the release profiles can be used to anticipate the release kinetics of other drugs loaded within the implants described here.

The architecture and topology of the 3D-printed implants were analysed using a Bruker SkyScan 1172 system μCT (Figure 3I–K). Cross-section reconstructions in the y–z plane of an implant containing

(Figure 3I) MB and (Figure 3J) IS were performed, and representative x–y cross-section of a 3D-printed implant was used for quantitative analysis. These images (Figure 3I,J) give an appreciation of the drug distribution within the cavity of the implant and show that the drug distribution is uniform for both MB and IS. The dimensional measurements calculated at different locations over the implant 3D volume for the core and shell of the samples are reported in Figure 3K and show that there is no significant ($p > 0.05$) difference in the size of the drug core for either drug. This indicates that the drugs were dispersed through the entire implant cavity and that the packing process did not damaged the implant structure.

Dissolution of the PVA "windows" in Implants B and E were visualised using OCT, digital microscopy and SEM and are shown in Figure 4A,B, respectively. It can be seen that complete dissolution of the PVA "window" in Implant B occurred after 25 min (Figure 4A1). Whereas, complete dissolution of the PVA "window" in Implant E took 35 min (Figure 4B1). Despite the "window" in Implant B being significantly larger than the "window" in Implant E, it fully dissolved more quickly. This may be explained by the reduced surface area-to-volume ratio of the "window" in Implant E, reducing the rate of dissolution for this implant. Goyanes et al. investigated the effect that the surface area-to-volume ratio had on the dissolution of PVA tablets and reported that a higher surface area to volume ratio resulted in tablets that dissolved more quickly [37]. It is important to note that the PVA "window" is designed to dissolve quickly to allow the drug to diffuse trough the generated "window". The "window" material can be tailored to achieve a delayed drug release. Additionally, in the last section of the manuscript, an alternative coating approach was described to prepare implants allowing sustained drug release over months. It is important to note that a quick-dissolving commercial PVA filament was used for this study. PVA is a biocompatible polymer [38], but commercial filaments can have potential excipients, such as plasticisers, that are not ideal for medical applications. However, the present work is a proof-of-concept study exploring the influence of the structure of the implant on the drug release kinetics. Accordingly, a commercial PVA was used as it was the quickest approach. However, future work will require the use of filaments prepared using pure biocompatible polymer. This approach opens the possibility of developing implants with delayed release by printing the implant windows with polymers with slower dissolution/disintegration kinetics such as cellulose derivatives [39,40].

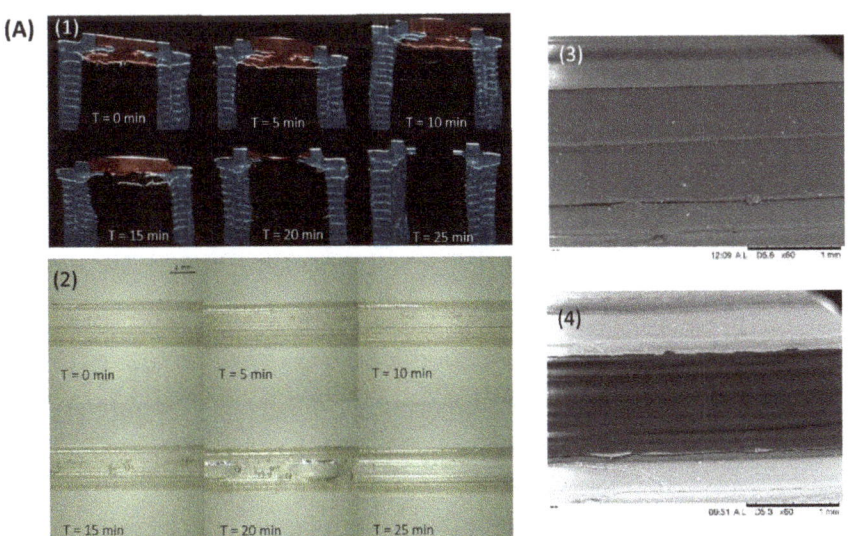

Figure 4. *Cont.*

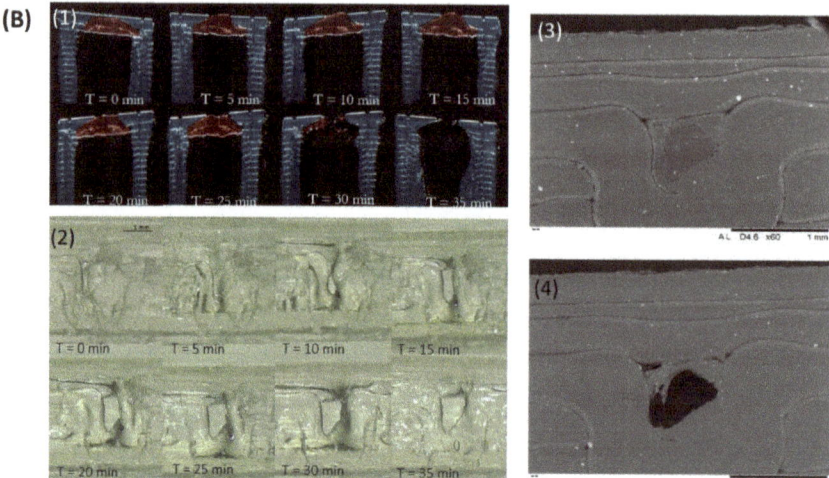

Figure 4. (**A**) Implant B (**1**) OCT images of poly(vinyl alcohol) (PVA) membrane dissolution in Implant B after emersion in phosphate buffered saline (PBS); (**2**) digital microscope images of poly(vinyl alcohol) (PVA) membrane dissolution in Implant B after emersion in PBS; SEM images of Implant B (**3**) before and (**4**) after dissolution. (**B**) (**1**) OCT images of poly(vinyl alcohol) (PVA) membrane dissolution in Implant E after emersion in PBS; (**2**) digital microscope images of poly(vinyl alcohol) (PVA) membrane dissolution in Implant E after emersion in PBS; SEM images of Implant E (**3**) before and (**4**) after dissolution.

To predict robustness of the designed implants, their break strength and degree of flexibility were evaluated. A very rigid implant is likely to break during insertion or in situ; therefore, a degree of flexibility is required, as well as sufficient strength to withstand insertion and remain mechanically strong enough for the duration of drug release. If an implant breaks or cracks, it is likely to cause an increase or a burst in the rate of drug release which would, in turn, cause undesirable side effects in the patient. The maximum force required for breaking the implants and the angle of bending at the break point were calculated for each implant configuration and shown in Figure 5.

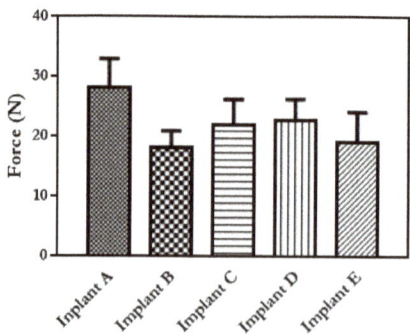

Figure 5. Force required to break each of the implant designs ($n = 5$, means + SD).

It can be seen from Figure 5 that there is no significant difference in the breaking force of Implants B–E (PLA implants). A significantly ($p < 0.5$) larger force was required to break Implant A (PVA), than was required for Implants B–E. This test was performed to evaluate if changing the design of the release "windows" from the implant has a direct influence on the mechanical properties of the resulting material. No mechanical tests directly comparable to those performed in this study have been performed on commercially available implantable drug delivery devices. However, mechanical testing of medical devices has been extensively reported. The results obtained here can be compared with the results reported by Horal et al. for 3D-printed PLA screws for orthopaedic applications [41]. In this case, PLA screws were manufactured and a three-point bending test was performed. The dimensions of these implants were similar to the ones described here (1–2 mm), and the forces applied during the bending tests were lower than the ones reported here (ranging between 0.5 and 10 N). These screws where designed for bone healing applications. Higher forces will be applied to bone screws than to implants designed to be implanted in soft tissue. Therefore, the implants presented here showed fracture forces higher than the forces that will be expected for soft tissue implants. As PLA has a long degradation time, up to 2 years [42], degradation of the implant structure would not be expected to have an effect on the mechanical properties during drug release or an effect on the release rate itself.

3.2. In Vitro Drug Release

MB has some inherent antibacterial activity; therefore, bacterial growth in the release media was not anticipated to be an issue for these implants [43]. However, SA was added to IS and IA release media to prevent microbial growth [23,44,45] over the course of the release experiment. The release profiles of MB from each of the five implant designs are shown in Figure 6. Implants made entirely from PVA (Implant A) had the most rapid drug release, with 100% of drug releasing within 24 h. As expected, Implants B and C showed significantly extended release profiles in comparison with Implant A, with release time being extended to over six days. Although, Implants B and C took the same time to reach 100% release, Implant C showed a more sustained release profile, which showed less variation. Implants D and E showed an extended release profile in comparison to the other implants and show that reducing the size and number of "windows" effectively prolongs release from this type of implant. The release profiles of MB from each of the PVA "window" implants were compared using similarity and difference factor (F_1/F_2), and the results are shown in Table 1. Implant A had a significantly different release profile to Implants B and C as the F_1 values were higher than 15 and the F_2 values were lower than 50. Implants B and C and Implants D and E also showed significantly different release profiles to each other. These results indicate that implant design has potential to modify the release profile of a loaded molecule by simply changing the design of the implant. Interestingly, implants with 1.0×1.0 mm "windows" were capable of providing drug release over 25 days. A sustained release profile like this can be useful for local antimicrobial therapy or for pain management after surgery [46,47]. In these cases, a prolonged release over a period of a few weeks can be extremely beneficial to prevent infections or for pain management. However, for prolonged applications alternative approaches need to be evaluated. For this purpose, coated implants were evaluated. This approach is described in Section 3.3 of the present manuscript.

The effect of drug properties on release from the designed implants was investigated by comparing the release profiles of MB (solubility 40 mg/mL [34]), with IS (solubility 100 mg/mL [35]) and IA (solubility 0.021 mg/mL [36]). The release profiles of IS from Implants B and E are shown in Figure 7A. The release rate of IS from Implant B was significantly increased in comparison to MB from the same implant. Complete IS release was achieved after just 80 min, whereas, 100% MB release took seven days. A similar increase in release rate is seen for Implant E, with 100% IS release achieved after six days and MB release after 25 days. These results show that obviously the implant design is not the only factor that contributes to change the release profile. The physicochemical properties of the drug loaded are important too. All in vitro releases were carried out under sink conditions; therefore, it is the dissolution rate of each of the drugs rather than solubility that is having an impact on drug release from the implant. Accordingly, changing the nature of the loaded molecule or including a formulation with a slower dissolution rate will provide an extra degree of control over the release profile.

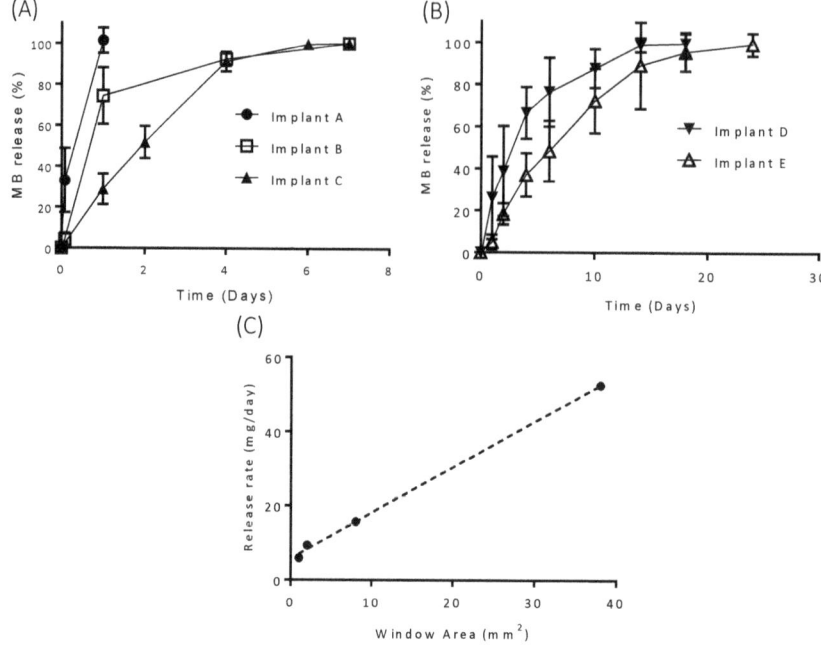

Figure 6. Release of methylene blue (MB) from (**A**) Implant A–C; (**B**) Implants D and E ($n = 3$, means ± SD) and (**C**) correlation between MB release rate and "window" area for the implants.

Table 1. Difference (F_1) and similarity (F_2) factor of each release profile for methylene blue (MB) release from poly(lactic acid) (PLA) implant with poly(vinyl alcohol) (PVA) "window" designs.

Curve 1	Curve 2	F_1	F_2
Implant A	Implant B	60.06	33.00
Implant A	Implant C	73.89	13.58
Implant B	Implant C	28.93	32.12
Implant D	Implant E	19.61	34.75

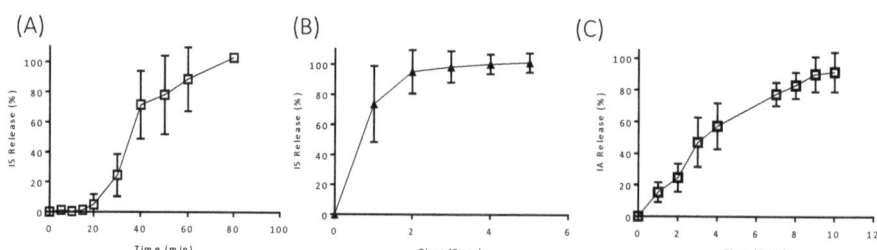

Figure 7. Release of (**A**) ibuprofen sodium (IS) from Implant B; (**B**) IS from Implant E and (**C**) release of ibuprofen acid (IA) from Implant B ($n = 3$, means ± SD).

IA release from Implant B is shown in Figure 7C. The release of this compound is significantly extended in comparison with MB and IS release from the same implant design, with release taking ten days in comparison to six days and 80 min for MB and IS, respectively. As mentioned previously, the release rate of this drug is slower due to its slower dissolution kinetics, confirming that the nature of the drug loaded need to be carefully considered for each application type.

Figure 8 shows the release profiles of MB and IS from Implant E into an agarose gel release model. Release is expected to be slower in the agarose gel when compared to the agitated vessel release model. Within the agitated vessel model, convection rapidly homogenises the drug within the release media, thus, maintaining the drug concentration gradient at the interface of the implant with the release media. However, living tissues exhibit different conditions than those applied in the in vitro agitated vessel method. The extracellular matrix that these formulations are likely to be in contact with after implantation behave more like a gel than like a bulk fluid [48]. Despite the existence of a large number of biorelevant media for simulating physiological fluids, there is still not an accepted standard for simulation of subcutaneous environment [48]. Agarose gels form a 3D structure linked by hydrogen bonds with pore sizes similar to those encountered in physiological tissue and have been suggested as a more realistic in vitro release model than bulk fluid [29,49]. Moreover, multiple research works have reported the suitability of agarose hydrogel as a good release medium simulating soft tissues [50–53].

Both drugs demonstrated progressive drug release over a prolonged period. Figure 8A,B shows the release obtained for MB-loaded implants. These results showed that the closest region (1.5 cm) to the implant reached a plateau in MB levels after seven days. However, in further regions the MB concentration increased over time up to 40 days for the further regions (4.5 cm). This shows that MB was continuously delivered over 40 days. This MB concentration increase is not due only to MB diffusion through the agarose gel, as the concentration always increased. This suggests that there was a constant MB release that took place over time. After 40 days no significant differences were found in the release obtained at different distances from the implant ($p > 0.05$). This indicated that MB concentration all over the agarose gel was equivalent and that there was no concentration gradient that will drive more release. Similar behaviour was observed for IS (Figure 8C,D) over a period of 21 days. These results confirm that the testing conditions had a substantial influence on the release results. Moreover, this set of results suggest that the selected implants can be used to provide drug release over periods of several weeks. Similarly, Hoang et al. investigated releases of ciprofloxacin hydrochloride and vancomycin hydrochloride from bone implants over 48 and 96 h, respectively and showed that release into an agarose model was extended when compared to release of the same drugs from the same implants into an agitated vial [29].

The releases achieved in this work range from just 80 min to over 25 days in an agitated vessel and over 40 days in an agarose gel model and show promise as drug delivery systems for prolonged drug delivery. The use of local anaesthetics (commonly, bupivacaine, lidocaine and procaine) to treat localised pain has many advantages when compared with the systemic administration of opioids [14]. Work has been carried out to optimise the drug delivery of these agents to achieve localised delivery and limit peripheral side effects. An implantable device that could locally deliver anaesthetic over days or weeks could be of benefit for delivery of these drugs. Currently, the majority of chemotherapeutic agents are delivery systemically. This allows the drug to distribute throughout the entire body, including to healthy tissues, causing adverse side effects [54]. Polymeric devices aiming to locally deliver cancer drugs have been investigated and aim to improve the delivery of these drugs by providing localised sustained delivery and, therefore, reduce the effect on healthy tissue. Salmoria et al. investigated the use of polymeric implant to locally deliver fluorouracil and showed a desirable release rate over 45 days [54]. Localised delivery of antibiotics may offer advantages over conventional oral delivery for localised conditions. Gimeno et al. showed promising delivery of antibiotics which could be tailored by changing the implant design, from rapid drug release within 20 h to longer release times around 200 h for the potential prevention of orthopaedic-implant-associated infections [15]. These examples highlight instances where the implants developed in this work could be used.

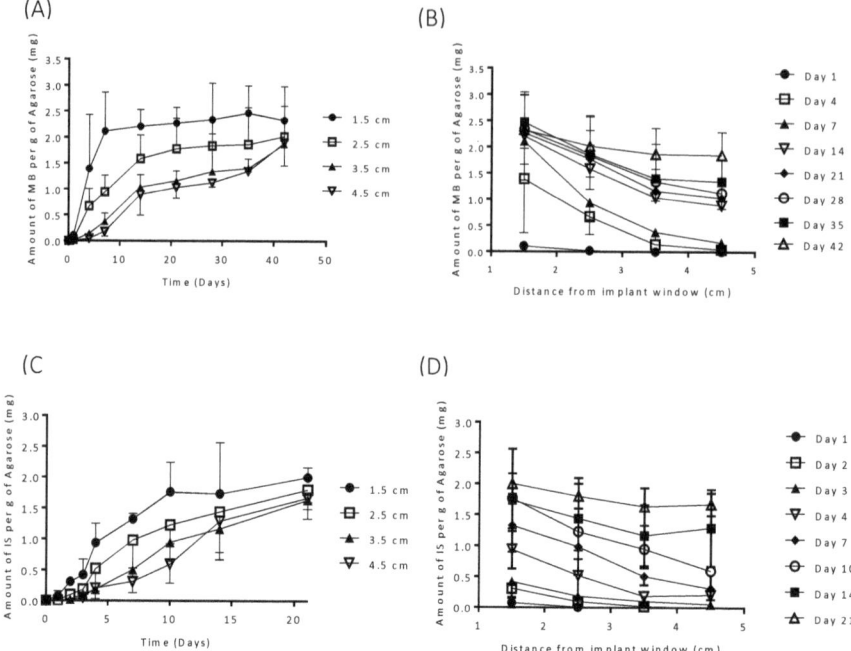

Figure 8. (**A** and **B**) MB and (**C** and **D**) IS releases from (**A**) Implant E into agarose gel ($n = 3$, means ± SD).

3.3. In Vitro Drug Release from Coated Implants

The results described in previous sections show that these implants can be used for sustained drug delivery over periods of several weeks. The treatment of some medical conditions, especially chronic conditions, can be improved significantly with drug delivery devices capable of providing drug release over prolonged periods of time. These periods of time range from months up to years for potent compounds such as hormones. Examples of this will be the treatment of chronic conditions or even pre-exposure prophylaxis of human immunodeficiency disease (HIV).

A good alternative to obtain implants with prolonged drug release profiles is to coat them with a membrane capable of sustaining drug release [55]. Accordingly, a simple dip coating procedure can be used to prepare implants with prolonged drug release profiles. Accordingly, a thin film covers the surface of the implant acting as a rate controlling membrane [9]. Figure 9 shows the release profile of MB from implants (Implant B) coated with a PCL-based formulation. It can be seen that the PCL rate controlling membrane is capable of providing sustained drug releases over periods of 300 days. Interestingly, non-coated equivalent implants showed MB release profiles extended over only four days (Figure 6). These results suggest that PCL coating could be an ideal approach for applications that require drug release over longer periods of time. PCL has been described previously as a good candidate to prepare rate controlling membranes for drug delivery applications [9]. PEG membranes have been used before to release tenofovir alafenamide for HIV pre-exposure prophylaxis [56]. These systems achieved prolonged releases between 100 and 200 days. Considering that tenofovir alafenamide shows a lower water solubility than MB, the system described has great potential for sustaining the release of hydrophilic molecules as MB showed up to 300 days of release.

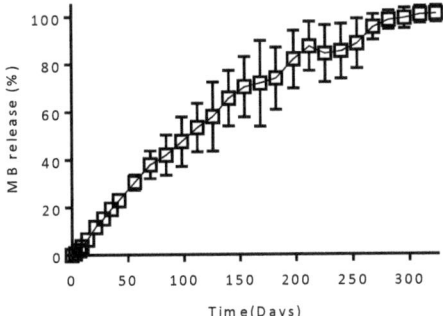

Figure 9. Release profile of methylene blue from Implant B with a PCL formulation coating ($n = 3$, means ± SD).

4. Conclusions

In this work, hollow 3D-printed implants with similar dimensions to those already available in the market were successfully produced. The flexibility of this manufacturing technique allowed five different implant designs to be easily designed and produced. This technique has the potential to allow personalisation of implantable drug delivery devices for individual patients and conditions. μCT confirmed consistent drug distribution within the implant and confirms the implants' suitability for a range of drug compounds. The mechanical properties of the designed implants were superior to those of other drug delivery systems. This work has shown that the release rate from these implants can be modified by changing the implant design but is also dependent on the properties of the compound contained within the implant. Finally, implant coating can provide an added degree of control over the release, with a PCL-based coating showing potential to extend expressively the release profile.

The results described in the present work demonstrate how 3D printing is a promising technology for drug eluting implant manufacture. Considering the simplicity of the technology described here, it can be easily transferred to a clinical setup, where implants could be designed on demand to fulfil patient's needs after surgery. These implants may be suited for delivery of drugs for localised treatment. For example, chemotherapy agents, antibiotics or localised anaesthetics. Alternatively, they could be tailored by coating them for prolonged drug delivery for the treatment of chronic conditions. This can be done due to the versatility of 3D printing technology.

Author Contributions: Conceptualisation, S.A.S. and E.L.; methodology, S.A.S., J.D.-R., and E.L.; investigation and formal analysis, S.A.S., J.D.-R., V.J.M., and E.M.; data curation, S.A.S., J.D.-R., and E.L.; writing, S.A.S., J.D.-R., and E.L.; writing—review and editing, E.L. and D.A.L.; funding acquisition, R.F.D.; and supervision, E.L. and R.F.D. All authors have read and agreed to the published version of the manuscript.

Funding: This work was financially supported by the Wellcome Trust (WT094085MA). Sarah A. Stewart is a PhD candidate funded by a Department for the Economy (Northern Ireland) studentship.

Conflicts of Interest: The authors declare no conflict of interest.

References

1. Rajgor, N.; Bhaskar, V.; Patel, M. Implantable drug delivery systems: An overview. *Syst. Rev. Pharm.* **2011**, *2*, 91. [CrossRef]
2. Langer, R. New methods of drug delivery. *Science* **1990**, *249*, 1527–1533. [CrossRef]
3. Dash, A.K.; Cudworth, G.C. Therapeutic applications of implantable drug delivery systems. *J. Pharmacol. Toxicol. Methods* **1998**, *40*, 1–12. [CrossRef]
4. Wang, Y.; Sun, L.; Mei, Z.; Zhang, F.; He, M.; Fletcher, C.; Wang, F.; Yang, J.; Bi, D.; Jiang, Y.; et al. 3D printed biodegradable implants as an individualized drug delivery system for local chemotherapy of osteosarcoma. *Mater. Des.* **2020**, *186*, 108336. [CrossRef]

5. Zhou, H.; Hernandez, C.; Goss, M.; Gawlik, A.; Exner, A. Biomedical imaging in implantable drug delivery systems. *Curr. Drug Targets* **2015**, *16*, 672–682. [CrossRef] [PubMed]
6. Fialho, S.L.; da Silva Cunha, A. Manufacturing techniques of biodegradable implants intended for intraocular application. *Drug Deliv.* **2005**, *12*, 109–116. [CrossRef] [PubMed]
7. Meng, E.; Hoang, T. Micro- and nano-fabricated implantable drug-delivery systems. *Ther. Deliv.* **2012**, *3*, 1457–1467. [CrossRef]
8. Rabin, C.; Liang, Y.; Ehrlichman, R.S.; Budhian, A.; Metzger, K.L.; Majewski-Tiedeken, C.; Winey, K.I.; Siegel, S.J. In vitro and in vivo demonstration of risperidone implants in mice. *Schizophr. Res.* **2008**, *98*, 66–78. [CrossRef]
9. Schlesinger, E.; Johengen, D.; Luecke, E.; Rothrock, G.; McGowan, I.; van der Straten, A.; Desai, T. A tunable, biodegradable, thin-film polymer device as a long-acting implant delivering tenofovir alafenamide fumarate for HIV pre-exposure prophylaxis. *Pharm. Res.* **2016**, *33*, 1649–1656. [CrossRef]
10. Stewart, S.; Domínguez-Robles, J.; Donnelly, R.; Larrañeta, E. Implantable polymeric drug delivery devices: Classification, manufacture, materials, and clinical Applications. *Polymers (Basel)* **2018**, *10*, 1379. [CrossRef]
11. Mansour, D. Nexplanon®: What Implanon® did next. *J. Fam. Plan. Reprod. Heal. Care* **2010**, *36*, 187–189. [CrossRef] [PubMed]
12. Palomba, S.; Falbo, A.; Di Cello, A.; Materazzo, C.; Zullo, F. Nexplanon: The new implant for long-term contraception: A comprehensive descriptive review. *Gynecol. Endocrinol.* **2012**, *28*, 710–721. [CrossRef] [PubMed]
13. Schlegel, P. A review of the pharmacokinetic and pharmacological properties of a once-yearly administered histrelin acetate implant in the treatment of prostate cancer. *BJU Int.* **2009**, *103*, 7–13. [CrossRef] [PubMed]
14. Bagshaw, K.R.; Hanenbaum, C.L.; Carbone, E.J.; Lo, K.W.; Laurencin, C.T.; Walker, J.; Nair, L.S. Pain management via local anesthetics and responsive hydrogels. *Ther. Deliv.* **2015**, *6*, 165–176. [CrossRef] [PubMed]
15. Gimeno, M.; Pinczowski, P.; Pérez, M.; Giorello, A.; Martínez, M.Á.; Santamaría, J.; Arruebo, M.; Luján, L. A controlled antibiotic release system to prevent orthopedic-implant associated infections: An in vitro Study. *Eur. J. Pharm. Biopharm.* **2015**, *96*, 264–271. [CrossRef]
16. Sun, H.; Mei, L.; Song, C.; Cui, X.; Wang, P. The in vivo degradation, absorption and excretion of PCL-based implant. *Biomaterials* **2006**, *27*, 1735–1740. [CrossRef] [PubMed]
17. Ulery, B.D.; Nair, L.S.; Laurencin, C.T. Biomedical applications of biodegradable polymers. *J. Polym. Sci. Part B Polym. Phys.* **2011**, *49*, 832–864. [CrossRef]
18. Kumari, A.; Yadav, S.K.; Yadav, S.C. Biodegradable polymeric nanoparticles based drug delivery systems. *Colloids Surfaces B Biointerfaces* **2010**, *75*, 1–18. [CrossRef]
19. Cockshott, I.D. Clinical pharmacokinetics of goserelin. *Clin. Pharmacokinet.* **2000**, *39*, 27–48. [CrossRef]
20. Park, E.J.; Amatya, S.; Kim, M.S.; Park, J.H.; Seol, E.; Lee, H.; Shin, Y.-H.; Na, D.H. Long-acting injectable formulations of antipsychotic drugs for the treatment of schizophrenia. *Arch. Pharm. Res.* **2013**, *36*, 651–659. [CrossRef]
21. Khaled, S.A.; Burley, J.C.; Alexander, M.R.; Roberts, C.J. Desktop 3D printing of controlled release pharmaceutical bilayer tablets. *Int. J. Pharm.* **2014**, *461*, 105–111. [CrossRef] [PubMed]
22. Barrett, S.E.; Teller, R.S.; Forster, S.P.; Li, L.; Mackey, M.A.; Skomski, D.; Yang, Z.; Fillgrove, K.L.; Doto, G.J.; Wood, S.L.; et al. Extended-duration MK-8591-eluting implant as a candidate for HIV treatment and prevention. *Antimicrob. Agents Chemother.* **2018**, *62*. [CrossRef] [PubMed]
23. Gunawardana, M.; Remedios-Chan, M.; Miller, C.S.; Fanter, R.; Yang, F.; Marzinke, M.A.; Hendrix, C.W.; Beliveau, M.; Moss, J.A.; Smith, T.J.; et al. Pharmacokinetics of long-acting tenofovir alafenamide (GS-7340) subdermal implant for HIV prophylaxis. *Antimicrob. Agents Chemother.* **2015**, *59*, 3913–3919. [CrossRef] [PubMed]
24. Domínguez-Robles, J.; Martin, N.; Fong, M.; Stewart, S.; Irwin, N.; Rial-Hermida, M.; Donnelly, R.; Larrañeta, E. Antioxidant PLA composites containing lignin for 3D printing applications: A potential material for healthcare applications. *Pharmaceutics* **2019**, *11*, 165. [CrossRef]
25. Mathew, E.; Domínguez-Robles, J.; Stewart, S.A.; Mancuso, E.; O'Donnell, K.; Larrañeta, E.; Lamprou, D.A. Fused deposition modeling as an effective tool for anti-infective dialysis catheter fabrication. *ACS Bbomaterials Sci. Eng.* **2019**, *5*, 6300–6310. [CrossRef]

26. Domínguez-Robles, J.; Mancinelli, C.; Mancuso, E.; García-Romero, I.; Gilmore, B.F.; Casettari, L.; Larrañeta, E.; Lamprou, D.A. 3D printing of drug-loaded thermoplastic polyurethane meshes: A potential material for soft tissue reinforcement in vaginal surgery. *Pharmaceutics* **2020**, *12*, 63. [CrossRef]
27. Donnelly, R.F.; Majithiya, R.; Singh, T.R.R.; Morrow, D.I.J.J.; Garland, M.J.; Demir, Y.K.; Migalska, K.; Ryan, E.; Gillen, D.; Scott, C.J.; et al. Design, optimization and characterisation of polymeric microneedle arrays prepared by a novel laser-based micromoulding technique. *Pharm. Res.* **2011**, *28*, 41–57. [CrossRef]
28. The British Pharmacopeia Commission British Pharmacopoeia. Available online: https://www.pharmacopoeia.com/bp-2020?date=2020-01-01 (accessed on 30 August 2019).
29. Hoang Thi, T.H.; Chai, F.; Leprêtre, S.; Blanchemain, N.; Martel, B.; Siepmann, F.; Hildebrand, H.F.; Siepmann, J.; Flament, M.P. Bone implants modified with cyclodextrin: Study of drug release in bulk fluid and into agarose gel. *Int. J. Pharm.* **2010**, *15*, 74–85. [CrossRef]
30. Larrañeta, E.; Martínez-Ohárriz, C.; Vélaz, I.; Zornoza, A.; Machín, R.; Isasi, J.R. In vitro release from reverse poloxamine/α-cyclodextrin matrices: Modelling and comparison of dissolution profiles. *J. Pharm. Sci.* **2014**, *103*, 197–206. [CrossRef]
31. Costa, P.; Sousa Lobo, J.M. Modeling and comparison of dissolution profiles. *Eur. J. Pharm. Sci.* **2001**, *13*, 123–133. [CrossRef]
32. Funk, S.; Miller, M.M.; Mishell, D.R.; Archer, D.F.; Poindexter, A.; Schmidt, J.; Zampaglione, E. Safety and efficacy of Implanon™, a single-rod implantable contraceptive containing etonogestrel. *Contraception* **2005**, *71*, 319–326. [CrossRef] [PubMed]
33. George, E.; Liacouras, P.; Rybicki, F.J.; Mitsouras, D. Measuring and establishing the accuracy and reproducibility of 3D printed medical models. *Radiographics* **2017**, *37*, 1424–1450. [CrossRef] [PubMed]
34. Drugbank Methylene Blue. Available online: https://www.drugbank.ca/drugs/DB09241 (accessed on 30 October 2019).
35. Sigma-Aldrich Ibuprofen Sodium Salt. Available online: https://www.sigmaaldrich.com/catalog/product/sial/i1892?lang=en&region=GB (accessed on 8 March 2019).
36. Drugbank Ibuprofen. Available online: https://www.drugbank.ca/drugs/DB01050 (accessed on 30 October 2019).
37. Goyanes, A.; Robles Martinez, P.; Buanz, A.; Basit, A.W.; Gaisford, S. Effect of geometry on drug release from 3D printed tablets. *Int. J. Pharm.* **2015**, *494*, 657–663. [CrossRef] [PubMed]
38. Chong, S.-F.; Smith, A.A.A.; Zelikin, A.N. Microstructured, functional PVA hydrogels through bioconjugation with oligopeptides under physiological conditions. *Small* **2013**, *9*, 942–950. [CrossRef] [PubMed]
39. Khizer, Z.; Akram, M.R.; Sarfraz, R.M.; Nirwan, J.S.; Farhaj, S.; Yousaf, M.; Hussain, T.; Lou, S.; Timmins, P.; Conway, B.R.; et al. Plasticiser-free 3D printed hydrophilic matrices: Quantitative 3D surface texture, mechanical, swelling, erosion, drug release and pharmacokinetic studies. *Polymers (Basel)* **2019**, *11*, 1095. [CrossRef] [PubMed]
40. Chai, X.; Chai, H.; Wang, X.; Yang, J.; Li, J.; Zhao, Y.; Cai, W.; Tao, T.; Xiang, X. Fused deposition modeling (FDM) 3D printed tablets for intragastric floating delivery of domperidone. *Sci. Rep.* **2017**, *7*, 2829. [CrossRef]
41. Horal, M. *3D printing implants for fracture healing studies in rat*; Lund University: Lund, Sweden, 2015.
42. Auras, R.; Lim, L.-T.; Selke, S.E.M.; Tsuji, H. *Poly(lactic acid): Synthesis, structures, properties, processing and applications*; Auras, R., Lim, L.-T., Selke, S.E.M., Tsuji, H., Eds.; John Wiley & Sons, Inc.: Hoboken, NJ, USA, 2010.
43. Fung, D.Y.C.; Miller, R.D. Effect of dyes on bacterial growth. *Appl. Microbiol.* **1973**, *25*, 793–799. [CrossRef]
44. Lichstein, H.C. Studies of the effect of sodium azide on microbic growth and respiration: III. The effect of sodium azide on the gas metabolism of B. subtilis and P. aeruginosa and the influence of pyocyanine on the gas exchange of a pyocyanine-free Strain of P. aerugino. *J. Bacteriol.* **1944**, *47*, 239–251. [CrossRef]
45. Herrera, L.C.; Tesoriero, M.V.; Hermida, L.G. In vitro release testing of PLGA microspheres with franz diffusion cells. *Dissolution Technol.* **2012**, *19*, 6–11. [CrossRef]
46. Kelm, J.; Regitz, T.; Schmitt, E.; Jung, W.; Anagnostakos, K. In vivo and in vitro studies of antibiotic release from and bacterial growth inhibition by antibiotic-impregnated polymethylmethacrylate hip spacers. *Antimicrob. Agents Chemother.* **2006**, *50*, 332–335. [CrossRef]
47. Liu, K.-S.; Chen, W.-H.; Lee, C.-H.; Su, Y.-F.; Liu, S.-J. Extended pain relief achieved by analgesic-eluting biodegradable nanofibers in the Nuss procedure: In vitro and in vivo studies. *Int. J. Nanomedicine* **2018**, *13*, 8355–8364. [CrossRef] [PubMed]

48. Leung, D.H.; Kapoor, Y.; Alleyne, C.; Walsh, E.; Leithead, A.; Habulihaz, B.; Salituro, G.M.; Bak, A.; Rhodes, T. Development of a convenient in vitro gel diffusion model for predicting the in vivo performance of subcutaneous parenteral formulations of large and small molecules. *AAPS PharmSciTech* **2017**, *18*, 2203–2213. [CrossRef] [PubMed]
49. Pernodet, N.; Maaloum, M.; Tinland, B. Pore size of agarose gels by atomic force microscopy. *Electrophoresis* **1997**, *18*, 55–58. [CrossRef] [PubMed]
50. Ye, F.; Larsen, S.W.; Yaghmur, A.; Jensen, H.; Larsen, C.; Østergaard, J. Drug release into hydrogel-based subcutaneous surrogates studied by UV imaging. *J. Pharm. Biomed. Anal.* **2012**, *71*, 27–34. [CrossRef] [PubMed]
51. Chen, X.; Astary, G.W.; Sepulveda, H.; Mareci, T.H.; Sarntinoranont, M. Quantitative assessment of macromolecular concentration during direct infusion into an agarose hydrogel phantom using contrast-enhanced MRI. *Magn. Reson. Imaging* **2008**, *26*, 1433–1441. [CrossRef]
52. McCabe, M. The diffusion coefficient of caffeine through agar gels containing a hyaluronic acid–protein complex. A model system for the study of the permeability of connective tissues. *Biochem. J.* **1972**, *127*, 249–253. [CrossRef]
53. Salloum, M.; Ma, R.H.; Weeks, D.; Zhu, L. Controlling nanoparticle delivery in magnetic nanoparticle hyperthermia for cancer treatment: Experimental study in agarose gel. *Int. J. Hyperth.* **2008**, *24*, 337–345. [CrossRef]
54. Salmoria, G.V.; Ghizoni, G.B.; Gindri, I.M.; Marques, M.S.; Kanis, L.A. Hot extrusion of PE/fluorouracil implantable rods for targeted drug delivery in cancer treatment. *Polym. Bull.* **2019**, *76*, 1825–1838. [CrossRef]
55. Launonen, V.; Vierimaa, O.; Kiuru, M.; Isola, J.; Roth, S.; Pukkala, E.; Sistonen, P.; Herva, R.; Aaltonen, L.A. Inherited susceptibility to uterine leiomyomas and renal cell cancer. *Proc. Natl. Acad. Sci. USA* **2001**, *98*, 3387–3392. [CrossRef]
56. Johnson, L.M.; Krovi, S.A.; Li, L.; Girouard, N.; Demkovich, Z.R.; Myers, D.; Creelman, B.; van der Straten, A. Characterization of a reservoir-style implant for sustained release of tenofovir alafenamide (TAF) for HIV pre-exposure prophylaxis (PrEP). *Pharmaceutics* **2019**, *11*, 315. [CrossRef]

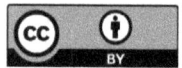

© 2020 by the authors. Licensee MDPI, Basel, Switzerland. This article is an open access article distributed under the terms and conditions of the Creative Commons Attribution (CC BY) license (http://creativecommons.org/licenses/by/4.0/).

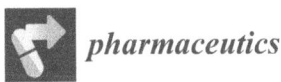

Article

Fabrication of Intragastric Floating, Controlled Release 3D Printed Theophylline Tablets Using Hot-Melt Extrusion and Fused Deposition Modeling

Bhupendra Raj Giri [1,†], Eon Soo Song [1,†], Jaewook Kwon [1], Ju-Hyun Lee [2], Jun-Bom Park [2] and Dong Wuk Kim [1,*]

1. College of Pharmacy & Research Institute of Pharmaceutical Sciences, Kyungpook National University, Daegu 41566, Korea; giribhupen77@gmail.com (B.R.G.); djstn0424@naver.com (E.S.S.); kjw11156@naver.com (J.K.)
2. College of Pharmacy, Sahmyook University, Seoul 01795, Korea; jelly_3004@naver.com (J.-H.L.); junji4@gmail.com (J.-B.P.)
* Correspondence: dkim17@knu.ac.kr; Tel.: +82-53-950-8579; Fax: +82-53-950-8557
† These authors contributed equally to this work.

Received: 27 December 2019; Accepted: 13 January 2020; Published: 17 January 2020

Abstract: This work presents a novel approach for producing gastro-retentive floating tablets (GRFT) by coupling hot-melt extrusion (HME) and fused deposition three-dimensional printing (3DP). Filaments containing theophylline (THEO) within a hydroxypropyl cellulose (HPC) matrix were prepared using HME. 3DP tablets with different infill percentages and shell thickness were developed and evaluated to determine their drug content, floating behavior, dissolution, and physicochemical properties. The dissolution studies revealed a relationship between the infill percentage/shell thickness and the drug release behavior of the 3DP tablets. All the developed GRFTs possessed the ability to float for 10 h and exhibited zero-order release kinetics. The drug release could be described by the Peppas–Sahlin model, as a combination of Fickian diffusion and swelling mechanism. Drug crystallinity was found unaltered throughout the process. 3DP coupled with HME, could be an effective blueprint to produce controlled-release GRFTs, providing the advantage of simplicity and versatility compared to the conventional methods.

Keywords: theophylline; hot-melt extrusion; fused deposition modeling 3D printing; gastro-retentive floating system; dissolution kinetics; controlled release

1. Introduction

The limitations of orthodox oral drug delivery systems such as fast emptying time and incomplete absorption due to physiological variations, particularly unpredictable gastrointestinal (GI) transit and emptying times as well as metabolic degradation in the lower GI tract, resulting in inferior pharmacokinetics with therapeutic failure for a few drugs [1]. This scenario has led to a scientific undertaking to identify better alternatives. The development of gastro-retentive drug delivery systems (GRDDS) was brought into the limelight in order to overcome the above constraints by retaining drugs in the stomach for an extended period, ensuring optimal bioavailability. Numerous strategies have been explored for GRDDS to slow the gastric emptying rate; for example, intra-gastric floating systems [2,3], bio-adhesives [4], swelling and expanding [5], and low/high-density systems [6]. The gastro-retentive floating tablet (GRFT) is a low-density system with enough buoyancy to remain afloat above the gastric content in the stomach for a prolonged and pre-determined period of time without interference from the normal peristalsis of the GI tract.

In general, GRFTs are categorized into effervescent and non-effervescent systems [7]. In the effervescent system, CO_2 air bubbles get liberated and entrapped into swollen hydrocolloids by the chemical reaction between effervescent agents such as magnesium carbonate, sodium bicarbonate, calcium carbonate, citric acid, etc., with gastric contents of the stomach that provides enough buoyancy for floating. Gas needs to be liberated and entrapped first; therefore, this system shows floating after a lag time, resulting in the risk of premature emptying of the dosage form from the stomach. In addition, unlike the swelling and mucoadhesive systems, the risk of gastric injuries, and unwanted side effects are low for floating devices [8]. On the other hand, the non-effervescent system uses a high percentage (20–75% w/w) of one or more gel-forming, highly swellable polymers into the tablet or capsule matrix to gain adequate buoyancy [7]. As a result, the drug release profile of dosage forms cannot be altered without adjusting the floating property and vice versa. In general, the conventional gastro-retentive systems always possess threats of floating lag time, premature gastric emptying, variable gastric retention time, and inconsistent drug release rate [9]. Therefore, to address the above challenges, a need is felt to develop a GRFTs system exploiting the novel 3DP and HME technologies that could stay afloat and releases the drug in a controlled manner.

3DP, also known as 'additive manufacturing' and 'rapid prototyping', is a manufacturing process used to create 3D physical objects by depositing materials in consecutive layers in the x, y, and z-axes with the aid of digital sketches obtained from a computer-aided design (CAD) software. Current 3DP technologies include (i) particle fusion-based methods, such as selective laser sintering (SLS), (ii) stereolithography (SLA), (iii) inkjet printing, and (iv) extrusion-based methods such as direct ink writing and fused deposition modeling (FDM). Among these, FDM is one of the most utilized and commercialized techniques for pharmaceutical applications due to its easy accessibility, efficiency, and cost-effectiveness, as well as its compatibility with a range of pharmaceutical thermoplastic polymers [10–13]. The starting material for FDM is produced via HME by blending the active pharmaceutical ingredients (APIs) with thermoplastic polymers to produce long, cylindrical, rod-shaped filaments. These filaments are fed into the heating nozzle, melted, and deposited layer-by-layer with FDM to produce the desired 3D shapes. The coupling of FDM and HME in one-unit operation has great potential for producing personalized dosage forms in-house for instant consumption. Thus, the combination is considered a revolutionary change in the context of pharmaceutical manufacturing [14].

More recently, a few studies have exploited novel 3DP technique to prolong gastric retention time of curcumin [15], acyclovir [16], amoxicillin [17], domperidone [18], riboflavin [19], and propranolol hydrochloride [20] however, the underlying drug release mechanism of 3D printed theophylline floating tablets remains unclear. Therefore, in this study, we aim to (i) develop controlled release THEO hollow tablets as intragastric floating devices by employing 3DP coupled with HME technology, and (ii) investigate the underlying drug release phenomenon from the 3DP THEO-HPC matrix tablets based on the mathematical modeling equations. The 3DP tablets with varying shell thickness and infill percentages were designed using 3D CAD software, and tablets were developed through an FDM 3D printer. Pharmaceutical grade hydroxypropyl cellulose (HPC) filaments need to be produced in-house with HME as no commercial HPC filaments are available. All the prepared 3DP GRFTs tablets could afloat for 10 h without showing any floating lag phase. Utilizing this approach could reduce the frequency of administration, minimize fluctuations in the plasma drug concentration with constant and steady drug release, and improve the overall therapeutic efficacy of THEO, leading to improved patient compliance and quality of life of patients. However, the in vivo analysis of the prepared dosage forms will be investigated in our future studies. To the best of our knowledge, this is the first work to exploit FDM 3DP paired with HME technology to develop a controlled release 3DP THEO-loaded HPC floating tablets.

2. Material and Methods

2.1. Materials

THEO was purchased from the Tokyo Chemical Industry Co. (Tokyo, Japan). HPC was donated by Hanmi Pharmaceutical Co. (Hwasung, Korea). Stearic acid (SA) was supplied by JUNSEI Chemical

Co. (Tokyo, Japan) and was used as a plasticizer. All the other chemicals were of reagent grade and were used without further purification.

2.2. Preparation of THEO-Loaded Filaments

THEO, HPC, and SA were evenly mixed at a weight ratio of 30:70:7 using a bench-top blender. The mixture was fed and extruded using a twin-screw extruder (Process 11, Thermo Fisher Scientific, Karlsruhe, Germany). The mixture was extruded at 150 °C for all zones with a standard screw configuration at a screw speed of 50 rpm. A 1.2-mm diameter rod-shaped die was used to prepare filaments. The brittleness and flexibility of the produced filaments were examined manually, and the filament diameter was measured in 5–10 cm intervals with a digital Vernier caliper.

2.3. Fabrication of FDM 3DP Tablets

Seven 3DP tablets (T1–T7) with different infill densities and shell thickness were produced using drug-loaded filaments via a standard FDM 3D printer (ANET-A8; Shenzhen Anet Technology Co. Ltd., Shenzhen, China). The 3DP tablets were created using the browser-based 3D design tool Tinkercad (Autodesk Inc., San Rafael, CA, USA), and the designed templates were exported as stereolithography (.stl) file into Cura v. 15.04.04 (Ultimaker B.V., Geldermalsen, The Netherlands). The selected geometry for the dosage form was a flat-faced cylindrical tablet with the dimensions X = 10.0 mm, Y = 10.0 mm, and Z = 5.0 mm. Cylinder-shaped tablets with different infill densities (0%, 10%, 20%, and 30%) and shell thickness (0, 0.4, 0.8, and 1.2 mm) (Table 1) were prepared to investigate the floating capability of the tablets. Other printer settings were as follows: standard resolution with the raft option deactivated and an extrusion temperature of 210 °C, speed of 20 mm/s while extruding, speed of 90 mm/s while traveling, and a layer height of 0.10 mm.

Table 1. Physical properties of the 3D printed floating tablets with varied infill densities and outside shell thickness.

Formulation	Infill (%)	Shell (mm)	Diameter (X, mm)	Diameter (Y, mm)	Thickness (Z, mm)	Weight (mg)
T1	30	0.8	10.54 ± 0.15	10.30 ± 0.17	4.63 ± 0.02	353.71 ± 8.78
T2	20	0.8	10.22 ± 0.04	10.25 ± 0.01	5.02 ± 0.37	326.30 ± 17.63
T3	10	0.8	10.52 ± 0.11	10.12 ± 0.09	4.74 ± 0.13	297.30 ± 5.35
T4	0	0.8	10.48 ± 0.40	10.41 ± 0.27	4.68 ± 0.04	273.70 ± 4.72
T5	20	1.2	10.40 ± 0.25	10.57 ± 0.14	5.09 ± 0.03	401.96 ± 8.75
T6	20	0.4	10.55 ± 0.14	10.46 ± 0.36	5.13 ± 0.03	322.95 ± 5.32
T7	20	0	10.55 ± 0.13	10.40 ± 0.16	5.17 ± 0.11	266.24 ± 3.50

2.4. Physicochemical Characterization

2.4.1. Determination of Drug Loading in 3DP Tablets

In order to determine the THEO content, each tablet or filament was cut into small pieces, weighed (approx. 0.1 g), and placed in a 100 mL volumetric flask containing methanol under magnetic stirring until complete dissolution to ensure complete drug release. Then the solution was diluted (100-fold), and the concentration of THEO was measured at UV 270 nm ($n = 3$).

2.4.2. Scanning Electron Microscopy (SEM)

The shape and surface morphology of the drug-loaded filaments and 3DP tablets were examined using SEM (SU8220; Hitachi; Tokyo, Japan) operating at an accelerated voltage of 5.0 kV. Samples were affixed onto a brass specimen holder using double-sided adhesive tape, and the samples were made electrically conductive by coating with platinum (6 nm/min) in a vacuum (0.8 Pa) for 4 min at 15 mA using an EmiTeck Sputter Coater (K575 K).

2.4.3. Differential Scanning Calorimetry (DSC)

A differential scanning calorimeter (TA DSC Q20; TA Instruments; Newcastle, DE, USA) was employed for thermal analysis. Approximately 5 mg of samples were weighed, sealed, and placed in an aluminum pan. The samples were heated from 50 °C to 300 °C at a constant temperature change rate of 10 °C/min under a nitrogen gas flow of 50 mL/min. All the measurement data were analyzed using the TA 2000 analysis software.

2.4.4. Powder X-Ray Diffraction (PXRD)

In order to evaluate the physical form of all the powder samples, a powder X-ray diffractometer (D/MAX-2500; Rigaku; Tokyo, Japan) equipped with a copper anode operated using Cu Kα radiation (1.54178 Å, 40 kV, and 40 mA). Samples were scanned from 5° to 50° using the step scan mode with a step size of 0.05°/s at room temperature and a 2θ diffraction angle to obtain the diffraction patterns.

2.5. In Vitro Dissolution and Floating Study

The floating behavior of the 3DP tablets was evaluated by placing the tablets in a transparent glass beaker containing 100 mL of 0.1 N HCl (pH 1.2) on a magnetic stirring at 50 rpm at room temperature. Furthermore, an in vitro drug release study was performed for all 3DP tablets using a USP type II dissolution apparatus (DT 620; ERWEKA; Heusenstamm, Germany). The tablets were placed in 900 mL of 0.1 M HCl medium maintained at 37 ± 0.5 °C and agitated at 50 rpm. Samples (2 mL) were extracted at predetermined intervals, and an equal amount of fresh media was immediately replenished to compensate for the loss during sampling. Prior to analysis, the collected samples were filtered with a PTFE membrane syringe filter Ø 0.45 µm and analyzed with a UV–vis spectrometer (UV-1800; Shimadzu, Kyoto, Japan) at 270 nm.

2.6. Dissolution Kinetics Studies

One of the primary goals of this work was the formulation of zero-order kinetics THEO loaded 3D tablets and understood the drug release mechanism of the gastro-retentive 3D dosage forms. Thus, various mathematical models such as Ritger–Peppes, Peppes–Sahlin, and zero-order release models were employed, and the correlation coefficient (R^2) was calculated. Dissolution data analysis was conducted by comparing the dissolution profiles while statistically applying the mathematical models to quantify and characterize the drug release from the 3D tablets.

3. Results and Discussion

3.1. Preparation of Drug-Loaded THEO Filaments

Material choice is a key aspect factor in FDM 3DP. Most of the pharmaceutical grade polymers used in the preparation of conventional oral dosage forms cannot be extruded with HME into the desired filaments for printing. In addition, only a few studies investigating cellulose and its derivatives for 3DP applications are available [21–23]. Hydroxypropyl cellulose (HPC), chemically known as cellulose 2-hydroxypropyl ether, is generally used as a thickening agent, tablet binder, film-coating, and extended release-matrix former in oral dosage forms [24]. It is a non-ionic, water-soluble, and pH-independent polymer, commercially available in a few grades with different viscosities and a molecular weight ranging from 50,000–1,250,000 g·mol^{-1} [25]. The low glass transition (T_g) temperature of HPC makes it pliable and easy to extrude through HME [26].

An HME-equipped with co-rotating twin-screw was used to extrude the mixtures of drug and cellulose polymer with a plasticizer to form long rod-shaped filaments. HME was carried out at 150 °C with a torque of 5–12 N/cm. The extruded HPC filaments loaded with THEO had a solid white appearance. Filaments with a consistent diameter in the range of 1.47 ± 0.01 mm and sufficient mechanical properties viz. strengths and flexibility suitable for FDM 3DP were produced with an HME die diameter of 1.2 mm. This increment in filament diameter compared to the HME die diameter (Ø 1.2 mm) is commonly known as the "die swell," corresponding to the effect of the heat and high shear stress generated during HME processing [27]. The HPC was subjected to a slightly higher temperature (150 °C) than its lower T_g value (105 °C) as well as high shear stress during mixing between the continuously rotating twin-screw and the wall of the barrel. Upon leaving the die, the polymer chains try to recover from the deformation applied by the co-rotating screw by "relaxing" and increasing their radius of gyration, resulting in the expansion of the filament diameter [27].

3.2. 3DP of THEO Dosage Forms

Cylindrical, hollow tablets with varying shell thickness and infill percentages were successfully printed via 3DP. The outer shell of the tablets kept the inner portion hollow (replaced with air) to ensure the tablets remained in a low-density state. The mechanical properties of the devices were found to be satisfactory, and the devices were not friable and were easy to handle. As presented in Table 1, the tablet weight was found to depend on both the shell thickness and infill percentage, with the former having a greater influence. As reported in previous literature, 3DP tablets have a plastic-like aspect with an incredibly high tablet strength, which is difficult to quantify with a conventional tablet hardness tester [28]. The friability of all the formulations was found to be zero, and it was difficult to separate the layers by applying force with sharp surfaces or human nails, without cutting the layers.

It is important to note that the 3DP temperature is significantly higher (210 °C) than the HME temperature (150 °C). This is due to the different heating rates of the two processes. During the preparation of filaments, the processing temperature is maintained for 5 min or longer. On the other hand, for successful printing, the filament needs to be in a semi-solid state, and therefore, the temperature is higher at the printer nozzle. The filament passes through the hot nozzle of the printer for a brief period at a much faster speed and, therefore, experiences the heat for a much shorter duration than during HME. The high temperature at the nozzle turns the filaments into a semi-solid state, which is followed by rapid fusion and quick solidification at room temperature. To attain such a rapid state change (from semi-solid to solid), the printers' temperature is usually elevated to around 210–250 °C. Interestingly, THEO-loaded HPC filaments were found to withstand this rise in temperature. The higher melting point of THEO (273 °C) compared to the 3D printer setting temperature (210 °C) allows the consistent flow of the semi-solid state filament from the printer's nozzle, and the low room temperature (25 °C) causes rapid solidification of the printed structure. However, lowering the nozzle temperature below 200 °C was found to increase the filament viscosity and cause poor material flow from the nozzle, resulting in the blockage of the printer nozzle, and finally, termination of the printing process.

3.3. Physicochemical State Characterization

3.3.1. Determination of Drug Loading

The chemical integrity of the drug in the 3DP tablets and filaments was analysed using a UV–vis spectrophotometer. Drug loading for the filaments was 302.83 ± 6.71 µg/mL (theoretical loading—300 µg/mL) and that for the printed tablets was 300.21 ± 1.49 µg/mL (theoretical amount—300 µg/mL), indicating no significant drug loss occurred during filament processing and tablet preparation. All the extruded filaments obtained in the present study showed appropriate characteristics for 3DP in terms of diameter, strength, flexibility, and brittleness.

3.3.2. Scanning Electron Microscopy (SEM)

SEM was used to investigate the topography of the extruded filament and the 3DP tablet structure. As depicted in Figure 1, the hot-melt extruded filament had a rod-shaped, robust, homogeneous smooth surface without a porous structure, indicating the absence of air pores and cavities in the filament. Figure 2A shows the pictures and SEM images of the 3DP THEO tablets with different infill percentages.

The tablet with the highest infill density (T1, 30% infill) contained numerous small holes with a dense mesh-like structure, whereas the structure appeared loose and contained larger air cavities as the infill percentages decreased (T2 20%, T3 10%, and a single large cavity was found in T4 with 0% infill). Figure 2B shows the layer-layer deposition structure of the printed tablet, suggesting the influence of shell thickness. As can be observed from the 3DP tablet pictures and SEM images, the tablet with high shell thickness (T5) had a compact rigid structure with a slightly smooth outer surface. However, upon reducing the shell thickness (from T5, 1.2 mm to T7, 0 mm), a loose gap appeared between the successive layers with increasing layer thickness, resulting in a coarse and rough outer surface.

Overall, all the prepared 3DP tablets were observed to have slightly uneven and rough external surfaces, among which, T7 shows the maximum roughness (Figure 2). This might be correlated with the 3D printer resolution and shell thickness. In 3DP technology, the nozzle moves in three dimensions, i.e., horizontally (XY axis), and the build platform goes vertically downwards (Z-axis) as the process continues. The XY resolution determines the physical area (length and breadth) of the 3DP objects and is generally found consistent whereas, the Z resolution that controls the layer thickness or layer height is fairly inconsistent [29]. Due to the reasons, the microscopic imaging of 3DP objects shows uneven, asymmetrical, and rough surfaces. However, post-processing or extra finishing steps might make the surface look smoother [29]. Further, a judicious selection of the FDM 3D printer, i.e., with higher resolution capabilities and performs well in all the three dimensions (XY and Z axis), could improve the quality of the printed object [30].

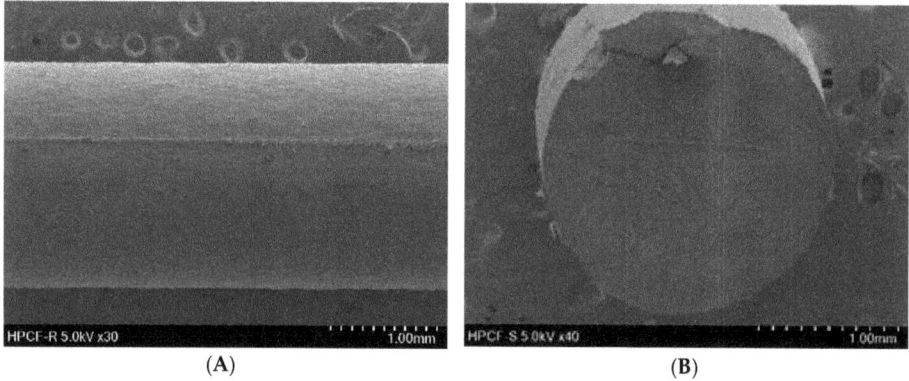

(A)   (B)

Figure 1. SEM images of hot-melt extruded filament. (**A**) Exterior appearance (30×) and (**B**) cross sectional shape (40×).

3.3.3. Differential Scanning Calorimetry (DSC)

DSC was conducted to examine changes in the crystallinity of the bulk materials, the extruded filament, and the 3DP tablet during the thermal processes. As shown in Figure 3, THEO had a strong endothermic peak at approximately 275 °C, corresponding to its melting point. However, with the introduction of HPC, DSC thermograms were absent for the physical mixture (PM), filament, and the subsequent 3DP tablet. The absence of these peaks in the DSC thermograpH may be due to the molecular dispersion of the THEO within the HPC polymer matrix, leading to reduced crystallinity that could not be detected with DSC. Therefore, PXRD was further employed for thermal analysis.

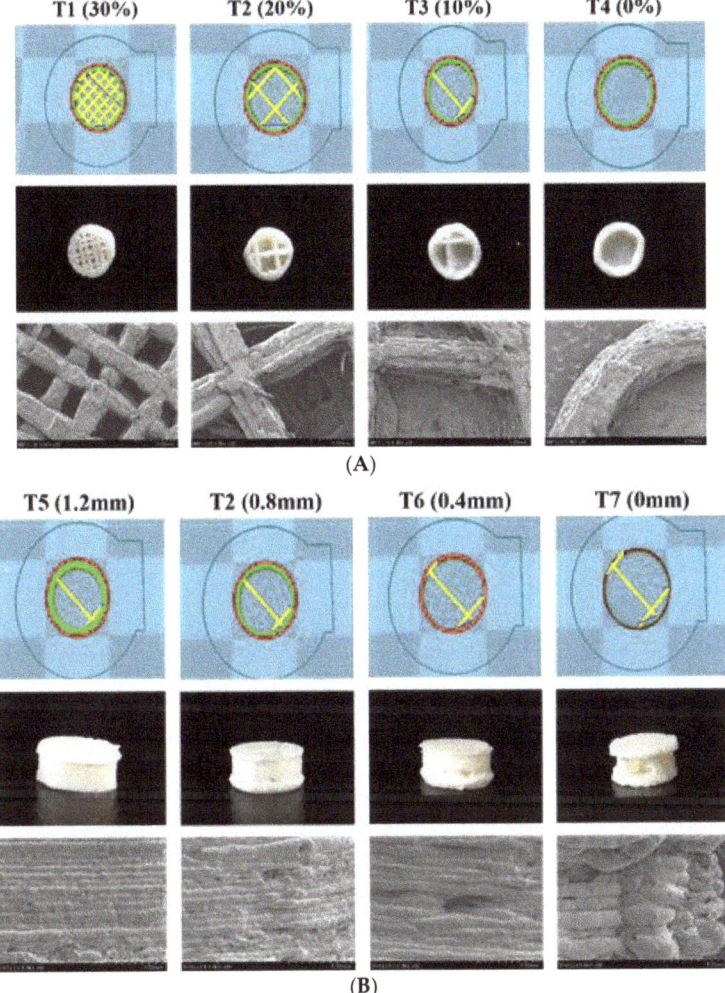

Figure 2. 3D tablet design templates, tablet photographs, and SEM images of 3D printed tablet surface with (**A**) constant shell thickness (0.8 mm), different infill percentages (T1 30%, T2 20%, T3 10%, and T4 0%) and (**B**) constant infill percentage (20%), different shell thickness (T5 1.2 mm, T2 0.8 mm, T6 0.4 mm, and T7 0 mm).

3.3.4. Powder X-Ray Diffraction (PXRD)

The use of high temperatures during HME and 3DP can lead to the degradation of thermolabile drugs and polymers. To further confirm the thermal properties of the samples, PXRD analysis was conducted. As illustrated in Figure 4, THEO showed numerous sharp diffraction peaks, with major peaks at $2\theta = 7, 12, 14,$ and 24 that corresponded to the expected diffraction patterns [31], suggesting a highly crystalline nature. Surprisingly, the PXRD results for the PM, filament, and 3DP tablets were quite different from the results obtained with the DSC thermogram. The PM, filament, and 3DP tablets showed numerous peaks, all with reduced intensities. This may be due to the fact that the low-resolution DSC thermogram could not show crystallinity below 2% [32,33]. These observations suggest that the THEO crystal had converted to a partially crystalline state, with molecular dispersion of the drug into the polymer matrix. One possible explanation of this observation is the homogeneous mixing of the active material and the amorphous polymer under the thermal processing conditions for HME and FDM 3DP. However, in this work, no significant thermal degradation was observed for both the filaments and 3DP tablets.

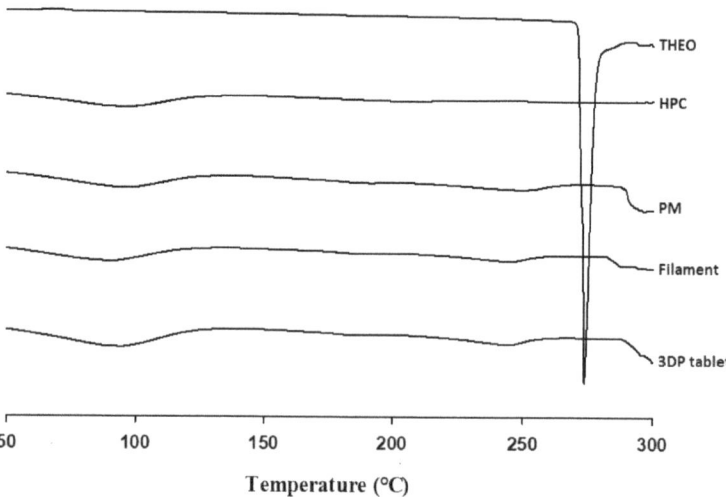

Figure 3. DSC curves of free THEO, hydroxypropyl cellulose (HPC), physical mixture (PM), THEO-HPC filament, and 3DP tablet. PM represents the physical mixture of THEO, HPC, and stearic acid (SA) at a 30:70:7 (*w/w/w*) ratio.

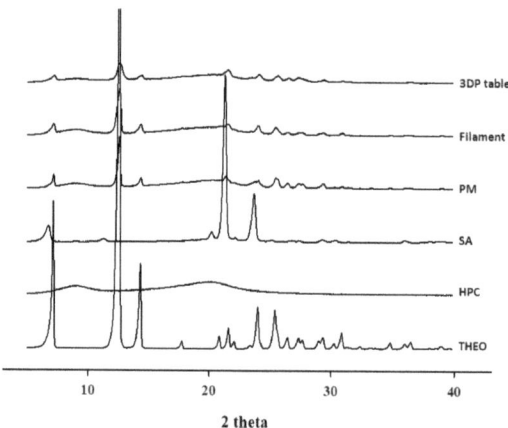

Figure 4. PXRD curves of 3DP tablet, THEO-HPC filament, PM, SA, HPC, and free THEO.

3.4. In Vitro Floating and Dissolution Study

The floating ability was influenced by the density of the 3DP tablets, which in turn was found to be associated with the infill percentage of the tablets. The 3DP tablet (T2) with a density of approximately 0.79 g/cm^3 was buoyant for more than 10 h (Figure 5), while the tablet with 60% infill sank to the bottom of the dissolution medium in less than 1 h (data not shown). Generally, tablets with lower infill percentages contain higher air content and, therefore, little to no floating lag time, owing to the low-density. In addition, the shell number did not show any marked differences in floating lag time for the 3DP tablets. Based on these observations, it can be inferred that the period of buoyancy for the 3DP tablets is closely related to their density, which in turn depends on the infill percentage.

In vitro dissolution studies for all seven formulations were performed in 0.1 N HCl (pH 1.2) to stimulate the gastric conditions of the stomach. In general, 0.1 N hydrochloric acid buffer (pH 1.2) is employed as the dissolution media to represent the acidic gastric fluid for gastro-retentive systems [16,18]. However, the dissolution test using a suitable biorelevant media, which seems to mimic the physiological in vivo dissolution better as compared to the buffer solutions may be worthy for future investigation [34]. The final run-out was over 90%, confirming that the drug was released at a relatively constant rate for 6 h before a plateau, with constant drug release thereafter (after 6 h). Figure 6A depicts the influence of infill percentage on the drug release profile of the 3DP THEO tablets. T1 (0.8 mm shell thickness and 30% infill) had a slow and extended drug profile compared with T4 (0.8 mm shell thickness and 0% infill). This could be mainly due to the large cavities/holes and large, loose gaps between the successive layers formed as the infill decreased. The higher porosity allows for quick penetration of the dissolution media into the tablet core, leading to rapid dissolution and diffusion of the drug from the THEO-HPC matrix. It has been reported that tablets with high infill percentages are harder and encounter a more intense retarding force that counteracts the positive effects of polymer dissolution, causing a delay in the drug release rate [35].

As illustrated in Figure 6B, the tablets with infill densities of 20% and varying shell thickness had different drug release rates. T2 (0.8 mm shell thickness, 20% infill), exhibited extended drug release rates because of its dense shell structure (as shown in SEM images, Figure 2B), while the tablets without shells (T7) exhibited fast drug release kinetics. This is mainly due to the thin and loose outer structure of T7, which dissociates promptly upon contact with the dissolution media, thus causing rapid drug release from the polymer matrix [35,36]. A large difference in drug release rate was observed with tablets having shell wall (T2, 0.8 mm) and without shell wall (T7, 0 mm); however, the difference was not that pronounced with tablets of different shell wall thickness (T2, T5, T6). Interestingly, the drug release profile of T5 (1.2 mm shell) was identical to the T6 (0.4 mm shell). Nevertheless, T2 (0.8 mm shell) displayed a slightly lower drug release rate compared to both T5 and T6, which might be possible due to the low printing resolution of the 3D printer (explained in Section 3.3.2).

Although the THEO 3DP tablets exceeded the tablet hardness limit on the hardness tester, the floating behavior and in vitro dissolution profile were found to be adequate, with 90% drug release over 8 h.

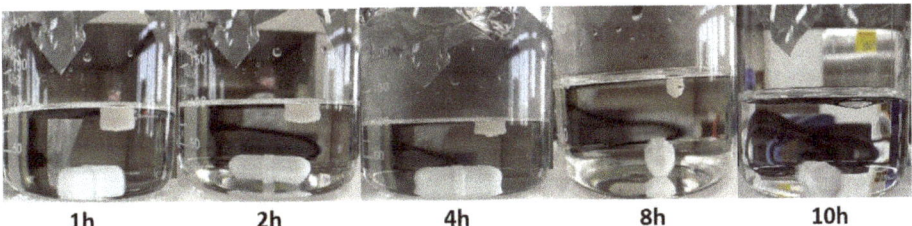

Figure 5. Photographs of 3DP tablet (T2) floating in dissolution medium (0.1 N HCl solution) at room temperature.

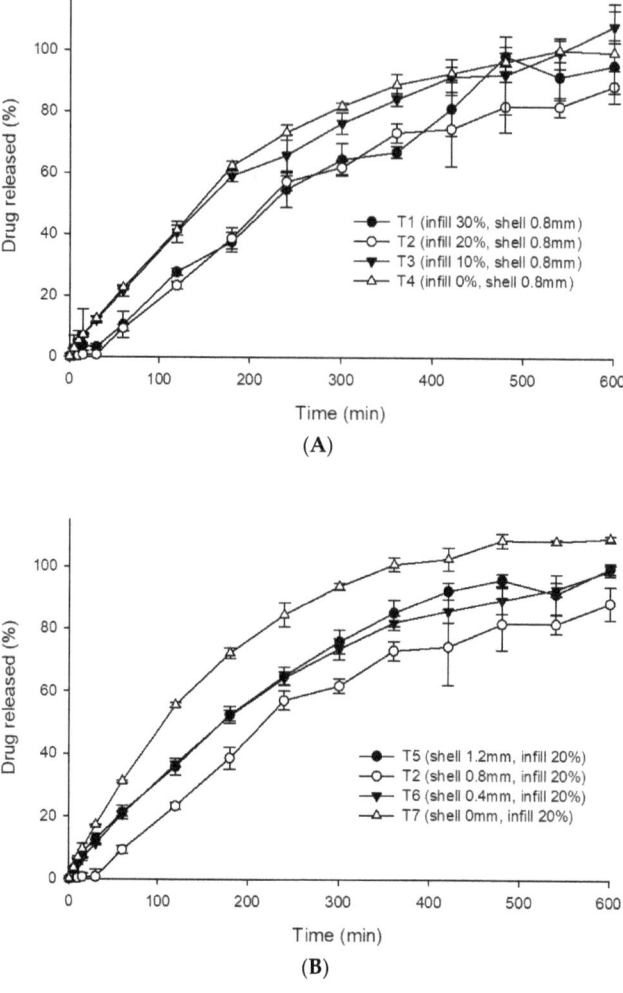

Figure 6. Drug release profiles of the 3DP tablets; (**A**) showing the influence of the infill percentages and (**B**) showing the influence of the shell thickness. Each value represents the mean ± standard deviation ($n = 3$).

3.5. Dissolution Kinetic Studies

Mathematical models are essential tools for describing and quantitatively analyzing in vitro/in vivo drug release kinetics, predicting the release profile, and ensuring the optimal design of dosage forms [37]. In 1961, Higuchi developed the most recognized and commonly used kinetic equation to describe the release profile of drugs dispersed in homogeneous matrix systems [38]. There are a few assumptions with the Higuchi model [39,40]:

1. The initial drug concentration in a matrix system is much higher than the drug solubility.
2. Drug diffusion is one-dimensional because edge effects are insignificant.
3. The thickness of the dosage form is much larger than the size of the suspended drug particles (macro or nanoparticles).
4. The swelling or dissolution of the polymer carrier is negligible.

5. The drug diffusion coefficient is constant.
6. Perfect sink conditions are achieved in the release medium.

The Higuchi equation can only be used for an ideal controlled-release system because the first assumption provides the basis for the explanation of the pseudo-steady state [40,41]. Further, the equation considers the drug diffusivity to be constant, which is only valid for polymers that do not swell upon contact with the dissolution medium. Generally, with 3DP tablets, the tablet matrix may show multidimensional diffusion, and the matrix swelling phenomena cannot be neglected. Therefore, the Higuchi model is not relevant for this study.

Thus, to find the dissolution mechanism, the in vitro dissolution data were fitted in the Ritger–Peppas model (also known as the power law). The power law is a more comprehensive semi-empirical equation that describes drug release from polymeric systems when the drug release phenomenon is not known or if more than one type of mechanism is involved [42,43]. The equation is as follows:

$$\frac{M_t}{M_\infty} = kt^n, \qquad (1)$$

where M_t is the cumulative amount of drug dissolved over time t, M_∞ is the total amount of drug contained in a dosage form at the beginning of the release process, k is a constant incorporating the structural modifications and geometrical characteristics of the device, and n is the release exponent (related to the drug release mechanism) [44].

It is generally recommended to use the first 60% of the drug release curve for statistical analysis [35]. Based on the release parameter (coefficient of determination, R^2), and the value of the release exponent (n), the mechanism by which the drug is released from the matrix system is proposed. For cylindrical tablets (Case I), $0.45 \leq n$ corresponds to a Fickian diffusion where the drug molecules are released due to a diffusion process. The solvent transport rate or diffusion phenomenon is more dominant than the polymeric chain relaxation process. When $n = 0.89$, the model is non-Fickian (Case II transport), and the drug release corresponds to zero-order release kinetics. The drug release primarily involves swelling or relaxation of polymeric chains in the drug-loaded matrix system. Moreover, if $0.45 < n < 0.89$, the model depicts non-Fickian or anomalous transport, and both diffusion and swelling mechanisms govern the drug release. At the end of Case II transport, a fast increase in the solvent absorption rate gives rise to the Super Case II transport model (when $n > 0.89$), during which the sorption process, tension, and breaking of the polymeric chains leading to drug release from the matrix system. Thus, the power law was applied to analyze the release profiles and the calculated data are listed in Table 2. T3 ($n = 0.89$, $R^2 = 0.98$), T4 ($n = 0.90$, $R^2 = 0.99$), T6 ($n = 0.84$, $R^2 = 0.98$) can be considered to exhibit Case II transport. The drug release kinetics from these tablets may be governed by the swelling of the polymer matrix. In addition, T5 ($n = 0.73$, $R^2 = 0.99$) and T7 ($n = 0.79$, $R^2 = 0.98$) exhibit an anomalous transport, whereas T1 ($n = 1.11$, $R^2 = 0.98$) and T2 ($n = 1.39$, $R^2 = 0.99$) potentially exhibit Super Case II transport. Overall, the drug release exponent varied from 0.73–1.39, suggesting that both the matrix swelling and diffusion mechanism were involved in governing drug release kinetics from the prepared 3D tablet matrix.

To analyze the approximate contribution of these mechanisms (diffusional and relaxational), Peppas–Sahlin developed the following kinetics model [45]:

$$\frac{M_t}{M_\infty} = k_1 t^m + k_2 t^{2m}, \qquad (2)$$

where k_1, k_2, and m are constants. The first term in the equation $k_1 t^m$ represents the Fickian diffusional contribution, whereas the second term $k_2 t^{2m}$ represents the Case II swelling contribution. The coefficient m is a purely Fickian diffusional exponent. The amount of drug release due to the Fickian mechanism (F) is calculated as follows:

$$F = \frac{1}{1 + \frac{k_2}{k_1} t^m} \qquad (3)$$

The ratio of both contributions can be calculated as:

$$\frac{R}{F} = \frac{k_2 t^m}{k_1} \quad (4)$$

Here, the diffusional contribution can be represented as a function of t^m, and the relaxational contribution as t^{2m}. The Peppas–Sahlin Equation (2) was applied to the dissolution profile of individually designed 3D tablets, and the ratio of relaxational contribution (R) over Fickian contribution (R/F) was calculated and plotted in Figure 7. Interestingly, though the correlation coefficients (R^2) for T1, T2, and T7 were good (close to 1), the value for k_1 was negative. A similar case was observed with the published report where the authors described the result as illogical and a possible consequence of the anomalous transport [35]. As shown in Figure 7, as the drug starts to dissolve in the T4 and T6, Fickian diffusion (F) decreases along with time, which indicates that the drug may be released as a result of polymer relaxation. The high mobility of carrier chains allowed easier solvent penetration into the tablet matrix, and the solvent diffusion rate was reduced below the relaxation rate. However, the R/F curve for T5 indicates that the influence of the swelling mechanism was significantly reduced due to the inclusion of Fickian diffusion in the drug release. Overall, the Peppas–Sahlin study revealed that both the swelling and diffusion mechanisms resulted in steady drug release from the 3DP tablets, and the swelling process had a relatively larger contribution during the entire drug release stage.

Table 2. In vitro dissolution parameters for the 3DP tablets.

Formulation	Ritger-Peppas Model		Linear Model		Peppas-Sahlin Model			
	Exponent, n	R^2	Slope, k	R^2	k_1	k_2	m	R^2
T1	1.11	0.9846	0.20	0.9876	−0.92	0.41	0.45	0.9814
T2	1.39	0.9927	0.19	0.9781	−0.55	0.13	0.56	0.9837
T3	0.89	0.9896	0.25	0.9519	0.80	0.20	0.52	1.0000
T4	0.90	0.9998	0.26	0.9422	0.87	0.01	0.73	0.9997
T5	0.73	0.9969	0.24	0.9708	1.20	0.02	0.63	0.9980
T6	0.84	0.9868	0.23	0.9594	0.40	0.45	0.44	0.9998
T7	0.79	0.9881	0.30	0.9043	−3.35	3.03	0.32	0.9894

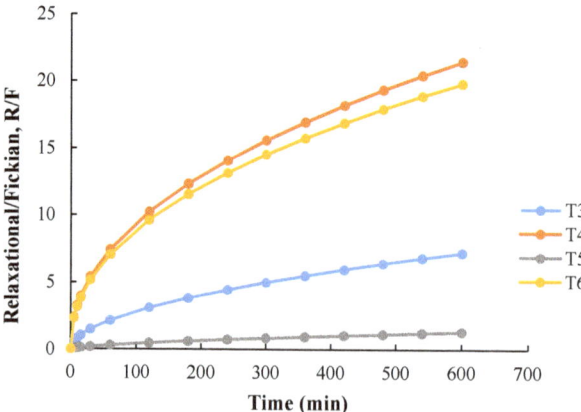

Figure 7. Swelling contribution (R) to the diffusion contribution (F), R/F ratio from T3, T4, T5, and T6.

Zero-Order Drug Release

Dosage forms that release the drug at a constant rate, resulting in a uniform drug plasma concentration, are desirable. Zero-order release can be represented by the equation:

$$M_t = M_o + kt, \tag{5}$$

where M_t is the cumulative amount of drug dissolved over time t, M_o is the initial amount of drug (most of the time, $M_o = 0$), and k is the zero-order release constant. As shown in the in vitro drug release curve (Figure 6), all seven formulations showed complete drug release within 10 h. The linear fitting of the in vitro drug release data is presented in Table 2. The linear regression (R^2) values, which were close to 1, indicated that the prepared dosage forms showed a good fit for the zero-order. As predicted, T3 ($R^2 = 0.95$), T4 ($R^2 = 0.94$), T5 ($R^2 = 0.97$), and T6 ($R^2 = 0.95$) showed a steady and constant linear regression curve (Figure 8). The zero-order linear fitting results for T3, T4, T5, and T6 were consistent with the outcomes of the Ritger–Peppas and Peppas–Sahlin models. Hence, it can be concluded that the coupling of 3DP with HME could be an effective approach to develop zero-order release GRFTs.

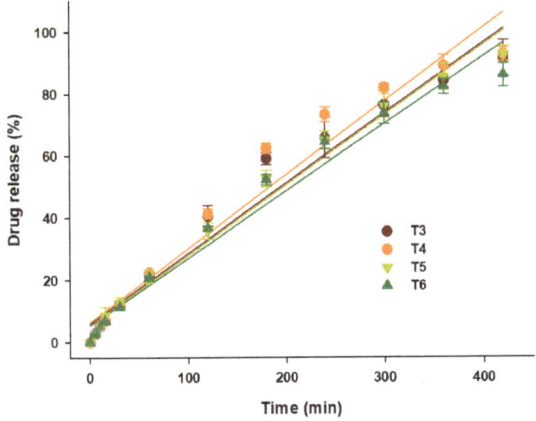

Figure 8. Linear fitting of drug release from T3, T4, T5, and T6 over 10 h.

4. Conclusions

THEO-loaded HPC filaments suitable for 3DP were successfully developed to produce 3DP intragastric floating tablets. The resulting 3D hollow tablets with different infill percentages and shell thickness showed sufficient buoyancy for approximately 10 h with zero-order drug release profiles, providing an alternative method to fabricate controlled-release intragastric floating drug delivery systems. Physical state characterization showed that the crystalline drug was molecularly dispersed within the cellulose matrix, resulting in reduced drug crystallinity. The infill density and shell thickness were found to be the key parameters for low-density, along with air entrapment in the inner core structure of the 3DP tablets, which altogether governs the in vitro drug release rate. Based on the Peppas–Sahlin model, both the swelling and diffusion phenomena were involved in the drug release process, with the former mechanism having a relatively larger contribution during the entire drug release stage. T3, T4, T5, and T6 had a constant and steady drug release profile with linear fitting, confirming that the drug release can be considered controlled (zero-order). Overall, this study demonstrates that the coupling of novel HME and FDM-based 3DP technologies could be an effective, efficient, and economical alternative to develop gastro-retentive dosage forms with better controlled-release rates as compared to the traditional pharmaceutical manufacturing. However, additional assessment for stability and in-vitro in-vivo correlation (IVIVC) studies of the 3DP floating formulations need to be further investigated. Despite considerable progress, 3DP technology is still in its early stages. Further innovations and development on product quality, novel structural design, better printing resolution, and proper regulatory mechanism, will facilitate this technology to become more practical in commercial manufacturing.

Author Contributions: Conceptualization—E.S.S. and D.W.K.; methodology and investigation—E.S.S., J.K., J.-H.L., J.-B.P. and D.W.K.; writing-original draft preparation—E.S.S., B.R.G. and D.W.K.; writing-review and editing—B.R.G. and D.W.K.; supervision, project administration, and funding acquisition—D.W.K. All authors have read and agreed to the published version of the manuscript.

Funding: This work was supported by the National Research Foundation (NRF) of South Korea grants funded by the South Korean government (MEST) (No. 2018R1D1A1B07050598).

Conflicts of Interest: The authors declare no conflicts of interest in this work.

References

1. Streubel, A.; Siepmann, J.; Bodmeier, R. Drug delivery to the upper small intestine window using gastroretentive technologies. *Curr. Opin. Pharmacol.* **2006**, *6*, 501–508. [CrossRef] [PubMed]
2. Shah, H.P.; Prajapati, S.T. Quality by design based development and optimization of novel gastroretentive floating osmotic capsules of clopidogrel bisulfate. *J. Pharm. Investig.* **2019**, *49*, 295–311. [CrossRef]
3. Lamichhane, S.; Park, J.B.; Sohn, D.H.; Lee, S. Customized Novel Design of 3D Printed Pregabalin Tablets for Intra-Gastric Floating and Controlled Release Using Fused Deposition Modeling. *Pharmaceutics* **2019**, *11*, 564. [CrossRef] [PubMed]
4. Chavanpatil, M.D.; Jain, P.; Chaudhari, S.; Shear, R.; Vavia, P.R. Novel sustained release, swellable and bioadhesive gastroretentive drug delivery system for ofloxacin. *Int. J. Pharm.* **2006**, *316*, 86–92. [CrossRef] [PubMed]
5. Klausner, E.A.; Lavy, E.; Friedman, M.; Hoffman, A. Expandable gastroretentive dosage forms. *J. Control. Release* **2003**, *90*, 143–162. [CrossRef]
6. Li, Z.; Xu, H.; Li, S.; Li, Q.; Zhang, W.; Ye, T.; Yang, X.; Pan, W. A novel gastro-floating multiparticulate system for dipyridamole (DIP) based on a porous and low-density matrix core: In vitro and in vivo evaluation. *Int. J. Pharm.* **2014**, *461*, 540–548. [CrossRef]
7. Pawar, V.K.; Kansal, S.; Asthana, S.; Chourasia, M.K. Industrial perspective of gastroretentive drug delivery systems: Physicochemical, biopharmaceutical, technological and regulatory consideration. *Expert Opin. Drug Deliv.* **2012**, *9*, 551–565. [CrossRef]
8. Arora, S.; Ali, J.; Ahuja, A.; Khar, R.K.; Baboota, S. Floating drug delivery systems: A review. *AAPS PharmSciTech* **2005**, *6*, E372–E390. [CrossRef]
9. Kim, S.; Hwang, K.M.; Park, Y.S.; Nguyen, T.T.; Park, E.S. Preparation and evaluation of non-effervescent gastroretentive tablets containing pregabalin for once-daily administration and dose proportional pharmacokinetics. *Int. J. Pharm.* **2018**, *550*, 160–169. [CrossRef]
10. Park, B.J.; Choi, H.J.; Moon, S.J.; Kim, S.J.; Bajracharya, R.; Min, J.Y.; Han, H.K. Pharmaceutical applications of 3D printing technology: Current understanding and future perspectives. *J. Pharm. Investig.* **2019**, *49*, 575–585. [CrossRef]
11. Guvendiren, M.; Molde, J.; Soares, R.M.D.; Kohn, J. Designing Biomaterials for 3D Printing. *ACS Biomater. Sci. Eng.* **2016**, *2*, 1679–1693. [CrossRef] [PubMed]
12. Ambrosi, A.; Pumera, M. 3D-printing technologies for electrochemical applications. *Chem. Soc. Rev.* **2016**, *45*, 2740–2755. [CrossRef] [PubMed]
13. Gross, B.C.; Erkal, J.L.; Lockwood, S.Y.; Chen, C.; Spence, D.M. Evaluation of 3D printing and its potential impact on biotechnology and the chemical sciences. *Anal. Chem.* **2014**, *86*, 3240–3253. [CrossRef]
14. Tan, D.; Maniruzzaman, M.; Nokhodchi, A. Advanced pharmaceutical applications of hot-melt extrusion coupled with fused deposition modelling (FDM) 3D printing for personalised drug delivery. *Pharmaceutics* **2018**, *10*, 203. [CrossRef] [PubMed]
15. Tagami, T.; Fukushige, K.; Ogawa, E.; Hayashi, N.; Ozeki, T. 3D printing factors important for the fabrication of polyvinylalcohol filament-based tablets. *Biol. Pharm. Bull.* **2017**, *40*, 357–364. [CrossRef] [PubMed]

16. Shin, S.; Kim, T.H.; Jeong, S.W.; Chung, S.E.; Kim, D.H.; Shin, B.S. Development of a gastroretentive delivery system for acyclovir by 3D printing technology and its in vivo pharmacokinetic evaluation in Beagle dogs. *PLoS ONE* **2019**, *14*, e0216875. [CrossRef]
17. Charoenying, T.; Patrojanasophon, P.; Ngawhirunpat, T.; Rojanarata, T.; Akkaramongkolporn, P.; Opanasopit, P. Fabrication of floating capsule-in-3D-printed devices as gastro-retentive delivery systems of amoxicillin. *J. Drug Deliv. Sci. Technol.* **2020**, *55*, 101393. [CrossRef]
18. Chai, X.; Chai, H.; Wang, X.; Yang, J.; Li, J.; Zhao, Y.; Cai, W.; Tao, T.; Xiang, X. Fused Deposition Modeling (FDM) 3D Printed Tablets for Intragastric Floating Delivery of Domperidone. *Sci. Rep.* **2017**, *7*, 2829. [CrossRef]
19. Fu, J.; Yin, H.; Yu, X.; Xie, C.; Jiang, H.; Jin, Y.; Sheng, F. Combination of 3D printing technologies and compressed tablets for preparation of riboflavin floating tablet-in-device (TiD) systems. *Int. J. Pharm.* **2018**, *549*, 370–379. [CrossRef]
20. Chen, D.; Xu, X.Y.; Li, R.; Zang, G.A.; Zhang, Y.; Wang, M.R.; Xiong, M.F.; Xu, J.R.; Wang, T.; Fu, H.; et al. Preparation and In vitro Evaluation of FDM 3D-Printed Ellipsoid-Shaped Gastric Floating Tablets with Low Infill Percentages. *AAPS PharmSciTech* **2020**, *21*, 6. [CrossRef]
21. Dai, L.; Cheng, T.; Duan, C.; Zhao, W.; Zhang, W.; Zou, X.; Aspler, J.; Ni, Y. 3D printing using plant-derived cellulose and its derivatives: A review. *Carbohydr. Polym.* **2019**, *203*, 71–86. [CrossRef]
22. Kempin, W.; Franz, C.; Koster, L.C.; Schneider, F.; Bogdahn, M.; Weitschies, W.; Seidlitz, A. Assessment of different polymers and drug loads for fused deposition modeling of drug loaded implants. *Eur. J. Pharm. Biopharm.* **2017**, *115*, 84–93. [CrossRef] [PubMed]
23. Zhang, J.; Feng, X.; Patil, H.; Tiwari, R.V.; Repka, M.A. Coupling 3D printing with hot-melt extrusion to produce controlled-release tablets. *Int. J. Pharm.* **2017**, *519*, 186–197. [CrossRef] [PubMed]
24. Kamel, S.; Ali, N.; Jahangir, K.; Shah, S.M.; El-Gendy, A.A. Pharmaceutical significance of cellulose: A review. *Express Polym. Lett.* **2008**, *2*, 758–778. [CrossRef]
25. Rowe, R.C.; Sheskey, P.; Quinn, M. *Handbook of Pharmaceutical Excipients*; Libros Digitales-Pharmaceutical Press: London, UK, 2009.
26. Sarode, A.; Wang, P.; Cote, C.; Worthen, D.R. Low-viscosity hydroxypropylcellulose (HPC) grades SL and SSL: Versatile pharmaceutical polymers for dissolution enhancement, controlled release, and pharmaceutical processing. *AAPS PharmSciTech* **2013**, *14*, 151–159. [CrossRef] [PubMed]
27. Crowley, M.M.; Zhang, F.; Repka, M.A.; Thumma, S.; Upadhye, S.B.; Battu, S.K.; McGinity, J.W.; Martin, C. Pharmaceutical applications of hot-melt extrusion: Part I. *Drug Dev. Ind. Pharm.* **2007**, *33*, 909–926. [CrossRef]
28. Goyanes, A.; Fina, F.; Martorana, A.; Sedough, D.; Gaisford, S.; Basit, A.W. Development of modified release 3D printed tablets (printlets) with pharmaceutical excipients using additive manufacturing. *Int. J. Pharm.* **2017**, *527*, 21–30. [CrossRef]
29. Lamichhane, S.; Bashyal, S.; Keum, T.; Noh, G.; Seo, J.E.; Bastola, R.; Choi, J.; Sohn, D.H.; Lee, S. Complex formulations, simple techniques: Can 3D printing technology be the Midas touch in pharmaceutical industry? *Asian J. Pharm. Sci.* **2019**, *14*, 465–479. [CrossRef]
30. Pietrzak, K.; Isreb, A.; Alhnan, M.A. A flexible-dose dispenser for immediate and extended release 3D printed tablets. *Eur. J. Pharm. Biopharm.* **2015**, *96*, 380–387. [CrossRef]
31. Räsänen, E.; Rantanen, J.; Jørgensen, A.; Karjalainen, M.; Paakkari, T.; Yliruusi, J. Novel identification of pseudopolymorphic changes of theophylline during wet granulation using near infrared spectroscopy. *J. Pharm. Sci.* **2001**, *90*, 389–396. [CrossRef]
32. Leuner, C.; Dressman, J. Improving drug solubility for oral delivery using solid dispersions. *Eur. J. Pharm. Biopharm.* **2000**, *50*, 47–60. [CrossRef]
33. Tran, P.H.L.; Tran, H.T.T.; Lee, B.J. Modulation of microenvironmental pH and crystallinity of ionizable telmisartan using alkalizers in solid dispersions for controlled release. *J. Control. Release* **2008**, *129*, 59–65. [CrossRef]
34. Klein, S. The use of biorelevant dissolution media to forecast the in vivo performance of a drug. *AAPS J.* **2010**, *12*, 397–406. [CrossRef] [PubMed]
35. Zhang, J.; Yang, W.; Vo, A.Q.; Feng, X.; Ye, X.; Kim, D.W.; Repka, M.A. Hydroxypropyl methylcellulose-based controlled release dosage by melt extrusion and 3D printing: Structure and drug release correlation. *Carbohydr. Polym.* **2017**, *177*, 49–57. [CrossRef] [PubMed]

36. Li, Q.; Guan, X.; Cui, M.; Zhu, Z.; Chen, K.; Wen, H.; Jia, D.; Hou, J.; Xu, W.; Yang, X.; et al. Preparation and investigation of novel gastro-floating tablets with 3D extrusion-based printing. *Int. J. Pharm.* **2018**, *535*, 325–332. [CrossRef] [PubMed]
37. Bruschi, M.L. (Ed.) 5-Mathematical models of drug release. In *Strategies to Modify the Drug Release from Pharmaceutical Systems*; Woodhead Publishing: Sawston, UK, 2015; pp. 63–86.
38. Higuchi, T. Rate of Release of Medicaments from Ointment Bases Containing Drugs in Suspension. *J. Pharm. Sci.* **1961**, *50*, 874–875. [CrossRef] [PubMed]
39. Omidian, H.; Park, K. Introduction to Hydrogels. In *Biomedical Applications of Hydrogels Handbook*; Ottenbrite, R.M., Park, K., Okano, T., Eds.; Springer: New York, NY, USA, 2010; pp. 1–16.
40. Siepmann, J.; Peppas, N.A. Modeling of drug release from delivery systems based on hydroxypropyl methylcellulose (HPMC). *Adv. Drug Deliv. Rev.* **2012**, *64*, 163–174. [CrossRef]
41. Siepmann, J.; Göpferich, A. Mathematical modeling of bioerodible, polymeric drug delivery systems. *Adv. Drug Deliv. Rev.* **2001**, *48*, 229–247. [CrossRef]
42. Peppas, N.A. Analysis of Fickian and non-Fickian drug release from polymers. *Pharm. Acta Helv.* **1985**, *60*, 110–111.
43. Peppas, N.A.; Narasimhan, B. Mathematical models in drug delivery: How modeling has shaped the way we design new drug delivery systems. *J. Control. Release* **2014**, *190*, 75–81. [CrossRef]
44. Korsmeyer, R.W.; Gurny, R.; Doelker, E.; Buri, P.; Peppas, N.A. Mechanisms of solute release from porous hydrophilic polymers. *Int. J. Pharm.* **1983**, *15*, 25–35. [CrossRef]
45. Peppas, N.A.; Sahlin, J.J. A simple equation for the description of solute release, III, Coupling of diffusion and relaxation. *Int. J. Pharm.* **1989**, *57*, 169–172. [CrossRef]

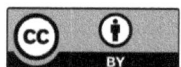

© 2020 by the authors. Licensee MDPI, Basel, Switzerland. This article is an open access article distributed under the terms and conditions of the Creative Commons Attribution (CC BY) license (http://creativecommons.org/licenses/by/4.0/).

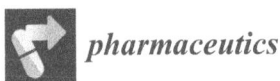

Article

Customized Novel Design of 3D Printed Pregabalin Tablets for Intra-Gastric Floating and Controlled Release Using Fused Deposition Modeling

Shrawani Lamichhane [1], Jun-Bom Park [2], Dong Hwan Sohn [1] and Sangkil Lee [1,*]

1. College of Pharmacy, Keimyung University, 1095 Dalgubeol-daero, Dalseo-gu, Daegu 42601, Korea; phr.shrawani@gmail.com (S.L.); dhsohn@kmu.ac.kr (D.H.S.)
2. College of Pharmacy, Samyook University, 815 Hwarang-ro, Nowon-gu, Seoul 01795, Korea; junji4@gmail.com
* Correspondence: skdavid@kmu.ac.kr; Tel.: +82-53-580-6655; Fax: +82-53-580-5164

Received: 11 October 2019; Accepted: 28 October 2019; Published: 30 October 2019

Abstract: Three-dimensional (3D) printing has been recently employed in the design and formulation of various dosage forms with the aim of on-demand manufacturing and personalized medicine. In this study, we formulated a floating sustained release system using fused deposition modeling (FDM). Filaments were prepared using hypromellose acetate succinate (HPMCAS), polyethylene glycol (PEG 400) and pregabalin as the active ingredient. Cylindrical tablets with infill percentages of 25%, 50% and 75% were designed and printed with the FDM printer. An optimized formulation (F6) was designed with a closed bottom layer and a partially opened top layer. Filaments and tablets were characterized by means of fourier-transform infrared spectroscopy (FTIR), differential scanning calorimetry (DSC), X-ray powder diffraction (XRPD), and thermogravimetric analysis (TGA). The results show that the processing condition did not have a significant effect on the stability of the drug and the crystallinity of the drug remained even after printing. A dissolution study revealed that drug release is faster in an open system with low infill percentage compared to closed systems and open systems with a high infill ratio. The optimized formulation (F6) with partially opened top layer showed zero-order drug release. The results show that FDM printing is suitable for the formulation of floating dosage form with the desired drug release profile.

Keywords: 3D printing; FMD; pregabalin; controlled release; gastric floating

1. Introduction

The concept of three-dimensional (3D) printing has been flourishing since the 1980s and has been applied to various fields as a tool for rapid prototyping, custom manufacturing and complex manufacturing [1]. Contrasting conventional manufacturing technique, 3D printing involves the fabrication of a 3D structure layer-by-layer from the bottom using a digital design, hence, it is also known as additive manufacturing [2,3]. From products as simple as hearing aids to high-tech parts of military jets, the scope of 3D printing is growing rapidly [4–6]. Furthermore, the excellence of this technology is not new in the medical and pharmaceutical sectors. From educational tools to surgical instruments to printed organs for transplantation, 3D printing is evolving as a new tool in the medical sector [7]. Likewise, FDA approval of the first 3D printed medicine in 2016 for the treatment of epilepsy has led to confidence that this technology can cause a paradigm shift in the field of pharmaceutics [3]. Several studies have been conducted and proven to show the suitability of using printing technology to develop different dosage forms with variable drug release profiles [4]. In recent years, numerous 3D printing technologies have been introduced and have been exploited for their respective advantages and disadvantages. Stereolithography was the first technology to be developed as a rapid prototyping technique [1], followed by fused deposition modeling (FDM), selective laser sintering (SLS) [8–11], and binder jet printing. Binder jet printing or inkjet printing was one of the first 3D printing technologies to be used in the preparation of drug delivery devices and one of the most widely studied technologies to date [12]. Most of the technologies involve a high temperature, which is one of the major drawbacks of these processes, especially in the case of pharmaceuticals. Nevertheless, this technology has provided a new method for the preparation of personalized medicine with an accurate and adjustable dose and customized drug release profiles. Moreover, complex formulations such as combined dosage forms with mixed release kinetics and complex designs have been carried out to achieve better patient compliance and better therapeutic outcomes. FDM, a technology developed in the late 1980s, is also one of the most widely studied technologies in pharmaceutics. This technology, based on material extrusion, involves melting of filaments and deposition of the melted materials in layers where they fuse together to fabricate a 3D structure [4,13]. For this method, the materials used should be thermostable, non-volatile and non-aerosolizing [14]. Commercially used polymers include polylactic acid or polylactide (PLA), polyvinyl alcohol (PVA) and acrylonitrile butadiene styrene (ABS) [3,15]; however, in the case of pharmaceuticals, polymers like Eudragit®, hydroxypropyl cellulose (HPC), and hypromellose® (HPMC) have been studied [16,17]. Initial studies also involved drug-loaded PVA filaments prepared by soaking commercial filaments in alcoholic drug solutions [18–21]. These studies proved the suitability of preparing various modified dosage forms using FDM technology, after which several pharmaceutical polymers along with suitable plasticizers were used to prepare filaments. Recently, a modification of fused deposition modeling has been introduced, known as direct powder extrusion, which works on a similar principle, minimizing the need to prepare filaments [22]. However, FDM technology is still being extensively studied in the field of drug delivery and dosage forms design [23,24]. One of the major advantages of this technology is its cost-effectiveness, along with its availability compared to other 3D printing technology. In contrast, FDM incorporates the deposition of materials vertically layer by layer, resulting in a step-like surface which appears relatively rougher compared to other technologies. Nevertheless, the resolution of printing does not affect the drug release mechanism; hence, it is suitable for the fabrication of desired dosage forms.

Pregabalin, a chemical analogue of neurotransmitter gamma-aminobutyric acid (GABA), is an $\alpha_2\delta$ receptor agonist which has analgesic, anticonvulsant and anxiolytic activities [25,26]. Immediate release formulations of pregabalin, available in different dosage strength, are approved by the FDA for the management of diabetic peripheral neuropathy, fibromyalgia, post-herpetic neuralgia, and also as adjunctive therapy for partial seizures [27]. However, pregabalin has a short elimination half-life of approximately 6 h [28]. Due to this reason, a commercial immediate release form must be administered 2–3 times a day. In 2017, the US FDA approved a sustained release of once daily tablets for the management of diabetic peripheral neuropathy and fibromyalgia. Controlled release pregabalin was found to be effective in reducing pain with a similar safety profile to that of immediate release pregabalin [29]. According to the biopharmaceutics classification system (BCS), pregabalin is a class I compound with high solubility and high permeability. Moreover, the drug has been proven to be mainly absorbed in the stomach and upper gastrointestinal tract [30]. Thus, one of the ways to decrease the frequency of administration has been to increase the gastric retention of the formulation. Among the various approaches for increasing the gastric retention time of the dosage form, only floating and swelling mechanisms have shown clinical evidence for prolonged gastric residence time at fed state. Floating gastro-retentive formulations can effectively minimize the risk of premature gastric emptying of swellable systems by floating above gastric juice and being away from the pylorus [27]. Previously, an intragastric floating tablets of domperidone was formulated using 3D technology. As FDM 3D technology requires filaments as the main material, hydroxy-propyl cellulose filaments loaded with domperidone were prepared using hot melt extruder and hollow tablets were made using a 3D printer. Printed tablets were studied for in vitro and in vivo floating time and drug release profile, which demonstrated a promising application of FDM technology to reduce the frequency of administration and improve patient compliance [31]. Moreover, various pharmaceutical grade filaments have been prepared in previous studies [17]. In this study, by combining these studies, we aimed to design a floating tablet of pregabalin with a controlled drug delivery profile using 3D printing. To the best of our knowledge, this is the first study to employ FDM technology to formulate a floating controlled release system using a novel shape of a tablet and pregabalin as a model drug.

2. Materials and Methods

2.1. Materials

Pregabalin and hypromellose (HPMC E4) were kindly donated from GL PharrmTech, Republic of Korea. Hot melt extrudable (HME) grade hypromellose (HPMC HME 15LV) was purchased from Colorcon, Seoul, Korea. Polyethylene glycol (PEG 400) was purchased from Yakuri pure chemicals Co., Ltd. (Kyoto, Japan). And hypromellose acetate succinate (HPMCAS, AQUOT AS-HG) was purchased from Shin-Etsu chemical Co., Ltd., Tokyo, Japan. Ammonium phosphate dibasic, sodium 1-octanesulfonate and polyvinyl alcohol (PVA) were purchased from Sigma-aldrich, Seoul, Republic of Korea. HPLC grade methanol and acetonitrile were purchased from Duksan chemicals, Seoul, Korea. Commercially available Lyrica® CR165 (Pfizer Inc., New York, NY, USA) was used as the reference product for the in vitro release study.

2.2. Preparation of Pregabalin-Loaded Filaments

Pregabalin-loaded filaments were prepared using Process 11 twin screw Hot Melt Extruder (Thermo scientific, Waltham, MA, USA) with nozzle diameter of 1.5 mm. Physical blends of active pharmaceutical ingredient (API) and polymers were prepared in a mixer and filaments were extruded at a temperature of 125 °C at a rotational speed of 10–20 rpm with a torque of 50–60 nm and used for the preparation of tablets.

2.3. Design and Printing of Tablets

Tablets were designed using Autodesk® 123D® design software version 1.1.4. (Autodesk, San Rafael, CA, USA) Cylindrical tablets were designed for preliminary studies and a novel shape of tablets was designed for optimized formulation. Printed tablets were then sliced using a slicing software Repetier host version 2.1.3 (Hot-World GmbH & Co. Willich, Germany) with an in-built slicer Cura engine. Finally, the tablets were printed using a Good bot 4025-MP FDM printer (3D Korea, Yongsin-ri, Republic of Korea) with a brass nozzle with a diameter of 0.2 mm. The printing temperature was 180 °C and the bed temperature was 50 °C, which remained constant for all the formulations. Various tablets were printed with different infill percentages as open or closed system. Open system tablets did not have a top and bottom layer, whereas closed system tablets had top and bottom layers of a thickness of 0.4 mm (Figure 1). Shell thickness was kept at 0.4 mm for open systems and 0.4 mm for closed systems. Tablet print speed including infill print speed and outer perimeter print speed were all maintained at 30 mm/s.

2.4. Characterization of Filaments and Tablets

2.4.1. Fourier Transform Infrared Spectroscopy (FTIR)

The FTIR spectra of pure pregabalin, HPMCAS-HG, PEG-400, physical mixture, filament and tablet were obtained using Nicolet iS10 (Thermo scientific, Waltham, MA, USA). The scan's frequency range was recorded as 400–4000 cm^{-1}.

2.4.2. X-ray Powder Diffractometry (XRPD)

The crystallinity of pure pregabalin and formulated filaments and tablets was characterized by X-ray diffraction using X-ray diffractometer D/Max-2500 (Rigaku, Japan) operating at 40 kV and 200 mA. The samples were analyzed from 2θ = 3 to 45° at a step of 0.02° and a scan speed of 0.5°/min.

2.4.3. Differential Scanning Calorimetry (DSC)

Pure pregabalin, physical mixture, filament and tablet were analyzed using DSC 4000 (Perkin–Elmer, Waltham, MA, USA) apparatus to study the effect of temperature. Samples were heated from 25 to 250 °C with a heating rate of 10 °C/min. Nitrogen gas was used as a purge gas with a flow rate of 20 mL/min. The degree of crystallinity (DOC) was calculated using the following Equation (1) [32]:

$$DOC(\%) = \frac{\Delta Hs}{\Delta Hp \times W} \times 100 \qquad (1)$$

where ΔHs and ΔHp are the melting enthalpy of the test samples and pure pregabalin respectively. W is the mass fraction of pregabalin in the formulation.

2.4.4. Thermogravimetric Analysis (TGA)

The thermal decomposition of API and formulations was carried by thermogravimetric analysis using a TA Q500 Auto-thermogravimetric analyzer (TA instruments, New Castle, DE, USA). Samples were heated from 25 to 250 °C with heating rate of 10 °C/min. Nitrogen gas was used as a purge gas with a flow rate of 40 mL/min.

2.4.5. Scanning Electronic Microscopy (SEM)

The surface morphology of filaments and tablets was studied by taking photographs using S-4800 SEM (Hitachi, Japan).

2.4.6. In Vitro Floating and Release Study

In vitro floating and in vitro release studies were conduction using the USP apparatus II paddle. Release study was carried out in accordance with the dissolution test of Korean pharmacopoeia. An amount of 500 mL of 0.06 N HCl buffer was used as dissolution media and temperature was set at 37 ± 0.5 °C with a rotational speed of 50 rpm. Samples were collected at predetermined times of 1, 2, 4, 6, 8, 12, and 24 h. Collected samples were filtered using 0.45 µm syringe filter and analysis was done using HPLC at 210 nm. The composition of the mobile phase was 0.04 M ammonium phosphate ((NH_4)$_2HPO_4$) buffer solution: acetonitrile: methanol = 84:5:11 containing 5 mM sodium 1-octanesulfonate, and a flow rate was adjusted (0.7 min/mL) so that the retention time of pregabalin was about 6.66 min. A column was a stainless-steel column with an internal diameter of about 4.6 mm and a length of about 250 mm, packed with 5 µm-octadecylsilyl silica gel for liquid chromatography. The release study results were fitted to various kinetic models such as Zero-order [33], First-order [34,35], Higuchi [36], and Hixon-Crowell [37]. Finally, the statistical analysis for comparison of the release profiles of optimized formulation (F6) and marketed formulation Lyrica® CR was done using a model independent approach: fit factor [38]. Moore and Flanner developed two equations to calculate the similarity and differences in the percentage (%) of drug dissolved per unit time between two dissolution profiles [39]. The similarity factor (f_2) gives the similarity in the percent (%) dissolution between the two curves, which is calculated as a logarithmic reciprocal of the square root transformation of the sum of the squared error as shown in Equation 2.

$$f_2 = 50 \times \log °\{[1 + (\frac{1}{n}) \sum_{t=1}^{n} (R_t - T_t)^2]^{-0.5} \times 100\} \qquad (2)$$

where R_t and T_t are the cumulative percentage of drug dissolved at each of the selected 'n' time points of the commercial and optimized formulation, respectively. In this study, we used similarity factor (f_2) to compare the dissolution profiles of optimized formulation and commercial product. The dissolution profiles are considered similar when f_2 is between 50 and 100.

3. Results and Discussion

3D printing with FDM technology requires filaments as the starting material, which have the desired composition of raw materials required to print the final object. Various commercial filament makers are available for this process. However, in our study, HME technology was used to prepare pregabalin-loaded filaments. HME technology has widely been used in pharmaceutics to prepare solid dispersions of drugs with poor solubility [40]. Nevertheless, HME has also been extensively used and studied to prepare various pharmaceutical grade filaments [17,41]. Different batches of filaments were prepared with various compositions, as mentioned in Table 1, and filaments were accepted based on the feasibility of extrusion during the HME process and printing, as mentioned in Table 2.

Table 1. Composition of filaments prepared.

Filaments	Pregabalin (%)	HPMCAS HG (%)	PEG 400 (%)	PVA (%)	HPMC E4 (%)	HPMC HME 15 LV (%)
FIL-1	-	-	-	-	100	-
FIL-2	-	-	-	10	90	-
FIL-3	-	-	10	-	90	-
FIL-4	25	-	10	-	-	65
FIL-5	25	-	5	-	-	70
FIL-6	50	20	10	-	-	20
FIL-7	25	65	10	-	-	-
FIL-8	50	40	10	-	-	-

Table 2. Properties of filaments obtained from the hot melt extruder.

Filaments	Result	Remarks
FIL-1	Difficulty in extrusion	High viscosity of polymer clogged extruder nozzle
FIL-2	Difficulty in printing	Filaments clogged print head due to gluey consistency after melting
FIL-3	Difficulty in printing	Filaments hardened with elevated temperature while printing
FIL-4	Difficulty in printing	Very flexible filaments
FIL-5	Difficulty in extrusion	Low concentration of plasticizer
FIL-6	Difficulty in printing	Very flexible filaments
FIL-7	Suitable for extrusion and printing	Filaments of enough strength and flow
FIL-8	Suitable for extrusion and printing	Filaments of enough strength and flow

Filament preparation and printing involves various process parameters that determine the result of the object to be printed. One of the variables that had a significant effect on the final printed object was the uniformity of the filament diameter. Commercially prepared filaments are available in 1.75 mm and 3 mm of diameters with deviations of ± 0.05 mm. However, prepared filaments were found to have a diameter of 1.5 mm, which is thinner than the commercially available and recommended filament size. Nevertheless, a slight change of print setting with filament diameter and flow rate of the filament from 100% to 120% made it possible to print out the tablets [42]. However, it is still important to have the filaments of a uniform diameter, as this will result in serious complications during extrusion. Under- or over-extrusion of the materials due to an inconsistent diameter of filaments is one of the major problems, along with difficulties associated with gripping of the filaments in the extruder, which causes coiling and breaking of the filament. Therefore, it is suggested to keep filament tolerance under ± 0.05 mm. For uniformity of the optimized filaments, we checked the thickness every 5-cm distance and the deviation was found to be ± 0.023. Another important parameter is the stiffness of the filaments. Filaments should have enough mechanical strength to not break in the feeding gear [41]. However, extremely flexible filaments also possess complications similar to an inconsistent diameter, such as under- or over-extrusion and coiling, along with stringing or oozing of extruded materials and weak infill.

In our case, these problems were solved by using direct a drive extruder instead of a bowden extruder, using low print speed and heated bed and also controlling the feed tension, extrusion temperature and retraction. Finally, the filament prepared with 40% HPMCAS, 50% API and 10% PEG 400 (FIL-8) was used as optimized filament. Tablets were printed according to the design shown in Figure 2. Tablets were found to have uniform weight with a deviation within the range (Table 3). The uniformity of the diameter of the filament affected the weight variation as well. Tablets prepared with uniform filaments resulted in uniform weight tablets. Printed tablets showed very high mechanical strength and were impossible to test using a conventional hardness tester and the friability was completely zero, which is common in case of various FDM printed formulations [37,38].

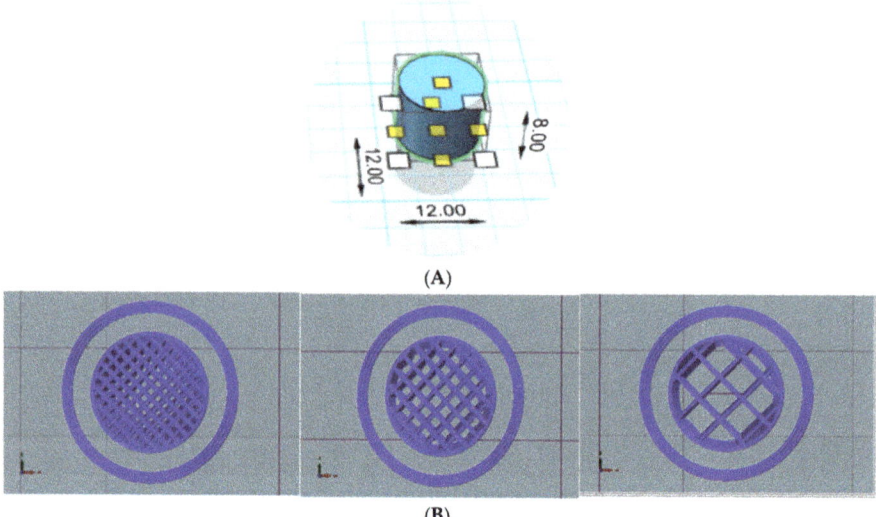

Figure 1. Design and internal structures of tablets. Design of preliminary cylindrical tablets (**A**) and slicing of tablets with infill percentages of 25%, 50% and 75%, left to right (**B**).

Table 3. Characteristics and evaluation of printed tablets.

Formulation	Dimension (mm)	Infill (%)	Shell Thickness (mm)	Weight (mg)	Density (g/cm^3)	Drug Content (mg)	Drug Loading (%)
F1	12 × 8	25	0.6	361.45 ± 0.35	0.40 ± 0.0003	168.22 ± 3.71	93.08 ± 1.54
F2	12 × 8	50	0.6	470.50 ± 8.48	0.52 ± 0.0091	227.75 ± 3.53	96.80 ± 1.26
F3	12 × 8	75	0.6	668.50 ± 27.57	0.74 ± 0.0304	322.75 ± 10.25	96.54 ± 3.22
F4	12 × 8	25	0.4	498.60 ± 4.52	0.55 ± 0.0050	235.95 ± 7.70	94.64 ± 3.03
F5	12 × 8	50	0.4	691.00 ± 14.14	0.76 ± 0.0156	335.47 ± 7.10	97.08 ± 2.06
F6	12 × 8	25	0.4	475.00 ± 2.57	-	234.90 ± 12.97	98.52 ± 5.40

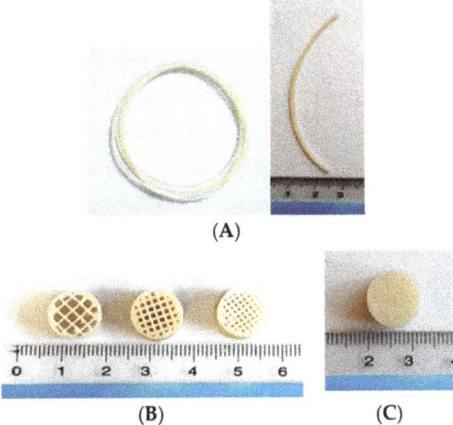

Figure 2. Prepared filaments and tablets. Drug loaded filaments (**A**), printed open system tablets with 25%, 50% and 75% infill left to right (**B**), and printed closed system tablet (**C**).

The FT-IR Spectrum of pure pregabalin and its physical mixture with polymers and different excipients are shown in Figure 3A. Pure pregabalin showed peaks at 2954.13 cm^{-1} (C–H stretch), 1642.69 cm^{-1} (N–H bend, NH$_2$ scissoring), 1544.23 cm^{-1} (N–O asymmetric stretch), 1469.62 cm^{-1} (C–H bend), 1333.18 cm^{-1} (N–O symmetric stretch), 1277.44 cm^{-1} (C–O stretch), and 932.16 cm^{-1} (O–H bend) which was similar to peaks found in previous study [43]. The physical mixture, prepared filament and tablets had almost superimposed peaks, except for few small changes in peaks 1642 cm^{-1} to 1643 cm^{-1}, 1544 cm^{-1} to 1546 cm^{-1} in the case of filament and 1545 cm^{-1} in the case of tablets, 1277 cm^{-1} to 1278 cm^{-1}, and 1469 cm^{-1} to 1468 cm^{-1} in case of tablets. This shows that there was no significant interaction between API and the polymers. To further study the interaction between polymers with API and the effect of mechanical and thermal processes on drug crystallinity, XRPD and DSC were used.

The XRPD pattern of pure pregabalin at 2 θ shows characteristic peaks at 4.7, 9.4, 18.20, 19.04, 19.75, 22.15, and 35.58 (Figure 3B). The characteristic peaks were also seen in the physical mixture, which was reduced in filaments and tablets. XRPD data reveals that pregabalin remained at least partly crystalline upon extrusion and printing which is in consistent with the results of DSC. The DSC graph shows the endothermic peak of pure pregabalin at 194.81 °C (Figure 3C). The endothermic had a negative shift to 175.10 °C in the physical mixture which further shifted to 161.82 °C and 161.46 °C. The degree of crystallinity was found to be 90%, 50% and 39% for the physical mixture, extruded filament and printed tablets, respectively. The extrusion process and printing seem to have had less effect on the crystallinity of pregabalin as the operating temperatures were lower than the melting point of API. FDM technology involves high temperatures in both the filaments-making process and the printing process. Although these processes require short exposure to high temperature, significant thermal degradation can be found in the case of thermolabile drugs and polymers [16,44]. The thermogravimetric analysis of API, physical mixture, filament and tablets were carried out as shown in Figure 3D. No significant mass loss was found from 115 to 125 °C (HME zone) and 180 °C (printing zone) for pure API, physical mixtures and filament. However, in the case of printed tablets, 2%–3% mass loss was found in the HME zone, while approximately 5% of mass loss was found in the printing zone. This could have been due to the repetitive exposure of printed tablets to high temperature, which resulted in the decomposition of polymers, causing weight loss.

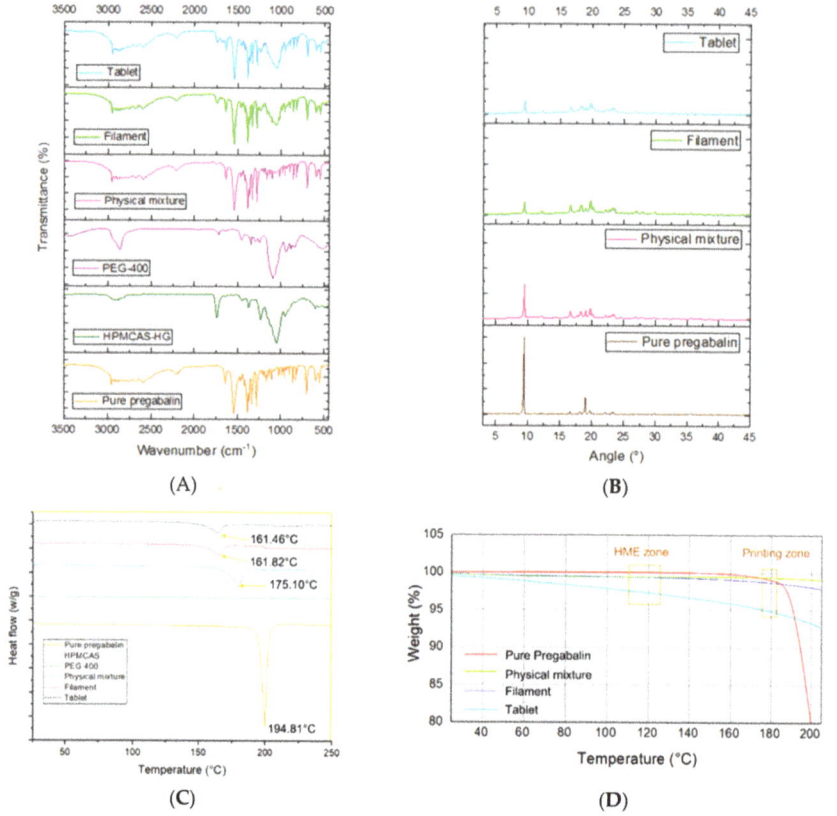

Figure 3. Physical characterization of printed tablets. Fourier-transform infrared spectroscopy (**A**), X-ray powder diffractometry (**B**), differential scanning calorimetry (**C**), and thermogravimetric analysis (**D**).

SEM imaging shows the surface morphology of filaments and tablets (Figure 4). Filaments showed an irregular surface due to the low extrusion temperature, which resulted in incomplete melting of the drug and remained in crystalline form [45]. Drug loaded filaments prepared by HME are relatively rougher compared to commercial filaments [20]. In the case of the printed tablets, we can see prominent printed layers and uniform layer height. Uniformity in layer height determines the overall uniformity of tablet. However, the roughness/smoothness of a tablet does not have any effect on the tablet floating and release properties.

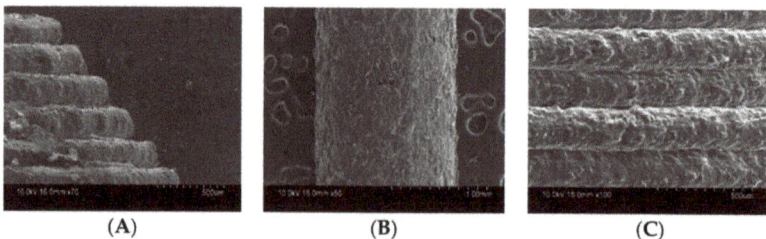

Figure 4. SEM image of filament and tablets. Outer surface of filament (**A**), side view of top layer (**B**), and center view of different layers (**C**).

In vitro floating study of open and closed systems with different infill ratios were carried out (Figure 5). In a previous study, floating capacity and duration were found to be dependent on the density of the tablets [31], whereas, in our study, the floating study revealed a very high correlation between the presence of top/bottom layer and the floating capacity, with a very minimum dependency on the density. All the open systems (F1–F3) failed to show floating properties and sank immediately to the bottom of the vessel (Figure 5A), whereas the closed systems (F4 and F5) showed excellent floating properties and remained floating for >24 h (Figure 5B). Open systems have void spaces where water enters and replaces the air inside and increases the density of the tablets, causing it to sink in the media (Figure 6). On the contrary, in the case of closed system, water penetrates at a very slow rate so that the void spaces inside the tablet help to retain the buoyancy of the printed tablets, which remained true for the optimized formulation (Figure 5C) with closed system and open space on one side of the tablet.

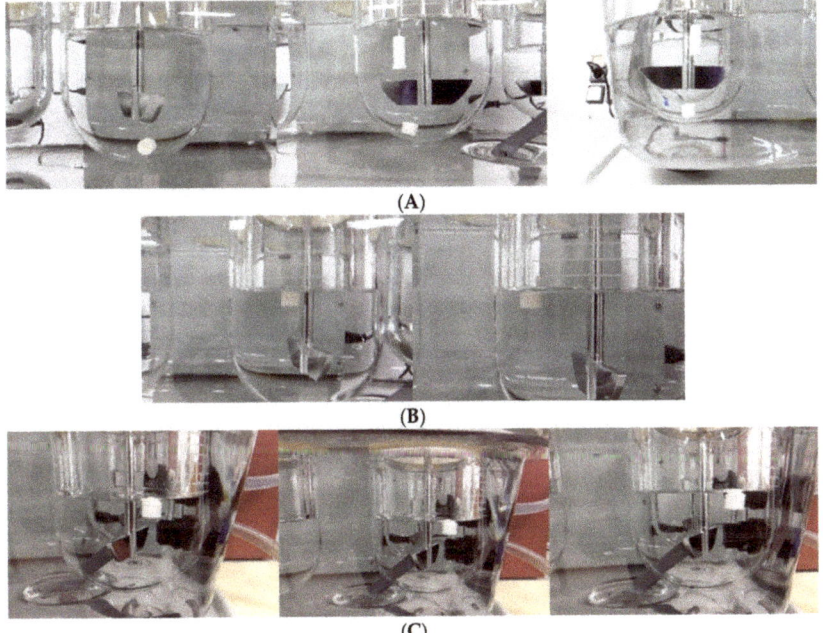

Figure 5. Floating study of prepared formulations. Open system (**A**), closed system (**B**), and optimized formulation (**C**) over 1, 8 and 24 h (left to right).

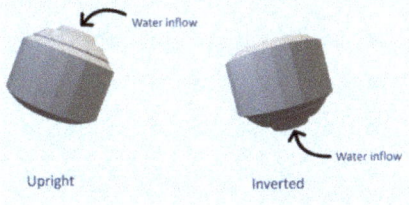

Figure 6. Floating mechanism of optimized formulation. The internal structure of tablet is composed of a grid infill with void space filled with air so that the tablet has low density, which helps in buoyancy of the tablet in media.

The release study of closed formulations F4–F5 showed a relationship between the internal structure of the printed tablet and the drug release rate (Figure 7A). 3D printing has unique characteristics whereby the infill percentage and the infill pattern can be changed [46]. Infill is the internal structure of the printed object which determines the mechanical strength of object in the general 3D printing process. However, in the case of pharmaceutical formulations, the infill percentage of the formulation has been shown to play a major role in the kinetics of drug release in a number of studies. Drug release was significantly higher in formulations with low infill percentages [18]. In this study, tablets with low infill percentages showed faster release compared to tablets with high infill percentage. However, there was incomplete drug release in the case of tablets with a higher infill ratio. However, in the case of open system formulations F1–F3, the infill ratio did not have significant effect on the drug release (Figure 7B). A similar trend was noted in a previous study as well [31]. In addition, drug release was more controlled in the case of closed systems compared to open systems in which peak drug release was obtained around 6–8 h. The compactness of the tablet and surface area interaction with the media played huge role in drug release. Open tablets with low infill have higher access of media compared to closed tablets and tablets with high infill. This facilitated a faster release of the drug from the system. Thus, the optimized formulation was designed to mimic the advantages of both open and close systems (Figure 8). One side of the tablet was closed, and the other side was partially opened, and the infill was maintained at 25%. Moreover, the geometry of the formulation has shown to control the drug release [47]. This unique design (F6) helped to achieve complete drug release (Figure 7C) while retaining its floating ability for 24 h. The closed bottom of the tablet helped the buoyancy of the tablet and the partially opened top layer allowed entry of water inside tablet in a controlled manner, which facilitated complete drug release over longer period which is in contrast to F1 although it had similar dimension and infill percentages. The use of polymer also plays role in controlling the release of drugs from a printed formulation [16,17]. In a previous study, formulation prepared with HPMCAS HG was not completely dissolved even after 24 h and drug release was pH-sensitive as the enteric polymer was distributed into the matrix rather than as a coating layer in conventional formulations [45]. This phenomenon contributed to the extended release in the case of our formulation as well.

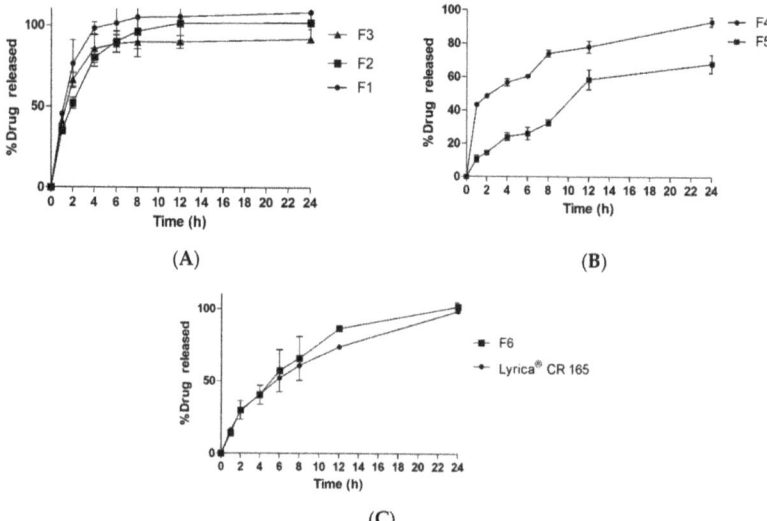

Figure 7. In vitro drug release study. Closed systems (**A**), open systems (**B**), and optimized formulation with commercial product (**C**).

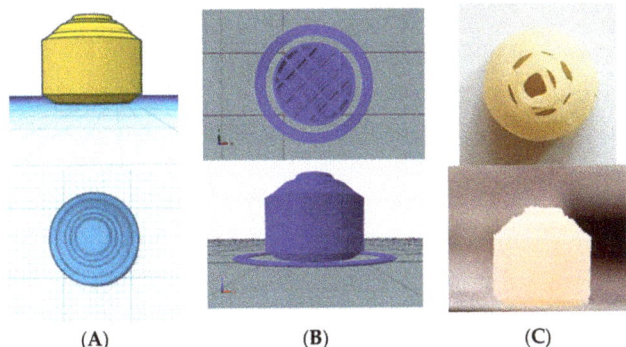

Figure 8. Top view and side view of optimized formulation. Design of unique shaped optimized formulation (**A**), slicing of tablets with 25% infill (**B**) and printed tablets (**C**).

To understand the release properties better, drug release data were fitted to different mathematical kinetic models (Figure 9). A single model could not define the drug release pattern from tablets and rather seemed to have a combination of different mechanisms. The regression value was found to be higher for the Zero-order and Higuchi models, suggesting that the release and diffusion rates were constant. Drug release for HPMCAS polymers have been found to be regulated by the drug diffusion and erosion polymer from the surface of the system [48]. Printed tablets did not show any changes in morphology and maintained their integrity during whole dissolution process.

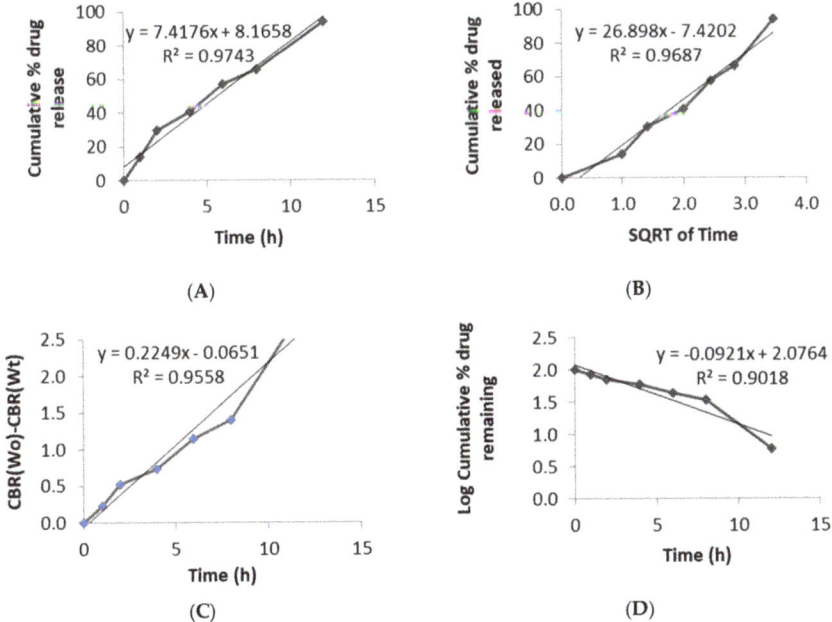

Figure 9. Drug release kinetics fitted to various models: Zero-order (**A**), Higuchi model (**B**), Hixon-Crowell model (**C**), and First-order (**D**).

Formulation F6 was compared to Lyrica® CR 165 mg, a marketed product of Pfizer, and release profiles were compared using similarity factor (f_2). The values of similarity factor (f_2) for the batch F6 showed a maximum of 65.32 (Table 4); hence, it was selected as optimum batch.

Table 4. Comparison of prepared formulations with commercialized products using similarity factor (f_2).

Formulations	F1	F2	F3	F4	F5	F6
Lyrica® CR 165	19.53	26.9	25.7	40.88	37.2	65.32

4. Conclusions

A uniquely shaped tablet was designed to formulate a floating gastro-retentive controlled release dosage form using FDM technology. This study proves the possibility of employing 3D printing technology to prepare a floating controlled release system of pregabalin. The feasibility of designing and printing tablets to meet a specific criterion using 3D printing technology has already been proven effective via various studies. Further development on design of formulations and resolution of printers to the extent where on-demand manufacturing and personalized medicine are possible will definitely change the future of pharmacotherapy.

Author Contributions: Conceptualization, S.L. (Shrawani Lamichhane), D.H.S. and S.L. (Sangkil Lee); methodology, S.L. (Shrawani Lamichhane), J.-B.P., D.H.S. and S.L. (Sangkil Lee); software, S.L. (Shrawani Lamichhane); formal analysis, S.L. (Shrawani Lamichhane); investigation, S.L. (Shrawani Lamichhane); resources, J.-B.P. and S.L. (Sangkil Lee); data curation, S.L. (Shrawani Lamichhane); writing—original draft preparation, S.L. (Shrawani Lamichhane); writing—review and editing, S.L. (Sangkil Lee); supervision, S.L. (Sangkil Lee); funding acquisition, S.L. (Sangkil Lee).

Funding: This research was supported by "Keimyung University Research Grant of 2017".

Acknowledgments: We would like to extend our deepest gratitude to GL PharmTech for providing us with raw materials.

Conflicts of Interest: The authors declare no conflict of interest.

References

1. Kodama, H. Automatic method for fabricating a three-dimensional plastic model with photo-hardening polymer. *Rev. Sci. Instrum.* **1981**, *52*, 1770–1773. [CrossRef]
2. Cohen, A.; Laviv, A.; Berman, P.; Nashef, R.; Abu-Tair, J. Mandibular reconstruction using stereolithographic 3-dimensional printing modeling technology. *Oral. Surg. Oral. Med. Oral. Pathol. Oral. Radiol. Endodontology* **2009**, *108*, 661–666. [CrossRef] [PubMed]
3. Trenfield, S.J.; Awad, A.; Goyanes, A.; Gaisford, S.; Basit, A.W. 3D Printing Pharmaceuticals: Drug Development to Frontline Care. *Trends Pharm. Sci.* **2018**, *39*, 440–451. [CrossRef] [PubMed]
4. Lamichhane, S.; Bashyal, S.; Keum, T.; Noh, G.; Seo, J.E.; Bastola, R.; Choi, J.; Sohn, D.H.; Lee, S. Complex formulations, simple techniques: Can 3D printing technology be the Midas touch in pharmaceutical industry? *Asian J. Pharm. Sci.* **2019**, *14*, 465–479. [CrossRef]
5. Attaran, M. The rise of 3-D printing: The advantages of additive manufacturing over traditional manufacturing. *Bus. Horiz.* **2017**, *60*, 677–688. [CrossRef]
6. Park, B.J.; Choi, H.J.; Moon, S.J.; Kim, S.J.; Bajracharya, R.; Min, J.Y.; Han, H.-K. Pharmaceutical applications of 3D printing technology: current understanding and future perspectives. *J. Pharm. Investig.* **2018**. [CrossRef]
7. Yao, R.; Xu, G.; Mao, S.-S.; Yang, H.-Y.; Sang, X.-T.; Sun, W.; Mao, Y.-L. Three-dimensional printing: review of application in medicine and hepatic surgery. *Cancer Biol. Med.* **2016**, *13*, 443.
8. Fina, F.; Goyanes, A.; Madla, C.M.; Awad, A.; Trenfield, S.J.; Kuek, J.M.; Patel, P.; Gaisford, S.; Basit, A.W. 3D printing of drug-loaded gyroid lattices using selective laser sintering. *Int. J. Pharm.* **2018**, *547*, 44–52. [CrossRef]
9. Fina, F.; Goyanes, A.; Gaisford, S.; Basit, A.W. Selective laser sintering (SLS) 3D printing of medicines. *Int. J. Pharm.* **2017**, *529*, 285–293. [CrossRef]

10. Fina, F.; Madla, C.M.; Goyanes, A.; Zhang, J.; Gaisford, S.; Basit, A.W. Fabricating 3D printed orally disintegrating printlets using selective laser sintering. *Int. Pharm.* **2018**, *541*, 101–107. [CrossRef]
11. Barakh Ali, S.F.; Mohamed, E.M.; Ozkan, T.; Kuttolamadom, M.A.; Khan, M.A.; Asadi, A.; Rahman, Z. Understanding the effects of formulation and process variables on the printlets quality manufactured by selective laser sintering 3D printing. *Int. J. Pharm.* **2019**, *570*, 118651. [CrossRef] [PubMed]
12. Wu, B.M.; Borland, S.W.; Giordano, R.A.; Cima, L.G.; Sachs, E.M.; Cima, M.J. Solid free-form fabrication of drug delivery devices. *J. Control. Release* **1996**, *40*, 77–87. [CrossRef]
13. Joo, Y.; Shin, I.; Ham, G.; Abuzar, S.M.; Hyun, S.-M.; Hwang, S.-J. The advent of a novel manufacturing technology in pharmaceutics: Superiority of fused deposition modeling 3D printer. *J. Pharm. Investig* **2019**. [CrossRef]
14. Norman, J.; Madurawe, R.D.; Moore, C.M.; Khan, M.A.; Khairuzzaman, A. A new chapter in pharmaceutical manufacturing: 3D-printed drug products. *Adv. Drug Deliv. Rev.* **2017**, *108*, 39–50. [CrossRef]
15. Goyanes, A.; Det-Amornrat, U.; Wang, J.; Basit, A.W.; Gaisford, S. 3D scanning and 3D printing as innovative technologies for fabricating personalized topical drug delivery systems. *J. Control. Release* **2016**, *234*, 41–48. [CrossRef]
16. Pietrzak, K.; Isreb, A.; Alhnan, M.A. A flexible-dose dispenser for immediate and extended release 3D printed tablets. *Eur. J. Pharm. Biopharm.* **2015**, *96*, 380–387. [CrossRef]
17. Melocchi, A.; Parietti, F.; Maroni, A.; Foppoli, A.; Gazzaniga, A.; Zema, L. Hot-melt extruded filaments based on pharmaceutical grade polymers for 3D printing by fused deposition modeling. *Int. Pharm.* **2016**, *509*, 255–263. [CrossRef]
18. Goyanes, A.; Buanz, A.B.M.; Basit, A.W.; Gaisford, S. Fused-filament 3D printing (3DP) for fabrication of tablets. *Int. J. Pharm.* **2014**, *476*, 88–92. [CrossRef]
19. Goyanes, A.; Chang, H.; Sedough, D.; Hatton, G.B.; Wang, J.; Buanz, A.; Gaisford, S.; Basit, A.W. Fabrication of controlled-release budesonide tablets via desktop (FDM) 3D printing. *Int. J. Pharm.* **2015**, *496*, 414–420. [CrossRef]
20. Skowyra, J.; Pietrzak, K.; Alhnan, M.A. Fabrication of extended-release patient-tailored prednisolone tablets via fused deposition modelling (FDM) 3D printing. *Eur. J. Pharm. Sci.* **2015**, *68*, 11–17. [CrossRef]
21. Jamróz, W.; Kurek, M.; Łyszczarz, E.; Szafraniec, J.; Knapik-Kowalczuk, J.; Syrek, K.; Paluch, M.; Jachowicz, R. 3D printed orodispersible films with Aripiprazole. *Int. J. Pharm.* **2017**, *533*, 413–420. [CrossRef] [PubMed]
22. Goyanes, A.; Allahham, N.; Trenfield, S.J.; Stoyanov, E.; Gaisford, S.; Basit, A.W. Direct powder extrusion 3D printing: Fabrication of drug products using a novel single-step process. *Int. J. Pharm.* **2019**, *567*, 118471. [CrossRef] [PubMed]
23. Carlier, E.; Marquette, S.; Peerboom, C.; Denis, L.; Benali, S.; Raquez, J.M.; Amighi, K.; Goole, J. Investigation of the parameters used in fused deposition modeling of poly(lactic acid) to optimize 3D printing sessions. *Int. J. Pharm.* **2019**, *565*, 367–377. [CrossRef] [PubMed]
24. Nober, C.; Manini, G.; Carlier, E.; Raquez, J.-M.; Benali, S.; Dubois, P.; Amighi, K.; Goole, J. Feasibility study into the potential use of fused-deposition modeling to manufacture 3D-printed enteric capsules in compounding pharmacies. *Int. J. Pharm.* **2019**, *569*, 118581. [CrossRef] [PubMed]
25. Rosenstock, J.; Tuchman, M.; LaMoreaux, L.; Sharma, U. Pregabalin for the treatment of painful diabetic peripheral neuropathy: A double-blind, placebo-controlled trial. *Pain* **2004**, *110*, 628–638. [CrossRef] [PubMed]
26. Crofford, L.J.; Rowbotham, M.C.; Mease, P.J.; Russell, I.J.; Dworkin, R.H.; Corbin, A.E.; Young Jr, J.P.; LaMoreaux, L.K.; Martin, S.A.; Sharma, U. Pregabalin for the treatment of fibromyalgia syndrome: results of a randomized, double-blind, placebo-controlled trial. *Arthritis Rheum* **2005**, *52*, 1264–1273. [CrossRef]
27. Kim, S.; Hwang, K.-M.; Park, Y.S.; Nguyen, T.-T.; Park, E.-S. Preparation and evaluation of non-effervescent gastroretentive tablets containing pregabalin for once-daily administration and dose proportional pharmacokinetics. *Int. J. Pharm.* **2018**, *550*, 160–169. [CrossRef]
28. Bockbrader, H.N.; Radulovic, L.L.; Posvar, E.L.; Strand, J.C.; Alvey, C.W.; Busch, J.A.; Randinitis, E.J.; Corrigan, B.W.; Haig, G.M.; Boyd, R.A. Clinical pharmacokinetics of pregabalin in healthy volunteers. *J. Clin. Pharmacol.* **2010**, *50*, 941–950. [CrossRef]
29. Huffman, C.L.; Goldenberg, J.N.; Weintraub, J.; Sanin, L.; Driscoll, J.; Yang, R.; Chew, M.L.; Scavone, J.M. Efficacy and Safety of Once-Daily Controlled-Release Pregabalin for the Treatment of Patients With Postherpetic Neuralgia. *Clin. J. Pain* **2017**, *33*, 569–578. [CrossRef]

30. Qin, C.; Wu, M.; Xu, S.; Wang, X.; Shi, W.; Dong, Y.; Yang, L.; He, W.; Han, X.; Yin, L. Design and optimization of gastro-floating sustained-release tablet of pregabalin: In vitro and in vivo evaluation. *Int. J. Pharm.* **2018**, *545*, 37–44. [CrossRef]
31. Chai, X.; Chai, H.; Wang, X.; Yang, J.; Li, J.; Zhao, Y.; Cai, W.; Tao, T.; Xiang, X. Fused deposition modeling (FDM) 3D printed tablets for intragastric floating delivery of domperidone. *Sci. Rep.* **2017**, *7*, 2829. [CrossRef] [PubMed]
32. Li, X.; Peng, H.; Tian, B.; Gou, J.; Yao, Q.; Tao, X.; He, H.; Zhang, Y.; Tang, X.; Cai, C. Preparation and characterization of azithromycin–Aerosil 200 solid dispersions with enhanced physical stability. *Int. J. Pharm.* **2015**, *486*, 175–184. [CrossRef] [PubMed]
33. Dash, S.; Murthy, P.N.; Nath, L.; Chowdhury, P. Kinetic modeling on drug release from controlled drug delivery systems. *Acta Pol. Pharm.* **2010**, *67*, 217–223. [PubMed]
34. Gibaldi, M.; Feldman, S. Establishment of sink conditions in dissolution rate determinations. Theoretical considerations and application to nondisintegrating dosage forms. *J. Pharm. Sci.* **1967**, *56*, 1238–1242. [CrossRef] [PubMed]
35. Bloomquist, C.J.; Mecham, M.B.; Paradzinsky, M.D.; Janusziewicz, R.; Warner, S.B.; Luft, J.C.; Mecham, S.J.; Wang, A.Z.; DeSimone, J.M. Controlling release from 3D printed medical devices using CLIP and drug-loaded liquid resins. *J. Control. Release* **2018**, *278*, 9–23. [CrossRef] [PubMed]
36. Higuchi, T. Mechanism of sustained-action medication. Theoretical analysis of rate of release of solid drugs dispersed in solid matrices. *J. Pharm. Sci.* **1963**, *52*, 1145–1149. [CrossRef] [PubMed]
37. Hixson, A.; Crowell, J. Dependence of reaction velocity upon surface and agitation. *Ind. Eng. Chem.* **1931**, *23*, 923–931. [CrossRef]
38. Anderson, N.; Bauer, M.; Boussac, N.; Khan-Malek, R.; Munden, P.; Sardaro, M. An evaluation of fit factors and dissolution efficiency for the comparison of in vitro dissolution profiles. *J. Pharm. Biomed. Anal.* **1998**, *17*, 811–822. [CrossRef]
39. Costa, P.; Lobo, J.M.S. Modeling and comparison of dissolution profiles. *Eur. J. Pharm. Sci.* **2001**, *13*, 123–133. [CrossRef]
40. Repka, M.A.; Battu, S.K.; Upadhye, S.B.; Thumma, S.; Crowley, M.M.; Zhang, F.; Martin, C.; McGinity, J.W. Pharmaceutical applications of hot-melt extrusion: Part II. *Drug Dev. Ind. Pharm.* **2007**, *33*, 1043–1057. [CrossRef]
41. Zhang, J.; Feng, X.; Patil, H.; Tiwari, R.V.; Repka, M.A. Coupling 3D printing with hot-melt extrusion to produce controlled-release tablets. *Int. J. Pharm.* **2017**, *519*, 186–197. [CrossRef] [PubMed]
42. Melocchi, A.; Parietti, F.; Loreti, G.; Maroni, A.; Gazzaniga, A.; Zema, L. 3D printing by fused deposition modeling (FDM) of a swellable/erodible capsular device for oral pulsatile release of drugs. *J. Drug Deliv. Sci. Technol.* **2015**, *30*, 360–367. [CrossRef]
43. Salaman, C.R.P.; Tesson, N.; Castano, M.T.; Romana, L.C. Crystalline forms of pregabalin and co-formers in the treatment of pain. European Patent EP 2 527 319 A1, 24 May 2011.
44. Goyanes, A.; Buanz, A.B.M.; Hatton, G.B.; Gaisford, S.; Basit, A.W. 3D printing of modified-release aminosalicylate (4-ASA and 5-ASA) tablets. *Eur. J. Pharm. Biopharm.* **2015**, *89*, 157–162. [CrossRef] [PubMed]
45. Goyanes, A.; Fina, F.; Martorana, A.; Sedough, D.; Gaisford, S.; Basit, A.W. Development of modified release 3D printed tablets (printlets) with pharmaceutical excipients using additive manufacturing. *Int. J. Pharm.* **2017**, *527*, 21–30. [CrossRef] [PubMed]
46. Moscato, S.; Bahr, R.; Le, T.; Pasian, M.; Bozzi, M.; Perregrini, L.; Tentzeris, M.M. Infill-dependent 3-D-printed material based on NinjaFlex filament for antenna applications. *IEEE Antennas Wirel. Propag. Lett.* **2016**, *15*, 1506–1509. [CrossRef]
47. Goyanes, A.; Martinez, P.R.; Buanz, A.; Basit, A.W.; Gaisford, S. Effect of geometry on drug release from 3D printed tablets. *Int. J. Pharm.* **2015**, *494*, 657–663. [CrossRef]
48. Reynolds, T.D.; Mitchell, S.A.; Balwinski, K.M. Investigation of the effect of tablet surface area/volume on drug release from hydroxypropylmethylcellulose controlled-release matrix tablets. *Drug Dev. Ind. Pharm.* **2002**, *28*, 457–466. [CrossRef]

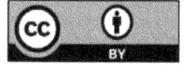

© 2019 by the authors. Licensee MDPI, Basel, Switzerland. This article is an open access article distributed under the terms and conditions of the Creative Commons Attribution (CC BY) license (http://creativecommons.org/licenses/by/4.0/).

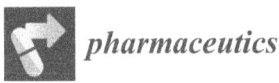

Article

Novel Gastroretentive Floating Pulsatile Drug Delivery System Produced via Hot-Melt Extrusion and Fused Deposition Modeling 3D Printing

Nagi Reddy Dumpa [1], Suresh Bandari [1] and Michael A. Repka [1,2,*]

1. Department of Pharmaceutics and Drug Delivery, School of Pharmacy, The University of Mississippi, Oxford, MS 38677, USA; ndumpa@go.olemiss.edu (N.R.D.); sbandari@olemiss.edu (S.B.)
2. Pii Center for Pharmaceutical Innovation & Instruction, The University of Mississippi, Oxford, MS 38677, USA
* Correspondence: marepka@olemiss.edu; Tel.: +1-662-915-1155; Fax: +1-662-915-1177

Received: 5 December 2019; Accepted: 6 January 2020; Published: 8 January 2020

Abstract: This study was performed to develop novel core-shell gastroretentive floating pulsatile drug delivery systems using a hot-melt extrusion-paired fused deposition modeling (FDM) 3D printing and direct compression method. Hydroxypropyl cellulose (HPC) and ethyl cellulose (EC)-based filaments were fabricated using hot-melt extrusion technology and were utilized as feedstock material for printing shells in FDM 3D printing. The directly compressed theophylline tablet was used as the core. The tablet shell to form pulsatile floating dosage forms with different geometries (shell thickness: 0.8, 1.2, 1.6, and 2.0 mm; wall thickness: 0, 0.8, and 1.6 mm; and % infill density: 50, 75, and 100) were designed, printed, and evaluated. All core-shell tablets floated without any lag time and exhibited good floating behavior throughout the dissolution study. The lag time for the pulsatile release of the drug was 30 min to 6 h. The proportion of ethyl cellulose in the filament composition had a significant ($p < 0.05$) effect on the lag time. The formulation (2 mm shell thickness, 1.6 mm wall thickness, 100% infill density, 0.5% EC) with the desired lag time of 6 h was selected as an optimized formulation. Thus, FDM 3D printing is a potential technique for the development of complex customized drug delivery systems for personalized pharmacotherapy.

Keywords: hot-melt extrusion; fused deposition modeling; 3D printing; floating systems; pulsatile release; chronotherapeutic delivery

1. Introduction

Maintaining a constant plasma drug concentration is not beneficial in all disease conditions. Some diseases may require pulse delivery of drugs to avoid unwanted adverse effects and drug exposure [1]. Certain diseases, such as bronchial asthma, angina pectoris, ulcers, and rheumatoid arthritis, are regulated by the circadian rhythm of the body and require drug administration at specific times of a day, particularly in the early morning hours. Such diseases require pulsatile drug delivery after a lag time to improve patient compliance and drug adherence. Pulsatile drug delivery systems (PDDS) provide a timely pharmacological effect to the patient, while preventing unwanted sustained drug exposure. PDDS does not interrupt patients normal sleep patterns following an evening dose of medication. Moreover, pulsatile systems can prevent detrimental drug–drug interactions without changing the administration schedule of patients taking multiple medications at the same time and can enhance patient compliance [2–4]. To address these issues, a drug delivery system that delivers a pulsatile release of drugs after a pre-determined lag time is necessary. Thus, drugs administered at bedtime would be released in the early morning hours and be available to alleviate the symptoms and improve the quality of life of the patients.

Various biological factors influence the transit time of drugs in the upper gastrointestinal tract and are a challenge to drugs that are locally active in the stomach, unstable at a high pH, or that have poor solubility in the lower parts of the gastrointestinal tract [5–7]. A strategy to increase the residence time of the drugs to overcome the above-mentioned drawbacks is necessary for optimal therapeutic outcomes. Numerous strategies have been used to increase the residence time of the dosage forms in the stomach, including mucoadhesive systems [8,9], high-density systems that sink to the bottom of the stomach [10], swelling systems [11] and floating systems [12–14]. Among these strategies, floating systems are considered superior as they do not interfere with the physiological activity of the gastrointestinal tract [15]. Floating systems are further subdivided into effervescent and non-effervescent floating systems. The effervescent systems use gas-forming agents, whereas the non-effervescent systems are formulated with gel-forming polymers or hollow microspheres [16].

Hot-melt extrusion (HME) is a well-known technique used in the plastic, rubber, and food industries. Over the last three decades, its use in drug delivery and research has tremendously increased owing to the advantages associated with this technology, such as high efficiency, solvent-free, innovative applications, and continuous manufacturing [17]. Although HME is most widely used in the preparation of amorphous solid dispersions, it is also used in the development of many innovative applications, such as taste masking, abuse-deterrent formulations, chronotherapeutic systems, topical formulations, semi-solid dosage forms, and co-amorphous systems [18–22]. Recently, the interest of researchers has shifted to additive manufacturing of pharmaceutical dosage forms where HME is combined with three-dimensional (3D) printing.

Three-dimensional printing is a process in which digitally controlled 3D objects are produced by the deposition of materials in a layer-by-layer manner [23]. Previously it was widely used in automobile, robotics, aerospace, and other industries for rapid prototyping purposes. Because of the widespread availability of commercial 3D printers and the recent FDA approval of the first 3D printed dosage form (Spritam), its use in pharmaceutical research has greatly increased [24]. The main reason for the increased attention of researchers on 3D printing is because of its potential to create complex, customized, and personalized-on-demand dosage forms. Recently, fused deposition modeling (FDM) 3D printing has been used in the preparation of various novel drug delivery systems, such as personalized vaginal progesterone rings [25], channeled tablets for superior disintegration and dissolution [26], personalized oral delivery devices [27], and topical nose-shaped device for the treatment of acne [28].

In this study, HME technology-paired FDM 3D printing and conventional direct compression methods were utilized to produce novel core-shell floating pulsatile tablets with a predetermined lag time of 6 h. Asthma is a chronic inflammatory condition of the airways and symptoms of this condition include shortness of breath, chest tightness and coughing, which are worsened at early morning hours due to regulation of the circadian rhythm. So, theophylline, which is widely used for the symptomatic treatment of chronic asthma, was chosen as a model drug. However, the in vivo performance of the developed drug delivery system will be investigated in our future studies. The aim of the developed drug delivery system is to achieve both floating characteristics and pulsatile release after the desired lag time to improve therapy and quality of life of patients with asthma.

2. Materials and Methods

2.1. Materials

Theophylline anhydrous (≥99% pure) was purchased from Sigma-Aldrich (St. Louis, MO, USA). Hydroxypropyl cellulose (HPC, Klucel LF) and ethyl cellulose (EC, Aqualon EC N14) were donated by Ashland Inc. (Covington, KY, USA). Croscarmellose sodium (Ac-Di-Sol®) and microcrystalline cellulose (Avicel PH® 102) were provided by FMC Biopolymer (Newark, DE, USA). Magnesium stearate was purchased from Alfa Aesar (Tewksbury, MA, USA). All other reagents and chemicals used were of analytical grade.

2.2. Thermogravimetric Analysis

A thermogravimetric analyzer (TGA 1-Pyris, PerkinElmer, Inc., Waltham, MA, USA) was used to determine the thermal degradation of the polymers at the temperature employed in HME and 3D printing techniques. The samples were loaded in aluminum pans and heated from 50 to 500 °C at a rate of 20 °C/min. Ultra-purified nitrogen was used as a purge gas at a flow rate of 25 mL/min. The data were collected and analyzed using the PerkinElmer Pyris™ software (Waltham, MA, USA), and the percent mass loss was calculated.

2.3. Preparation of the Filaments Using HME

An 11 mm twin-screw co-rotating hot-melt extruder (Process 11 Thermo Fisher Scientific, Waltham, DE, USA) was used to prepare the filaments required for 3D printing of the floating pulsatile tablets. The standard screw configuration with 3 mixing zones was employed at 50 rpm screw speed in this study. After the filaments exited from the extruder die, a conveyor belt was used to straighten and collect the filaments for easy processing into the 3D printer. Two formulations, HPC alone (100% w/w) or in combination with EC (99.5 w/w % HPC, 0.5% w/w EC)) were mixed in a V-shell blender (Maxiblend®, Globe Pharma, New Brunswick, NJ, USA) for 15 min and used for fabrication of the filaments. A temperature of 165 °C was set in all the eight heating zones and torque inside the barrel was observed between 4–5 Nm during the extrusion process. After the extrusion process, the filaments obtained were stored in a desiccator to avoid moisture pickup before they were used for 3D printing of the tablets. The filaments stored outside the desiccator absorbed moisture more quickly compared to the ones stored in the desiccator.

2.4. Mechanical Characteristics of Hot-Melt Extruded Filaments

The mechanical properties of the extruded filaments (flexibility or ductility and brittleness) are the critical parameters that are used to determine the suitability of the filaments for FDM 3D printing (Repka-Zhang test). Texture analyzer (TA-XT2i analyzer and Texture Technologies, Hamilton, MA, USA) were used to evaluate the mechanical properties of the filaments. The filaments were cut into a length of 5 mm and placed on the bottom flat surface of the texture analyzer. The top blade part of the texture analyzer was moved down until it penetrated the filament (0.6 mm) to create a 35% deformation in the shape of the filament. Testing for each single filament formulation was repeated 6 times. The force required to deform the filament was measured and analyzed using Exponent software version 6.1.5.0 (Stable Micro Systems, Godalming, UK). The parameters for the test were as follows: pre-test speed, 10 mm/s; test speed, 5 mm/s; and post-test speed 10 mm/s (Figure 1). The force applied by the feeding gears of the FDM 3D printer on the filament during the feeding process could be co-related with the force applied by the texture analyzer. This provides preliminary data for the assessment of the 3D printability of extruded filaments.

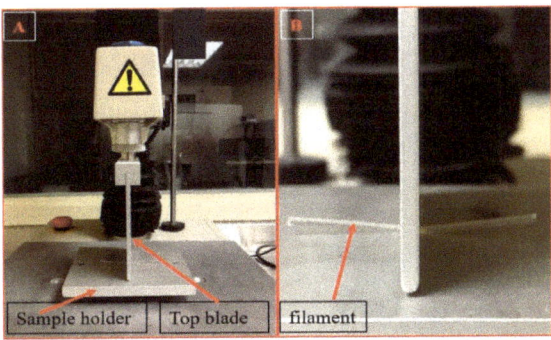

Figure 1. Texture analyzer set up (**A**) and stiffness test of the extruded filaments (**B**).

2.5. Preparation of the Core Tablets by Direct Compression

Theophylline (57% *w/w*), croscarmellose sodium (8% *w/w*), microcrystalline cellulose (34% *w/w*) and magnesium stearate (1% *w/w*) were sifted using a #30 sieve and blended using V-shell blender (Maxiblend®, Globe Pharma, New Brunswick, NJ, USA) for 10 min. The blended physical mixture (175 mg) equivalent to 100 mg of theophylline was compressed into tablets using 8 mm round flat punches by a single punch press (MCTMI, GlobePharma Inc., New Brunswick, NJ, USA).

2.6. 3D Printing of Pulsatile Floating Tablets

Initially, the hollow tablets were designed using Autodesk® Tinkercad™ free online software (Autodesk, CA, USA) and saved into 3D printer readable stl. format files. The stl. files were then imported into Ultimaker Cura software (Cura version 4.0, Ultimaker, Geldermalsen, Netherlands). Hot-melt extruded filaments were loaded into an FDM 3D printer (Prusa i3 3D desktop printer, Prusa Research, Prague, Czech Republic), which has an E3D v6 Hot End and a 0.4 mm nozzle and the floating tablets were printed. All the tablets were designed to have the same dimensions (14.5 mm diameter and 7 mm height) but with different shell thicknesses, wall (outer shell) thicknesses, and infill densities (Table 1). The tablets were printed at a nozzle temperature of 190 °C. The other settings used for 3D printing were as follows: bed temperature, 60 °C; nozzle traveling speed, 50 mm/s; layer height, 0.10 mm; and printing speed, 50 mm/s.

The structural parameters of a dosage form that were altered in FDM 3D printing were shell thickness, wall thickness (outer shell) and infill density. The shell can be defined as the total width of the perimeter of the dosage form, whereas the wall was a part of the shell that had different infill patterns and compact structures compared to the inner core. Alteration in the infill density changes the porosity of the structure of the dosage form. The wall has the same composition as that of the shell, but the printing pattern is different from the shell. Firstly, pure HPC filaments were used to print the hollow tablets with four different shell thicknesses (0.8, 1.2, 1.6, and 2.0 mm) as shown in Figure 2A. To tassess the lag time, in vitro release studies were conducted for floating tablets of plain HPC and HPC with different concentrations of ethyl cellulose (0.5 to 10 *w/w* %). Secondly, to assess the effect of wall thickness and % infill density of the shell on the drug release profiles, tablets with three different wall thickness (outer shell) (0, 0.8, and 1.6 mm) as shown in (Figure 2B), and three different % infill densities (50, 75, and 100) as shown in (Figure 2C) were printed using the filament containing 0.5% EC. The impact of infill density can only be assessed without a wall. So, a wall thickness of 0 mm was used while printing the tablets with different infill densities.

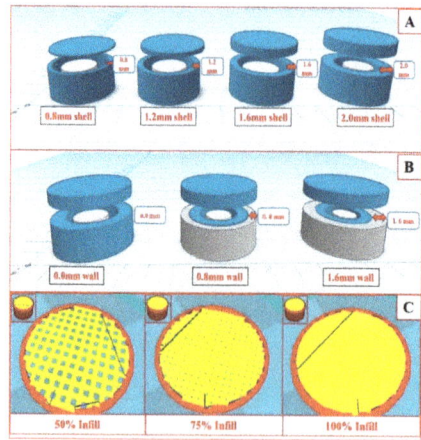

Figure 2. Graphical images of the floating tablets with different shell thickness (**A**), wall thickness (**B**), and infill density (**C**).

2.7. Loading Capacity and Buoyancy of the 3D Printed Floating Tablets

The printed tablets should remain buoyant in the gastric fluid in the stomach until the pulse release of the drugs occurs. Theoretically, an object can float when the buoyancy force exerted by the fluid is more than the opposite force by gravity (Archimedes' principle), i.e., if the total force acting vertically on the object is positive. To attain this, the total density of the dosage form should be less than the density of the gastric contents (reported as ~1.004 g/mL) [1]. Based on this principle, the maximum amount of the drug that can be loaded in the proposed floating system and can remain buoyant in the gastric fluid was calculated.

2.8. In Vitro Floating Study and Refloating Ability

The in vitro floating study of the 3D printed floating tablets was performed using a United States Pharmacopeia (USP II) dissolution test apparatus (Hanson SR8-plus™; Hanson Research, Chatsworth, CA, USA). The media was 900 mL of 0.1 N HCl maintained at 37 ± 0.5 °C and the paddle speed was set at 50 rpm. To determine the re-floating ability of the printed tablets, tablets were immersed in the dissolution medium for 5 s per hour using a glass rod during the floating study. The test was performed in triplicate. To obtain clear images of the floating tablets, the tablets were transferred to 500 mL glass beakers filled with the dissolution media and the photographs were captured at 0, 2, 4, and 6 h [29,30].

2.9. Scanning Electron Microscopy (SEM)

The surface morphology of the extruded filaments and 3D printed floating tablets were studied with a JOEL JSM 5610LV scanning electron microscope (SEM) (JOEL, Peabody, MA, USA) with an accelerating voltage of 5 kV. All the samples were placed on the SEM stubs and adhered by using double-adhesive tape. The samples were sputter-coated with gold under an argon atmosphere using a Hummer 6.2 Sputter Coater (Ladd Research Industries, Williston, VT, USA) prior to imaging.

2.10. In Vitro Drug Release Study

The drug release characteristics of the 3D printed floating tablets were determined using a United States Pharmacopeia (USP II) dissolution test apparatus (Hanson SR8-plus™; Hanson Research, Chatsworth, CA, USA). The dissolution media was 900 mL of 0.1 N HCl maintained at 37 ± 0.5 °C, and the paddle speed was set at 50 rpm (29). The samples were collected at the pre-determined time intervals and analyzed for drug content using a UV/VIS spectrophotometer (GENESYS 180, Thermo Scientific) at a wavelength of 272 nm. The calibration curve of $y = 0.0556x + 0.008$ was acquired with an r^2 value of 0.9996. Each test was carried out in triplicate and the collected data were plotted as percentage cumulative drug release versus time.

2.11. Statistical Analysis

Statistical analysis was performed by one-way analysis of variance (ANOVA) with Student-Newman-Keuls post-hoc testing using GraphPad Prism 5 software (GraphPad Software, San Diego, CA, USA) with $p \leq 0.05$ as the level of significance.

3. Results and Discussion

3.1. Thermal Analysis of the Polymers

The thermal degradation behaviors of HPC and EC are analyzed using thermogravimetric analyzer. From the results and literature reports, it was observed that the percentage loss in the mass was <1% at the temperature (190° C) used for 3D printing of the tablets [31]. A significant mass loss of the polymers was observed at temperatures >250 °C, implying that the polymers were stable during the HME and 3D printing processes.

3.2. Filament Preparation and Characterization

Different pharmaceutical-grade polymers were recently investigated for FDM 3D printing of the tablets for various applications. From the available pharmaceutical-grade polymers suitable for FDM 3D printing [27,29], HPC was utilized for the preparation of domperidone sustained release intragastric floating tablets. In this study, HPC was chosen for fabrication of the filaments required as feedstock materials for the development of 3D printed floating pulsatile tablets. In the preliminary studies, EC was added at different concentrations (10%, 5%, 2.5%, and 1%) to HPC to prolong the lag time for the pulsatile drug release characteristics. After all the EC concentrations were studied, the lag time observed was >8 h. The developed tablets with 0.5% EC exhibited a desired lag time of 6 h.

During the HME process, the filaments exiting the extruder die were coiled in irregular shapes and were difficult to process through the 3D printer. Therefore, a conveyor belt was used to straighten the filaments for easy loading into the 3D printer. After solidification, the filaments were coiled and stored in a desiccator to prevent moisture uptake. The filaments that absorbed moisture became soft and squeezed between the feeding gears of the 3D printer. This is because, after moisture absorption, the flexibility of the filaments increased, preventing the melted material from pushing through the heater. Further, the inflow of materials from the printer nozzle was irregular.

After fabrication of the filaments using the HME technique, the mechanical properties of these extruded filaments were tested using a texture analyzer and compared with those of the commercially available polylactic acid (PLA) filaments, which have optimum mechanical properties suitable for FDM 3D printing. For a filament to be considered suitable for FDM 3D printing, it should not either break or be curved aside by the feeding gears during the feeding process because this might result in an inadequate flow of materials through the nozzle. If the filament is too brittle it may get broken by the gears and if it is too flexible it may curve away from the feeding gears because the materials cannot be pushed through the narrow 0.4 mm nozzle of the 3D printer. For this reason, there should be a balance between the brittleness and the flexibility of the filaments.

Even though PLA is considered as a reference material for comparing the mechanical properties of the filaments in 3D printing, it is interesting to note that filaments with a lower stiffness (breaking stress and force) than the PLA filament were good enough for the FDM 3D printing process. This may be due to a variation in the force applied by the gears of the different 3D printers during feeding of the filaments into the 3D printer. In this study (Figure 3), the force required to create a 35% deformation in the shape of the filament was considered as the maximum force that the filaments could withhold during the feeding process without any breaking or squeezing phenomenon in the feeder. Pure HPC and HPC + EC require a lower force of 8500 g and 7409 g, respectively, as compared to that of the reference material PLA (25,630 g). However, these filaments did not show any breaking or squeezing problems during the printing process, which resulted in the fabrication of high-quality floating tablets.

In a study conducted by Chai et al. [29], the authors developed intragastric sustained release floating tablets of domperidone using HPC EXF as matrix polymer for the fabrication of filaments. The authors used 10% (w/w) domperidone in the filament composition. The fabricated filaments exhibited the desired mechanical properties suitable for FDM 3D printing. Similar results were observed in the current study. In the earlier study, filaments fabricated using HPC EF and HPC HF grades with 30% paracetamol were not suitable for FDM 3D printing [32]. The filaments produced using both HPC EF and HPC HF were too soft. This may be due to the relatively high drug load of 30% (w/w) paracetamol, which acted as a plasticizer and softened the filaments. These studies indicate the significance of drug loading and the properties of drugs in the fabrication of filaments to be utilized in FDM 3D printing.

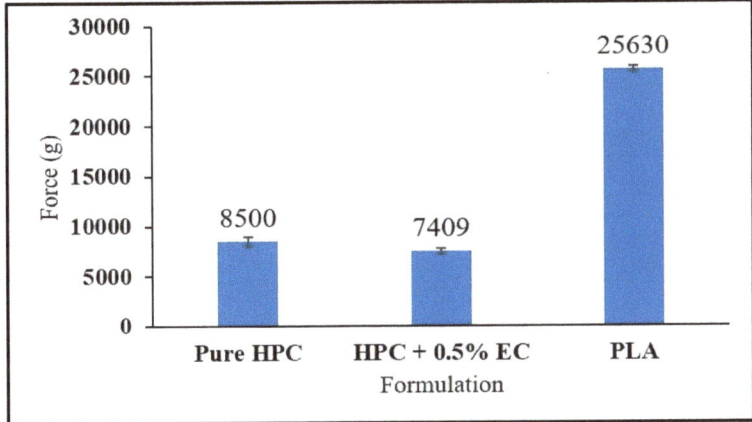

Figure 3. Force values of stiffness test of the hot-melt extruded filaments (error bars represent mean ± S.D).

3.3. Physical Properties of the Compressed Tablets

After performing preliminary experiments with different ratios of theophylline and other ingredients, the composition (theophylline (57% w/w), croscarmellose sodium (8% w/w), microcrystalline cellulose (34% w/w), and magnesium stearate (1% w/w)) was selected to prepare immediate-release theophylline tablets. All the compressed theophylline tablets demonstrated acceptable uniformity in weight (175.09 ± 5.76 mg), thickness (2.90 ± 0.16 mm), and hardness (4.27 ± 0.70 kp). The disintegration time was <1 min and the tablets showed 100% drug release within 30 min.

3.4. 3D Printing of the Floating Tablets

The physical properties of all the printed floating tablets are enumerated in Table 1. 3D printing of the floating pulsatile tablets was achieved in three steps (Figure 4). In the first step, 80% of the tablet shells were printed and the printer was paused. In the second step, the directly compressed core tablets were placed in the 80% printed shell and the final printing was resumed to form a completely sealed floating tablet. This process resulted in the printing of tablets without any structural defects. The thicknesses of the top and bottom were the same as the shell thickness of all the prepared tablets. The tablets printed without any wall had rough surfaces and structural defects in some of the tablets, whereas the surfaces of the tablets with walls were smooth and no structural deformities were observed during the printing process.

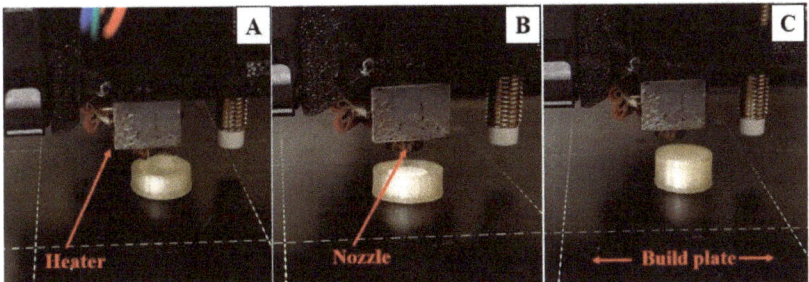

Figure 4. Eighty percent of the printed empty shell of a floating tablet (**A**), placement of a compressed tablet in the shell (**B**), and a completely sealed floating tablet (**C**).

Table 1. Physical properties of the 3D printed floating tablets.

Filament 1 (100% (w/w) HPC)					
Shell Thickness (mm)	Wall Thickness (mm)	Infill Density (%)	Weight (mg)	Density (mg/mm^3)	Floating Duration (h)
0.8 mm	0.8 mm	100	633.13 ± 11.20	0.55 ± 0.01	1.50 ± 0.21
1.2 mm	0.8 mm	100	774.67 ± 12.06	0.67 ± 0.01	3.00 ± 0.16
1.6 mm	0.8 mm	100	868.67 ± 18.72	0.75 ± 0.02	3.50 ± 0.08
2.0 mm	0.8 mm	100	1088.66 ± 7.37	0.94 ± 0.01	4.00 ± 0.12
Filament 2 (0.5%EC (w/w), 99.5% HPC)					
Shell Thickness (mm)	Wall Thickness (mm)	Infill Density (%)	Weight (mg)	Density (mg/mm^3)	Floating Duration (h)
2.0 mm	1.6 mm	100	1086.33 ± 6.66	0.94 ± 0.01	6.00 ± 0.09
	0.8 mm	100	1080.67 ± 10.69	0.93 ± 0.01	5.00 ± 0.13
	0.0 mm	100	1080.00 ± 16.82	0.93 ± 0.01	4.50 ± 0.26
		75	902.33 ± 8.39	0.78 ± 0.01	2.00 ± 0.22
		50	648.67 ± 9.87	0.56 ± 0.01	0.50 ± 0.19

3.5. Loading Capacity and Buoyancy of the 3D Floating Tablets

For a tablet to remain buoyant in the gastric fluid [1],

$$F_{Buoyancy} \geq F_{Gravity}. \tag{1}$$

Equation (1) above can also be represented as follows:

$$\rho L \cdot V_{max}\, g \geq (m_s + m_t)\, g \tag{2}$$

where ρL is the density of gastric fluid, V_{max} is the maximum volume of liquid displaced (i.e., the volume of floating pulsatile tablet, V_t), g is the acceleration due to gravity, m_s is the mass of shell, and m_t is the mass of the compressed tablet. Equation (2) is simplified as Equation (3):

$$\rho L \cdot V_t \geq (m_s + m_t), \tag{3}$$

where ρL is the density of the gastric fluid i.e., 1 g/cm^3, and mass of shell (m_s) + mass of compressed tablet (m_t) is the total mass of the floating tablet (M_t). So, Equation (3) was further simplified as Equation (4) as follows:

$$(\rho L \cdot V_t) - m_s \geq m_t. \tag{4}$$

The volume of the floating tablet (V_t) can be calculated from its dimensions. The optimized floating tablet shell had a weight of 913 mg and a volume of 1155 mm^3. So, the maximum weight of the compressed core tablet that can be accommodated was 242 mg. In our study, we used a compressed core tablet with a total weight of 175 mg, which is equivalent to 100 mg of theophylline. By optimizing the composition of the core compressed tablets for an immediate-release profile, any drug that is a suitable candidate for a floating pulsatile release system can be delivered with this proposed pulsatile floating tablet.

3.6. Floating and Refloating Abilities of the Printed Tablets

All the tablets placed in the dissolution media floated immediately without any lag time. The floating ability of the printed tablets was highly correlated with their density as reported in the previous literature [28]. Tablets with a density of >1 mg/mm^3 sunk to the bottom of the dissolution vessels. The density of the printed tablets ranged from 0.548–0.941 mg/mm^3. Tablets with high shell thickness and high infill had higher densities. No difference in the density was observed between the tablets with various wall thicknesses with 100% infill density ($p < 0.005$). When the tablets were immersed in the dissolution media to see their refloating ability, they rose to the top of the dissolution vessel immediately without any lag time. All the tablets showed good refloating ability without any loss of structural integrity. The images of the floating tablets obtained at different time points during the dissolution study are shown in Figure 5.

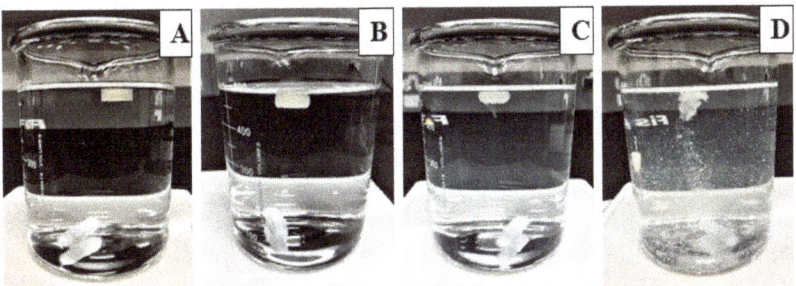

Figure 5. Images of the floating tablets taken at different time points during the dissolution study in 0.1 N HCl: 0 h (**A**), 2 h (**B**), 4 h (**C**), and 6 h (**D**).

3.7. Surface Morphology

The surface morphology of the extruded filaments, cross-sectional structure, and surface of the floating tablets are shown in Figure 6. The surface of the extruded filament was smooth and homogeneous without any deformities, suggesting suitability for 3D printing. Filaments that have rough or irregular surfaces will not feed smoothly into the 3D printer and result in irregular shaped tablets. The cross-sectional structure of the floating tablets showed multiple single layers printed side by side to form the shell. The surface of the 100% infill 3D printed tablets showed close adjacent layers without any gaps.

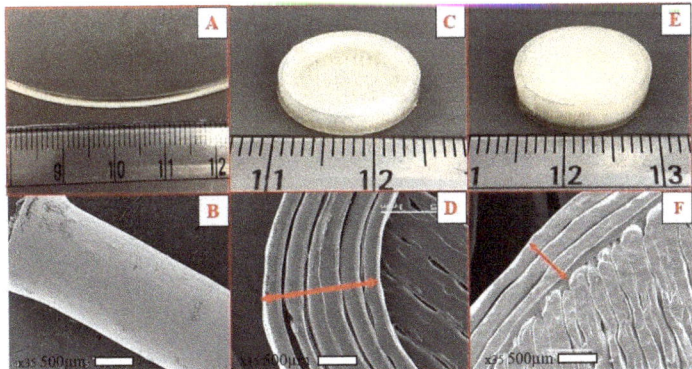

Figure 6. Digital images and representative SEM images of the hot-melt extrusion (HME) filament (**A,B**), the cross-sectional structure of the floating tablet showing shell (**C,D**), and surface morphology of a 100% infill 3D printed tablet (**E,F**).

3.8. In Vitro Dissolution Study

The dissolution behavior of the 3D printed floating tablets is shown in Figure 7. From the dissolution data, it was observed that both the tablet geometry and addition of EC into HPC had a significant effect on the drug release profiles ($p < 0.05$). The tablets with higher shell thicknesses had integrity for a longer period of time before the pulse release of API into the dissolution media as compared to tablets with a lower thickness (Figure 7A). The tablets with a shell thickness of 2.0 mm (highest) demonstrated pulse release at the end of 4 ± 0.12 h, whereas those with a shell thickness of 0.8 mm (lowest) showed drug release in 1.5 ± 0.21 h. The tablets with a shell thickness of 1.2 mm and 1.6 mm showed a lag time of 3 ± 0.16 and 3.5 ± 0.08 h, respectively, before complete drug release. Similar results have been reported in the literature on the effects of shell thickness. In a previous study conducted by Maroni et al., the authors printed two-compartment capsular devices, each compartment with different thicknesses and reported that the duration of the lag phase for the pulse release of drugs increased proportionally with an increase in the compartment thickness [33]. This phenomenon can be caused by a higher shell thickness that prevents the entry of the dissolution media into the core for a longer time. The addition of EC to the formulation increased the threshold time for complete drug release (Figure 7B). The tablets with 2.0 mm shell thickness, which had an EC of 0.5%, showed pulse release at the end of 5 ± 0.13 h.

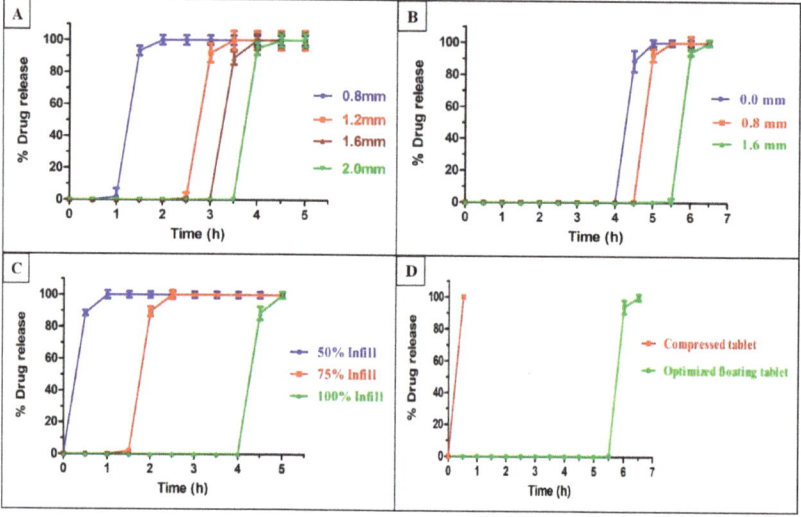

Figure 7. In vitro release profiles of the floating tablets with different shell thicknesses in 0.1 N HCl (**A**), different wall thicknesses (**B**), different fill densities (**C**), and optimized floating tablets and compressed tablets (**D**). Error bars represent mean ± S.D.

To assess the effect of the wall thickness and infill density of shell on the pulse release of drug, tablets with three different wall thicknesses (0.0, 0.8, and 1.6 mm) and three infill densities were studied (50%, 75%, and 100%). The tablets with higher wall thicknesses prevented the entry of the dissolution media more effectively than those with low wall thicknesses. This is attributed to the closed, compact structure of the wall. This observation was consistent with the results of a previous study [34]. The tablets with 100% infill densities demonstrated pulse release at the end of 4.5 ± 0.26 h, followed by 75% infill (2 ± 0.22 h), and 50% infill (0.5 ± 0.19) (Figure 7C). The higher porosity of lower infill density has a higher surface area and allows easy entry of the dissolution media into the core, resulted in a faster release of API. Yang et al. [35] and Chen et al. [36], who used FDM 3D printing for the development of controlled release dosage forms, reported that a higher fill density caused a reduction in the total surface area and resulted in slower drug release from the dosage forms.

All the prepared floating tablets exhibited a pulse release of drug with different threshold times varying from 30 min to 6 h. The tablets with a specific geometrical structure (2 mm shell, 1.6 mm wall, 100% infill) with 0.5% EC (Figure 7D) were considered optimized formulations for pulsatile release of drugs after 6 h for effective chronotherapeutic treatment of asthma.

4. Conclusions

Floating pulsatile tablets with the desired lag time for pulse release of theophylline were successfully developed with the proposed HME coupled 3D printing technique. The geometrical properties of the tablets (shell and wall thickness and infill density) and EC showed significant ($p < 0.05$) effect on the lag time. Thus, the lag time can be varied from 30 min to 6 h based on the requirements. The proposed floating pulsatile system showed high potential to deliver drugs that need high residence time in the stomach and the pulsatile release of theophylline. This strategy reduces unwanted adverse effects and improves patient compliance. In addition, thermolabile drugs can be delivered through this system as the inner core tablet is not exposed to high temperatures involved in the FDM 3D printing process. In conclusion, HME coupled 3D printing is a novel technique to develop low-cost customized drug dosage forms for personalized pharmacotherapy. However, dosage forms fabricated using FDM 3D printing technology need to overcome the challenges in terms of regulatory concerns. Therefore, these floating systems need to be further assessed in in vivo conditions to demonstrate their suitability for patient use.

Author Contributions: N.R.D. and S.B.; conceptualized the study, investigation and rough draft provided by N.R.D.; initial review and editing by S.B.; supervision and manuscript editing by M.A.R. All authors have read and agreed to the published version of the manuscript.

Funding: This project was partially supported by Grant Number P30GM122733-01A1, funded by the National Institute of General Medical Sciences (NIGMS) a component of the National Institutes of Health (NIH) as one of its Centers of Biomedical Research Excellence (COBRE).

Acknowledgments: Authors acknowledge the Pii Center for Pharmaceutical Innovation & Instruction.

Conflicts of Interest: The authors declare no conflict of interest.

References

1. Thitinan, S.; McConville, J.T. Development of a gastroretentive pulsatile drug delivery platform. *J. Pharm. Pharmacol.* **2012**, *64*, 505–516. [CrossRef]
2. Jain, D.; Raturi, R.; Jain, V.; Bansal, P.; Singh, R. Recent technologies in pulsatile drug delivery systems. *Biomatter* **2011**, *1*, 57–65. [CrossRef] [PubMed]
3. Sunil, S.A.; Srikanth, M.V.; Rao, N.S.; Uhumwangho, M.U.; Latha, K.; Murthy, K.V.R. Chronotherapeutic drug delivery systems: An approach to circadian rhythms diseases. *Curr. Drug Deliv.* **2011**, *8*, 622–633. [CrossRef]
4. Maroni, A.; Zema, L.; Del Curto, M.D.; Loreti, G.; Gazzaniga, A. Oral pulsatile delivery: Rationale and chronopharmaceutical formulations. *Int. J. Pharm.* **2010**, *398*, 1–8. [CrossRef] [PubMed]
5. Streubel, A.; Siepmann, J.; Bodmeier, R. Gastroretentive drug delivery systems. *Expert Opin. Drug Deliv.* **2006**, *3*, 217–233. [CrossRef]
6. Worsøe, J.; Fynne, L.; Gregersen, T.; Schlageter, V.; Christensen, L.A.; Dahlerup, J.F.; Rijkhoff, N.J.; Laurberg, S.; Krogh, K. Gastric transit and small intestinal transit time and motility assessed by a magnet tracking system. *BMC Gastroenterol.* **2011**, *11*, 145. [CrossRef]
7. Butreddy, A.; Dudhipala, N. Enhancement of Solubility and Dissolution Rate of Trandolapril Sustained Release Matrix Tablets by Liquisolid Compact Approach. *Asian J. Pharm.* **2015**, *9*, 1.
8. Amin, L.; Ahmed, T.; Mannan, A. Development of Floating-Mucoadhesive Microsphere for Site Specific Release of Metronidazole. *Adv. Pharm. Bull.* **2016**, *6*, 195–200. [CrossRef] [PubMed]
9. Preda, M.; Leucuta, S.E. Oxprenolol-loaded bioadhesive microspheres: Preparation and in vitro/in vivo characterization. *J. Microencapsul.* **2003**, *20*, 777–789. [CrossRef]
10. Garg, R.; Gupta, G. Progress in Controlled Gastroretentive Delivery Systems. *Trop. J. Pharm. Res.* **2008**, *7*, 1055–1066. [CrossRef]
11. Chen, J.; Park, H.; Park, K. Synthesis of superporous hydrogels: Hydrogels with fast swelling and superabsorbent properties. *J. Biomed. Mater. Res.* **1999**, *44*, 53–62. [CrossRef]
12. Almutairy, B.K.; Alshetaili, A.S.; Ashour, E.A.; Patil, H.; Tiwari, R.V.; Alshehri, S.M.; Repka, M.A. Development of a floating drug delivery system with superior buoyancy in gastric fluid using hot-melt extrusion coupled with pressurized CO_2. *Pharmazie* **2016**, *71*, 128–133. [PubMed]

13. Reddy, A.B.; Reddy, N.D. Development of Multiple-Unit Floating Drug Delivery System of Clarithromycin: Formulation, in vitro Dissolution by Modified Dissolution Apparatus, in vivo Radiographic Studies in Human Volunteers. *Drug Res.* **2017**, *67*, 412–418. [CrossRef] [PubMed]
14. Lalge, R.; Thipsay, P.; Shankar, V.K.; Maurya, A.; Pimparade, M.; Bandari, S.; Zhang, F.; Murthy, S.N.; Repka, M.A. Preparation and evaluation of cefuroxime axetil gastro-retentive floating drug delivery system via hot melt extrusion technology. *Int. J. Pharm.* **2019**, *566*, 520–531. [CrossRef]
15. Vo, A.Q.; Feng, X.; Morott, J.T.; Pimparade, M.B.; Tiwari, R.V.; Zhang, F.; Repka, M.A. A novel floating controlled release drug delivery system prepared by hot-melt extrusion. *Eur. J. Pharm. Biopharm.* **2016**, *98*, 108–121. [CrossRef]
16. He, W.; Li, Y.; Zhang, R.; Wu, Z.; Yin, L. Gastro-floating bilayer tablets for the sustained release of metformin and immediate release of pioglitazone: Preparation and in vitro/in vivo evaluation. *Int. J. Pharm.* **2014**, *476*, 223–231. [CrossRef]
17. Tiwari, R.V.; Patil, H.; Repka, M.A. Contribution of hot-melt extrusion technology to advance drug delivery in the 21st century. *Expert Opin. Drug Deliv.* **2016**, *13*, 451–464. [CrossRef]
18. Pimparade, M.B.; Morott, J.T.; Park, J.-B.; Kulkarni, V.I.; Majumdar, S.; Murthy, S.N.; Lian, Z.; Pinto, E.; Bi, V.; Dürig, T.; et al. Development of taste masked caffeine citrate formulations utilizing hot melt extrusion technology and in vitro-in vivo evaluations. *Int. J. Pharm.* **2015**, *487*, 167–176. [CrossRef] [PubMed]
19. Maddineni, S.; Battu, S.K.; Morott, J.; Soumyajit, M.; Repka, M.A. Formulation optimization of hot-melt extruded abuse deterrent pellet dosage form utilizing design of experiments. *J. Pharm. Pharmacol.* **2014**, *66*, 309–322. [CrossRef]
20. Lakshman, J.P.; Cao, Y.; Kowalski, J.; Serajuddin, A.T.M. Application of Melt Extrusion in the Development of a Physically and Chemically Stable High-Energy Amorphous Solid Dispersion of a Poorly Water-Soluble Drug. *Mol. Pharm.* **2008**, *5*, 994–1002. [CrossRef]
21. Bhagurkar, A.M.; Angamuthu, M.; Patil, H.; Tiwari, R.V.; Maurya, A.; Hashemnejad, S.M.; Kundu, S.; Murthy, S.N.; Repka, M.A. Development of an Ointment Formulation Using Hot-Melt Extrusion Technology. *AAPS PharmSciTech* **2016**, *17*, 158–166. [CrossRef]
22. Dumpa, N.R.; Sarabu, S.; Bandari, S.; Zhang, F.; Repka, M.A. Chronotherapeutic Drug Delivery of Ketoprofen and Ibuprofen for Improved Treatment of Early Morning Stiffness in Arthritis Using Hot-Melt Extrusion Technology. *AAPS PharmSciTech* **2018**, *19*, 2700–2709. [CrossRef]
23. Goole, J.; Amighi, K. 3D printing in pharmaceutics: A new tool for designing customized drug delivery systems. *Int. J. Pharm.* **2016**, *499*, 376–394. [CrossRef] [PubMed]
24. Trenfield, S.J.; Awad, A.; Goyanes, A.; Gaisford, S.; Basit, A.W. 3D Printing Pharmaceuticals: Drug Development to Frontline Care. *Trends Pharmacol. Sci.* **2018**, *39*, 440–451. [CrossRef]
25. Fu, J.; Yu, X.; Jin, Y. 3D printing of vaginal rings with personalized shapes for controlled release of progesterone. *Int. J. Pharm.* **2018**, *539*, 75–82. [CrossRef] [PubMed]
26. Sadia, M.; Arafat, B.; Ahmed, W.; Forbes, R.T.; Alhnan, M.A. Channelled tablets: An innovative approach to accelerating drug release from 3D printed tablets. *J. Control. Release* **2018**, *269*, 355–363. [CrossRef] [PubMed]
27. Liang, K.; Carmone, S.; Brambilla, D.; Leroux, J.-C. 3D printing of a wearable personalized oral delivery device: A first-in-human study. *Sci. Adv.* **2018**, *4*, 2544. [CrossRef] [PubMed]
28. Goyanes, A.; Det-Amornrat, U.; Wang, J.; Basit, A.W.; Gaisford, S. 3D scanning and 3D printing as innovative technologies for fabricating personalized topical drug delivery systems. *J. Control. Release* **2016**, *234*, 41–48. [CrossRef] [PubMed]
29. Chai, X.; Chai, H.; Wang, X.; Yang, J.; Li, J.; Zhao, Y.; Cai, W.; Tao, T.; Xiang, X. Fused Deposition Modeling (FDM) 3D Printed Tablets for Intragastric Floating Delivery of Domperidone. *Sci. Rep.* **2017**, *7*, 2829. [CrossRef]
30. Li, Q.; Guan, X.; Cui, M.; Zhu, Z.; Chen, K.; Wen, H.; Jia, D.; Hou, J.; Xu, W.; Yang, X.; et al. Preparation and investigation of novel gastro-floating tablets with 3D extrusion-based printing. *Int. J. Pharm.* **2018**, *535*, 325–332. [CrossRef]
31. Meena, A.; Parikh, T.; Gupta, S.S.; Serajuddin, T.M. Investigation of thermal and viscoelastic properties of polymers relevant to hot melt extrusion II: Cellulosic polymers. *J. Excip. Food Chem.* **2014**, *5*, 46–55.
32. Zhang, J.; Xu, P.; Vo, A.Q.; Bandari, S.; Yang, F.; Durig, T.; Repka, M.A. Development and evaluation of pharmaceutical 3D printability for hot melt extruded cellulose-based filaments. *J. Drug Deliv. Sci. Technol.* **2019**, *52*, 292–302. [CrossRef]

33. Maroni, A.; Melocchi, A.; Parietti, F.; Foppoli, A.; Zema, L.; Gazzaniga, A. 3D printed multi-compartment capsular devices for two-pulse oral drug delivery. *J. Control. Release* **2017**, *268*, 10–18. [CrossRef]
34. Zhang, J.; Yang, W.; Vo, A.Q.; Feng, X.; Ye, X.; Kim, D.W.; Repka, M.A. Hydroxypropyl methylcellulose-based controlled release dosage by melt extrusion and 3D printing: Structure and drug release correlation. *Carbohydr. Polym.* **2017**, *177*, 49–57. [CrossRef] [PubMed]
35. Yang, Y.; Wang, H.; Li, H.; Ou, Z.; Yang, G. 3D printed tablets with internal scaffold structure using ethyl cellulose to achieve sustained ibuprofen release. *Eur. J. Pharm. Sci.* **2018**, *115*, 11–18. [CrossRef] [PubMed]
36. Chen, D.; Xu, X.Y.; Li, R.; Zhang, G.A.; Zhang, Y.; Wang, M.R.; Xiong, M.F.; Xu, J.R.; Wang, T.; Hu, Q.; et al. Preparation and In vitro Evaluation of FDM 3D-Printed Ellipsoid-Shaped Gastric Floating Tablets with Low Infill Percentages. *AAPS PharmSciTech* **2020**, *21*, 6. [CrossRef] [PubMed]

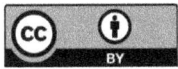

© 2020 by the authors. Licensee MDPI, Basel, Switzerland. This article is an open access article distributed under the terms and conditions of the Creative Commons Attribution (CC BY) license (http://creativecommons.org/licenses/by/4.0/).

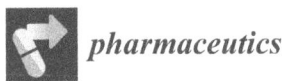

Article
3D-Printed Solid Dispersion Drug Products

Suet Li Chew [1], Laura Modica de Mohac [1,2] and Bahijja Tolulope Raimi-Abraham [1,*]

1. Drug Delivery Group, Institute of Pharmaceutical Science, Faculty of Life Sciences and Medicine, King's College London, Franklin-Wilkins Building, 150 Stamford Street, London SE1 9NH, UK; suet.chew@kcl.ac.uk (S.L.C.); laura.1.modica_de_mohac@kcl.ac.uk (L.M.d.M.)
2. Department of Sciences for Health Promotion and Mother-Child Care "G. D'Alessandro", University of Palermo, 90100 Palermo, Italy
* Correspondence: Bahijja.Raimi-Abraham@kcl.ac.uk; Tel.: +020-7836-5454

Received: 14 October 2019; Accepted: 5 December 2019; Published: 11 December 2019

Abstract: With the well-known advantages of additive manufacturing methods such as three-dimensional (3D) printing in drug delivery, it is disappointing that only one product has been successful in achieving regulatory approval in the past few years. Further research and development is required in this area to introduce more 3D printed products into the market. Our study investigates the potential of fixed dose combination solid dispersion drug products generated via 3D printing. Two model drugs—fluorescein sodium (FS) and 5-aminosalicylic acid (5-ASA)—were impregnated onto a polyvinyl alcohol (PVA) filament, and the influence of solvent choice in optimal drug loading as well as other influences such as the physicochemical and mechanical properties of the resultant filaments were investigated prior to development of the resultant drug products. Key outcomes of this work included the improvement of filament drug loading by one- to threefold due to solvent choice on the basis of its polarity and the generation of a 3D-printed product confirmed to be a solid dispersion fixed dose combination with the two model drugs exhibiting favourable in vitro dissolution characteristics.

Keywords: 3D printing; amorphous solid dispersion; additive manufacturing; poor solubility; fixed dose combination

1. Introduction

A fixed-dose combination (FDC) product is a single dosage form that incorporates two or more active pharmaceutical ingredients (APIs) [1,2]. Between 2013 and 2018, the European Medicines Agency (EMA) approved 66 FDCs, most of which were antiretrovirals for human immunodeficiency virus (HIV) infections [3]. FDC products have several advantages over conventional medicinal products, namely, greater efficacy (43%, $n = 33$) and compliance (18%, $n = 14$) [4–7]. However, disadvantages have been highlighted, such as a reduction in medication adherence (24%–26%) in some cases [8,9].

The use of three-dimensional (3D) printing in drug delivery is still in its infancy compared to traditional technologies; however, research and development is rapidly expanding in this area due to the benefits of 3D printing to develop personalized patient-specific dosage forms with tailored release profiles [10–13]. Traditional powder direct compression techniques to generate FDC medicinal products is not suitable [14–19]. Currently, the only regulatory approved (by the Food and Drug Administration (FDA)) 3D printed medicinal product is the oro-dispersible levetiracetam tablet, Spritam developed by Aprecia Pharmaceuticals in 2015 [20]. The number of regulatory approved 3D printed drug products remains limited due to the number of printers available to comply with good manufacture practice (GMP), high variability of 3D printers, and end product quality [21–24]. Fused deposition modelling (FDM) uses heat to melt thermoplastic polymers into the molten state and the object to be printed is designed by computer-aided drafting, which enables it to be printed layer-by-layer as the printer nozzle deposits the extrudate [15,25]. FDM 3D printing has been explored extensively in the development of medicinal products and, more specifically, FDC products. FDM 3D printing is capable of producing drug products with multiple active pharmaceutical ingredients in various compartments, which is advantageous in developing patient-centric formulations to reduce multiple daily dosing, therefore improving patient compliance and therapeutic efficiency [26–28].

The use of solid dispersion technology has been explored in FDM 3D printing [26]. In the study described here, we firstly explored the influence of solvent type on filament (polyvinyl alcohol (PVA)) drug loading using the drug impregnation method. We then manufactured solid dispersion FDC 3D printed dosage forms using the drug-solvent-filament combination, which gave the highest drug loading. Physicochemical characterization of the filaments was conducted and an evaluation of filament and FDC mechanical properties by way of hardness and tensile strength were also evaluated. In vitro drug dissolution studies on the FDC 3D printed dosage forms were also conducted [29,30].

Several studies have used the drug impregnation method to load drugs onto polymer filaments for 3D printing. In the case of PVA filaments, this is commonly done by soaking the filament in a highly saturated drug solution. However, this method can result in low drug-loading (<2% w/w) due to slow drug diffusion into polymer [17,24,29–31]. The general drug-loading differences using different solvents such as ethanol (EtOH) and methanol (MeOH) for this filament drug loading method still remains relatively unknown. Studies conducted on 3D-printed FDC often separate APIs into different compartments such as the DuoCaplet design by Goyanes et al. [23]. The potential of FDM-printed monolithic FDC design, by incorporating two APIs into the same polymer filament, is yet to be investigated in terms of ability to independently tailor the different APIs release. This study aimed to explore the potential of increasing drug-loading efficiency by altering solvent choice, and to study the in vitro dissolution profiles of the FDM-printed monolithic FDC tablet developed. Fluorescein sodium (FS) and 5-aminosalicyclic acid (5-ASA) were chosen as model drugs due to their proven FDM-printability [29,30]. PVA was selected as main polymer as it is the only commercially extruded polymer filament that would dissolve in vivo [29].

2. Materials and Methods

2.1. Materials

Fluorescein sodium salt (FS, 376.27 g/mol, decomposition temperature = 315–395 °C), absolute ethanol, and methanol ≥99.8% were manufactured by Sigma-Aldrich, United Kingdom. Dimethyl sulfoxide (DMSO) was purchased from Honeywell. 5-Aminosalicyclic acid (5-ASA, 153.14 g/mol, decomposition temperature = 280 °C) purchased from FLUKA was donated by University College London School of Pharmacy. Polyvinyl alcohol (PVA) filament, 1.75 mm diameter, was purchased from RS-Pro. Phosphate buffer (pH 6.8) tablets were purchased from Millipore Corporation.

2.2. Methods

2.2.1. Filament Preparation

Drug-containing filaments were prepared using the method described by Goyanes et al. [29,30]. In brief, 5 m of PVA filament was soaked in the drug-solvent mixture (100 mL) and stirred magnetically at 470 rpm for 24 h. The drug-loaded filaments were then heated (60 °C) in an oven (Pickstone Ovens, Island Scientific, Isle of Wight, UK) to facilitate rapid solvent evaporation (≈2 h). Resultant filaments were protected from light and moisture with aluminum foil and desiccants, respectively. Tagami et al. [31] suggested that this method of drug load requires the use of a saturated drug solution. Therefore, the drug concentrations chosen were based on drug concentrations (of FS and 5-ASA) used in previous studies [29,30]. Table 1 outlines the solvents, drug choices, and concentrations for the preparation of drug-loaded and solvent-soaked filaments. The names of the filament samples are included in brackets.

Table 1. Solvent, drug, and drug concentrations used.

Active Pharmaceutical Ingredient (API)	Ethanol (EtOH)	Methanol (MeOH)	Dimethyl Sulfoxide (DMSO)
		PVA	
Fluorescein sodium (FS)	2.0% w/v (FS-EtOH)	2.5% w/v (2.5%FS-MeOH)	2.5% w/v (FS-DMSO)
5-aminosalicyclic acid (5-ASA)	1.0% w/v (5-ASA-EtOH)	1.25% w/v (5-ASA-MeOH)	1.25% w/v (5-ASA-DMSO)
FS and 5-ASA		2.5% w/v FS and 1.25% w/v 5-ASA (FDC-MeOH)	

2.2.2. Solid State Characterization of Filaments

X-Ray Powder Diffration

Structural characterization of filaments produced was conducted using a D/Max-BR diffractometer (RigaKu, Tokyo, Japan) with Cu Kα radiation operating at 40 kV and 15 mA (Cu Kalpha radiation) over the 2θ range 10–50° with a step size of 0.02° at 2°/min.

2.2.3. 3D-Printed Drug Product Design and Optimization

Tablets were designed using TinkerCAD and were then imported as stl. format into MakerBot Desktop Beta (V3.10.1.1389) (MakerBot Industries. Brooklyn, NY, USA). Tablets were printed with PVA filament and drug loaded filaments using a MakerBot Replicator 2X (MakerBot Inc., Brooklyn, NY USA) with the following dimensions 10.45 × 10.54 × 1.2 mm [30]. Printer settings were standard resolution, 230 °C extrusion and 20 °C platform temperature, 100% hexagonal infill with raft option deactivated when printing drug-loaded tablets but activated for blank PVA tablets [24]. Printed tablets were assessed for weight uniformity.

2.2.4. Morphology Studies

Scanning Electron Microscopy

Hitachi S5000 Emission Gun (FEG) (Hitachi, Maidenhead, UK) with Tungsten Tip (25 kV) was used to examine gold-coated (10 nm thickness) PVA tablet. Images were captured using secondary electron detector from ×70 to ×10.9 K magnification.

2.2.5. Crushing Strength

The crushing strength tests were conducted using a C50 Tablet Hardness and Compression tester (Engineering System, Nottingham, United Kingdom) on PVA and drug-loaded filaments. Figure 1 shows the sample orientation in the tester. Filament hardness was recorded as mean crushing strength (kg).

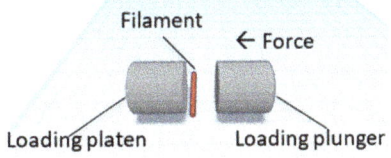

Figure 1. Orientation of filaments between loading plunger and platen. Increasing force was applied by loading plunger towards the platen. Direction of force is indicated by the arrow (←).

2.2.6. Solubility, Drug Content, and In Vitro Drug Dissolution Studies

Solubility Studies

Solubility studies were conducted on FS and 5-ASA dissolved in the in vitro dissolution media, pH 6.8 phosphate buffer, and PVA solutions. Different amounts of PVA filament were dissolved in pH 6.8 phosphate buffers to prepare PVA-pH 6.8 solutions. Excess API (either FS or 5-ASA) was added to PVA solutions and vigorously stirred for 72 h at 37 ± 0.5 °C at 150 rpm. The saturated solutions were then filtered using a 0.45 µm membrane, and the API concentration in the filtrate was determined spectrophotometrically at 330 nm for 5-ASA and 490 nm for FS.

Calculation of Drug Content in PVA Filaments

Drug-loaded filaments were dissolved in pH 6.8 phosphate buffer and assayed spectrophotometrically (Perkin Elmer Lambda 35 Spectrophotometer) (PerkinElmer, Inc. Waltham, MA, USA) at 330 nm for 5-ASA and 490 nm for FS. PVA did not interfere with the UV analysis. Drug content was calculated using Equation (1) below.

$$\text{Drug} - \text{content}\ (\%\ w/w) = \left(\frac{\text{Weight of drug (g)}}{\text{Weight of filament (g)}}\right) \times 100 \qquad (1)$$

In Vitro Drug Dissolution Studies

In vitro dissolution studies were conducted in pH 6.8 phosphate buffer (small intestine) at 37 ± 0.5 °C and a rotational speed of 100 rpm under non-sink conditions to observe any supersaturation effect from the solid dispersion products generated. At predetermined intervals, samples were withdrawn and filtered through a 0.45 µm filter and the filtrate was analysed spectrophotometrically at 330 nm for 5-ASA and 490 nm for FS.

2.2.7. Statistical Analysis

Unpaired two-tailed t-test was performed using SigmaPlot V14.0 (Systat Software Inc. Berkshire, UK) with 95% significance level. $p < 0.05$ was regarded as significant.

3. Results

3.1. Solvent Choice Optimization

Solvents of increasing polarity: DMSO < EtOH < MeOH were investigated for their drug-loading efficiency into PVA filaments. Model drugs FS and 5-ASA are both polar; dissolving in solvents of higher polarity allows for generation of a larger concentration gradient for drug diffusion into the polymer (PVA) filament, therefore giving higher drug-loading in the presence of solvents of a higher polarity [32,33].

Table 2 shows mean drug content of the drug-impregnated filaments. DMSO completely solubilized PVA; therefore, the results below are based only on EtOH and MeOH. Coefficient of variation (%CV) ranged from 0.2% to 13.5%, highlighting the issue of non-uniform drug loading with soaking method, requiring further soaking apparatus choice selection.

Table 2. Mean drug-content (% w/w) of drug-loaded filaments prepared via drug impregnation method.

Solvents	Drug-Loaded Filaments	Drug Loading (% w/w)
Ethanol	FS-EtOH	1.19 ± 0.161
	5-ASA-EtOH	0.10 ± 0.001
Methanol	FS-MeOH	4.89 ± 0.449
	5-ASA-MeOH	0.17 ± 0.007
	FDC-MeOH	FS: 6.16 ± 0.197 5-ASA: 2.97 ± 0.362

Comparing single-drug-loaded filaments, MeOH was found to significantly increase drug loading compared to EtOH, irrespective of drugs ($p < 0.05$), fitting the hypothesis. The ratio of FS drug loading between MeOH and EtOH was approximately 4:1, whereas the ratio was smaller but statistically significant for 5-ASA (approximately 1.5:1 between MeOH and EtOH). Despite using the same drug concentration, 5-ASA content in FDC-MeOH filament was significantly higher ($\approx$17 fold) than 5-ASA content in 5-ASA-MeOH filament ($p < 0.01$). MeOH was chosen to prepare FDC filament for the rest of the study due to its improved drug loading.

3.2. Filament Characterization

3.2.1. Filament Hardness

It is expected that filament mechanical properties, hardness in particular, will change after drug impregnation, especially as most of the solvents used have the potential to degrade PVA [23]. Changes to filament properties can influence printability [34]. The crushing strength is frequently used in the pharmaceutical industry to describe the resistance of tablets to the application of a compression load [35]. In this study, we used the crushing strength to provide an indication of the changes in filament strength after soaking in EtOH and MeOH. Interestingly, the PVA filament crushing strength (kg) of 46.13 ± 0.89 kg decreased when the PVA filament was soaked (without the presence of the APIs) in EtOH and MeOH to 10.25 ± 1.04 kg and 10.78 ± 0.48kg, respectively. For single-drug-loaded filament, both FS-EtOH and 5-ASA-EtOH filaments had crushing strengths of 14.93 ± 1.74 kg and 14.65 ± 0.81 kg, respectively, however, these values significantly increased ($p < 0.01$) for MeOH-loaded drug filaments, FS-MeOH (25.34 ± 1.52 kg), and 5-ASA-MeOH (22.78 ± 1.21 kg). The crushing strength of FDC-MeOH filament was 16.77 ± 1.12 kg, similar to API-EtOH filaments ($p > 0.05$).

3.2.2. Solid State Characterization of Filaments

X-Ray Powder Diffraction (XRPD) studies were conducted to determine any potential physico-chemical changes to the API such as crystalline-amorphous transformation. XRPD diffractograms of raw materials of 5-ASA (Figure 2A) and FS (Figure 2B) both showed characteristic Bragg's peaks, as confirmed by Groom et al. and Banic-Tomisic et al. [36,37]. XRPD studies on PVA filament, (Figure 2C) PVA-MeOH (Figure 2D), and FDC-MeOH filament (Figure 2E) showed characteristic amorphous halo with no evidence of crystalline API peaks.

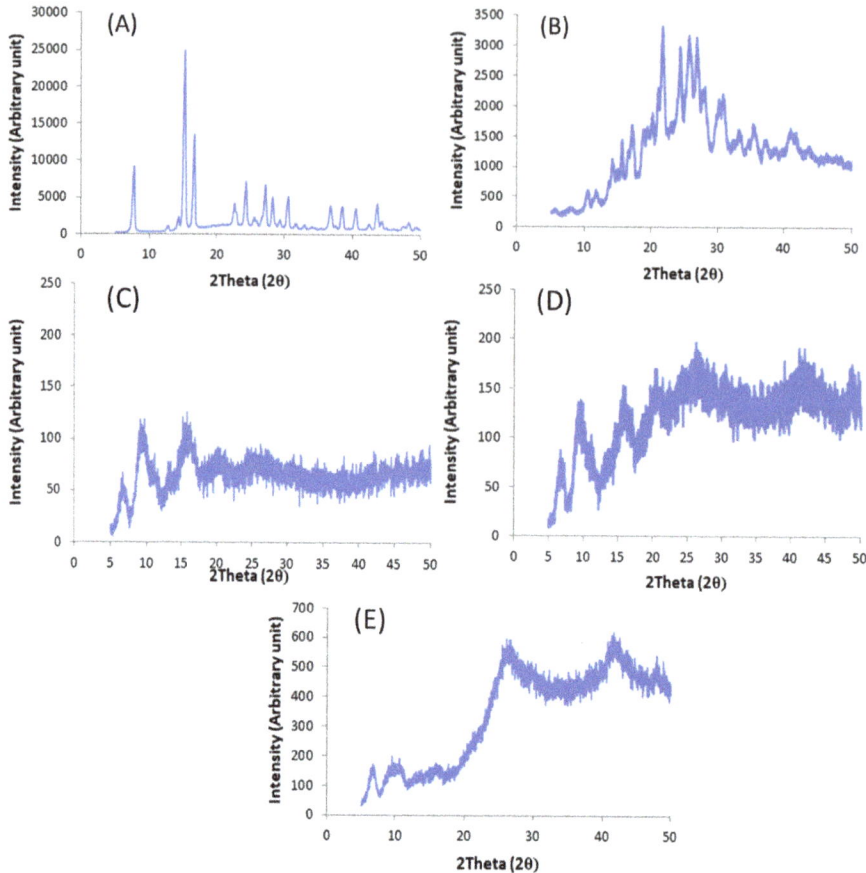

Figure 2. X-ray powder diffractograms of (**A**) 5-ASA, (**B**) FS, (**C**) blank polyvinyl alcohol (PVA) filament, (**D**) PVA-MeOH filament, and (**E**) FDC-MeOH filament data. Samples were scanned from 10–50° 2θ (stepwise: 0.02°, at 2°/min). Please note that different y-axis scales were used.

3.3. Characterization of 3D-Printed Dosage Forms

Morphology Studies

Layer-by-layer building of object via molten polymer fusion onto previously solidified extrudate layer during printing was expected to give extrudate-stacking appearance [38]. SEM images of a representative 3D printed dosage form is shown in Figure 3. Figure 3 clearly shows multiple voids on the dosage form surface, moreover, the dosage form obtained shows extrudate-stacking as expected and previously identified with FDM-printed dosage forms [25]. Representative images of printed products are provided in Figure 4.

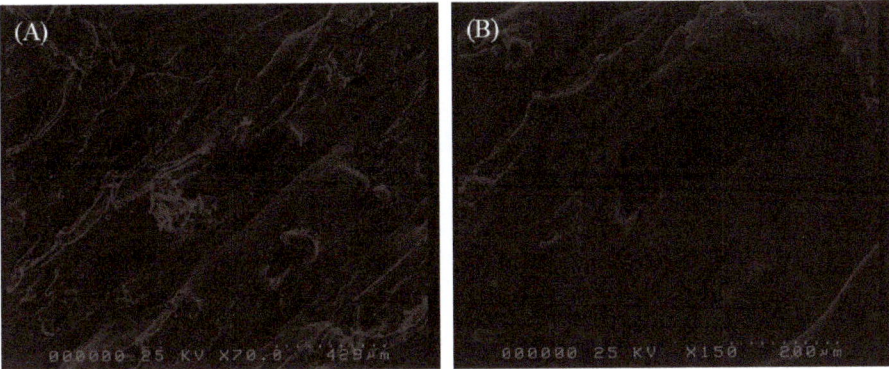

Figure 3. Surface morphology of PVA tablet (top view) at (**A**) ×70 and (**B**) ×150 magnification.

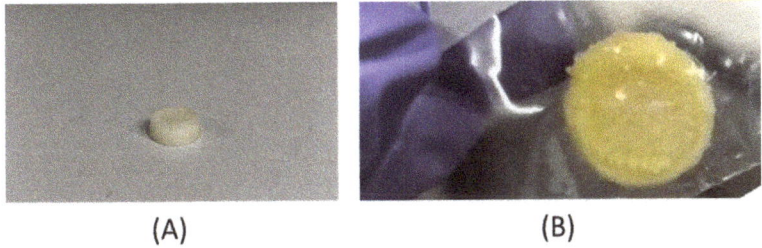

Figure 4. Representative image (**A**) printed PVA product and (**B**) three-dimensional (3D)-printed fixed-dose combination (FDC) drug product with dimensions 10.45 × 10.54 × 3.79 mm.

3.4. In Vitro Dissolution

Saturated solubility of FS and 5-ASA was determined in in vitro dissolution medium at increasing PVA concentration. FS and 5-ASA saturated solubility in pH 6.8 phosphate buffer was 385.82 and 2.98 mg/mL, respectively. In the presence of increased PVA concentration (0.6% *w/v* and 0.4% *w/v*), FS and 5-ASA saturated solubility was 465.75 and 1.60 mg/mL, respectively.

FS and 5-ASA raw materials achieved complete dissolution within 5 min (data not shown); therefore, Figure 5 shows dissolution profiles of the 3D-printed FDC-MeOH product. Amorphous solid dispersion (ASD) formulations are known to experience rapid dissolution before recrystallizing at a rate corresponding to PVA concentration, acting as a crystallization inhibitor [39–41]. The 3D-printed FDC-MeOH product dissolution showed characteristic ASD spring-and-parachute dissolution profile of both FS and 5-ASA. Peak concentration was achieved at $t = 30$ min for 5-ASA (8.36 ± 0.06 µg/mL), corresponding to a dissolution rate of 16.71 µg/mL/h and $t = 45$ min for FS (19.24 ± 0.24 µg/mL).

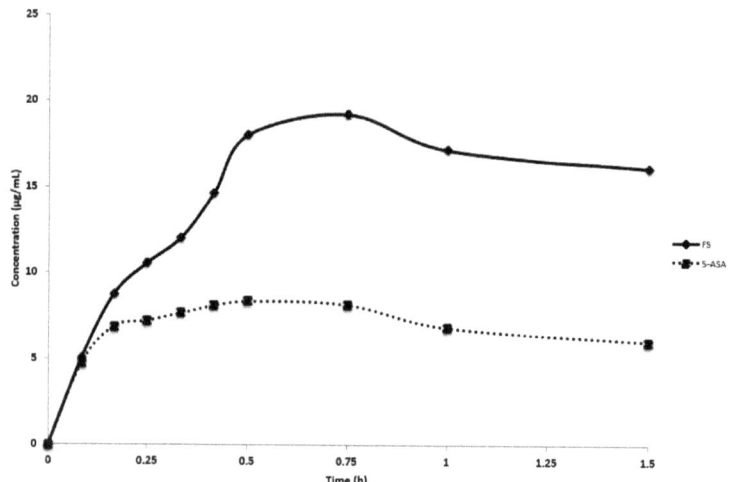

Figure 5. In vitro dissolution profile of 3D-printed FDC-MeOH dosage form in phosphate buffer pH 6.8. Error bars representing standard deviations.

4. Discussion

The main aim of this study was to investigate the effect of different solvent in loading drugs on printable PVA filament. The impregnation method used has already been used in studies by Goyanes et al. where drug contents for 5-ASA- and FS-loaded PVA filaments were 0.063 ± 0.001% *w/w* and 0.29 ± 0.01% *w/w*, respectively [29,30]. In our study, we were able to achieve approximately three-fold and one-fold higher FS and 5-ASA drug-loading, respectively, compared to the studies of Goyanes et al. In particular, it was noted that MeOH-loaded drug filaments had significant improvement in drug-loading of polar FS and 5-ASA compared to EtOH, highlighting the importance of matching solvent drug polarity when using the drug impregnation method. Apart from solvent polarity, drug dielectric constant, solubility, as well as temperature and hygroscopicity can affect drug loading [42]. The presence of FS may have altered MeOH dielectric constant, facilitating H^+ ion dissociation from 5-ASA, and increasing 5-ASA solubility in MeOH; this proposed synergistic effect requires further investigation [43–46].

Our findings on changes in filament hardness before and after drug impregnation showed that drug and solvent molecules can interpose between polymer chains, weakening polymer–polymer interaction and increasing chains movements, resulting in reducing PVA filament hardness by more than 50% after drug-loading and solvent-soaking [47–49]. Because plasticizing effect has previously been found to increase with plasticizer concentration, FDC-MeOH filament, having significantly higher drug loading compared to single-drug filaments, resulted in lower hardness compared to other MeOH-loaded filaments.

The drug dissolution profile of the FDM-printed monolithic FDC tablet (FS and 5-ASA) was evaluated. The advantage of this drug product as a solid dispersion is based on the water-soluble matrix that provides activation energy to drive crystallization [28,50–53]. As drug release from PVA is also regulated by polymer dissolution, all printed tablets in the current study also exhibited spring-and-parachute profile with crystallization inhibited depending on PVA concentration.

The reason for rapid supersaturation resulting in higher maximum concentration could be that the system had insufficient time to induce crystallization when transformation from stable to metastable supersaturation state was quick [54,55]. In the current study, 5-ASA released from the the 3D-printed drug product had initial rapid de-supersaturation; however, the rate declined alongside with the reduction of 5-ASA in the system. This could be because polymer has a greater precipitation inhibitory effect at lower supersaturation [56–58].

5. Conclusions

The use of FDM 3DP technology in the pharmaceutical industry is hindered by several formulation challenges, which the current study aimed to address. This study investigated the solvent influence on optimal drug filament impregnation with an identification that MeOH possessed superior properties compared to EtOH for FS and 5-ASA. Using this method and solvent choice, reasonable drug loading of both FS and 5-ASA onto a single PVA filament was achieved. A 3D-printed solid dispersion FDC drug product was successfully designed and characterized with favourable release profiles and behaviours. Further studies using clinically relevant drugs would be advantageous for the advancement of the work in this area.

Author Contributions: Conceptualization, L.M.d.M. and B.T.R.-A.; Methodology, S.L.C., L.M.d.M. and B.T.R.-A.; Software, S.L.C., L.M.d.M. and B.T.R.-A.; Validation, B.T.R.-A.; Formal analysis, S.L.C.; Investigation, S.L.C.; Resources, B.T.R.-A.; Data curation, S.L.C.; Writing—original draft preparation, S.L.C.; Writing—review and editing, L.M.d.M. and B.T.R.-A.; Supervision, L.M.d.M. and B.T.R.-A.; Project administration, L.M.d.M. and B.T.R.-A.

Funding: This research received no external funding.

Acknowledgments: The authors would like to thank Alvaro Goyanes and Simon Gaisford of University College London (UCL), School of Pharmacy, for providing raw material 5-aminosalicyclic acid, and Gareth Williams (UCL, School of Pharmacy) for X-ray powder diffraction results.

Conflicts of Interest: The authors declare no conflict of interest.

References

1. Desai, D.; Wang, J.; Wen, H.; Li, X. Timmins P. Formulation design, challenges, and development considerations for fixed dose combination (FDC) of oral solid dosage forms. *Pharm. Dev. Technol.* **2013**, *18*, 1265–1276. [CrossRef] [PubMed]
2. EMA/CHMP/158268/2017, (CHMP) C for HMP. *Guideline on Clinical Development of Fixed Combination Medicinal Products.* 2017. Available online: https://www.ema.europa.eu/en/documents/scientific-guideline/guideline-clinical-development-fixed-combination-medicinal-products-revision-2_en.pdf (accessed on 2 October 2018).
3. Kavanagh, O.N.; Albadarin, A.B.; Croker, D.M.; Healy, A.M.; Walker, G.M. Maximising success in multidrug formulation development: A review. *J. Control. Release* **2018**, *283*, 1–19. [CrossRef] [PubMed]
4. Sawicki-Wrzask, D.; Thomsen, M.; Bjerrum, O.J. An Analysis of the Fixed-Dose Combinations Authorized by the European Union, 2009–2014. *Ther. Innov. Regul. Sci.* **2015**, *49*, 553–559. [CrossRef] [PubMed]
5. Bangalore, S.; Kamalakkannan, G.; Parkar, S.; Messerli, F.H. Fixed-Dose Combinations Improve Medication Compliance: A Meta-Analysis. *Am. J. Med.* **2007**, *120*, 713–719. [CrossRef] [PubMed]
6. FDA. *Fixed Dose Combinations, Co-Packaged Drug Products, and Single-Entity Versions of Previously Approved Antiretrovirals for the Treatment of HIV*; Center for Drug Evaluation and Research (CDER): Rockville, MD, USA, 2006.
7. TheKing'sFund. Polypharmacy and Medicines Optimisation: Making it Safe and Sound. Published 2013. Available online: https://www.kingsfund.org.uk/publications/polypharmacy-and-medicines-optimisation (accessed on 6 December 2018).
8. Rea, F.; Corrao, G.; Merlino, L.; Mancia, G. Early cardiovascular protection by initial two-drug fixed-dose combination treatment vs. monotherapy in hypertension. *Eur. Heart J.* **2018**, *39*, 3654–3661. [CrossRef] [PubMed]
9. Pourkavoos, N. Unique Risks, Benefits, and Challenges of Developing Drug-Drug Combination Products in a Pharmaceutical Industrial Setting. *Comb. Prod. Ther.* **2012**, *2*, 2. [CrossRef]
10. Jamróz, W.; Szafraniec, J.; Kurek, M.; Jachowicz, R. 3D Printing in Pharmaceutical and Medical Applications—Recent Achievements and Challenges. *Pharm. Res.* **2018**, *35*, 176. [CrossRef]

11. Richey, R.H.; Hughes, C.; Craig, J.V.; Shah, U.U.; Ford, J.L.; Barker, C.E.; Peak, M.; Nunn, A.J.; Turner, M.A. A systematic review of the use of dosage form manipulation to obtain required doses to inform use of manipulation in paediatric practice. *Int. J. Pharm.* **2017**, *518*, 155–166. [CrossRef]
12. Shastry, B.S. Pharmacogenetics and the concept of individualized medicine. *Pharmacogenom. J.* **2006**, *6*, 16–21. [CrossRef]
13. Acosta-Vélez, G.F. 3D Pharming: Direct Printing of Personalized Pharmaceutical Tablets. *Polym. Sci.* **2016**, *2*. [CrossRef]
14. Konta, A.; García-Piña, M.; Serrano, D. Personalised 3D Printed Medicines: Which Techniques and Polymers Are More Successful? *Bioengineering* **2017**, *4*, 79. [CrossRef] [PubMed]
15. Norman, J.; Madurawe, R.D.; Moore, C.M.V.; Khan, M.A.; Khairuzzaman, A. A new chapter in pharmaceutical manufacturing: 3D-printed drug products. *Adv. Drug Deliv. Rev.* **2017**, *108*, 39–50. [CrossRef] [PubMed]
16. Khaled, S.A.; Burley, J.C.; Alexander, M.R.; Yang, J.; Roberts, C.J. 3D printing of five-in-one dose combination polypill with defined immediate and sustained release profiles. *J. Control. Release* **2015**, *217*, 308–314. [CrossRef] [PubMed]
17. Goyanes, A.; Robles Martinez, P.; Buanz, A.; Basit, A.W.; Gaisford, S. Effect of geometry on drug release from 3D printed tablets. *Int. J. Pharm.* **2015**, *494*, 657–663. [CrossRef] [PubMed]
18. Kadry, H.; Al-Hilal, T.A.; Keshavarz, A.; Alam, F.; Xu, C.; Joy, A.; Ahsan, F. Multi-purposable filaments of HPMC for 3D printing of medications with tailored drug release and timed-absorption. *Int. J. Pharm.* **2018**, *544*, 285–296. [CrossRef] [PubMed]
19. Sadia, M.; Isreb, A.; Abbadi, I.; Isreb, M.; Aziz, D.; Selo, A.; Timmins, P.; Alhnan, M.A. From 'fixed dose combinations' to 'a dynamic dose combiner': 3D printed bi-layer antihypertensive tablets. *Eur. J. Pharm. Sci.* **2018**, *123*, 484–494. [CrossRef] [PubMed]
20. Wang, J.; Goyanes, A.; Gaisford, S.; Basit, A.W. Stereolithographic (SLA) 3D printing of oral modified-release dosage forms. *Int. J. Pharm.* **2016**, *503*, 207–212. [CrossRef]
21. Feuerbach, T.; Kock, S.; Thommes, M. Characterisation of fused deposition modeling 3D printers for pharmaceutical and medical applications. *Pharm. Dev. Technol.* **2018**, *23*, 1136–1145. [CrossRef]
22. Tran, T.Q.; Chinnappan, A.; Lee, J.K.Y.; Loc, N.H.; Tran, L.T.; Wang, T.; Vijay Kumar, V.; Jayathilaka, W.A.D.M.; Ji, D.; Doddamani, M.; et al. 3D Printing of Highly Pure Copper. *Metals* **2019**, *9*, 756. [CrossRef]
23. Goyanes, A.; Wang, J.; Buanz, A.; Martínez-Pacheco, R.; Telford, R.; Gaisford, S.; Basit, A.W. 3D Printing of Medicines: Engineering Novel Oral Devices with Unique Design and Drug Release Characteristics. *Mol. Pharm.* **2015**, *12*, 4077–4084. [CrossRef]
24. Skowyra, J.; Pietrzak, K.; Alhnan, M.A. Fabrication of extended-release patient-tailored prednisolone tablets via fused deposition modelling (FDM) 3D printing. *Eur. J. Pharm. Sci.* **2015**, *68*, 11–17. [CrossRef] [PubMed]
25. Rahman, Z.; Barakh Ali, S.F.; Ozkan, T.; Charoo, N.A.; Reddy, I.K.; Khan, M.A. Additive Manufacturing with 3D Printing: Progress from Bench to Bedside. *AAPS J.* **2018**, *20*, 101. [CrossRef] [PubMed]
26. Solanki, N.G.; Tahsin, M.; Shah, A.V.; Serajuddin, A.T.M. Formulation of 3D Printed Tablet for Rapid Drug Release by Fused Deposition Modeling: Screening Polymers for Drug Release, Drug-Polymer Miscibility and Printability. *J. Pharm. Sci.* **2018**, *107*, 390–401. [CrossRef] [PubMed]
27. Alhnan, M.A.; Okwuosa, T.C.; Sadia, M.; Wan, K.-W.; Ahmed, W.; Arafat, B. Emergence of 3D Printed Dosage Forms: Opportunities and Challenges. *Pharm. Res.* **2016**, *33*, 1817–1832. [CrossRef] [PubMed]
28. Modica de Mohac, L.; Keating, A.; de Fátima Pina, M.; Raimi-Abraham, B. Engineering of Nanofibrous Amorphous and Crystalline Solid Dispersions for Oral Drug Delivery. *Pharmaceutics* **2018**, *11*, 7. [CrossRef] [PubMed]
29. Goyanes, A.; Buanz, A.B.M.; Hatton, G.B.; Gaisford, S.; Basit, A.W. 3D printing of modified-release aminosalicylate (4-ASA and 5-ASA) tablets. *Eur. J. Pharm. Biopharm.* **2015**, *89*, 157–162. [CrossRef]
30. Goyanes, A.; Buanz, A.B.M.; Basit, A.W.; Gaisford, S. Fused-filament 3D printing (3DP) for fabrication of tablets. *Int. J. Pharm.* **2014**, *476*, 88–92. [CrossRef]
31. Tagami, T.; Fukushige, K.; Ogawa, E.; Hayashi, N.; Ozeki, T. 3D Printing Factors Important for the Fabrication of Polyvinylalcohol Filament-Based Tablets. *Biol. Pharm. Bull.* **2017**, *40*, 357–364. [CrossRef]
32. Hayes, A.W.; Kruger, C.L. *Hayes' Principles and Methods of Toxicology*; CRC Press: Boca Raton, FL, USA, 2014.
33. Hassan, S.; Adam, F.; Abu Bakar, M.R.; Abdul Mudalip, S.K. Evaluation of solvents' effect on solubility, intermolecular interaction energies and habit of ascorbic acid crystals. *J. Saudi Chem. Soc.* **2019**, *23*, 239–248. [CrossRef]

34. Babagowda Kadadevara Math, R.S.; Goutham, R.; Srinivas Prasad, K. Study of Effects on Mechanical Properties of PLA Filament which is blended with Recycled PLA Materials. *IOP Conf. Ser. Mater. Sci. Eng.* **2018**, *310*, 012103. [CrossRef]
35. Fell, J.T.; Newton, J.M. Determination of Tablet Strength by the Diametral-Compression Test. *J. Pharm. Sci.* **1970**, *59*, 688–691. [CrossRef] [PubMed]
36. Banić-Tomišić, Z.; Kojić-Prodić, B.; Širola, I. Hydrogen bonds in the crystal packings of mesalazine and mesalazine hydrochloride. *J. Mol. Struct.* **1997**, *416*, 209–220. [CrossRef]
37. Groom, C.R.; Bruno, I.J.; Lightfoot, M.P.; Ward, S.C. The Cambridge Structural Database. *Acta Crystallogr. Sect. B Struct. Sci. Cryst. Eng. Mater.* **2016**, *72*, 171–179. [CrossRef] [PubMed]
38. Michael ARepka Nigel Langley, J.D. *Melt Extrusion: Materials, Technology and Drug Product Design (AAPS Advances in the Pharmaceutical Sciences Series Book*; Springer Science & Business Media: Berlin, Germany, 2013. [CrossRef]
39. Wlodarski, K.; Zhang, F.; Liu, T.; Sawicki, W.; Kipping, T. Synergistic Effect of Polyvinyl Alcohol and Copovidone in Itraconazole Amorphous Solid Dispersions. *Pharm. Res.* **2018**, *35*, 16. [CrossRef]
40. Konno, H.; Handa, T.; Alonzo, D.E.; Taylor, L.S. Effect of polymer type on the dissolution profile of amorphous solid dispersions containing felodipine. *Eur. J. Pharm. Biopharm.* **2008**, *70*, 493–499. [CrossRef]
41. Konno, H.; Taylor, L.S. Influence of Different Polymers on the Crystallization Tendency of Molecularly Dispersed Amorphous Felodipine. *J. Pharm. Sci.* **2006**, *95*, 2692–2705. [CrossRef]
42. Gupta, D.; Jassal, M.; Agrawal, A.K. The electrospinning behavior of poly(vinyl alcohol) in DMSO–water binary solvent mixtures. *RSC Adv.* **2016**, *6*, 102947–102955. [CrossRef]
43. Paruta, A.N.; Sciarrone, B.J.; Lordi, N.G. Correlation between solubility parameters and dielectric constants. *J. Pharm. Sci.* **1962**, *51*, 704–705. [CrossRef]
44. ThermoFisher. *Kaolin Asp® 400p Safety Data Sheet*; Emirates U.A.: Fair Lawn, NJ, USA, 2012; pp. 8–10.
45. Åkerlöf, G. Dielectric constants of some organic solvent-water mixtures at various temperatures. *J. Am. Chem. Soc.* **1932**, *54*, 4125–4139. [CrossRef]
46. Chernyak, Y. Dielectric constant, dipole moment, and solubility parameters of some cyclic acid esters. *J. Chem. Eng. Data* **2006**, *51*, 416–418. [CrossRef]
47. Mohsin, M.; Hossin, A.; Haik, Y. Thermomechanical properties of poly(vinyl alcohol) plasticized with varying ratios of sorbitol. *Mater. Sci. Eng. A* **2011**, *528*, 925–930. [CrossRef]
48. Goyanes, A.; Chang, H.; Sedough, D.; Hatton, G.B.; Wang, J.; Buanz, A.; Gaisford, S.; Basit, A.W. Fabrication of controlled-release budesonide tablets via desktop (FDM) 3D printing. *Int. J. Pharm.* **2015**, *496*, 414–420. [CrossRef] [PubMed]
49. Choi, J.; Jang, B.N.; Park, B.J.; Joung, Y.K.; Han, D.K. Effect of Solvent on Drug Release and a Spray-Coated Matrix of a Sirolimus-Eluting Stent Coated with Poly(lactic-co-glycolic acid). *Langmuir* **2014**, *30*, 10098–10106. [CrossRef] [PubMed]
50. Raimi-Abraham, B.T.; Mahalingam, S.; Edirisinghe, M.; Craig, D.Q.M. Generation of poly(N-vinylpyrrolidone) nanofibres using pressurised gyration. *Mater. Sci. Eng. C* **2014**, *39*, 168–176. [CrossRef] [PubMed]
51. Modica de Mohac, L.; de Fátima Pina, M.; Raimi-Abraham, B.T. Solid microcrystalline dispersion films as a new strategy to improve the dissolution rate of poorly water soluble drugs: A case study using olanzapine. *Int. J. Pharm.* **2016**, *508*, 42–50. [CrossRef]
52. Sun, D.D.; Lee, P.I. Probing the mechanisms of drug release from amorphous solid dispersions in medium-soluble and medium-insoluble carriers. *J. Control. Release* **2015**, *211*, 85–93. [CrossRef]
53. Baghel, S.; Cathcart, H.; O'Reilly, N.J. Polymeric Amorphous Solid Dispersions: A Review of Amorphization, Crystallization, Stabilization, Solid-State Characterization, and Aqueous Solubilization of Biopharmaceutical Classification System Class II Drugs. *J. Pharm. Sci.* **2016**, *105*, 2527–2544. [CrossRef]
54. Sun, D.D.; Lee, P.I. Evolution of Supersaturation of Amorphous Pharmaceuticals: The Effect of Rate of Supersaturation Generation. *Mol. Pharm.* **2013**, *10*, 4330–4346. [CrossRef]
55. Craig, D.Q.M. The mechanisms of drug release from solid dispersions in water-soluble polymers. *Int. J. Pharm.* **2002**, *231*, 131–144. [CrossRef]
56. Ilevbare, G.A.; Liu, H.; Edgar, K.J.; Taylor, L.S. Inhibition of solution crystal growth of ritonavir by cellulose polymers—Factors influencing polymer effectiveness. *CrystEngComm* **2012**, *14*, 6503. [CrossRef]

57. Megrab, N.A.; Williams, A.C.; Barry, B.W. Oestradiol permeation through human skin and silastic membrane: Effects of propylene glycol and supersaturation. *J. Control. Release* **1995**, *36*, 277–294. [CrossRef]
58. Curatolo, W.; Nightingale, J.A.; Herbig, S.M. Utility of Hydroxypropylmethylcellulose Acetate Succinate (HPMCAS) for Initiation and Maintenance of Drug Supersaturation in the GI Milieu. *Pharm. Res.* **2009**, *26*, 1419–1431. [CrossRef] [PubMed]

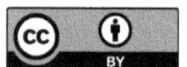

© 2019 by the authors. Licensee MDPI, Basel, Switzerland. This article is an open access article distributed under the terms and conditions of the Creative Commons Attribution (CC BY) license (http://creativecommons.org/licenses/by/4.0/).

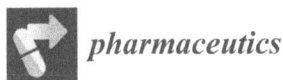

Article

Fused Deposition Modeling 3D Printing: Test Platforms for Evaluating Post-Fabrication Chemical Modifications and In-Vitro Biological Properties

Petra Arany [1], Eszter Róka [1,2], Laurent Mollet [3], Anthony W. Coleman [3], Florent Perret [2], Beomjoon Kim [4], Renátó Kovács [5], Adrienn Kazsoki [6], Romána Zelkó [6], Rudolf Gesztelyi [7], Zoltán Ujhelyi [1], Pálma Fehér [1], Judit Váradi [1], Ferenc Fenyvesi [1], Miklós Vecsernyés [1] and Ildikó Bácskay [1,*]

[1] Department of Pharmaceutical Technology, Faculty of Pharmacy, University of Debrecen, Nagyerdei körút 98, H-4032 Debrecen, Hungary; arany.petra@pharm.unideb.hu (P.A.); eszter.roka@gmail.com (E.R.); ujhelyi.zoltan@pharm.unideb.hu (Z.U.); feher.palma@pharm.unideb.hu (P.F.); varadi.judit@pharm.unideb.hu (J.V.); fenyvesi.ferenc@pharm.unideb.hu (F.F.); vecsernyes.miklos@pharm.unideb.hu (M.V.)

[2] ICBMS, UMR 5246, Université Lyon 1, F69622 Villeurbanne, France; florent.perret@univ-lyon1.fr

[3] LMI CNRS UMR 5615, Université Lyon 1, 69622 Villeurbanne, France; laurent.mollet@univ-lyon1.fr (L.M.); anthony.coleman@univ-lyon1.fr (A.W.C.)

[4] LIMMS/CNRS-IIS UMI 2820, Institute of Industrial Science, The University of Tokyo, Tokyo 153-8505, Japan; bjoonkim@iis.u-tokyo.ac.jp

[5] Department of Medical Microbiology, Faculty of Medicine and Faculty of Pharmacy, University of Debrecen, Nagyerdei körút 98, H-4032 Debrecen, Hungary; kovacs.renato@med.unideb.hu

[6] University Pharmacy Department of Pharmacy Administration, Faculty of Pharmacy, University of Semmelweis, Hőgyes Endre utca 7-9, H-1092 Budapest, Hungary; kazsoki.adrienn@pharma.semmelweis-univ.hu (A.K.); zelko.romana@pharma.semmelweis-univ.hu (R.Z.)

[7] Department of Pharmacology and Pharmacotherapy, University of Debrecen, Nagyerdei körút 98, H-4032 Debrecen, Hungary; gesztelyi.rudolf@pharm.unideb.hu

* Correspondence: bacskay.ildiko@pharm.unideb.hu; Tel.: +36-5241-1717 (ext. 54034)

Received: 6 May 2019; Accepted: 10 June 2019; Published: 13 June 2019

Abstract: 3D printing is attracting considerable interest for its capacity to produce prototypes and small production runs rapidly. Fused deposit modeling (FDM) was used to produce polyvalent test plates for investigation of the physical, chemical, and in-vitro biological properties of printed materials. The polyvalent test plates (PVTPs) are poly-lactic acid cylinders, 14 mm in diameter and 3 mm in height. The polymer ester backbone was surface modified by a series of ramified and linear oligoamines to increase its hydrophilicity and introduce a positive charge. The chemical modification was verified by FT-IR spectroscopy, showing the introduction of amide and amine functions, and contact angle measurements confirmed increased hydrophilicity. Morphology studies (SEM, optical microscopy) indicated that the modification of PVTP possessed a planar morphology with small pits. Positron annihilation lifetime spectroscopy demonstrated that the polymeric free volume decreased on modification. An MTT-based prolonged cytotoxicity test using Caco-2 cells showed that the PVTPs are non-toxic at the cellular level. The presence of surface oligoamines on the PVTPs reduced biofilm formation by *Candida albicans* SC5314 significantly. The results demonstrate that 3D printed objects may be modified at their surface by a simple amidation reaction, resulting in a reduced propensity for biofilm colonization and cellular toxicity.

Keywords: fused deposition modeling; polylactic acid; chemical modification; MTT assay; biofilm formation

1. Introduction

Three-dimensional (3D) printing has become one of the major innovative technologies of recent years, and has led to a revolution in personalized medication using medical devices [1] and modified-release products [2]. The first solid dosage form (Spritam) of a medication printed by 3D technology was approved by the FDA in 2015. Nowadays, 3D printing methods may support the development of personalized medicine and therapy, for example in cardiac and orthopedic surgeries [3]. This innovative technique has also attracted significant attention in dental and plastic surgeries [4]. There are other technologies that are also being used for biomedical applications; for instance, fused deposition modeling (FDM) or stereolithography (SLA) [5]. Obviously, the first is used to prepare medical devices for surgical implantation, but is still onerous and highly expensive, whilst the second is cheap and suitable for prototyping devices both for biomedical analytical usage and clinical prototyping, such as drug patches [6]. For both FDM and SLA, commercial polymers or pre-polymers are now widely available, but little or nothing is known about their behavior in terms of bacterial colonization or biofilm formation, and indeed whether the printing process itself has an effect on the bio-properties of the post-printed structures remains to be clarified.

The concept of 3D printing in the medical field is aimed at designing anatomically correct prototypes using different imaging techniques, such as MRI, CT, and so forth, in which these pictures are transformed into file formats for 3D printers [7]. The possibility of producing individualized implants and oral drug formulations holds potential for a variety of different medical purposes. The use of 3D printing in the chemical sciences has expanded rapidly because different synthesis processes can be automatically controlled by, for instance, robot technics [8]. Glatzel et al. reported that a robotic setup may produce 3D printed antibacterial assays, which may promote new opportunities in the development of laboratory practice [9]. PLA-based implants are widely used due to their advantageous biodegradability and favorable cytocompatibility properties [10]. They also have good thermal plasticity and suitable mechanical properties [11]. Scaffold modifications/functionalizations have a great impact on the morphology and cytocompatibility of medical devices or 3D printed medicines. Side chain modifications may result in different surface properties [12]. Similarly, the use of surface absorption of polymers may allow modulation of the chemical and biological properties of 3D printed scaffolds, as in the very recent paper of Thire et al. on the use of polydopamine absorption onto 3D printed PLA scaffolds [13].

In a slightly earlier article, surface modification and the anti-microbial properties of the obtained systems were demonstrated. The previously utilized methods provided access to coated surfaces, however such systems can be expected to wear over time, which may limit their utility. Direct chemical modification of the polymers forming 3D printed objects would seem to be of interest, as the actual surface of the object is changed and not coated [14].

Of the available methods to characterize printed and modified PLA objects, FT-IR will definitively show the presence of new chemical functions, but intensities of the IR bands may be weak in the case of surface changes. Contact angle measurements will provide information on the hydrophilicity and hydrophobicity of the surface, and when correlated with FT-IR allow rapid characterization of surface chemical modifications. Scanning electron microscopy is an appropriate method for characterization of porosity and pore size of the surface of implants. Values of positron lifetimes and the corresponding intensities measured by positron annihilation lifetime spectroscopy may be connected with the size and the structural defects of implants [15].

To reach the general market with 3D printed implants, these devices must meet all standards and regulations defined by different authorities [16]. Biocompatibility investigation is a compulsory test of implantable devices. The ISO 10993-5 standard determines the parameters of the required cytotoxicity test. The main requirement is the time of contact duration: In the case of limited exposure the duration time is less than 24 h, and for prolonged exposure 1–30 days of investigation is required. Contact periods of longer than 30 days is regulated as requiring long-term studies [17]. Caco-2 cells are mainly used as a monolayer, rather than individual cells, however several assays are performed prior to reaching complete integrity, such as the end point or noninvasive cell viability assays (MTT assay, LDH test, real-time cell electronic sensing assay (RT-CES), etc.) [18]. MTT assay is a broadly used, rapid colorimetric method to measure the in-vitro cytotoxicity of certain compounds on cell lines or primary cells. It is usually performed in 96-well plates, thus is a high throughput method, which excludes cell counting. For decades it was considered as evident that MTT is transformed in the mitochondria, however in the last few years, doubts have arisen regarding the mitochondrial localization of the formazan formation [19].

Microbial biofilm formation could be a risk factor of implanted devices, potentially resulting in unpredictable complications [20]. These microbial biofilm formations may contribute to causing an inflammatory response and result in subsequent operations, such as dental operations. The ability of *Candida albicans* to form biofilms on medical devices could be a key property that enhances its ability to cause disease in humans [21]. Here, the use of chemical modification may allow inhibition of microbial biofilm formation, or may enhance such surface colonization. Interestingly, both growth inhibition and enhancement can be of considerable use to the researcher. A key point in such a modification is the presence of reactive ester groups in many of the polymers used in 3D printing, thus polylactic acid (PLA) and polyethylene terephthalate (PET) are based on polymers with ester backbones, whereas poly(methyl methacrylate) (PMMA) has ester side chain functions.

Many studies have been published on 3D printed implants and dosage forms, however, the connections between the chemical structures, structural parameters, and cytocompatibility results have not been well characterized yet. The objectives of our study were to find connections between the abovementioned parameters in case of chemically modified PLA based 3D printed polyvalent test plates platforms, or PVTPs. Various amines were used for the post fabrication chemistry to form active amide functionalities along the surface of 3D printed PVTP structures.

The structural parameters of the samples were evaluated using Fourier transform infrared (FTIR) spectroscopy, contact angle measurements, scanning electron microscopy (SEM), surface roughness measurement, and positron annihilation lifetime spectrometry (PALS). A cytotoxicity test based on an MTT assay on Caco-2 cells and investigation of biofilm formation with *Candida albicans* were performed to certify the cytocompatibility of the PVTPs. The work is a first step towards chemical functionalization of FDM and SLA 3D printed objects and also the study of the cytocompatibility of generic structures, and shows that simple structures can be produced rapidly and cheaply by 3D printing for use in biological experiments.

2. Materials and Methods

General: All chemicals were purchased from Sigma-Aldrich, Saint Quentin Fallavier, France and used without further purification. Deionized water was obtained using a Millipore (Merck Millipore Direct-Q 5 UV, Millipore SAS, Molsheim, France. 3D printer filaments were purchased from MakerShop Le Mans, France and stored under dry, dark conditions at room temperature.

2.1. Implant Manufacturing and Side Chain Modification

2.1.1. 3D Printing Technique

The PVTPs were obtained using ColorFabb PLA Naturel filament of 2.85 mm [22]. PLA-PVTPs were printed using either a Lulzbot Taz 5 or a Lulzbot Mini 3D printer (Aleph Objects Inc., London UK). The print conditions are summarized in Table 1, below.

Table 1. Printing characteristics for the plates and plate arrays used in the current work.

Printer	Lulzbot Mini	Lulzbot Taz 5
Filament Type	PLA	PLA
Source	Maker Shop France	Maker Shop France
Filament Diameter; mm	2.85	2.85
Extruder Nozzle Diameter; µm	350	350
Infill Percentage	100	100
Extrusion Temperature (°C)	215	215
Bed Temperature (°C)	60	60
Layer Thickness µm	50	75
Print Speed mm/s	50	50

The PVTPs were designed using the Inventor program. The PVTP size was 14 mm diameter and 3 mm thickness. Batches of 25 were printed on the Lulzbot Mini and 50 on the Lulzbot Taz 3D printer. As with all FDM printing, initially adhesion happens to the print bed surface then to the previously printed layers, hence the importance of using the correct bed temperature for each source of filament [23].

2.1.2. PLA PVTP Modification

The amidation reagents used were ethylene diamine (ED), triethylenetetramine (TET), N-methyl-1,3-propanediamine (NMePrN bis(aminopropyl)amine (BAPA), 2,2′ (ethylenedioxy)diethylamine (NPEGN), and tris(2-aminoethyl) amine (Tris). A total of 1000 mL 1 M solution of each amidation reagent was prepared in deionized water. No coupling reagents were added, as prior work using adenosine monophosphate had shown clean functionalization under the above conditions [24].

The PVTPs were placed in an in-house reactor, in this case a glass beaker, and 100 mL of the reactant solution was added. The use of beakers allows objects of dimensions up to 70 mm diameter and 50 mm height to be modified using low volatility reagents in closed aqueous conditions. The tops were closed and the system agitated on a rocking incubator for 24 h at 20 °C. The PVTPs were then isolated in a glass funnel and washed five times with 500 mL of deionized water. Finally, the implants were dried in air, under dust free conditions. The PVTPs were kept in air-tight containers prior to use [25].

2.2. Material Structure Characterisation

2.2.1. FT Infra-Red Spectroscopy

Fourier transform infrared (FTIR) spectra of the PLA derivatives were recorded at room temperature by using an IRAffinity-1S FTIR spectrometer (SHIMADZU, Noisiel, France in the wave number range of 600–4000 cm^{-1}. For these measurements, the samples were directly put on the attenuated total reflectance (ATR)-FTIR module (Miracle 10) and spectra recorder in the transmittance (%) mode [26].

2.2.2. Contact Angle Measurement

Contact angle measurements were performed on a Kruss goniometer using DSA3 software (Lyon; France). A total of 10 µL of deionized water was deposited on the surface of the PVTP, and the droplet shape was imaged. The contact angle was determined using the internal Kruss software. Measurements were carried out a minimum of ten times for each PVTP, and the results were the average of the measurements [27].

2.2.3. Scanning Electron Microscopy

SEM images were taken with a field emission-scanning electron microscope FE-SEM S-5000 (Hitachi Ltd., Tokio, Japan. Before SEM observation, 4 nm of palladium was deposited by atomic layer deposition on the treated surfaces, and they were put under vacuum overnight [28].

2.2.4. Surface Roughness Measurement

The PVTPs were imaged using a VHX 6000 optical microscope (Keyence, Jonage, France, and the images were treated with the internal software to generate line profiles [29].

2.2.5. Positron Annihilation Lifetime Spectrometry

For positron lifetime measurements, a positron source made of carrier-free ^{22}NaCl was used, for which the activity was around 106 Bq. The active material was sealed between two very thin Kapton® foils. The source was put between two pieces of implant. Lifetime spectra were measured with a fast–fast coincidence system based on BaF2/XP2020Q detectors and Ortec® electronics. Three parallel spectra were measured from each sample. The spectra were evaluated by the RESOLUTION computer code. Three lifetime components were found in all samples, and the longest component was identified as positronium triplet state (o-Ps) lifetime [30].

2.3. Cytotoxicity Experiments

2.3.1. Cytotoxicity PLA-Based PVTPs Sterilization

PLA-based PVTPs were immersed in 70% (v/v) ethanol in a laminar air flow (LAF) cabinet for 12 h, and were taken into sterile mull paper individually for drying [31].

2.3.2. Cell Culture

The colon adenocarcinoma (Caco-2) cell line was received from the European Collection of Cell Cultures (ECACC, Salisbury, United Kingdom, catalogue No.86010202). Caco-2 cell line is a well-established cell culture in our laboratory. As it can be seen in the article of Nemes et al. the cell culture is used in based on the same protocol. We state that the Caco-2 cell line provenance is from ECACC. Cells were seeded in plastic cell culture flasks (Thermo Fisher Scientific Inc., Budapest, Hungary in DMEM medium supplemented with 3.7 g/L NaHCO$_3$, 10% (v/v) heat-inactivated fetal bovine serum (FBS), 1% (v/v) non-essential amino acids solution, 1% (v/v) L-glutamine, 100 IU/mL penicillin, and 100 µg/mL streptomycin at 37 °C in an atmosphere of 5% CO$_2$. For the cytotoxic experiment, cells between 20–40 in passage number were used. The culture media was replaced with fresh media every three or four days [32].

2.3.3. MTT Cell Viability Test

Cells were seeded on flat bottom 96-well tissue culture plates at a density of 10^4 or 3×10^4 cells/well. After sterilization of the test samples separately, they were put in sterile centrifuge tubes and immersed in 2 mL of the DMEM medium. The samples were stored in a cell incubator at 37 °C. The test was performed on the 4th, 8th, and 12th day, while the samples were stored under the same conditions. The first step of the MTT assay was to remove the culture media from the cells, then the cells were treated with 200 µL of the test sample solution and incubated for 30 min. After the incubation time, the samples were removed and the cells were washed with 200 µL PBS solution/well. Then, the cells were incubated with 0.5 mg/mL MTT dye. Finally, the formazan crystals were dissolved in acidic isopropanol (isopropanol: 1.0 N hydrochloric acid = 25:1). The absorbance was measured at 570 nm against a 690 nm reference with a FLUOstar OPTIMA Microplate Reader (BMG LABTECH, Offenburg, Germany). Cell viability was expressed as the percentage of the untreated control [33].

2.3.4. Biofilm Formation

In brief, aliquots of 500 µL of standardized SC5314 cell suspension (1×10^6 cells/mL) in Roswell Park Memorial Institute (RPMI) 1640 medium (Sigma Laboratories Ltd., Budapest, Hungary) were added into flat bottom 12-well tissue culture plates containing implants (diameter of 1.6 cm), and incubated at 37 °C for 24 h [34]. Afterwards, the samples were taken into a new 12-well plate and incubated with 0.1% crystal violet solution for 10 min, and the bounded crystal violet was dissolved with 30% acetic acid. The dissolved solution was taken into a flat bottom 96-well tissue culture plate, and absorbance was measured at 540 nm in an Anthos HTII spectrophotometer (Anthos, Salzburg, Austria) [35].

2.4. Statistical Analysis

Data were analyzed using GraphPad Prism (version 7.0; GraphPad Software Inc., La Jolla, CA, USA) and presented as means ± standard deviations (S.D) of triplicates. Comparison of the groups was performed by a one-way ANOVA in STATISTICA software version 13. 2. (Statsoft, Tulsa, OKUSA) at a confidence level of 95%; results were regarded as significant at $p < 0.05$. All experiments were carried out in triplicate and repeated at least three times.

3. Results

3.1. Implant Manufacturing and Side Chain Modification

In our experiments, PLA filaments were pre-formed with a localized heating cylinder so the filaments were melted. Then, the filament was 3D printed at 215 °C through a 0.4 mm stainless steel nozzle, using a layer height of 50 µm or 75 µm. The infill used was 100%, ensuring that porosity arises from the small spaces between the extruded filaments and any cavities between individual polymer molecules in the extruded filament. An infill of 100% also ensures high mechanical strength and that the reactant solution does not enter the printed PVTP and break down inter-layer cohesion. These 3D printed PLA polymer PVTPs of 14 mm diameter and 3 mm height provided the base for chemical modification, as shown in Figure 1.

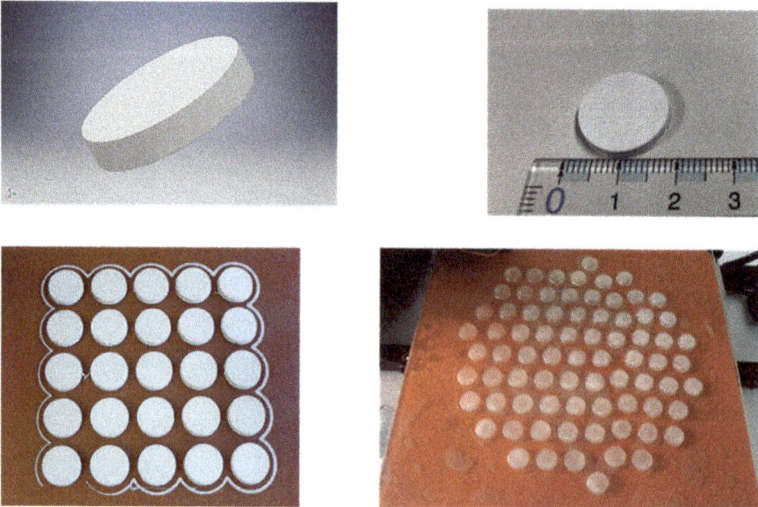

Figure 1. Top left STL (standard tessellation language) file format view of the polyvalent test plate (PVTP), top right printed PVTP showing size, bottom left 25 PVTP print batch on Lulzbot Mini, and bottom right 50 PVTP print batch on Lulzbot Taz 5.

PLA PVTPs were chemically modified using different amines as side chains. This is unique to our study, because these 3D printed PLA PVTPs containing amine side chains have not been previously achieved. The concept of our modifications is based on the work of Haddad et al. [25]. The chemical reaction used in the surface modification is given in Figure 2A, and the structures of the modified PVTPs are presented in Figure 2B. PLA as a base polymer has advantageous mechanical properties and thermoplastic properties [36]. Due to these favorable attributes, it has been widely used in FDM based 3D printing processes.

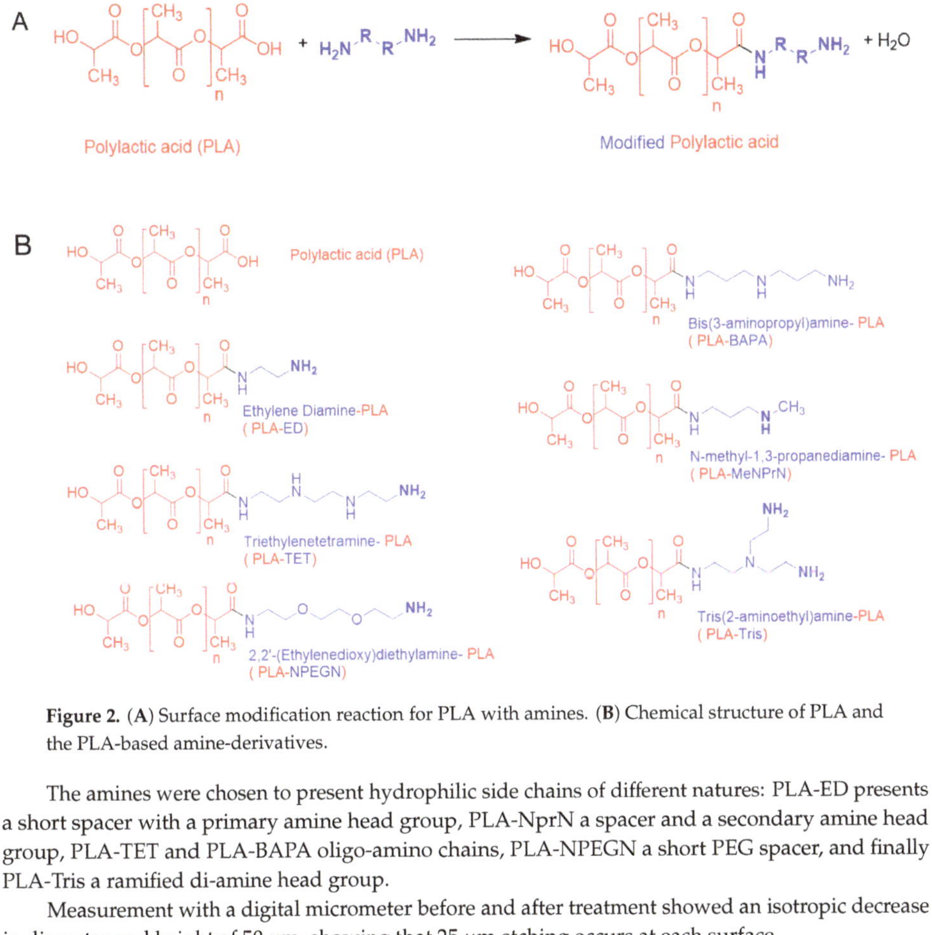

Figure 2. (**A**) Surface modification reaction for PLA with amines. (**B**) Chemical structure of PLA and the PLA-based amine-derivatives.

The amines were chosen to present hydrophilic side chains of different natures: PLA-ED presents a short spacer with a primary amine head group, PLA-NprN a spacer and a secondary amine head group, PLA-TET and PLA-BAPA oligo-amino chains, PLA-NPEGN a short PEG spacer, and finally PLA-Tris a ramified di-amine head group.

Measurement with a digital micrometer before and after treatment showed an isotropic decrease in diameter and height of 50 µm, showing that 25 µm etching occurs at each surface.

3.2. Material Structure Characterization

3.2.1. FT-IR Characterization of Chemical Modifications

The FT-IR spectra of PLA unmodified and PLA-ED are given in Figure 3, and FT-IR spectra for all modified PVTPs are given in Appendix A, Figures A1–A7. As expected, the spectrum of PLA is characterized by a weak C–H stretch band at 3000 cm^{-1} and a very strong C=O ester stretch at 1750 cm^{-1}. For PLA-ED, additional C=O amide bands are observed at 1550 cm^{-1} and 1650 cm^{-1}, and the presence of an amide stretch can only come from the formation of a covalent bond between the PLA polymer and the ethylene diamine. This is further confirmed by the presence of an N–H amide stretch band at 3300 cm^{-1}. As expected from the fact that only surface modification is occurring, the intensities are much lower than that of the ester C=O band.

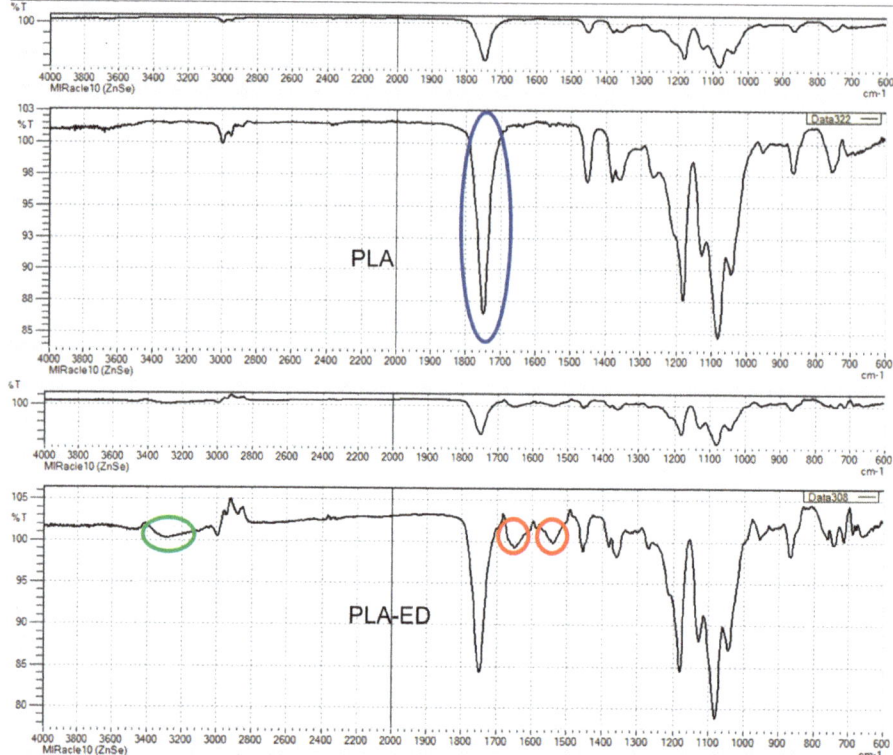

Figure 3. FT-IR spectra of PVTPs of PLA and PLA-ED. The ester C=O band is highlighted by a blue oval, the amide C=O bands by red circles, and the amide NH band by a green oval. From the presence of only the ester C=O stretch in PLA and the presence of both C=O amide and NH amide bands in the PLA-ED spectra, it is clear that the amide functionalization reaction has occurred, as was previously observed by time of flight secondary ion mass spectrometry (TOF-SIMS) for the surface modification of poly-ethylene-terephthalate (PET) by adenosine mono-phosphate (AMP) under the same conditions as in the current study [24].

3.2.2. Contact Angle Measurement

The contact angle values obtained are given in Figure 4. The contact angle measurement results can be sorted based on a decreasing volume: PLA PVTP without water wash = PLA PVTP with water wash > PLA-MeNprN > PLA-ED > PLA-NPEGN > PLA-BAPA > PLA-Tris > PLA-TET. The contact angle values of our PVTPs were between 26.5 ± 3.0° and 69 ± 0.1°, showing that all the PVTPs are hydrophilic and that the chemical modification by introduction of polar oligo-amine functions results in increasing hydrophilicity. As expected, the unmodified PVTPs show the highest contact angles.

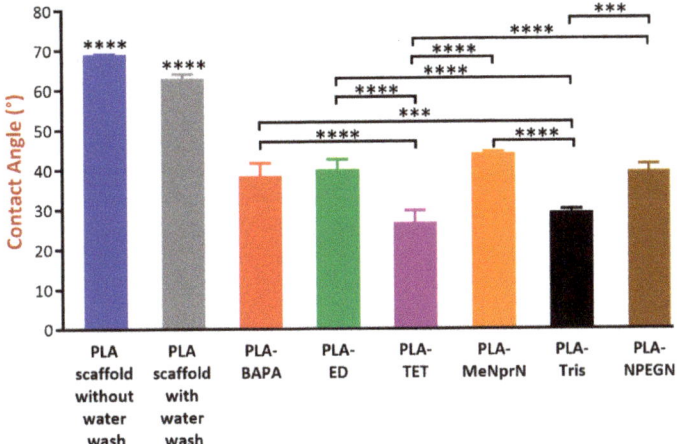

Figure 4. Contact angle values for the various PLA and chemically modified PVTPs. Data are expressed as means ± SD. Experiments were performed in triplicate, $n = 3$. Contact angle (°) values can be sorted in a decreasing order: PLA PVTP without water wash (69 ± 0.1°) = PLA PVTP with water wash (69 ± 0.1°) > PLA-MeNprN (45 ± 1.3°) > PLA-ED (41 ± 0.3°) > PLA-NPEGN (40 ± 1.1°) > PLA-BAPA (39 ± 0.5°) > PLA-Tris (30 ± 1.2°) > PLA-TET (26.5 ± 3.0°). The PLA PVTP with and without water wash have statistically significant differences in the contact angle values in comparison with the modified PLA based samples. PLA-TET and PLA-Tris modifications have statistically significantly lower results in comparison with the other modified PLA based samples. Error bars represent SD; *, **, and *** indicate statistically significant differences at $p < 0.05$, $p < 0.01$, and $p < 0.001$, respectively. In general, surfaces with contact angles of less than 90° are considered hemato-compatible.

3.2.3. Scanning Electron Microscopy

The surface of the PLA PVTP and its modifications were tested using a scanning electron microscope. In our study, both the untreated surface and the deionized water washed surfaces had the general aspect of a stepped surface, with some small deviation from planarity for the untreated surface. After washing the surface appeared smoother, correlating with the change in the contact angle. For the six treated surfaces shown in Figure 5 below (C:PLA-BAPA, D:PLA-ED, G:PLA-Tris, and H:PLA-NPEGN), all appeared flattened with respect to the initial surface, however all showed a large number of indentations. PLA-Tris showed ca 1 μm pore diameters. In the case of the TET modified surface, the overall aspect was close to that of the untreated printed surface, and small indentations were visible with diameters of ca 100–200 nm. Finally, in the case of the MeNprN modified surface, etching appeared to have occurred and the surface was separated into iceberg-like systems overlying a flat surface. This confirms that the surface of the 3D printed PLA PVTPs had been modified, which confirms the formation of separated plates on the printed surface.

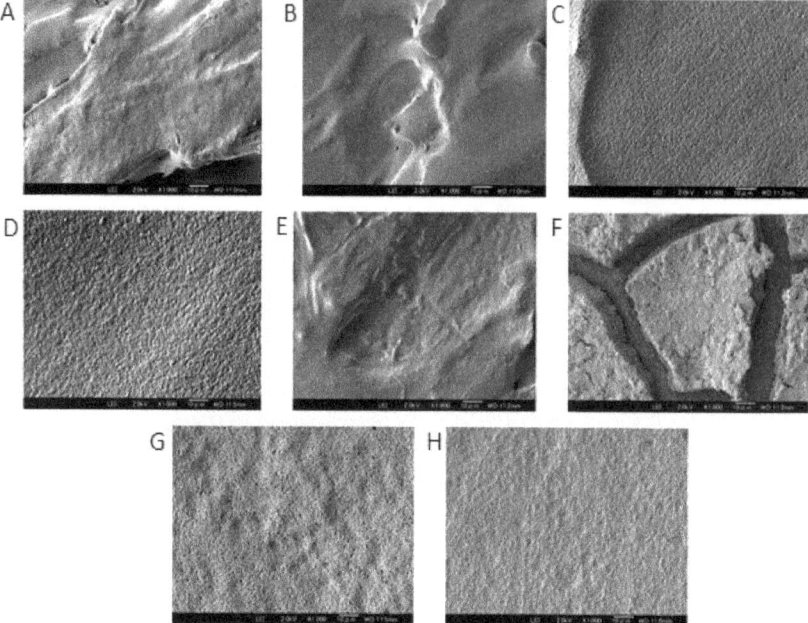

Figure 5. Surface morphology, and pore structure of the 3D printed PLA PVTPs were characterized using scanning electron microscopy (SEM). Magnification is ×1000, scale bar is 90 μm. (**A**) PLA with no treatment, (**B**) PLA with water wash, (**C**) PLA-BAPA, (**D**) PLA-ED, (**E**) PLA-TET, (**F**) PLA-MeNprN, (**G**) PLA-Tris, and (**H**) PLA-NPEGN.

3.2.4. Optical Microscopy Roughness Measurement

In Figure 6, line sections for PVTPs of unmodified PLA, PLA-Ed, and PLA-NPEGN are given, and other modifications of line sections can be seen in Appendix B, Figures A8–A10. These were obtained using a Keyence VHX 6000 optical microscope. Using the internal image processing program, Rz values of 29 μm for PLA, 3 μm for PLA-ED, and 6 μm for PLA-NPEGN were observed. The values of the PLA results from the presence of a void of about 20 μm between two extruded polymer filaments, and small depressions at 400 μm intervals arising from other filaments, were less than 5 μm in depth. The surfaces of modified PVTPs were generally quite flat with small pits and protrusions present in the modified samples, which was in agreement with the morphology observed using SEM. No systematically repeated depressions at 400 μm distances were observed. This was in agreement with the observation that 25 μm was etched from the PVTP during modification.

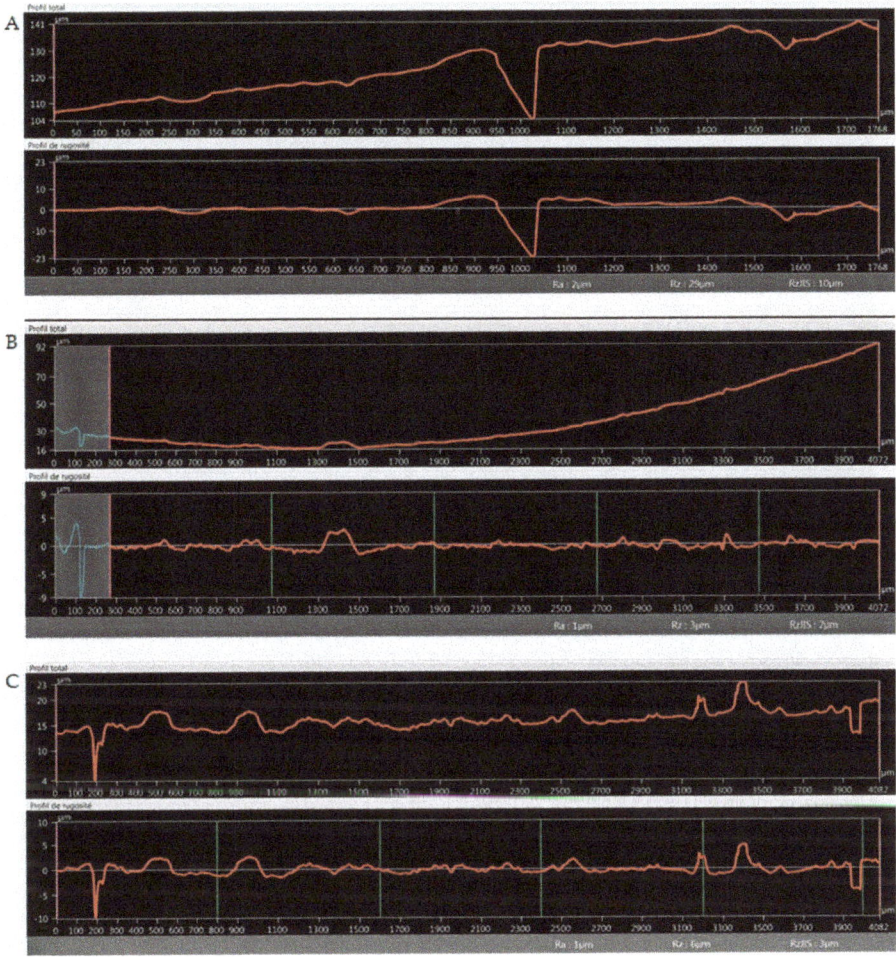

Figure 6. Line sections through printed PVTPs. (**A**) PLA unmodified 1768 μm length, (**B**) PLA-ED 4082 μm length, and (**C**) PLA-NPEGN 4082 μm. Rz values of 29 μm for PLA, 3 μm for PLA-ED, and 6 μm for PLA-NPEGN are observed.

3.2.5. Positron Annihilation Lifetime Spectrometry

Figure 7 illustrates the average discrete o-Ps lifetime values of various samples. The higher lifetime values indicate higher free volume holes between the polymeric chains, and also residual space between filaments. The results showed that the modified polymeric bases (BAPA through NPEGN) were of similar o-Ps lifetimes, thus were free volume holes, while the PLA PVTP represented significantly higher o-Ps lifetimes. Based on our results, after the modification, PLA-ED and PLA-Tris contained the most free volume in their structures. PLA-MeNprN had the least free volume in its structure. The latter could be explained by the fact that through modification, the amines could be built into the polymeric chains, resulting in smaller free volumes between chains and especially between polymer molecules in the filaments.

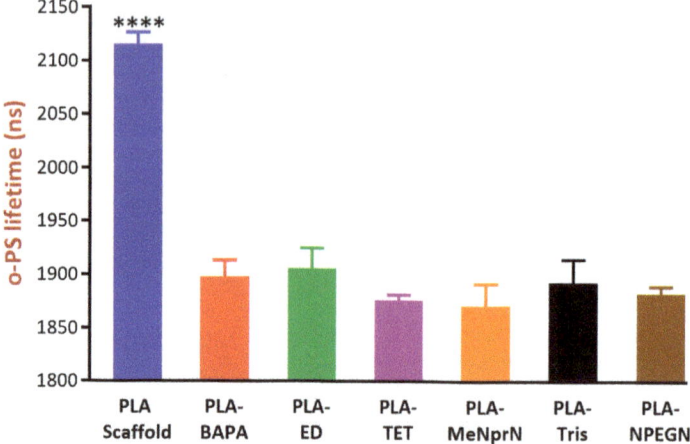

Figure 7. Average discrete positronium triplet state (o-Ps) lifetimes of various samples. A higher o-Ps lifetime represents higher free volume holes in the structure of the PLA based PVTPs. Values are presented as means ± SD. Experiments were performed in triplicate, $n = 3$. PLA PVTP has statistically significantly different o-PS lifetime values compared to the modified PLA based samples. In comparison, there is not a statistically significant different between the modified samples. BAPA = polylactic acid-bis(3-aminopropyl)amine; ED = polylactic acid-ethylenediamine; TET = polylactic acid-triethylenetetramine; MeNprN = polylactic acid-N-methyl-1,3-propanediamine; Tris = polylactic acid-tris(2-aminoethyl) amine; and NPEGN = polylactic acid-2,2'-(Ethylenedioxy)diethylamine. Error bar represents SD; **** indicate statistically significant differences at $p < 0.0001$.

3.3. Cytocompatibility Experiments

3.3.1. MTT Cell Viability Test

A prolonged cell viability test was utilized in our work to gain information about the cytocompatibility of our PLA PVTPs. The samples were incubated in the cell culture medium for four, eight, and 12 days, and the Caco-2 cells were treated by this medium [37,38]. This method differs from the original MTT assay because the inhibitory concentration (IC_{50}) was not measured, but the cell viability was calculated in comparison with a negative (DMME medium). In the works of Kinnari and Chessa et al., Caco-2 cell lines were the gold standard for the cytotoxicity examinations of orthopedic and breast implants [39,40]. Caco-2 cell lines are a model of the intestinal barrier, because numerous attributes are the same as in the mature enterocyte.

The results are expressed as the percentage of negative or untreated control (Co−). As a positive control (Co+) Triton-X 100 (10% w/v) solubilizing agent was used, which resulted in significant differences from the other examined samples. We compared cytotoxic values and found none of the samples decreased significantly in cell viability compared to the untreated control (Figure 8.) Based on our MTT assay, PLA-TET cytotoxicity did not decrease under 100% in comparison with the negative control. PLA-ED, PLA-BAPA, PLA-Tris, and PLA-NPEGN cell viability values were higher than 90% in the case of prolonged exposure. Based on the ISO 10993-5:2009(E) standard, if the relative cell viability is higher than 70% in comparison with the control group (100%), the materials can be considered non-cytotoxic [41]. According to this regulation, all our PLA PVTPs qualified as cytocompatible.

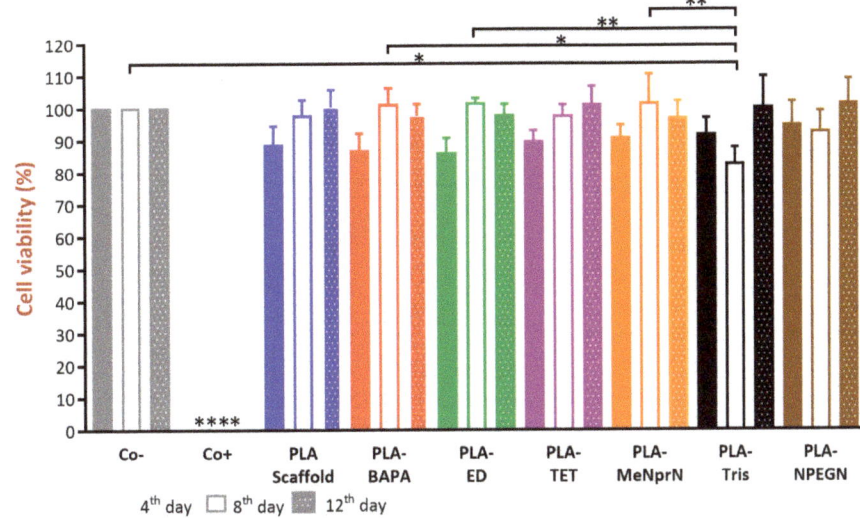

Figure 8. Prolonged cytotoxicity effects of the PLA based chemically modified PVTPs on CaCo-2 cells determined by an MTT cell viability test on the 4th, 8th, and 12th days. Cell viability was expressed as the percentage of untreated control in the case of PLA-based chemically modified PVTPs. The positive control was Triton X 100 (10% w/v), which has significantly different cell viability results compared to the Co− and the examined samples. Data are means of three independent experiments ± S.D. We compared cytotoxic values and found none of the samples decreased significantly in cell viability compared to the untreated control. Error bars represent SD; *, **, and **** indicate statistically significant differences at $p < 0.05$, $p < 0.01$, and $p < 0.001$, respectively.

3.3.2. Biofilm Formation

Our experiments were based on the fact that the formed biofilm can be visualized with a crystal violet (CV) stain, and the absorbance of the dye can be measured. The measured absorbance values were in correlation with the amount of biofilm in the implants [34,42]. All of the results of biofilm formation were under a 0.24 absorbance value. PLA PVTP and BAPA modification result in significantly higher absorbance results than other modifications. MeNprN has higher absorbance results than 0.05, but TET, Tris, NPEGN, and ED have lower absorbance results than 0.05. In comparison with the other PVTPs, ED resulted in the smallest absorbance value. (Figure 9). According to the classification from Marcos-Zambrano et al., low biofilm forming ability occurs with absorbance values under 0.44, moderate biofilm forming ability occurs between absorbance values of 0.44–1.17, and high absorbance forming ability occurs with absorbance values above 1.17. Based on this classification, all of our implants showed low biofilm forming ability [43]. There are some significant differences among the chemically modified PLA PVTPs because PLA-ED resulted in the lowest biofilm formation, however PLA-BAPA and PLA PVTP represented the highest biofilm formation.

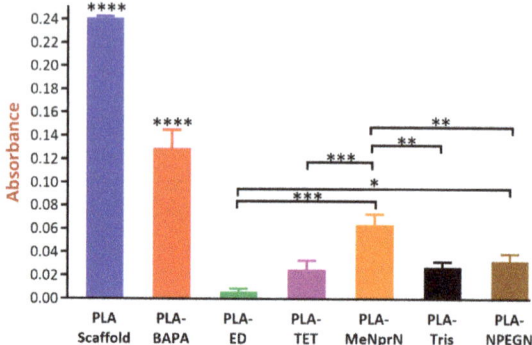

Figure 9. Biofilm formation results are presented as an absorbance value plotted against the examined samples, and all absorbance results were under 0.24. Values are presented as means ± S.D. Experiments were performed in triplicate, $n = 3$. PLA PVTP and BAPA modification have significantly higher absorbance results than other modifications. MeNprN has higher absorbance results than 0.05 but TET, Tris, NPEGN, and ED have lower absorbance results than 0.05. In comparison with the other PVTPs, ED resulted in the smallest absorbance value. Error bars represent SD; *, **, ***, and **** indicate statistically significant differences at $p < 0.05$, $p < 0.01$, $p < 0.001$, and $p < 0.0001$, respectively.

4. Discussion

Nowadays, 3D printing technologies for medical purposes are mainly focusing on bioprinting, dental applications, orthopedic applications, and development of modified release oral drug delivery systems [2]. In our study, morphological characterization and in-vitro anti-fungal and cytocompatibility tests of chemically modified PLA-based 3D printed PVTPs are presented. In our research, surface modification of PLA polymer using oligoamines introduced better anti-infective properties to the polymer without altering its other properties, however in the paper by Tappa et al., addition of anti-infective agents was associated with a decrease in the mechanical properties of PLA, even though it retained its anti-infective properties [44].

Polyvalent test plates were designed for investigation of the physical, chemical, and in-vitro biological properties of FDM printed materials, thus the term polyvalent in this article refers to the use of a single structure for testing of a wide range of properties. The advantage of such a PVTP was the exclusion of effects due to differing geometries, and enabling of the direct comparison between test results. A polyvalent can be used in many situations—chemistry, physics, mechanics, biology, and cell growth, and even biofilm formation.

The reason the printed PVTPs were chemically modified was to increase their favorable surface properties and biocompatibilities. These chemical modifications were verified by FT-IR spectroscopy, showing introduction of amide and amine functions. The FT-IR data was upgraded, highlighting the bands corresponding to the ester C=O, amide C=O, and N-H stretches. The intensities of the amide C=O and N-H are relatively weak as they are surface bonds. Other methods are able to show amide formation, but none are applicable to surface modification. For example, 13C NMR would not detect C at less than 0.1% [45]. Other methods would not show the formation of covalent bonds.

There is clear evidence for the influence of surface topographical and wetting characteristics on macromolecular and cellular levels at implant interfaces [46]. The polymer ester backbone was surface modified by a series of ramified and linear oligoamines to increase the hydrophilicity of the PVTP surfaces and introduce positive charge. These hydrophilic surface modifications were certified by contact angle measurement, which is crucial based on work by Song et al. because wettability of PVTPs may be affected by chemical modification [47]. However, as ethylene diamine is a small and highly water soluble molecule, it would be expected to be washed off the surface. This is not the case, as the contact angle remains constant after washing vigorously. The surface wettability of biomaterials determines the biological events at the biomaterial/host interface [46]. Wettability is modulated by surface chemistry, as was shown in our work and in the articles of Nasrin et al. and Mi et al., because a large range of solid characterization methods can be used for the qualification of different 3D printed polymers in these articles [28,48]. There is also evidence regarding the pH dependence of the contact angle, but the method is as yet not fully proved [49].

The roughness of our PLA based PVTPs was determined by scanning electron microscopy. However, the result of surface scanning depends on many parameters (i.e., the applied filters, the evaluation areas, etc.). The assessment of micron, submicron, and nano-roughness of different implant surfaces is inevitable. Nevertheless, there are only a few standardized methods for the correct determination of implant surfaces [46], although the prediction of the biological performance of different implants in the human body is essential.

Positron annihilation spectroscopy (PALS) measures the supramolecular structure of polymeric-based implants, which can give correct information about the pore sizes and the porosity of the surfaces. Approximately the upper 100 µm of the surface can be examined with this method, and deviations can be seen in a nano-dimensional range. This method is based on one of Einstein's principles, and the detected o-Ps lifetime values are in correlation with the free volume holes of the samples, which enables the comparison of the loaded and unloaded delivery bases. The latter could be useful in the characterization of amorphous solid dispersions or solutions [50].

Comparing the results of PALS and SEM experiments, PLA-ED, PLA-TET, and PLA-Tris all showed high free volumes and the presence of numerous pits. For PLA-ED and PLA-Tris these were ca 1 µm in diameter, and for PLA-TET these pits were ca 100–200 nm in diameter. However, for MeNprN, few pits were present and the free volume was much reduced. Thus, there appeared to be a direct relationship between the free volume measured by PALS and the presence of large numbers of pits observed by SEM.

PLA showed good biocompatibility results and was biodegradable through hydrolytic degradation [47]. Our samples were stored in DMEM medium at 37 °C until the end of the 12th day, and these extracts were measured on days four, eight, and 12 on the Caco-2 cells. The incubation period was 30 min. The cytotoxicity test was harmonized with the ISO 10993-5 standard, but the incubation period was shorter [41]. There is clear evidence that PLA degrades into lactic acid and glycolic acid during storage, and different factors (pH, molecular weight, etc.) can influence this degradation [51]. Many studies have dealt with the degradation of PLA polymers, so the main focus of our study was not the investigation of PLA degradation but the cytotoxic and biofilm formation effects of the modified PLA samples stored in DMEM medium, where the samples may degrade. In vitro cytotoxicity methods can be the first filter in the assessment of cytocompatibility, because the assay is sensitive, efficiently adaptable, and well reproducible [52]. MTT assay is a highly efficient screening test because only the viable cells are able to convert the dye through their mitochondrial enzymes. Van Tonder et al. revealed that the MTT dye alteration to formazan salt depends on the cells' metabolic rate and number of mitochondria [19]. In spite of this limitation of MTT assay, it is still the most reliable and quickest test for the assessment of cytocompatibility [53]. Ramot et al. revealed that PLA can provoke an inflammatory reaction through implantation [54]. Silva et al., however, certified our result because they pointed out that these inflammatory responses, as adverse reactions caused by PLA samples, are extremely rare [55]. Based on the results of the MTT test our PLA samples proved to be cytocompatible.

Biofilm formation is also a compulsory element of cytocompatibility examination, based on the paper by Yang et al. In this research, 3D printed polylactide-*co*-glycolide and hydroxyapatite PVTPs were examined [56]. Biofilm formation can be associated with long-term implantation, which can lead to infections and antimicrobial resistance [34]. During implantation any kind of infection could be dangerous, because it may result in serious inflammation and the rejection of implants. However, biofilm formation can alter the structure of PLA and may cause liberation of different APIs in the case of 3D printed medicine, for example [54]. In our study, biofilm formation was performed with *Candida albicans* SC5314 reference isolate, because one of the most common biofilm forming fungi are *Candida* spp. [34] and other species of *Candida* can cause serious invasive candidiasis, with a mortality rate of about 45% [57]. Ideally, the measured absorbance is zero, which means that no kind of biofilm is formed on the implant by the reference isolate. According to the evaluation of biofilm formation, the chemically modified PLA-PVTPs are biocompatible.

In our paper, we demonstrated the importance of surface characterization and cytocompatibility investigations of 3D printed PLA- PVTPs and chemically modified PLA-based PVTPs. The amines as side chains can favorably alter the surface properties, wettability, and biofilm formation of PLA PVTP. Low biofilm formation ability and favorable cytocompatibility profiles were also presented in the case of prolonged exposure. There are connections between the type and the other properties of PLA PVTPs. Overall, the properties of 3D printing materials can be dramatically enhanced by the modification of base polymers. These implants may ensure a high possibility for the incorporation of different antimicrobial APIs. According to these results, PLA-ED, PLA-Tris, and PLA-TET PVTPs can show favorable surface and anti-infective properties. Therefore, these samples were selected for further in-vivo and/or human studies.

5. Conclusions

To conclude, we have successfully printed 3D PVTPs in runs of up to 50 units, and these have then been chemically functionalized at the surface by various amine head groups. The surface characterization confirms the modification. The various types of PVTP show no toxicity. Finally, we note that a suitable choice of the head group allows *Candida albicans* biofilm formation to be reduced by a factor of ten. Based on these in-vitro tests (MTT and biofilm formation tests), it can be concluded that more than one assay should be used to determine cytotoxicity, so as not to over or underestimate the cytocompatibility of 3D printed PVTPs. However, cytotoxicity data alone are not necessarily predictive of in-vivo issues, but alongside other experiments (contact angle, PALS, and SEM results) the in-vivo compatibility data may be estimated. This work is being extended to other functionalizations, including anionic head groups and other polymers such as PET or PMMA.

Author Contributions: P.A., made the cell culture experiments, and carried out the statistical analysis and wrote the methods in the article. F.P., designed the 3D printing samples and designed the chemical structure figures. A.W.C. designed the article and the structure of 3D printed implants, and made contact angle experiments. I.B. conceived and designed the overall project and wrote the introduction and discussion part of manuscript. E.R., was responsible for cell culture. Z.U., made the MTT cytotoxicity experiment, P.F. evaluated the cytotoxicity data. J.V., controlled the abstract and the introduction part. F.F., controlled and qualified the data. M.V., was responsible for figure drawings. Furthermore, designed and performed prolonged MTT assay. R.G. carried out statistical analysis. R.K., designed and performed the biofilm formation studies. A.K. was responsible for PALS examination. R.Z., controlled PALS experiments. L.M., controlled and validated 3D printing process. B.K. carried out, SEM experiments. All authors read and approved the final manuscript.

Funding: The research was financed by the Higher Education Institutional Excellence Program of the Ministry of Human Capacities in Hungary, within the framework of the Research and Development on Therapeutic purposes thematic program of the University of Debrecen. 20428-3/2018/FEKUTSTRAT. The project was supported by the EFOP-3.6.1-16-2016-00022. The project is co-financed by the European Union and the European Social Fund. The project was supported by the Gedeon Richter's Talentum Foundation (1103 Budapest, Gyömrői út 19-21 Hungary).

Conflicts of Interest: The authors declare no conflict of interest.

Appendix A

FT-IR spectra of polyvalent test platforms (PVTP).

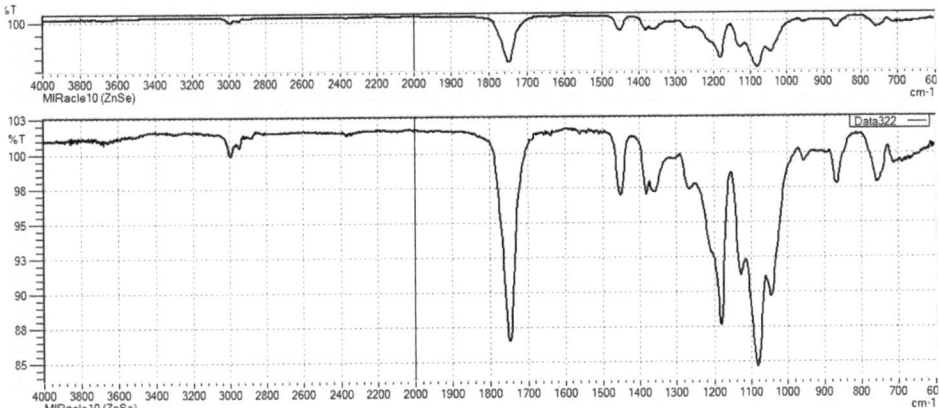

Figure A1. PLA.

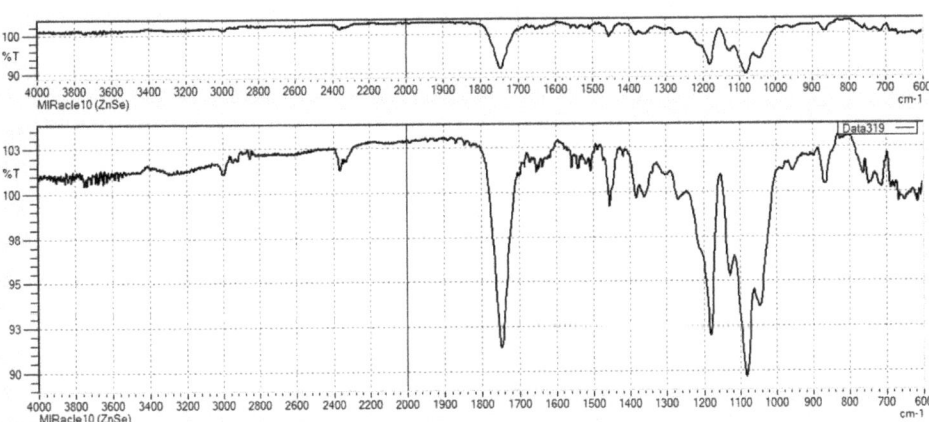

Figure A2. PLA-BAPA.

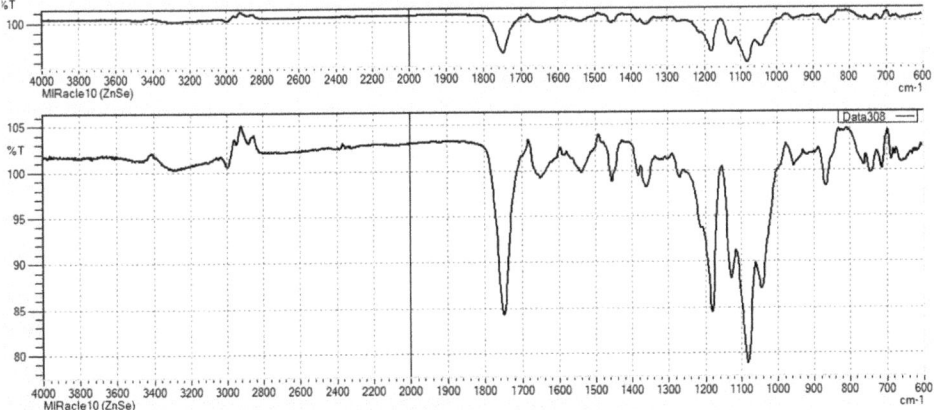

Figure A3. PLA-ED.

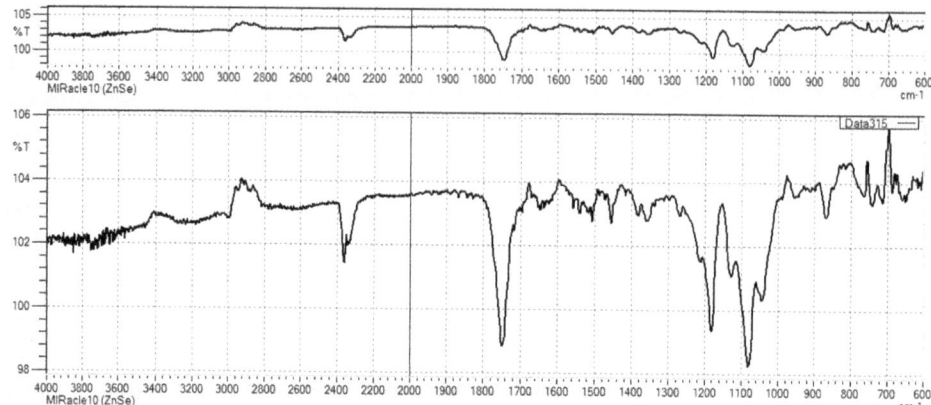

Figure A4. PLA-TET.

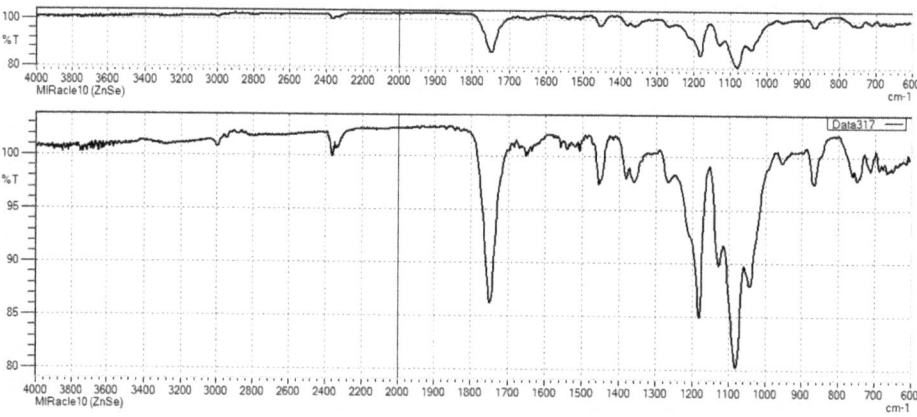

Figure A5. PLA-MeNprN.

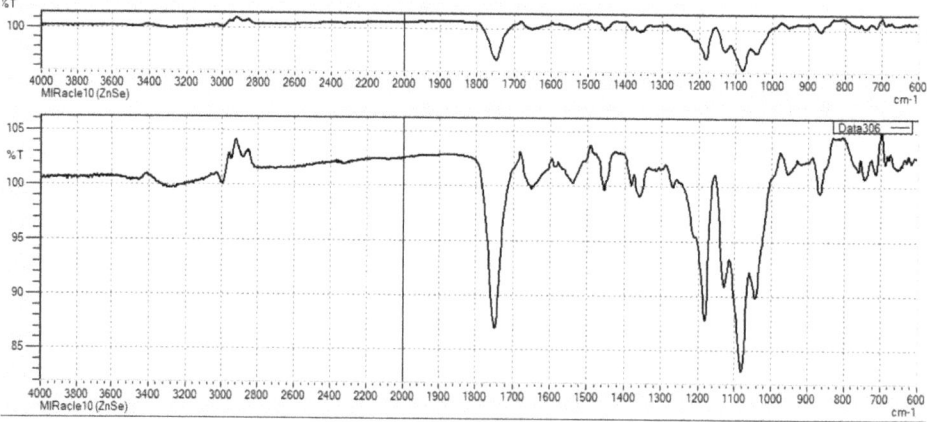

Figure A6. PLA-Tris.

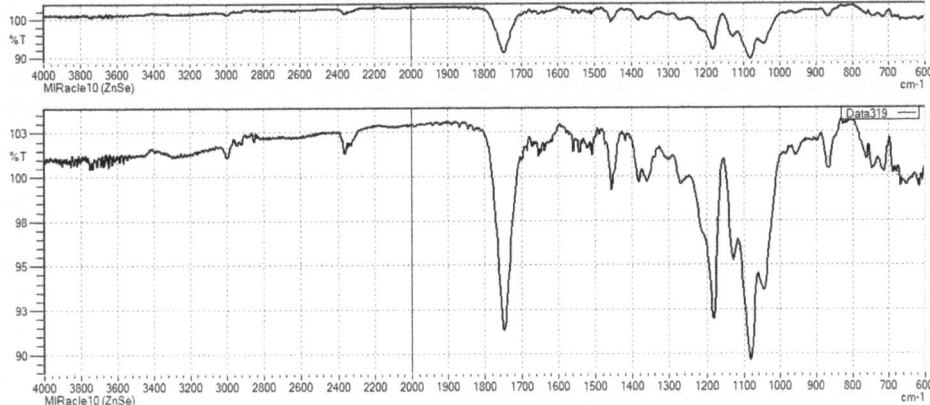

Figure A7. PLA-NPEGN.

Appendix B

Line sections through printed PVTPs.

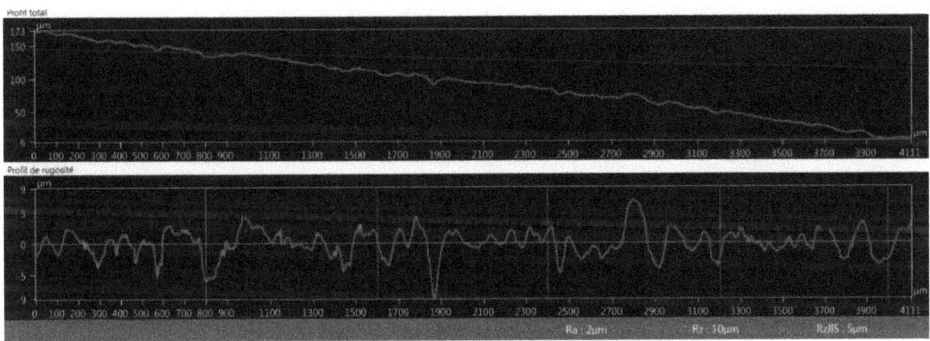

Figure A8. Line section PLA-MeNPrN.

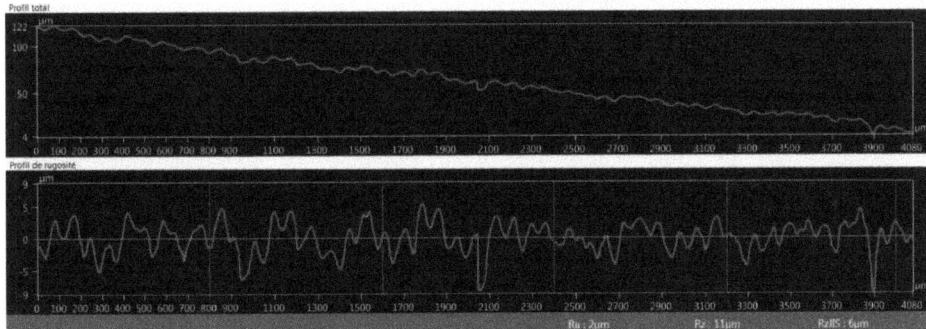

Figure A9. Line section PLA-BAPA.

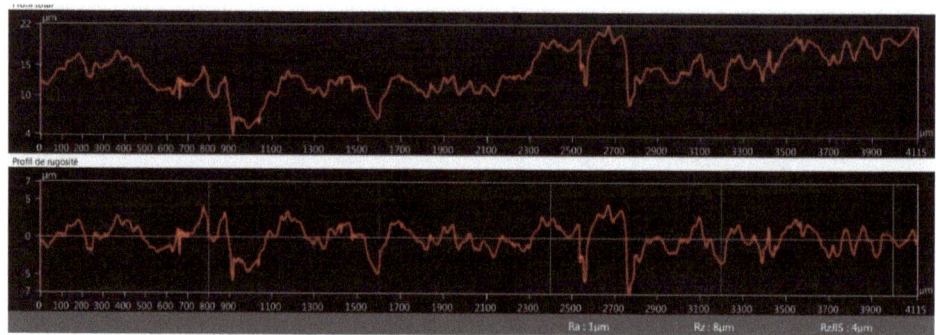

Figure A10. Line section PLA-Tris.

References

1. Li, Z.; Jia, S.; Xiong, Z.; Long, Q.; Yan, S.; Hao, F.; Liu, J.; Yuan, Z. 3D-printed scaffolds with calcified layer for osteochondral tissue engineering. *J. Biosci. Bioeng.* **2018**, *126*, 389–396. [CrossRef] [PubMed]
2. Boetker, J.; Water, J.J.; Aho, J.; Arnfast, L.; Bohr, A.; Rantanen, J. Modifying release characteristics from 3D printed drug-eluting products. *Eur. J. Pharm. Sci.* **2016**, *90*, 47–52. [CrossRef] [PubMed]
3. Kiraly, L. Three-dimensional modelling and three-dimensional printing in pediatric and congenital cardiac surgery. *Transl. Pediatr.* **2018**, *7*, 129–138. [CrossRef] [PubMed]
4. Martelli, N.; Serrano, C.; Van Den Brink, H.; Pineau, J.; Prognon, P.; Borget, I.; El Batti, S. Advantages and disadvantages of 3-dimensional printing in surgery: A systematic review. *Surgery* **2016**, *159*, 1485–1500. [CrossRef] [PubMed]
5. Tappa, K.; Jammalamadaka, U. Novel biomaterials used in medical 3D printing techniques. *J. Funct. Biomater.* **2018**, *9*, 17. [CrossRef]
6. Luzuriaga, M.A.; Berry, D.R.; Reagan, J.C.; Smaldone, R.A.; Gassensmith, J.J. Biodegradable 3D printed polymer microneedles for transdermal drug delivery. *Lab Chip* **2018**, *18*, 1223–1230. [CrossRef]
7. Aldaadaa, A.; Owji, N.; Knowles, J. Three-dimensional Printing in Maxillofacial Surgery: Hype versus Reality. *J. Tissue Eng.* **2018**, *9*. [CrossRef]
8. Kitson, P.J.; Glatzel, S.; Cronin, L. The digital code driven autonomous synthesis of ibuprofen automated in a 3D-printer-based robot. *Beilstein J. Org. Chem.* **2016**, *12*, 2776–2783. [CrossRef]
9. Glatzel, S.; Hezwani, M.; Kitson, P.J.; Gromski, P.S.; Schürer, S.; Cronin, L. A PorTable 3D Printer System for the Diagnosis and Treatment of Multidrug-Resistant Bacteria. *Chem* **2016**, *1*, 494–504. [CrossRef]
10. Diomede, F.; Gugliandolo, A.; Cardelli, P.; Merciaro, I.; Ettorre, V.; Traini, T.; Bedini, R.; Scionti, D.; Bramanti, A.; Nanci, A.; et al. Three-dimensional printed PLA scaffold and human gingival stem cell-derived extracellular vesicles: A new tool for bone defect repair. *Stem Cell Res. Ther.* **2018**, *9*, 104–125. [CrossRef]
11. Barbeck, M.; Serra, T.; Booms, P.; Stojanovic, S.; Najman, S.; Engel, E.; Sader, R.; Kirkpatrick, C.J.; Navarro, M.; Ghanaati, S. Analysis of the in vitro degradation and the in vivo tissue response to bi-layered 3D-printed scaffolds combining PLA and biphasic PLA/bioglass components—Guidance of the inflammatory response as basis for osteochondral regeneration. *Bioact. Mater.* **2017**, *2*, 208–223. [CrossRef] [PubMed]
12. Jackson, R.J.; Patrick, P.S.; Page, K.; Powell, M.J.; Lythgoe, M.F.; Miodownik, M.A.; Parkin, I.P.; Carmalt, C.J.; Kalber, T.L.; Bear, J.C. Chemically Treated 3D Printed Polymer Scaffolds for Biomineral Formation. *ACS Omega* **2018**, *3*, 4342–4351. [CrossRef] [PubMed]
13. Teixeira, B.N.; Aprile, P.; Mendonça, R.H.; Kelly, D.J.; Thiré, R.M. Evaluation of bone marrow stem cell response to PLA scaffolds manufactured by 3D printing and coated with polydopamine and type I collagen. *J. Biomed. Mater. Res. Part B Appl. Biomater.* **2019**, *107*, 37–49. [CrossRef] [PubMed]
14. Vargas-Alfredo, N.; Dorronsoro, A.; Cortajarena, A.L.; Rodríguez-Hernández, J. Antimicrobial 3D Porous Scaffolds Prepared by Additive Manufacturing and Breath Figures. *ACS Appl. Mater. Interfaces* **2017**, *9*, 37454–37462. [CrossRef] [PubMed]

15. Pach, K.; Filipecki, J.; Golis, E.; Yousef, E.S.; Boyko, V. Measurements of Defect Structures by Positron Annihilation Lifetime Spectroscopy of the Tellurite Glass 70TeO$_2$-5XO-10P$_2$O$_5$-10ZnO-5PbF$_2$ (X = Mg, Bi$_2$, Ti) Doped with Ions of the Rare Earth Element Er^3. *Nanoscale Res. Lett.* **2017**, *12*, 304. [CrossRef] [PubMed]
16. Morrison, R.J.; Kashlan, K.N.; Flanangan, C.L.; Wright, J.K.; Green, G.E.; Hollister, S.J.; Weatherwax, K.J. Regulatory Considerations in the Design and Manufacturing of ImplanTable 3D-Printed Medical Devices. *Clin. Transl. Sci.* **2015**, *8*, 594–600. [CrossRef] [PubMed]
17. Pizzoferrato, A.; Ciapetti, G.; Stea, S.; Cenni, E.; Arciola, C.R.; Granchi, D.; Savarino, L. Cell culture methods for testing biocompatibility. *Clin. Mater.* **1994**, *15*, 173–190. [CrossRef]
18. Sambuy, Y.; De Angelis, I.; Ranaldi, G.; Scarino, M.L.; Stammati, A.; Zucco, F. The Caco-2 cell line as a model of the intestinal barrier: Influence of cell and culture-related factors on Caco-2 cell functional characteristics. *Cell Biol. Toxicol.* **2005**, *21*, 1–26. [CrossRef] [PubMed]
19. van Tonder, A.; Joubert, A.M.; Cromarty, A.D. Limitations of the 3-(4,5-dimethylthiazol-2-yl)-2,5-diphenyl-2H-tetrazolium bromide (MTT) assay when compared to three commonly used cell enumeration assays. *BMC Res. Notes* **2015**, *8*, 47. [CrossRef]
20. Galdiero, M.; Larocca, F.; Iovene, M.R.; Francesca, M.; Pieretti, G.; D'Oriano, V.; Franci, G.; Ferraro, G.; D'Andrea, F.; Nicoletti, G.F. Microbial Evaluation in Capsular Contracture of Breast Implants. *Plast. Reconstr. Surg.* **2018**, *141*, 23–30. [CrossRef]
21. Salari, S.; Sadat Seddighi, N.; Ghasemi Nejad Almani, P. Evaluation of biofilm formation ability in different Candida strains and anti-biofilm effects of Fe$_3$O$_4$-NPs compared with Fluconazole: An in vitro study. *J. Mycol. Med.* **2018**, *28*, 23–28. [CrossRef] [PubMed]
22. Gomaa, Y.A.; Garland, M.J.; McInnes, F.J.; Donnelly, R.F.; El-Khordagui, L.K.; Wilson, C.G. Microneedle/nanoencapsulation-mediated transdermal delivery: Mechanistic insights. *Eur. J. Pharm. Biopharm.* **2014**, *86*, 145–155. [CrossRef] [PubMed]
23. Stansbury, J.W.; Idacavage, M.J. 3D printing with polymers: Challenges among expanding options and opportunities. *Dent. Mater.* **2016**, *32*, 54–64. [CrossRef] [PubMed]
24. Tauran, Y.; Tarhan, M.C.; Mollet, L.; Gerves, J.B.; Fujit, H.; Collard, D.; Perret, F.; Desbrosses, M.; Leon, D. Elucidating the mechanism of the considerable mechanical stiffening of DNA induced by the couple Zn^{2+}/Calix[4]arene-1,3-O-diphosphorous acid. *Sci. Rep.* **2018**, *8*, 1226. [CrossRef] [PubMed]
25. Haddad, T.; Noel, S.; Liberelle, B.; El Ayoubi, R.; Ajji, A.; De Crescenzo, G. Fabrication and surface modification of poly lactic acid (PLA) scaffolds with epidermal growth factor for neural tissue engineering. *Biomatter* **2016**, *6*, e1231276. [CrossRef]
26. Yildirimer, L.; Seifalian, A.M.; Butler, P.E. Surface and mechanical analysis of explanted Poly Implant Prosthèse silicone breast implants. *Br. J. Surg.* **2013**, *100*, 761–767. [CrossRef]
27. Tham, C.Y.; Abdul Hamid, Z.A.; Ahmad, Z.; Ismail, H. Surface Modification of Poly(lactic acid) (PLA) via Alkaline Hydrolysis Degradation. *Adv. Mater. Res.* **2014**, *970*, 324–327. [CrossRef]
28. Nasrin, R.; Biswas, S.; Rashid, T.U.; Afrin, S.; Jahan, R.A.; Haque, P.; Rahman, M.M. Preparation of Chitin-PLA laminated composite for implantable application. *Bioact. Mater.* **2017**, *2*, 199–207. [CrossRef]
29. Shalabi, M.M.; Gortemaker, A.; Van't Hof, M.A.; Jansen, J.A.; Creugers, N.H.J. Implant surface roughness and bone healing: A systematic review. *J. Dent. Res.* **2006**, *85*, 496–500. [CrossRef]
30. Kazsoki, A.; Szabó, P.; Süvegh, K.; Vörös, T.; Zelkó, R. Macro- and microstructural tracking of ageing-related changes of papaverine hydrochloride-loaded electrospun nanofibrous buccal sheets. *J. Pharm. Biomed. Anal.* **2017**, *143*, 62–67. [CrossRef]
31. Seyednejad, H.; Gawlitta, D.; Kuiper, R.V.; De Bruin, A.; Van Nostrum, C.F.; Vermonden, T.; Dhert, W.J.A.; Hennink, W.E. In vivo biocompatibility and biodegradation of 3D-printed porous scaffolds based on a hydroxyl-functionalized poly(ε-caprolactone). *Biomaterials* **2012**, *33*, 4309–4318. [CrossRef]
32. Nemes, D.; Ujhelyi, Z.; Arany, P.; Peto, A.; Feher, P.; Varadi, J.; Fenyvesi, F.; Vecsernyes, M.; Bacskay, I. Biocompatibility investigation of different pharmaceutical excipients used in liquid dosage forms. *Pharmazie* **2018**, *73*, 16–18. [PubMed]
33. Ujhelyi, Z.; Fenyvesi, F.; Váradi, J.; Fehér, P.; Kiss, T.; Veszelka, S.; Deli, M.; Vecsernyés, M.; Bácskay, I. Evaluation of cytotoxicity of surfactants used in self-micro emulsifying drug delivery systems and their effects on paracellular transport in Caco-2 cell monolayer. *Eur. J. Pharm. Sci.* **2012**, *47*, 564–573. [CrossRef] [PubMed]

34. Pierce, C.G.; Uppuluri, P.; Tristan, A.R.; Wormley, F.L., Jr.; Mowat, E.; Ramage, G.; Lopez-ribot, J.L. A simple and reproducible 96 well plate-based method for the formation of fungal biofilms and its application to antifungal susceptibility testing. *Nat. Protoc.* **2009**, *3*, 1494–1500. [CrossRef]
35. O'Toole, G.A. Microtiter Dish Biofilm Formation Assay. *J. Vis. Exp.* **2011**, e2437. [CrossRef] [PubMed]
36. Xu, W.; Pranovich, A.; Uppstu, P.; Wang, X.; Kronlund, D.; Hemming, J.; Öblom, H.; Moritz, N.; Preis, M.; Sandler, N.; et al. Novel biorenewable composite of wood polysaccharide and polylactic acid for three dimensional printing. *Carbohydr. Polym.* **2018**, *187*, 51–58. [CrossRef]
37. Wang, J.; Witte, F.; Xi, T.; Zheng, Y.; Yang, K.; Yang, Y.; Zhao, D.; Meng, J.; Li, Y.; Li, W.; et al. Recommendation for modifying current cytotoxicity testing standards for biodegradable magnesium-based materials. *Acta Biomater.* **2015**, *21*, 237–249. [CrossRef]
38. Shiraishi, R.; Hirayama, N. Cytotoxicity associated with prolonged room temperature storage of serum and proposed methods for reduction of cytotoxicity. *J. Virol. Methods* **2015**, *225*, 16–22. [CrossRef]
39. Kinnari, T.J.; Soininen, A.; Esteban, J.; Zamora, N.; Alakoski, E.; Kouri, V.P.; Lappalainen, R.; Konttinen, Y.T.; Gomez-Barrena, E.; Tiainen, V.M. Adhesion of staphylococcal and Caco-2 cells on diamond-like carbon polymer hybrid coating. *J. Biomed. Mater. Res. Part A* **2008**, *86*, 760–768. [CrossRef]
40. Chessa, D.; Ganau, G.; Spiga, L.; Bulla, A.; Mazzarello, V.; Campus, G.V.; Rubino, S. Staphylococcus aureus and Staphylococcus epidermidis Virulence Strains as Causative Agents of Persistent Infections in Breast Implants. *PLoS ONE* **2016**, *11*, e0146668. [CrossRef]
41. ISO/EN10993-5. *Biological Evaluation of Medical Devices—Part 5: Tests for in Vitro Cytotoxicity*, 3rd ed.; International Organization of Standardization: Geneva, Switzerland, 2009.
42. Finkel, J.S.; Mitchell, A.P. Genetic Control of Candida Albicans Biofilm Development. *Natl. Reviiew Microbiol.* **2011**, *9*, 109–118. [CrossRef] [PubMed]
43. Marcos-Zambrano, L.J.; Escribano, P.; Bouza, E.; Guinea, J. Production of biofilm by Candida and non-Candida spp. isolates causing fungemia: Comparison of biomass production and metabolic activity and development of cut-off points. *Int. J. Med. Microbiol.* **2014**, *304*, 1192–1198. [CrossRef]
44. Tappa, K.; Jammalamadaka, U.; Weisman, J.; Ballard, D.; Wolford, D.; Pascual-Garrido, C.; Wolford, L.; Woodard, P.; Mills, D. 3D Printing Custom Bioactive and Absorbable Surgical Screws, Pins, and Bone Plates for Localized Drug Delivery. *J. Funct. Biomater.* **2019**, *10*, 17. [CrossRef] [PubMed]
45. Wishart, D.S.; Bigam, C.G.; Yao, J.; Abildgaard, F.; Dyson, H.J.; Oldfield, E.; Markley, J.L.; Sykes, B.D. ^{1}H, ^{13}C and ^{15}N chemical shift referencing in biomolecular NMR. *J. Biomol. NMR* **1995**, *6*, 135–140. [CrossRef] [PubMed]
46. Rupp, F.; Liang, L.; Geis-Gerstorfer, J.; Scheideler, L.; Hüttig, F. Surface characteristics of dental implants: A review. *Dent. Mater.* **2018**, *34*, 40–57. [CrossRef]
47. Song, F.; Ma, L.; Fan, J.; Chen, Q.; Zhang, L.; Li, B.Q. Wetting behaviors of a nano-droplet on a rough solid substrate under perpendicular electric field. *Nanomaterials* **2018**, *8*, 340. [CrossRef]
48. Mi, H.Y.; Salick, M.R.; Jing, X.; Jacques, B.R.; Crone, W.C.; Peng, X.F.; Turng, L.S. Characterization of thermoplastic polyurethane/polylactic acid (TPU/PLA) tissue engineering scaffolds fabricated by microcellular injection molding. *Mater. Sci. Eng. C* **2013**, *33*, 4767–4776. [CrossRef]
49. Holmes-Farley, S.R.; Reamey, R.H.; McCarthy, T.J.; Deutch, J.; Whitesides, G.M. Acid-base behavior of carboxylic acid groups covalently attached at the surface of polyethylene: The usefulness of contact angle in following the ionization of surface functionality. *Langmuir* **1985**, *1*, 725–740. [CrossRef]
50. Sebe, I.; Szabó, B.; Zelkó, R. Positron Annihilation Lifetime Spectrometry (PALS) and its pharmaceutical applications. *Acta Pharm. Hung.* **2012**, *82*, 23–32.
51. Wurm, M.C.; Möst, T.; Bergauer, B.; Rietzel, D.; Neukam, F.W.; Cifuentes, S.C.; von Wilmowsky, C. In-vitro evaluation of Polylactic acid (PLA) manufactured by fused deposition modeling. *J. Biol. Eng.* **2017**, *11*, 1–9. [CrossRef]
52. Johnson, H.J.; Northup, S.J.; Darby, T.D. Biocompatibility test procedures for materials evaluation in vitro. II. Objective methods of toxicity assessment. *J. Biomed. Mater. Res.* **1984**, *19*, 489–508. [CrossRef] [PubMed]
53. Gaucher, S.; Jarraya, M. Technical note: Comparison of the PrestoBlue and LDH release assays with the MTT assay for skin viability assessment. *Cell Tissue Bank.* **2015**, *16*, 325–329. [CrossRef] [PubMed]
54. Ramot, Y.; Haim-Zada, M.; Domb, A.J.; Nyska, A. Biocompatibility and safety of PLA and its copolymers. *Adv. Drug Deliv. Rev.* **2016**, *107*, 153–162. [CrossRef] [PubMed]

55. da Silva, D.; Kaduri, M.; Poley, M.; Adir, O.; Krinsky, N.; Shainsky-Roitman, J.; Schroeder, A. Biocompatibility, biodegradation and excretion of polylactic acid (PLA) in medical implants and theranostic systems. *Chem. Eng. J.* **2018**, *340*, 9–14. [CrossRef]
56. Yang, Y.; Yang, S.; Wang, Y.; Yu, Z.; Ao, H.; Zhang, H.; Qin, L.; Guillaume, O.; Eglin, D.; Richards, R.G.; et al. Anti-infective efficacy, cytocompatibility and biocompatibility of a 3D-printed osteoconductive composite scaffold functionalized with quaternized chitosan. *Acta Biomater.* **2016**, *46*, 112–128. [CrossRef]
57. Antinori, S.; Milazzo, L.; Sollima, S.; Galli, M.; Corbellino, M. Candidemia and invasive candidiasis in adults: A narrative review. *Eur. J. Intern. Med.* **2016**, *34*, 21–28. [CrossRef]

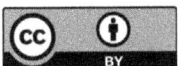

© 2019 by the authors. Licensee MDPI, Basel, Switzerland. This article is an open access article distributed under the terms and conditions of the Creative Commons Attribution (CC BY) license (http://creativecommons.org/licenses/by/4.0/).

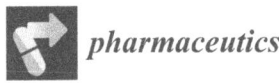

Article

Antioxidant PLA Composites Containing Lignin for 3D Printing Applications: A Potential Material for Healthcare Applications

Juan Domínguez-Robles, Niamh K. Martin, Mun Leon Fong, Sarah A. Stewart, Nicola J. Irwin, María Isabel Rial-Hermida, Ryan F. Donnelly and Eneko Larrañeta *

School of Pharmacy, Queen's University Belfast, 97 Lisburn Road, Belfast BT9 7BL, UK; j.dominguezrobles@qub.ac.uk (J.D.-R.); nmartin24@qub.ac.uk (N.K.M.); mfong03@qub.ac.uk (M.L.F.) sstewart35@qub.ac.uk (S.A.S.); n.irwin@qub.ac.uk (N.J.I.); mariaisabel.rial@usc.es (M.I.R.-H.); r.donnelly@qub.ac.uk (R.F.D.)
* Correspondence: e.larraneta@qub.ac.uk; Tel.: +44-(0)28-9097-2360

Received: 7 March 2019; Accepted: 2 April 2019; Published: 4 April 2019

Abstract: Lignin (LIG) is a natural biopolymer with well-known antioxidant capabilities. Accordingly, in the present work, a method to combine LIG with poly(lactic acid) (PLA) for fused filament fabrication applications (FFF) is proposed. For this purpose, PLA pellets were successfully coated with LIG powder and a biocompatible oil (castor oil). The resulting pellets were placed into an extruder at 200 °C. The resulting PLA filaments contained LIG loadings ranging from 0% to 3% (w/w). The obtained filaments were successfully used for FFF applications. The LIG content affected the mechanical and surface properties of the overall material. The inclusion of LIG yielded materials with lower resistance to fracture and higher wettabilities. Moreover, the resulting 3D printed materials showed antioxidant capabilities. By using the 2,2-diphenyl-1-picrylhydrazyl (DPPH) method, the materials were capable of reducing the concentration of this compound up to ca. 80% in 5 h. This radical scavenging activity could be potentially beneficial for healthcare applications, especially for wound care. Accordingly, PLA/LIG were used to design meshes with different designs for wound dressing purposes. A wound healing model compound, curcumin (CUR), was applied in the surface of the mesh and its diffusion was studied. It was observed that the dimensions of the meshes affected the permeation rate of CUR. Accordingly, the design of the mesh could be modified according to the patient's needs.

Keywords: 3D printing; fused filament fabrication; lignin; antioxidant materials; wound dressing

---

1. Introduction

The interest in additive manufacturing (commonly known as 3D printing) for biomedical applications has increased significantly during the last decade [1]. Among all the different types of 3D printing, fused filament fabrication (FFF) is the most commonly used [2]. In FFF, a polymer filament is heated and extruded through a small nozzle and subsequently solidified on a build plate [3]. FFF gained popularity quickly after the RepRap project in 2005 [4]. This project was focused on developing low cost do-it yourself FFF printers [4]. Accordingly, different biomedical and pharmaceutical applications of additive manufacturing have been described during the last decade [1,5,6]. These applications include drug delivery systems, prosthetics or implantable devices [1,5–7]. The most common material used for FFF is poly(lactic acid) (PLA). This is due to its processability for extrusion applications, high mechanical strength and low coefficient of thermal expansion [8]. Moreover, PLA is a renewable, biodegradable and biocompatible polymer [7,9]. These properties make this material ideal for pharmaceutical and biomedical applications.

To provide extra features to PLA, different strategies have been followed. The combination of PLA with other molecules that can give added value to the final composite material for healthcare applications have been explored in the past [10]. One of the potential scenarios is the incorporation of molecules with antioxidant properties to PLA. The unrestrained production of free radicals and reactive oxygen species is linked with the onset of diseases such as rheumatoid arthritis, atherosclerosis or cancer [11]. Accordingly, the development of antioxidant compounds/materials can contribute to reduce the concentration of these compounds [12]. Moreover, it has been shown that the excess of reactive oxygen species prevents wound healing [13,14]. Accordingly, antioxidants have been proposed as a way to control oxidative stress in wounds to accelerate their healing.

The use of antioxidant compounds for 3D printing applications has not been extensively explored in the past. Van Lith et al. proposed the use of stereolithography (an alternative to FFF 3D printing technology) to create bioresorbable antioxidant vascular stents [15]. The stents provided antioxidant capabilities that are beneficial to reduce oxidative stress Another application of antioxidant compounds for 3D printing applications was described by Lücking et al. [16]. In this work, another type of 3D printing, selective laser sintering, was used to prepare materials containing antioxidant to enhance cell proliferation [16]. They used UV-stable polyamide 12 material with antioxidant properties. However, the nature of the antioxidant compound was not disclosed.

An interesting renewable and natural compound with antioxidant properties is lignin (LIG). LIG is a biopolymer present in the support tissues of vascular plants and provides chemical and mechanical protection from external stresses [17]. Moreover, it has been reported that LIG presents antioxidant and antimicrobial properties [18–21]. Among other alternatives, LIG-based materials have attracted the attention of researchers [17,22–27]. Considering that LIG is the second most abundant polymer on Earth [17,24], the applications of LIG to develop new materials are unexploited as only a 2% of the total LIG production (ca. 70 million tons) is reused for specialty products [17]. The rest is used as burning fuel or treated as a waste [17,28]. Due to its high availability and its antimicrobial and antioxidant properties, LIG has potential for biomedical applications. These are not the only advantages as LIG is a relatively cheap to obtain with prices ca. €33 per ton [29]. To date, the biomedical applications of this biopolymer, remain relatively unexplored. A few scientific articles can be found describing its use to prepare coatings, nanoparticles or hydrogels [21,30–32] for potential medical applications.

In the present work, we propose the combination of LIG with PLA to create filament that can be used for healthcare FFF applications. These compounds were combined via hot melt extrusion. The resulting composite materials were characterized and successfully used for fused deposition modeling applications. This approach has potential for multiple applications but in the present study we hypothesized that it can be used for wound dressing applications. The antioxidant properties of the material could potentially enhance wound healing. The resulting polymeric composite material has antioxidant properties and do not rely on the release of an antioxidant agents. Accordingly, the material can provide localized and prolonged antioxidant activity. Finally, the proposed method is simple and allows combination of PLA with LIG and additional molecules such as antibiotics. In this way, the resulting material can have advanced properties. For the present work we selected tetracycline (TC) as in this way the material can be used to prevent wound infections.

2. Materials and Methods

2.1. Materials

Ingeo PLA 3D850 biopolymer (PLA pellets) was purchased from NatureWorks LCC (Minnetonka, MN, USA). This PLA grade (3D850) has been specifically developed for FFF applications, having an excellent processability and printability.

LIG sample (BioPiva 100) was a softwood Kraft LIG acquired from UPM (Helsinki, Finland). This LIG sample was used as provided (63–68% dry matter content). However, the higher moisture content of this sample was considered for any following calculations. An important part of the characterization of this aromatic polymer was kindly provided from the supplier. Klason LIG content (TAPPI T 222 om-02) was around 92% of the dry matter and acid-soluble LIG (TAPPI UM 250) was around 4% of the dry matter. On the other hand, the total amount of carbohydrates (SCAN-CM 71:09) accounted for around 2% of the dry matter and the content of inorganic particles (internal method, 700 °C) accounted for around 1% of the dry matter. Molar mass of this LIG sample was 5000—6000 Da. Finally, the particle size (median d_{50}) was around 20 µm and it was analyzed using a Mastersizer 3000 (Malvern, UK).

Castor oil used to attach LIG and TC to the pellets surface was purchased from Ransom Naturals Ltd. (England, UK). TC was acquired from Honeywell Fluka™ (Leicestershire, UK). To perform the release study, Hydroxypropyl-methyl cellulose (HPMC) was acquired by Colorcon Limited (Dartford, UK), ascorbic acid (AA) was provided by DSM (Heerlen, the Netherlands), tween 80 (T80) was obtained from Tokyo Chemical Industry UK Ltd. (Oxford, UK) and curcumin (CUR), the model drug used in this study, was purchased from Cayman Chemical (Michigan, USA). Finally, poly(vinyl alcohol) (PVA) filament was obtained from Ultimaker B.V., The Netherlands (Diameter: 2.85 mm; Melting Temperature: 163 °C).

Staphylococcus aureus (ATCC 6538; LGC Standards, Middlesex, UK) were maintained on cryopreservative beads in 10% glycerol at −80 °C and cultivated in Mueller Hinton broth (MHB) at 37 °C when required for the microbiological assessments.

2.2. LIG-PLA Pellets Production

The method used to produce these LIG-PLA coated pellets was previously described by Weisman et al. [10]. Briefly, 50 mL Falcon tube was filled with PLA pellets (40 g). Then, castor oil (40 µL) was added into the tube and it was vortexed until the pellets were properly coated. Subsequently, these castor oil covered pellets were placed into a new 50 mL Falcon tube and the LIG or LIG and tetracycline powder were added, and it was vortexed again. Different batches containing 0.5%, 1%, 2% and 3% (w/w) of LIG coating and 1% and 2% (w/w) of LIG and TC, respectively, were prepared. Additionally, castor oil covered PLA pellets and only PLA pellets were used as control samples to make the filaments.

2.3. Extrusion of Filaments

The Next 1.0 filament extruder (3devo, Utrecht, The Netherlands) was used to prepare the different filaments. The temperature was adjusted through a control panel positioned at the side of the extruder and it was between 170 and 190 °C, due to the existence of 4 heaters. Moreover, the extruder speed was established at 5.0 rpm and the fan speed was 70%. Additionally, 2.85 mm was selected as the diameter of the extruded filaments.

2.4. Fused Filament Fabrication

Once the filaments were extruded, discs and squares were 3D-printed using an Ultimaker 3 (Ultimaker B.V., Geldermalsen, The Netherlands) FFF system and Cura® software between 185 and 205 °C. The Ultimaker 3 FFF system was equipped with two extruders containing a 0.4 mm nozzle. It is important to note that this equipment is a RepRap Open Source FFF equipment [4]. Thermogravimetric analyses were performed to ascertain the stability of LIG at the process temperatures (data not shown), showing that a small amount of LIG was degraded during the process (ca. 3%).

2.5. Material Characterization

2.5.1. Microscopy

The morphologies of the materials prepared using FFF as well as the filaments and pellets were assessed using a Leica EZ4 D digital microscope (Leica, Wetzlar, Germany).

2.5.2. Contact Angle Measurement

The influence of the LIG on the contact angle of water with the surface of the 3D printed materials (squares) was assessed using an Attension Theta equipment (Attension Theta, Biolin Scientific, Gothenburg, Sweden). OneAttension software analyzed results to give an indication of the wettability of the surface. Measurements were performed in triplicate.

2.5.3. Thermal Properties

The glass transition temperature (T_g) of the 3D printed materials as well as the pure materials (PLA, LIG, tetracycline and castor oil) was measured using DSC Q100 differential scanning calorimeter (TA instruments, Bellingham, WA, USA). Scans were run from 30 to 300 °C at 10 °C/min under a nitrogen flow rate of 10 mL/min.

2.5.4. Stability Study

For the degradation experiments, the 3D printed discs were incubated at 37 °C in screw-capped vials containing 3 mL of phosphate-buffered saline (PBS) (pH = 7.4) over a period of 30 days. The specimens incubated were run in triplicate. After different interval times, the discs were separated from the degradation medium and the excess of it was removed with a tissue paper and subsequently they were dried at 80 °C in an oven for 5 min. The degradation medium or PBS was replaced after each time interval and the mass loss was measured.

2.5.5. Mechanical Properties

The break strength of the different filaments extruded were evaluated using a TA.XTplus texture analyzer (Stable Micro Systems, Surrey, UK) in compression mode. Pieces of filaments of 2 cm were cut and used for the test. Then, these samples were placed on two aluminum blocks (with 1 cm of separation) and a tapered aluminum probe (5.5 cm in length with a blunt end of radius 1.0 mm) was moved towards the pieces of filaments. The probe moved at a speed of 2 mm·s^{-1} with a maximum distance of travel of 5 mm. The filament failure force was assumed to be the peak maximum of the force-distance curve.

2.6. PLA-LIG Mesh Production and CUR Release for Potential Wound Healing Applications

Different 3D printed meshes (0.4 mm thickness) made using the filament containing 2% of LIG were used for CUR permeation experiments. Figure 1 shows the different types of meshes that were prepared and their dimensions. Moreover, combined meshes were prepared using a two layered distribution (0.4 mm each layer). The first layer contained a PLA/LIG mesh and the second layer was printed using PVA. For these purpose, horizontal diffusion cell system was used with some modifications. Each side of the system was employed as an individual replicate for the different mesh systems. Curcumin was used as the model drug for this test. Films were prepared with HPMC and CUR. For his purpose, a solution containing 10% (w/w) of HPMC and an excess of CUR was prepared in ethanol-water (70% ethanol). The solution was centrifuged to remove the non-dissolved CUR. Subsequently, films were casted using this solution. Then, a 1 cm diameter cork-borer was employed to cut this film into discs, which were placed together the different 3D printed meshes in the cells. Then, each cell of the system was filled with 3 mL of a solution containing 10% (w/v) of Tween 80 and 1 mg/mL of ascorbic acid prepared in PBS, which was stirred and thermostatically maintained at 37 ± 1 °C. Samples (≤0.5 mL) were removed from the sampling arms of the cells at predetermined time intervals and replace with fresh release media. The concentration of CUR was evaluated using a UV-visible plate reader (PowerWave XS Microplate Spectrophotometer, Bio-Tek, Winooski, VT, USA) at a wavelength of 425 nm.

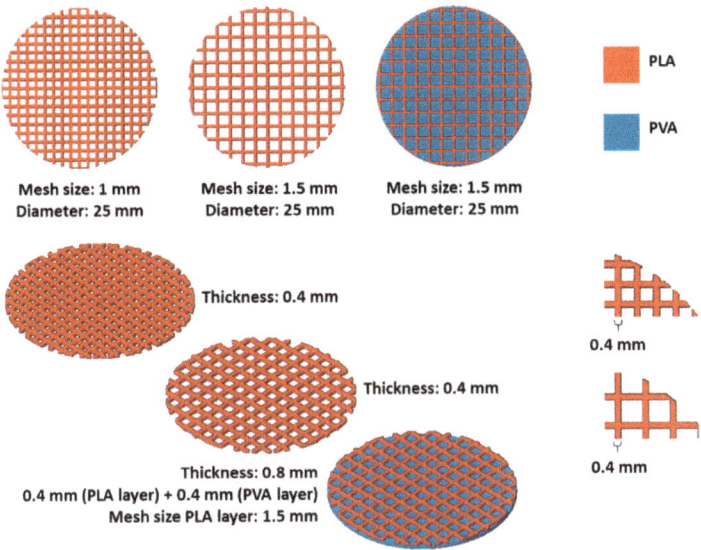

Figure 1. Scheme of the different meshes produced using FFF.

2.7. Antioxidant Activity

DPPH (2,2-diphenyl-1-picrylhydrozyl) radical was employed to measure the antioxidant activity of 3D printed materials based on the radical scavenging property of the LIG [33]. Briefly, 3 mL of a DPPH solution dissolved in methanol (23.6 mg/L) was added to the 3D printed samples (a square of 1 cm × 1 cm × 0.1 cm) placed in a 24-well plate. A control sample of 23.6 mg/L of DPPH in methanol was also measured. The samples were then incubated in the dark for 300 min at room temperature. At predetermined time intervals (each 60 min), 300 μL samples were collected and the well was immediately replenished with an equivalent volume of methanol. The absorbance of the different solutions was measured at 517 nm in triplicate using a UV–vis plate reader (PowerWave XS Microplate Spectrophotometer, Bio-Tek, Winooski, VT, USA). The residual DPPH content in the solution was calculated using Equation (1)

$$\text{Residual DPPH content (\%)} = 100 - 100\,(A_0 - A_1/A_0) \tag{1}$$

where A_0 is the absorbance of the control sample and A_1 is the absorbance in the presence of the sample at any time. Decreased absorbance of the reaction indicates a stronger DPPH radical scavenging activity.

2.8. Antimicrobial Properties

The in vitro microbiological analysis was performed according to the previous published works [34,35]. In brief, a bacterial suspension of S. aureus (1×10^8 cfu mL^{-1}) in PBS and supplemented with 0.5% TSB (pH 7), was diluted (1:100) with PBS containing 0.5% TSB. Replicate samples of 3D printed squares (1 cm × 1 cm × 0.1 cm) were placed in individual wells of a 24-well plate and then aliquots of 1 mL of the diluted bacterial suspension with a density of 1×10^6 cfu mL^{-1} was added completely covering the 3D printed squares. The plate was continuously shaken in an orbital incubator at 37 °C for 24 h. Then the samples were removed from the 24-well plate containing the bacterial suspension and the non-adherent bacteria were removed by several washing steps, first in PBS (1 × 10 mL), and then in quarter-strength Ringer's solution (QSRS) (3 × 10 mL) [36]. After the wash step, 3D printed squares were transferred into fresh QSRS (5 mL), sonicated (15 min) and vortexed (30 s) to remove adherent bacteria. The sonication technique has previously been demonstrated not to affect bacterial viability or morphology [37]. A viable count of the QSRS was performed by the Miles and Misra serial dilution technique [38] followed by plating onto Mueller–Hinton agar to enumerate the previously adhered bacteria per sample.

2.9. Statistical Analysis

All data were expressed as mean ± standard deviation. Data were compared using a one-way analysis of variance (ANOVA), with Tukey's HSD post-hoc test. In all cases, $p < 0.05$ was the minimum value considered acceptable for rejection of the null hypothesis.

3. Results

3.1. PLA and LIG Composite Material Preparation and Characterization

The antioxidant capabilities of LIG have been reported multiple times in the past. Considering the potential health benefits associated with antioxidant materials, LIG has potential to be combined with 3D printable biocompatible polymers for biomedical applications. For this purpose, PLA was selected as the ideal material to be combined with LIG. It has been extensively used for FFF 3D printing applications and it is biocompatible and biodegradable [7,9].

Hot melt extrusion was used to combine LIG and PLA to form a composite material. PLA was supplied in pellet form while LIG was supplied in powder form. To get a homogeneous mixture of both types of materials, a coating approach was used. Castor oil was used to coat the PLA pellets and, subsequently, LIG powder was added to the mixture. This method was described before to combine PLA with chemotherapeutic and antibiotic drugs. Figure 2A shows the image of the LIG coated pellets containing LIG concentrations ranging from 0.5% to 3% (w/w). When higher amounts of LIG were added, the pellets showed a higher coating degree. TC, an antibiotic compound with reported antioxidant capabilities, was combined with PLA and LIG. These pellets contained a 2% (w/w) of TC and 1% (w/w) of LIG. The coating of these pellets was homogeneous, as it can be seen in Figure 2A. Finally, 3% was the maximum LIG loading that was evaluated, as, in this case, the pellets were completely coated by LIG powder (Figure 2A).

PLA was combined with LIG and TC successfully using hot melt extrusion. Figure 2B shows fragments of the obtained filaments. Moreover, the filaments were successfully used for FFF application, as sshown in Figure 2C. Squares (1 cm × 1 cm) were successfully printed using the PLA/LIG composites. However, the filaments could be used successfully to prepare more complex geometries as it is illustrated in Figure 2D.

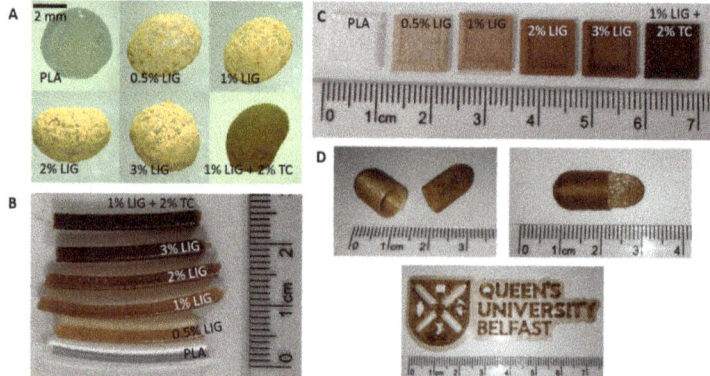

Figure 2. Photographs of: PLA and PLA coated pellets (**A**); LIG and TC containing PLA filaments (**B**); LIG and TC containing 1 cm × 1 cm squares prepared using 3D printing (**C**); and different shapes printed using the filament containing 2% (w/w) LIG (**D**).

The proposed method is a good alternative to combine PLA and LIG, as it provided a good mixture of both components and did not require the use of any solvents. In the past, LIG and PLA have been combined using a casting method [39]. This method requires the use of solvents that could present toxicity issues for healthcare applications.

LIG/PLA filaments showed lower resistance to fracture than PLA filaments. Figure 3A shows that the presence of LIG in the material reduced the maximum load that the materials can resist before fracture. There were no significant differences between the maximum load obtained for materials containing 0% and 0.5% (w/w) of LIG ($p = 0.506$). Interestingly, the maximum load dropped when the LIG content was increased from 0.5% to 1% (w/w) ($p < 0.05$). Moreover, when the LIG content reached 3%, the resulting materials showed higher resistance to fracture ($p < 0.05$).

The surface properties of the 3D printed materials were evaluated. Figure 3B shows the contact angle of water with the material surface. Interestingly, there were no significant differences between the contact angles obtained for PLA + castor oil and the materials containing up to 1% of LIG ($p > 0.05$). Castor oil did not influence in the contact angle of the materials. The obtained contact angles for PLA and PLA/castor oil showed no significant differences between them ($p = 0.995$). However, the materials showed a noticeable reduction in their wettability when the LIG content was increased up to 2% (w/w). The measured contact angle between materials containing 2% and 3% of LIG were significantly lower than the previously described materials ($p < 0.05$). Additionally, the obtained contact angles for these materials showed similar values.

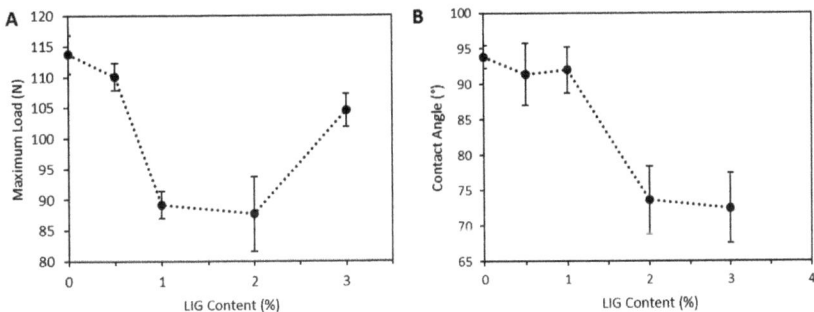

Figure 3. Maximum load before fracture for LIG containing filaments ($n = 5$) (**A**); and contact angle of water with the surface of 3D printed materials obtained using PLA/LIG composites ($n = 4$) (**B**).

The materials were analyzed using FTIR spectroscopy (data not shown). No differences were observed in the spectra of pure PLA and LIG containing materials. This is due to the lower LIG loading within the materials. DSC measurements were performed to evaluate the interaction between LIG and PLA. Figure 4A shows the DSC thermograms of LIG, PLA, castor oil and the 3D printed PLA/LIG composites. This figure shows that PLA/LIG composites showed the same transitions that can be observed for PLA. The first transition observed was a glass transition (T_g) at ca. 65 °C. PLA melting point was observed at ca. 180 °C. When LIG was incorporated into the material, a reduction in the T_g was observed (Figure 4B,C). The materials containing 0.5% and 1% of LIG showed almost the same T_g value as pure PLA. However, when LIG loading increased up to 2%, a T_g reduction was observed (Figure 4B,C). Composite materials containing 3% of LIG showed similar behavior. Interestingly, the melting temperature of the materials was not affected by the LIG presence. Finally, the stability studies showed that the materials did not lose weight after 30 days in PBS ($p < 0.05$) (data not shown).

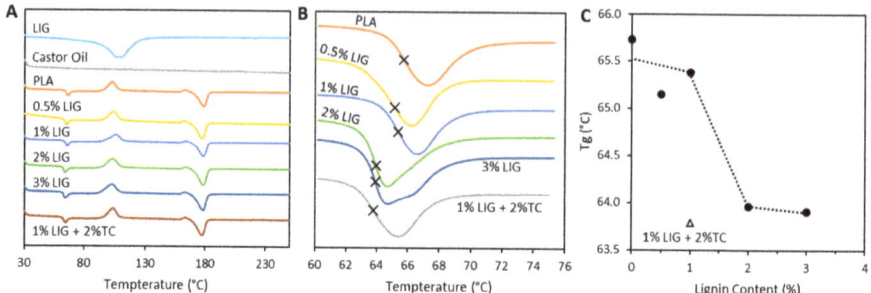

Figure 4. DSC thermograms obtained for LIG, PLA, castor oil and the resulting PLA/LIG and TC composites (**A**); expanded view of the thermogram between 60 and 76 °C (**B**); and T_g variation as a function of the LIG content (**C**).

3.2. PLA and LIG Composite Antioxidant and Antimicrobial Properties

Figure 5A shows the radical scavenging activity of PLA/LIG 3D printed composites. The presence of LIG in the material gave the material antioxidant properties. PLA and PLA + castor oil based materials did not show a DPPH concentration reduction over time. Moreover, materials containing LIG showed higher radical scavenging activity as the presence of DPPH decreased over time. This indicates that the presence of LIG provides the antioxidant activity to the materials. As expected, materials with higher LIG content showed higher antioxidant activity as they were more efficient in reducing the DPPH concentration over time.

It has been reported previously that LIG has antimicrobial activity. Accordingly, the antimicrobial capabilities of the 3D printed materials were evaluated by studying bacterial adhesion. The adhesion of *S. aureus* to the material was evaluated (Figure 5B). When comparing the bacterial adhesion of PLA/castor oil (blank) and the 3D printed material containing 1% (w/w) LIG, there were no significant differences ($p = 0.980$). Accordingly, it can be established that the presence of 1% (w/w) LIG did not provide any antimicrobial capabilities to the material. Moreover, similar results were obtained for higher concentrations of LIG ($p > 0.05$) (data not shown). Accordingly, we can establish that the selected concentrations of LIG were not adding any antimicrobial capabilities to the composite materials. However, the addition of the TC showed significant reductions in bacterial adherence (Figure 5B) ($p = 0.001$). TC is an antibiotic compound and accordingly can reduce the bacterial load attached to the surface of the material.

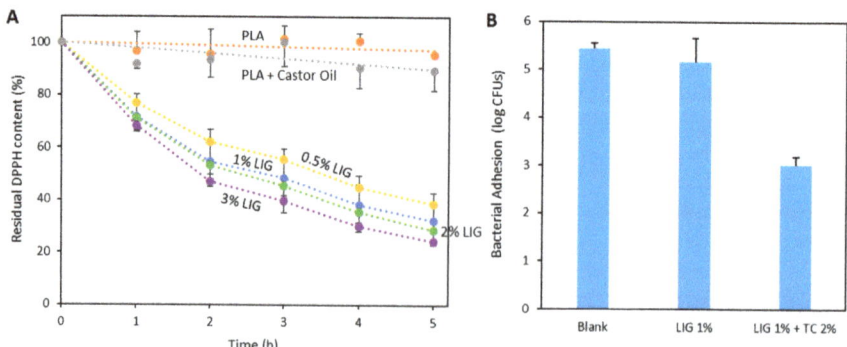

Figure 5. Residual DPPH content as a function of time for the LIG containing composites ($n = 3$) (**A**); and bacterial adhesion to the PLA/LIG and PLA/LIG/TC composites ($n = 3$) (**B**).

3.3. 3D Printed PLA and LIG Composite Meshes for Potential Wound Healing Applications

As described previously, antioxidant materials can be extremely beneficial for healthcare applications such as wound healing. Accordingly, the proposed materials can be easily integrated in wound dressings. For this purpose, 3D printed meshes were prepared using PLA/LIG composite materials. These meshes can provide mechanical protection to the wound while providing antioxidant activity. Due to their design, soluble patches containing drugs can be applied to the surface of the mesh. The drug can diffuse through the mesh pores to the wound. An experimental setup was prepared to evaluate the delivery of an antioxidant and wound healing model compound, CUR (Figure 6A). Two different types of meshes were prepared containing two different grid sizes (1 and 1.5 mm) (Figure 6B). As shown in Figure 6B, the materials were flexible and thus could adapt to the surface of the wound.

Figure 6C shows the permeation of CUR through the meshes. The 1.5 mm meshes provided a slower CUR release than the control (CUR containing film alone). This effect was more substantial when the mesh size was reduced to 1 mm (Figure 6D). Moreover, the release rate could be delayed by combining the mesh with a soluble PVA film. The PVA film could be printed in combination with the LIG/PLA mesh using fuse deposition modeling equipment equipped with a dual extruder. Figure 6C shows how the incorporation of a PVA film with a LIG/PLA mesh delayed CUR release.

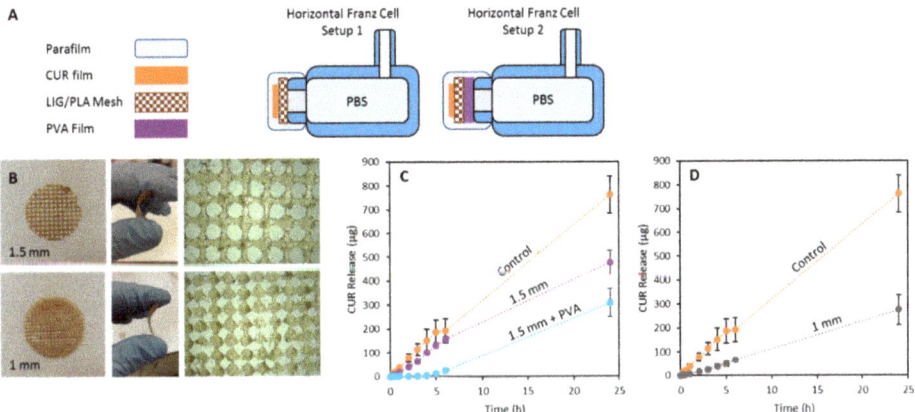

Figure 6. Experimental setup used to measure drug diffusion trough the 3D printed meshes (**A**); photographs of the 3D printed meshes made of PLA and 2% (w/w) LIG (**B**); and CUR release through 1.5 mm (**C**) and 1 mm (**D**) 3D printed meshes ($n = 3$).

4. Discussion

Human population growth and industrial development are generating an increasing demand for polymeric materials. The majority of these types of materials are derived from the petrochemical industry and, accordingly, they have an enormous impact on the environment [40]. Therefore, the scientific community is developing green and sustainable alternatives to the traditional polymeric materials [17]. As mentioned previously, LIG has potential to be used as a functional additive due to its interesting properties.

The antioxidant properties of LIG can be used for potential healthcare related applications such as wound healing. Reactive oxygen species are strongly linked to the pathogenesis of chronic wounds [41]. Accordingly, as antioxidant materials contribute to reduce the concentration of these species, they have potential to be applied as wound healing materials. Moreover, it has been shown that LIG nanofibrous dressings contribute to wound healing [42].

PLA is a biocompatible and biodegradable material. Accordingly, by combining it with LIG materials, added value can be obtained. Due to the flexibility of PLA for 3D printing applications, the resulting composite materials can be produced in any shape. This allows physicians to prepare dressing for patients on demand modifying the size and shape. Finally, due to the biodegradable nature of PLA, the combination of PLA and LIG yields green materials.

The present work showed that PLA and LIG can be combined easily by coating PLA pellets with LIG. Other alternatives to prepare PLA/LIG composites have been explored but they require organic solvents or more complex equipment such as twin screws extruders [39,43,44].

Ye et al. described a method to prepare LIG/PLA composites by using a casting method. In this work, they achieved higher LIG loadings [39]. The composite materials described in that work showed similar properties to those described in this paper. Their PLA-based composites showed a contact angle reduction for the composites containing higher LIG loadings [39]. In the present work, the 3D printed composites containing 3% (w/w) and 2% (w/w) of LIG showed contact angles of ca. 75° (Figure 3B). In contrast, Ye et al. reported loadings of up to 20% (w/w) to obtain a similar effect. Accordingly, LIG improve the wettability of the materials. Moreover, Ye et al. did not report any T_g changes for the composites. In the present work, materials containing LIG contents $\geq$2% (w/w) showed a T_g reduction (Figure 4). Accordingly, it can be established that small amounts of LIG can contribute to change PLA chain mobility within the glass transition region [43]. Similar behavior was observed by Kai et al. [45].

Moreover, the mechanical properties of the resulting material showed that the produced LIG containing filaments showed lower resistance to load than pure PLA. However, this effect was not obvious for composites containing 3% (w/w) of LIG. In this case, the materials showed an increase in the maximum load before fracture.

The antioxidant properties of LIG-containing 3D printed materials were evaluated by using the DPPH assay (Figure 5A). Similarly, Kai et al. investigated the antioxidant properties of PLA and LIG nanofibers [45]. They obtained DPPH concentration reductions up to ca. 60% after 72 h [45]. However, in the present study, after 5 h, the DPPH concentration reduction was ca. 80%. Moreover, these nanofibers contained up to 50% (w/w) LIG. Accordingly, the materials described in the present papers showed a more efficient antioxidant capability. There are a wide variety of antioxidant compounds described in the literature, such as resveratrol or curcumin. However, these compounds are generally expensive. Considering that LIG can be considered a reduced cost additive [29], the combination of PLA with LIG is a more viable option to obtain antioxidant 3D printable composites. Finally, there are a wide variety of wood-based filaments for FFF. These products are made using PLA, ABS or similar polymers combined with wood particles or sawdust [46]. The antioxidant compounds from wood need to be isolated before they can have its effect [47]. Therefore, the direct combination of LIG with PLA seems to be the best approach to obtain low-cost green 3D printable biomaterials with antioxidant properties.

The present method used to obtain LIG containing filaments for 3D printing application can be used to incorporate multiple compounds. It was demonstrated that an antibiotic, TC, can be incorporated into the filaments (Figure 2). Accordingly, the materials containing 2% (w/w) of TC showed effective reduction of S. aureus adhesion to the materials (Figure 5B). Moreover, LIG did not show any antibacterial activity in this case. It has been reported in the past that LIG can be added to materials to provide antibacterial activity against Gram-positive (S. aureus) and Gram-negative (P. mirabilis) bacteria [21]. However, the present study showed that LIG did not provide antibacterial activity at the selected concentrations. Accordingly, LIG and TC can be combined effectively with PLA to provide antioxidant and antimicrobial activities. This combination of molecules is extremely beneficial for wound dressings for chronic wounds as the materials can contribute to wound healing and to prevent infections.

Finally, the selected materials can be easily shaped as meshes (Figure 6B). These meshes can be adapted to the wound site due to their flexibility while providing some degree of protection. Moreover, the mesh design can be used to administer therapeutic compounds through the pores to the wound surface. In the present work, we used CUR as a model molecule. CUR has been extensively used for wound healing purposes [48]. Accordingly, films containing CUR were prepared and its permeation through the meshes was studied (Figure 6C,D). As expected, the permeation of CUR through the meshes was slower than the dissolution of a disc containing CUR alone. Moreover, permeation through the 1.5 mm meshes was quicker than the permeation through 1 mm ones. By controlling the geometry, the permeation rate can be controlled. Accordingly, this can be adapted to the needs of the patients.

Modern FFF systems contain a two-nozzle configuration that can be used to prepare devices containing two different materials. In the present work, we designed a combined patch that contained a PVA film in contact with the release medium. In this way, a delayed release was obtained (Figure 6C). This PVA film could play a double role, providing a moist environment to the wound while delaying and controlling the CUR release. It has been reported previously that a moist wound environment improves the wound closure while reducing pain and scar formation [49].

Overall, the present paper describes a simple method to combine an antioxidant renewable compound, LIG, with PLA for 3D printing applications. A potential scenario for this material is as a wound dressing material due to the antioxidant activity of the composite material that can contribute to wound closure. Due to the low price of 3D printing equipment and its versatility, these materials can be used in hospitals to print wound dressings for patients on demand.

There are more potential applications for these environmentally-friendly materials. A clear example of this is food packaging. There are some antioxidants on the market that can be combined with plastics for food packaging [50,51]. Antioxidant packaging can be used to improve the condition and increase the shelf-life of packaged food. Due to the enhanced cell proliferation on antioxidant materials [16], these materials can be used for tissue culture applications or even for regenerative medicine. Due to the versatility of FFF, complex geometries can be prepared such as scaffolds. However, before this type of materials can be implanted into humans, the safety of lignin-based materials should be evaluated. It has been reported before that LIG-based materials are biocompatible [45] but more studies should be performed.

Author Contributions: Conceptualization, J.D.-R. and E.L.; methodology, J.D.-R., E.L., M.I.R.-H. and N.J.I.; investigation and formal analysis, M.L.F., N.K.M. and S.A.S.; data curation, E.L. and J.D.-R.; writing, E.L. and J.D.-R.; writing—review and editing, E.L. and S.A.S.; and supervision, E.L. and R.F.D.

Funding: This work was supported by the Wellcome Trust Biomedical Vacation Scholarship (SS 213361/Z/18/Z) and the Society for Applied Microbiology Student Placement Scholarship.

Conflicts of Interest: The authors declare no conflict of interest.

References

1. Capel, A.J.; Rimington, R.P.; Lewis, M.P.; Christie, S.D.R. 3D Printing for Chemical, Pharmaceutical and Biological Applications. *Nat. Rev. Chem.* **2018**, *2*, 422–436. [CrossRef]
2. McIlroy, C.; Olmsted, P.D. Disentanglement Effects on Welding Behaviour of Polymer Melts during the Fused-Filament-Fabrication Method for Additive Manufacturing. *Polymer* **2017**, *123*, 376–391. [CrossRef]
3. Goyanes, A.; Buanz, A.B.; Basit, A.W.; Gaisford, S. Fused-Filament 3D Printing (3DP) for Fabrication of Tablets. *Int. J. Pharm.* **2014**, *476*, 88–92. [CrossRef] [PubMed]
4. Baumann, F.; Bugdayci, H.; Grunert, J.; Keller, F.; Roller, D. Influence of Slicing Tools on Quality of 3D Printed Parts. *Comput. Aided Des. Appl.* **2016**, *13*, 14–31. [CrossRef]
5. Jamroz, W.; Szafraniec, J.; Kurek, M.; Jachowicz, R. 3D Printing in Pharmaceutical and Medical Applications—Recent Achievements and Challenges. *Pharm. Res.* **2018**, *35*, 176. [CrossRef] [PubMed]
6. Trenfield, S.J.; Awad, A.; Goyanes, A.; Gaisford, S.; Basit, A.W. 3D Printing Pharmaceuticals: Drug Development to Frontline Care. *Trends Pharmacol. Sci.* **2018**, *39*, 440–451. [CrossRef] [PubMed]
7. Stewart, A.S.; DomÃnguez-Robles, J.; Donnelly, F.R.; LarraÃ±eta, E. Implantable Polymeric Drug Delivery Devices: Classification, Manufacture, Materials, and Clinical Applications. *Polymers* **2018**, *10*, 1379. [CrossRef]

8. Chiulan, I.; Frone, A.N.; Brandabur, C.; Panaitescu, D.M. Recent Advances in 3D Printing of Aliphatic Polyesters. *Bioengineering* **2017**, *5*, 2. [CrossRef] [PubMed]
9. Farah, S.; Anderson, D.G.; Langer, R. Physical and Mechanical Properties of PLA, and their Functions in Widespread Applications—A Comprehensive Review. *Adv. Drug Deliv. Rev.* **2016**, *107*, 367–392. [CrossRef]
10. Weisman, J.A.; Nicholson, J.C.; Tappa, K.; Jammalamadaka, U.; Wilson, C.G.; Mills, D.K. Antibiotic and Chemotherapeutic Enhanced Three-Dimensional Printer Filaments and Constructs for Biomedical Applications. *Int. J. Nanomed.* **2015**, *10*, 357–370. [PubMed]
11. Barapatre, A.; Aadil, K.R.; Tiwary, B.N.; Jha, H. In Vitro Antioxidant and Antidiabetic Activities of Biomodified Lignin from Acacia Nilotica Wood. *Int. J. Biol. Macromol.* **2015**, *75*, 81–89. [CrossRef] [PubMed]
12. van Lith, R.; Gregory, E.K.; Yang, J.; Kibbe, M.R.; Ameer, G.A. Engineering Biodegradable Polyester Elastomers with Antioxidant Properties to Attenuate Oxidative Stress in Tissues. *Biomaterials* **2014**, *35*, 8113–8122. [CrossRef] [PubMed]
13. Dhall, S.; Do, D.; Garcia, M.; Wijesinghe, D.S.; Brandon, A.; Kim, J.; Sanchez, A.; Lyubovitsky, J.; Gallagher, S.; Nothnagel, E.A.; et al. A Novel Model of Chronic Wounds: Importance of Redox Imbalance and Biofilm-Forming Bacteria for Establishment of Chronicity. *PLoS ONE* **2014**, *9*, e109848. [CrossRef] [PubMed]
14. Dhall, S.; Do, D.C.; Garcia, M.; Kim, J.; Mirebrahim, S.H.; Lyubovitsky, J.; Lonardi, S.; Nothnagel, E.A.; Schiller, N.; Martins-Green, M. Generating and Reversing Chronic Wounds in Diabetic Mice by Manipulating Wound Redox Parameters. *J. Diabetes Res.* **2014**, *2014*, 562625. [CrossRef] [PubMed]
15. van Lith, R.; Baker, E.; Ware, H.; Yang, J.; Farsheed, A.C.; Sun, C.; Ameer, G. 3D-Printing Strong High-Resolution Antioxidant Bioresorbable Vascular Stents. *Adv. Mater. Technol.* **2016**, *1*, 1600138. [CrossRef]
16. Lücking, T.H.; Sambale, F.; Schnaars, B.; Bulnes-Abundis, D.; Beutel, S.; Scheper, T. 3D-Printed Individual Labware in Biosciences by Rapid Prototyping: In Vitro Biocompatibility and Applications for Eukaryotic Cell Cultures. *Eng. Life Sci.* **2015**, *15*, 57–64. [CrossRef]
17. Kai, D.; Tan, M.J.; Chee, P.L.; Chua, Y.K.; Yap, Y.L.; Loh, X.J. Towards Lignin-Based Functional Materials in a Sustainable World. *Green Chem.* **2016**, *18*, 1175–1200. [CrossRef]
18. Thakur, V.K.; Thakur, M.K. Recent Advances in Green Hydrogels from Lignin: A Review. *Int. J. Biol. Macromol.* **2015**, *72*, 834–847. [CrossRef] [PubMed]
19. Sánchez, R.; Espinosa, E.; Domínguez-Robles, J.; Loaiza, J.M.; Rodríguez, A. Isolation and Characterization of Lignocellulose Nanofibers from Different Wheat Straw Pulps. *Int. J. Biol. Macromol.* **2016**, *92*, 1025–1033. [CrossRef] [PubMed]
20. Liu, D.; Li, Y.; Qian, Y.; Xiao, Y.; Du, S.; Qiu, X. Synergistic Antioxidant Performance of Lignin and Quercetin Mixtures. *ACS Sustain. Chem. Eng.* **2017**, *5*, 8424–8428. [CrossRef]
21. Larrañeta, E.; Imízcoz, M.; Toh, J.X.; Irwin, N.J.; Ripolin, A.; Perminova, A.; Domínguez-Robles, J.; Rodríguez, A.; Donnelly, R.F. Synthesis and Characterization of Lignin Hydrogels for Potential Applications as Drug Eluting Antimicrobial Coatings for Medical Materials. *ACS Sustain. Chem. Eng.* **2018**, *6*, 9037–9046. [CrossRef] [PubMed]
22. Pucciariello, R.; Bonini, C.; D'Auria, M.; Villani, V.; Giammarino, G.; Gorrasi, G. Polymer Blends of Steam-Explosion Lignin and Poly(E-Caprolactone) by High-Energy Ball Milling. *J. Appl. Polym. Sci.* **2008**, *109*, 309–313. [CrossRef]
23. Dong, X.; Dong, M.; Lu, Y.; Turley, A.; Jin, T.; Wu, C. Antimicrobial and Antioxidant Activities of Lignin from Residue of Corn Stover to Ethanol Production. *Ind. Crops Prod.* **2011**, *34*, 1629–1634. [CrossRef]
24. Kai, D.; Low, Z.W.; Liow, S.; Abdul Karim, A.; Ye, H.; Jin, G.; Li, K.; Loh, X.J. Development of Lignin Supramolecular Hydrogels with Mechanically Responsive and Self-Healing Properties. *ACS Sustain. Chem. Eng.* **2015**, *3*, 2160–2169. [CrossRef]
25. Domínguez-Robles, J.; Sánchez, R.; Díaz-Carrasco, P.; Espinosa, E.; García-Domínguez, M.T.; Rodríguez, A. Isolation and Characterization of Lignins from Wheat Straw: Application as Binder in Lithium Batteries. *Int. J. Biol. Macromol.* **2017**, *104*, 909–918. [CrossRef] [PubMed]
26. Azadfar, M.; Gao, A.H.; Bule, M.V.; Chen, S. Structural Characterization of Lignin: A Potential Source of Antioxidants Guaiacol and 4-Vinylguaiacol. *Int. J. Biol. Macromol.* **2015**, *75*, 58–66. [CrossRef] [PubMed]
27. Kai, D.; Zhang, K.; Jiang, L.; Wong, H.Z.; Li, Z.; Zhang, Z.; Loh, X.J. Sustainable and Antioxidant Lignin-Polyester Copolymers and Nanofibers for Potential Healthcare Applications. *ACS Sustain. Chem. Eng.* **2017**, *5*, 6016–6025. [CrossRef]

28. Stewart, D. Lignin as a Base Material for Materials Applications: Chemistry, Application and Economics. *Ind. Crops Prod.* **2008**, *27*, 202–207. [CrossRef]
29. Jönsson, A.S.; Wallberg, O. Cost Estimates of Kraft Lignin Recovery by Ultrafiltration. *Desalination* **2009**, *237*, 254–267. [CrossRef]
30. Domínguez-Robles, J.; Peresin, M.S.; Tamminen, T.; Rodríguez, A.; Larrañeta, E.; Jääskeläinen, A.S. Lignin-Based Hydrogels with "super-Swelling" Capacities for Dye Removal. *Int. J. Biol. Macromol.* **2018**, *115*, 1249–1259. [CrossRef]
31. Figueiredo, P.; Lintinen, K.; Kiriazis, A.; Hynninen, V.; Liu, Z.; Bauleth-Ramos, T.; Rahikkala, A.; Correia, A.; Kohout, T.; Sarmento, B.; et al. In Vitro Evaluation of Biodegradable Lignin-Based Nanoparticles for Drug Delivery and Enhanced Antiproliferation Effect in Cancer Cells. *Biomaterials* **2017**, *121*, 97–108. [CrossRef] [PubMed]
32. Erakovic, S.; Jankovic, A.; Tsui, G.C.; Tang, C.Y.; Miskovic-Stankovic, V.; Stevanovic, T. Novel Bioactive Antimicrobial Lignin Containing Coatings on Titanium obtained by Electrophoretic Deposition. *Int. J. Mol. Sci.* **2014**, *15*, 12294–12322. [CrossRef] [PubMed]
33. Qazi, S.S.; Li, D.; Briens, C.; Berruti, F.; Abou-Zaid, M.M. Antioxidant Activity of the Lignins Derived from Fluidized-Bed Fast Pyrolysis. *Molecules* **2017**, *22*, 372. [CrossRef] [PubMed]
34. Larrañeta, E.; Henry, M.; Irwin, N.J.; Trotter, J.; Perminova, A.A.; Donnelly, R.F. Synthesis and Characterization of Hyaluronic Acid Hydrogels Crosslinked using a Solvent-Free Process for Potential Biomedical Applications. *Carbohydr. Polym.* **2018**, *181*, 1194–1205. [CrossRef] [PubMed]
35. McCoy, C.P.; Irwin, N.J.; Brady, C.; Jones, D.S.; Carson, L.; Andrews, G.P.; Gorman, S.P. An Infection-Responsive Approach to Reduce Bacterial Adhesion in Urinary Biomaterials. *Mol. Pharm.* **2016**, *13*, 2817–2822. [CrossRef] [PubMed]
36. Wang, R.; Neoh, K.G.; Shi, Z.; Kang, E.T.; Tambyah, P.A.; Chiong, E. Inhibition of Escherichia Coli and Proteus Mirabilis Adhesion and Biofilm Formation on Medical Grade Silicone Surface. *Biotechnol. Bioeng.* **2012**, *109*, 336–345. [CrossRef]
37. Jones, D.S.; McGovern, J.G.; Woolfson, A.D.; Gorman, S.P. Role of Physiological Conditions in the Oropharynx on the Adherence of Respiratory Bacterial Isolates to Endotracheal Tube Poly(Vinyl Chloride). *Biomaterials* **1997**, *18*, 503–510. [CrossRef]
38. Miles, A.A.; Misra, S.S.; Irwin, J.O. The Estimation of the Bactericidal Power of the Blood. *J. Hyg.* **1938**, *38*, 732–749. [CrossRef] [PubMed]
39. Ye, H.; Zhang, Y.; Yu, Z. Effect of Desulfonation of Lignosulfonate on the Properties of Poly(Lactic Acid)/Lignin Composites. *Bioresources* **2017**, *12*, 4810–4829. [CrossRef]
40. Thompson, R.C.; Moore, C.J.; vom Saal, F.S.; Swan, S.H. Plastics, the Environment and Human Health: Current Consensus and Future Trends. *Philos. Trans. R. Soc. Lond. B. Biol. Sci.* **2009**, *364*, 2153–2166. [CrossRef] [PubMed]
41. Moseley, R.; Walker, M.; Waddington, R.J.; Chen, W.Y. Comparison of the Antioxidant Properties of Wound Dressing Materials—Carboxymethylcellulose, Hyaluronan Benzyl Ester and Hyaluronan, Towards Polymorphonuclear Leukocyte-Derived Reactive Oxygen Species. *Biomaterials* **2003**, *24*, 1549–1557. [CrossRef]
42. Reesi, F.; Minaiyan, M.; Taheri, A. A Novel Lignin-Based Nanofibrous Dressing Containing Arginine for Wound-Healing Applications. *Drug Deliv. Transl. Res.* **2018**, *8*, 111–122. [CrossRef] [PubMed]
43. Wang, X.; Jia, Y.; Liu, Z.; Miao, J. Influence of the Lignin Content on the Properties of Poly(Lactic Acid)/Lignin-Containing Cellulose Nanofibrils Composite Films. *Polymers* **2018**, *10*, 1013. [CrossRef]
44. Li, H.; Legros, N.; Ton-That, M.; Rakotovelo, A. PLA-Thermoplastic Lignin Blends. *Plast. Eng.* **2013**, *69*, 60–64. [CrossRef]
45. Kai, D.; Ren, W.; Tian, L.; Chee, P.L.; Liu, Y.; Ramakrishna, S.; Loh, X.J. Engineering Poly(Lactide)-Lignin Nanofibers with Antioxidant Activity for Biomedical Application. *ACS Sustain. Chem. Eng.* **2016**, *4*, 5268–5276. [CrossRef]
46. Kariz, M.; Sernek, M.; Obućina, M.; Kuzman, M.K. Effect of Wood Content in FDM Filament on Properties of 3D Printed Parts. *Mater. Today Comm.* **2018**, *14*, 135–140. [CrossRef]

47. Meullemiestre, A.; Kamal, I.; Maache-Rezzoug, Z.; Chemat, F.; Rezzoug, S.A. Antioxidant Activity and Total Phenolic Content of Oils Extracted from Pinus Pinaster Sawdust Waste. Screening of Different Innovative Isolation Techniques. *Waste Biomass Valorization* **2014**, *5*, 283–292. [CrossRef]
48. Tejada, S.; Manayi, A.; Daglia, M.; Nabavi, S.F.; Sureda, A.; Hajheydari, Z.; Gortzi, O.; Pazoki-Toroudi, H.; Nabavi, S.M. Wound Healing Effects of Curcumin: A Short Review. *Curr. Pharm. Biotechnol.* **2016**, *17*, 1002–1007. [CrossRef]
49. Ajalloueian, F.; Tavanai, H.; Hilborn, J.; Donzel-Gargand, O.; Leifer, K.; Wickham, A.; Arpanaei, A. Emulsion Electrospinning as an Approach to Fabricate PLGA/Chitosan Nanofibers for Biomedical Applications. *Biomed. Res. Int.* **2014**, *2014*, 475280. [CrossRef]
50. Cherif Lahimer, M.; Ayed, N.; Horriche, J.; Belgaied, S. Characterization of Plastic Packaging Additives: Food Contact, Stability and Toxicity. *Arab. J. Chem.* **2017**, *10*, S1938–S1954. [CrossRef]
51. Addivant's Weston 705 Antioxidant Gains Food Contact Approval in Mercosur Region. *Addit. Polym.* **2018**, *2018*, 3–4. [CrossRef]

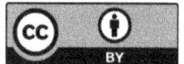

© 2019 by the authors. Licensee MDPI, Basel, Switzerland. This article is an open access article distributed under the terms and conditions of the Creative Commons Attribution (CC BY) license (http://creativecommons.org/licenses/by/4.0/).

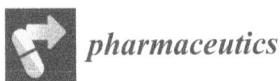

Article

3D Printing of Drug-Loaded Thermoplastic Polyurethane Meshes: A Potential Material for Soft Tissue Reinforcement in Vaginal Surgery

Juan Domínguez-Robles [1,†], Caterina Mancinelli [1,2,†], Elena Mancuso [3], Inmaculada García-Romero [4], Brendan F. Gilmore [1], Luca Casettari [2], Eneko Larrañeta [1,*] and Dimitrios A. Lamprou [1,*]

1. School of Pharmacy, Queen's University Belfast, Lisburn Road 97, Belfast BT9 7BL, UK; j.dominguezrobles@qub.ac.uk (J.D.-R.); c.mancinelli3@campus.uniurb.it (C.M.); b.gilmore@qub.ac.uk (B.F.G.)
2. Department of Biomolecular Sciences, University of Urbino Carlo Bo, Piazza del Rinascimento 6, 61029 Urbino, Italy; luca.casettari@uniurb.it
3. Nanotechnology and Integrated Bio-Engineering Centre (NIBEC), Ulster University, Jordanstown Campus, Jordanstown BT37 0QB, UK; e.mancuso@ulster.ac.uk
4. Wellcome-Wolfson Institute for Experimental Medicine, Queen's University Belfast, Belfast BT9 7BL, UK; I.Garcia-Romero@qub.ac.uk
* Correspondence: e.larraneta@qub.ac.uk (E.L.); d.lamprou@qub.ac.uk (D.A.L.)
† These authors contributed equally to this work.

Received: 20 December 2019; Accepted: 9 January 2020; Published: 13 January 2020

Abstract: Current strategies to treat pelvic organ prolapse (POP) or stress urinary incontinence (SUI), include the surgical implantation of vaginal meshes. Recently, there have been multiple reports of issues generated by these meshes conventionally made of poly(propylene). This material is not the ideal candidate, due to its mechanical properties leading to complications such as chronic pain and infection. In the present manuscript, we propose the use of an alternative material, thermoplastic polyurethane (TPU), loaded with an antibiotic in combination with fused deposition modelling (FDM) to prepare safer vaginal meshes. For this purpose, TPU filaments containing levofloxacin (LFX) in various concentrations (e.g., 0.25%, 0.5%, and 1%) were produced by extrusion. These filaments were used to 3D print vaginal meshes. The printed meshes were fully characterized through different tests/analyses such as fracture force studies, attenuated total reflection-Fourier transform infrared, thermal analysis, scanning electron microscopy, X-ray microcomputed tomography (µCT), release studies and microbiology testing. The results showed that LFX was uniformly distributed within the TPU matrix, regardless the concentration loaded. The mechanical properties showed that poly(propylene) (PP) is a tougher material with a lower elasticity than TPU, which seemed to be a more suitable material due to its elasticity. In addition, the printed meshes showed a significant bacteriostatic activity on both *Staphylococcus aureus* and *Escherichia coli* cultures, minimising the risk of infection after implanting them. Therefore, the incorporation of LFX to the TPU matrix can be used to prepare anti-infective vaginal meshes with enhanced mechanical properties compared with current PP vaginal meshes.

Keywords: 3D printing; fused deposition modelling; extrusion; vaginal meshes; mechanical properties; drug release; anti-infective devices; pelvic organ prolapse; stress urinary incontinence

1. Introduction

Pelvic organ prolapse (POP) and stress urinary incontinence (SUI), are two very common disorders affecting 30–40% of women worldwide, mainly with the increase in age [1]. Since the population is growing gradually older, with the passage of time there will be an increase in the incidence of POP of 46% between 2010 and 2050 [2]. Although they are not lethal diseases, these two pathologies negatively influence the quality of life of women, including their social, sexual, physical and psychological well-being [1,3]. The implantation of meshes to reinforce soft tissue defects and provide an additional support to prolapsed organs and viscera is a common approach to treat POP and SUI [4].

Vaginal meshes are commonly made of poly(propylene) (PP) or polyester, materials that are already used for hernia repair [5,6]. These materials are safe for hernia repair, but their safety was not properly tested for pelvic floor applications [5]. However, they were approved by the US FDA [5,6]. Since approval, multiple cases of complications associated to vaginal meshes have been reported [7]. The main problem for these meshes is the different structure and motility of the pelvic floor when compare with the abdominal wall. In addition to this, important movements and morphological changes occur during a woman's life, and as a result, the material used to repair the pelvic floor must be not only biocompatible, but also able to tolerate the stress and tension associated with such a dynamic environment and at the same time flexible and elastic [5].

PP is the main polymer used for the production of synthetic meshes for POP surgery due to its chemical stability and non-biodegradable property [8]. However, complications such as adhesion to the viscera and high inflammatory response found in the repair of the pelvic floor [8] have led researchers to study alternative solutions. Biodegradable/bioresorbable polymers, such as poly(caprolactone) or poly(lactic acid) (PLA), have been used for mesh implant application with mixed results [9–11]. In some cases, this type of implants can display mechanical failures due to their degradation. For example, PLA_{94} can present mechanical problems after 8 months [11]. Accordingly, non-biodegradable polymers seem to be a safer approach. Recently, it was reported that poly(urethane)-based meshes were safer and more suitable than PP for vaginal meshes production [12,13]. Accordingly, polyurethane-based polymers seem to be the ideal candidate for this application.

In addition to safer materials, new manufacturing methods can provide benefit to the resulting medical devices. A potential technology to produce the aforementioned meshes is 3D printing. This technology allows clinicians to prepare devices adapted to patient's anatomy and requirements [14–17]. Furthermore, a wide range of materials can be used for 3D printing applications. These materials include PLA, PP or nylon. PLA has been extensively used for biomedical applications and for 3D printing applications [18–20]. PLA is one of the most widely used materials for 3D printing (specifically for fused deposition modelling) [20,21]. However, as described before, due to its biodegradable nature, it is not the ideal candidate for vaginal mesh preparation. Interestingly, poly(urethane), a promising material for pelvic floor surgery, has been used before for 3D printing applications [14].

The flexibility of 3D printing also allows to combine polymeric materials with drugs to prepare drug eluting devices [14,19,22]. This is extremely useful for implantable devices that have a relatively high risk of infection [14,19,23]. If the device is loaded with antibiotics this will prevent bacterial colonisation of its surface preventing infections [14,19]. There are a wide variety of techniques within 3D printing technology [16]. In the present work, fused deposition modelling (FDM) was used. This technique relies on the extrusion of a polymeric filament trough a hot nozzle to prepare objects. To combine the polymers with drugs within the filament hot melt extrusion (HME) is needed. For this purpose, a drug substance and the selected polymer are melted inside a rotating screw to mix them and subsequently extrude them to form a filament [15]. This filament will be subsequently used for FDM applications.

The aim of this work is to develop a new generation of vaginal mesh implants. For this purpose, meshes will be prepared using thermoplastic poly(urethane) (TPU) and they will be loaded with an antibacterial agent, levofloxacin (LFX) (a drug commonly used to treat urinary infections), using fused deposition modelling (FDM). This technique is the most common type of 3D printing. Three different filaments of TPU containing 0.25%, 0.5%, and 1% of LFX were prepared through single hot-melt extruder in order to be used for the 3D Printing FDM process. Mechanical strength, drug release and antimicrobial properties were evaluated to confirm the efficiency of the meshes.

2. Materials and Methods

2.1. Materials

Elastollan® thermoplastic polyurethane (TPU) 80A pellets were used for this study and kindly provided by DistruPol Ltd. (A Univar Company, Co., Dublin, Ireland). Castor oil was purchased from Ransom, LFX ((S)-9-fluoro-2,3-dihydro-3-methyl-10-(4-methylpiperazin-1-yl)-7-oxo-7H-pyrido[1,2,3-de]-1,4-benzoxazine-6-carboxylic acid) >98% was obtained by Sigma–Aldrich, and the phosphate buffered saline (PBS) tablets pH 7.4 from Merck. The PP filament (2.85 mm diameter) was purchased from Verbatim (Tokyo, Japan).

2.2. Preparation of Thermoplastic Poly(urethane) (TPU) Filaments Containing Levofloxacin (LFX)

In order to 3D print meshes, filaments were prepared using the Hot-Melt Extrusion (HME) technique by combining the TPU with LFX. An oil method was used to ensure a homogeneous distribution of the drug on the pellet's surface. TPU pellets (30 g) were placed in 50 mL Falcon tubes and castor oil (30 µL) was added and vortexed for a few min in order for the pellets to be covered homogeneously by the oil. The pellets were transferred to a new 50 mL Falcon tubes to avoid drug wastage that could remain attached due to excess oil on the wall of the previous tubes, as previously reported [14]. Then, LFX was added in ratio of 0.25% w/w and the tube was vortexed in order to coat the pellets. Finally, the coated pellets were introduced in the filament extruder (3Devo, Utretch, The Netherlands) using an extrusion speed range of 3–5 rpm and a filament diameter of 2.85 mm. The temperature was regulated directly during the extrusion over four heaters between 170 °C and 200 °C. The same procedure was performed for preparing filaments containing 0.5% and 1% of LFX. The filament formed using only TPU, which used for the preparation of blank meshes, was manufactured introducing directly the pellets into the extruder. Formulations with their compositions to manufacture the filaments are presented in the Table 1.

Table 1. Composition of TPU filaments containing LFX.

Formulations	TPU (g)	Castor Oil (µL)	LFX (g)
TPU	30	-	-
0.25% LFX	30	30	0.075
0.50% LFX	30	30	0.15
1.00% LFX	30	30	0.3

2.3. Preparation of 3D Printed Meshes Containing LFX

Meshes were printed with the drug-loaded and unloaded filaments that previously prepared with the extruder, using an Ultimaker 3 (Ultimaker B.V., Geldermalsen, The Netherlands) fused filament fabrication (FFF) system, furnished of two extruders with a 0.4 mm nozzle, and Cura®software 3.0 (Ultimaker B.V., Geldermalsen, The Netherlands). Different models were designed through a CAD-based software. For the TPU meshes, the layer height was set at 0.1 mm with the in-fill setting on the software at 100%. The printing temperature was set at 190 °C and the printing speed was 12 mm/s. However, for the PP meshes, the printing temperature was set between 195 °C and 208 °C and the printing speed was 25 mm/s. These PP meshes were manufactured using the filament obtained from Verbatim (Tokyo, Japan).

2.4. Characterization of 3D Printed Meshes

2.4.1. Mechanical Properties

Meshes with 50 mm × 10 mm size were printed, and the fracture force was studied with TA.XTplus texture analyser (Stable Micro Systems, Surrey, UK). Each sample was vertically fixed with two clamps, with a distance between them of 40 mm, and stretched at a rate of 5 mm/s up to 200 mm. The experiment was repeated 4 times for each sample. The force/displacement curves were recorded, and different parameters were obtained. The elastic limit of the resulting meshes were obtained using the 0.2% offset method [24]. Additionally, the tensile stiffness was calculated from the force/displacement curves as the slope of the initial linear region [25].

2.4.2. Fourier Transform Infrared (FT-IR) Spectroscopy

The Fourier Transform Infrared (FT-IR) spectra of 1 cm × 1 cm meshes were recorded through a Spectrum Two™ instrument (Perkin Elmer, Waltham, MA, USA). The spectra were recorded between 4000 cm^{-1} and 600 cm^{-1} applying a resolution of 4 cm^{-1}; total of 32 scans were collected.

2.4.3. Thermogravimetric Analysis (TGA)

As the elastomer was subjected to high temperatures during the 3D-printing process, the thermal degradation behaviour of the polymer was examined. Thermogravimetric analysis (TGA) was performed to measure the weight loss of the TPU meshes containing LFX. For this purpose, a small fragment of these meshes (3 mg and 10 mg) was used. TGA was performed using a Q500 Thermogravimetric analysis (TA instruments, Bellingham, WA, USA). Scans were run at room temperature to 550 °C, at a speed rate of 10 °C/min under a nitrogen flow rate of 50 mL/min.

2.4.4. Scanning Electron Microscopy (SEM)

Scanning electron microscopy was used in order to investigate the surface morphologies of the 1 cm × 1 cm 3D-printed meshes containing 0.25%, 0.5% and 1% of LFX compared with the blank mesh, using samples before and after a 14-day release study. The meshes were examined using a Hitachi TM3030 SEM (Tokyo, Japan), and images were taken with a magnification of 50×, 60×, 80×, 300× and 500×. Additionally, a Leica EZ4 D digital microscope (Leica, Wetzlar, Germany) was used to examine the presence or not of drug aggregates within the extruded materials.

2.4.5. X-ray Microcomputed Tomography (μCT)

X-ray Microcomputed Tomography imaging was performed on 3D printed meshes using the same approach previously reported [14]. Briefly, all the samples were analysed by using a Bruker Skyscan 1275 (Bruker μCT, Kontich, Belgium), with a Hamamatsu L11871 source (40 kV, 250 μA). The meshes were mounted vertically on dental wax and positioned at 57.5 mm from the source, where camera to source distance was 286 mm. No filter was applied for an exposure time of 49 ms. The images generated were 1536 × 1944 pixels with a resolution of 17 μm per pixel. A total of 1056 images were taken in 0.2° steps around one hemisphere of the sample, with an average of 3 frames taken at each rotation step. Attenuation thresholding was conducted manually, in order to eliminate speckle around the samples. The same thresholding was applied within Bruker's CTAn software v.1.18, where the samples were further processed.

2.5. In Vitro Drug Release Studies

The release profile for the LFX was defined conducting release studies that allowed calculating the amount of drug eluted from the LFX-loaded meshes. Each sample was placed in Eppendorf's with 2 mL of PBS. Subsequently the Eppendorf's were located in a shaking incubator at 37 °C at 40 rpm. After 1, 2, 4, 24, 48, 72, 96 and 120 h the sample was removed from the tube, dried and relocated in a new Eppendorf containing 2 mL of fresh PBS. Further studies performed also in new samples for 7 and 14 days. The concentration of LFX was calculated after measuring the UV absorbance of the solution taken from the Eppendorf's with a UV–visible plate reader (PowerWave XS Microplate Spectrophotometer, Bio-Tek, Winooski, VT, USA) at a wavelength of 292 nm as previously reported [26]. For each concentration (control, 0.25%, 0.5% and 1%), 1 cm × 1 cm meshes were used in series of 4.

2.6. In Vitro Microbiological Analysis

Printed meshes (1 cm × 1 cm × 0.1 cm) were tested for inhibitory effect on bacterial cultures of *Staphylococcus aureus* NCTC 10788 (Gram-positive) and *Escherichia coli* NSM59 (Gram-negative). *E. coli* and *S. aureus* are examples of bacteria that can cause a variety of community-and hospital-acquired infections. This in vitro microbiological analysis was performed according to a previous published work, with some modifications [14]. Briefly, bacteria were grown overnight at 37 °C in Mueller–Hinton (MH) broth. For each bacterium, 50 µL of the overnight culture were added to 5 mL of MH soft agar. This mixture was vortexed and then poured on top of the MH agar plate. Finally, meshes were placed in the centre of the plate and incubated for 24 h at 37 °C. The inhibition zone caused for both bacterial strains was then measured in mm. Moreover, inoculated plates for each bacterial strain were also incubated as a positive control. The results were expressed as mean ± standard deviation of 5 replicates.

2.7. Statistical Analysis

Quantitative data were expressed as a mean ± standard deviation, $n \geq 3$. The statistical analysis was performed using a one-way analysis of variance (ANOVA), $p < 0.05$ was considered to be statistically significant.

3. Results

3.1. Preparation and Characterisation of TPU Filaments and Meshes Containing LFX

The extrusion of the TPU pellets containing the different LFX concentrations were used to produce smooth and flexible filaments of 2.85 mm in diameter (Figure 1A). The resulting materials contained different amounts of LFX ranging from 0.25% to 1% (w/w). All the filaments prepared using hot-melt extrusion showed the same translucent colour. No visible aggregates of drug were seen within the extruded materials. Considering that LFX is a white solid, this suggests that the antibiotic was mixed with the molten TPU within the extrusion process. Moreover, the results suggest that TPU and LFX can be mixed properly using a single screw extruder following the pellet coating method. Otherwise, more complicated equipment—such as a twin-screw extruder—will be required to mix the drug and the polymer properly.

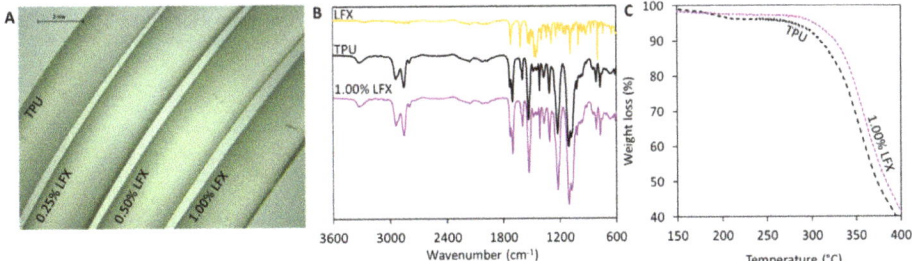

Figure 1. Microscopy image of the thermoplastic polyurethane (TPU) and levofloxacin (LFX)-loaded TPU filaments (**A**). FTIR spectra of LFX, TPU and TPU containing 1% of LFX (**B**). TGA of TPU and TPU containing 1% LFX (**C**).

FT-IR and TGA were used to try to establish if there was any interaction between TPU and LFX. The FT-IR spectra of the materials containing LFX showed the same peaks as the blank TPU (Figure 1B). The drug loadings selected for the present work were too low to be able to produce any changes in FT-IR spectra. However, TGA measurements (Figure 1C) show that when LFX was combined with TPU using hot melt extrusion, the resulting material presented different thermal degradation behaviour. Filaments containing LFX started to degrade at higher temperatures than the blank TPU filaments. In order to compare both materials, the onset temperatures (T_{onset}) were measured. T_{onset} denotes the temperature at which the weight loss begins (5% weight loss). The onset temperature for TPU was 280 °C, while the recorded onset temperature for TPU containing 1% of LFX was 303 °C. As mentioned before this temperature differences can be attributed to interactions between the TPU and the LFX.

The TPU filaments previously described were used to prepare different types of surgical meshes. These designs were prepared using Computer Aided Software and subsequently prepared using fused deposition modelling. Figure 2A shows the designs used to prepare the meshes with their dimensions. Moreover, Figure 2C shows some 1 × 1 cm mesh prototypes produced using the filaments described in Section 3.1. As expected, all these prototypes presented the same appearance as LFX was completely mixed with the TPU. These resulting meshes are flexible as can be seen in Figure 2B. These results can be corroborated by using SEM (Figure 2D). The microscopy images showed that all the resulting meshes showed the same structure and no signs of drug aggregation within the surface of the devices.

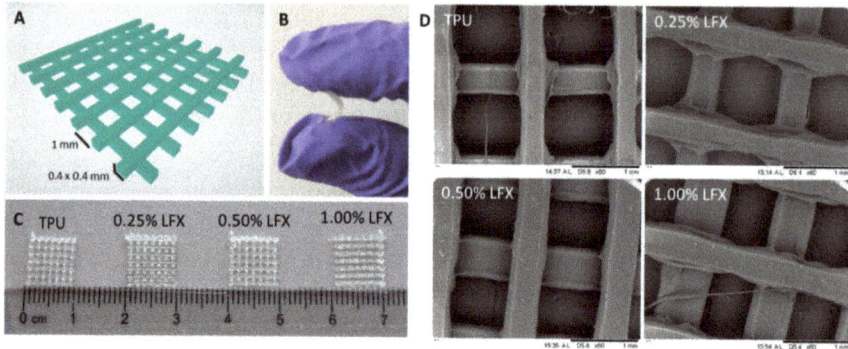

Figure 2. CAD 3D image of the two layer meshes with its dimensions (**A**). Representative image showing the flexibility of a TPU-based mesh (**B**). Image of TPU and TPU loaded with LFX 3D printed meshes (**C**). SEM images of TPU and LFX loaded TPU 3D printed meshes (**D**).

The 3D printed samples were analysed by using a Bruker Skyscan 1172 system (Figure 3), in order to investigate samples' topology as well as drug distribution within their architecture. As it could be seen in Figure 3B–D, the incorporation of LFX did not affect the 3D printed mesh morphology, which resulted very similar for all the analysed samples and comparable to the one of pure TPU80 (Figure 3A).

In addition, as shown in the representative reconstruction images, the meshes exhibited the same topology. Particularly, even at the highest concentration of LFX (Figure 3D), no traces of particles were detected within the printed meshes, thus indicating a uniform distribution of the drug, regardless the concentration tested. Moreover, according to this outcome it was further demonstrated the effectiveness of the manufacturing process from drug incorporation to 3D printed sample fabrication.

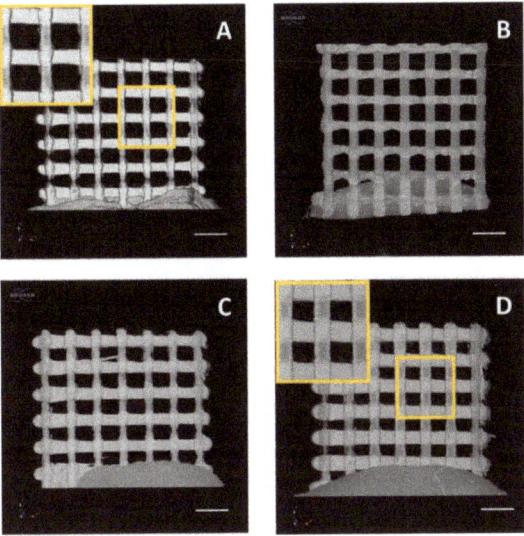

Figure 3. μCT reconstructions in the xz plane of pure TPU80 mesh (**A**) and TPU80 mesh loaded with 0.25% (**B**), 0.5% (**C**) and 1% (**D**) of LFX (scale bar = 2 mm).

3.2. Mechanical Characterisation of LFX 3D Printed Meshes

The mechanical properties of two-layered mesh implants prepared using fused deposition modelling were measured. Figure 4 shows representative force/displacement graphs for the prepared meshes. All the TPU-based meshes showed similar profiles. The first region of the graph showed elastic behaviour (initial linear section of the graph), and then when higher forces were applied the meshes showed plastic deformation (see Figure 4A,B). It is important to note that though they did not fully break under the testing conditions (200 mm of elongation), in some cases they show some minor fractures during the last stages of the test (Figure 4B). However, this does not happen consistently in all the meshes. This was observed only in two cases. It is important to note that these partial fractures happened after the mesh elongated more than three times its original size. On the other hand, meshes made of PP were prepared to compare the obtained results with the material typically used for mesh implant manufacturing. PP showed a different mechanical behaviour than TPU-based meshes. PP meshes failed during the test as they showed a clear and reproducible fracture point (Figure 4A).

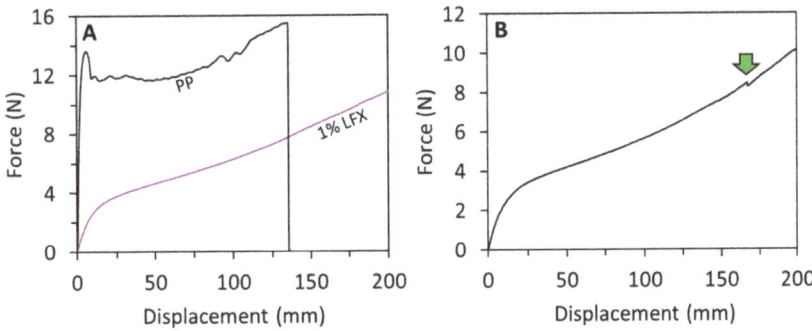

Figure 4. Force/displacement graphs obtained for TPU meshes containing 1% LFX and PP meshes (**A**). Force/displacement graph showing a small fracture for a TPU-based mesh (**B**). The arrow indicates the fracture point.

The elastic limit and the tensile stiffness were evaluated from the force/displacement curves. The elastic limit was measured from the force/displacement curves using the 0.2% offset method. This value represents the force required to produce a 0.2% of plastic deformation of the meshes. All TPU-based meshes showed elastic limits around 1 N (Table 2). Moreover, a statistical analysis showed that there were no significant differences between all these values ($p > 0.05$). These results suggest that LFX loadings of up to 1% (w/w) did not alter the mechanical properties of TPU. This is important for future applications, as TPU was selected due to its elasticity as opposed to conventional PP meshes. Polypropylene meshes showed significantly higher elastic limit than the TPU-based meshes ($p < 0.05$). This is consistent with the nature of the material that is not an elastic material as opposed to TPU. Finally, the tensile stiffness of the mesh implants was evaluated. Again, the results showed that all TPU-based meshes showed equivalent values of tensile stiffness ca. 0.4 N/mm ($p > 0.05$). Moreover, PP meshes showed significantly higher values of tensile stiffness ($p < 0.05$). These values showed that PP required higher forces to elongate within the elastic region of the material. Accordingly, PP is a tougher material with lower elasticity. Again, TPU seems a more suitable approach for mesh implant manufacture due to its elasticity.

Table 2. Mechanical properties obtained for the 3D printed meshes formed by two layers.

	LFX Content (%)	Elastic Limit (N)	Tensile Stiffness (N/mm)	Fracture Force (N)	Elongation at Break (mm)
TPU	0.00	1.2 ± 0.4	0.44 ± 0.12	-	-
LFX 0.25%	0.25	1.0 ± 0.2	0.32 ± 0.06	-	-
LFX 0.50%	0.50	1.1 ± 0.1	0.37 ± 0.04	-	-
LFX 1.00%	1.00	1.3 ± 0.2	0.45 ± 0.08	-	-
PP	0.00	6.5 ± 0.2	6.05 ± 0.83	15. 42 ± 0.66	129 ± 7

3.3. LFX Release from 3D Printed Meshes

Figure 5 shows the LFX release from 3D printed meshes. Figure 5A shows the LFX released as a function of time for the 3D printed meshes. The prepared meshes are capable of providing sustained release of LFX for at least 3 days. Additionally, it can be seen that all the release profiles showed the similar shapes. The total amount of LFX released after 5 days (Figure 5B) increased with drug loading. However, there is a significant increase in the drug loading when the LFX loading increased from 0.25% to 0.5% ($p > 0.05$). When drug loading increased from 0.5% to 1% a small increment in drug release was observed. However, statistical analysis revealed that this different is not statistically significant ($p < 0.05$). Accordingly, it can be hypothesised that LFX could be interacting with TPU within the meshes, preventing a higher drug release. This is consistent with the results described in Section 3.1. These results are more obvious when the release was expressed as percentage of the initial drug loading (Figure 5C). This graph showed some interesting results. The percentage of drug release increase with drug loading up to a maximum. This maximum was obtained for meshes containing 0.5% of LFX. Subsequently, the percentage of drug release decreases when drug loading was increased up to 1% ($p < 0.05$). This showed that LFX/TPU interactions are taking place and reducing drug release.

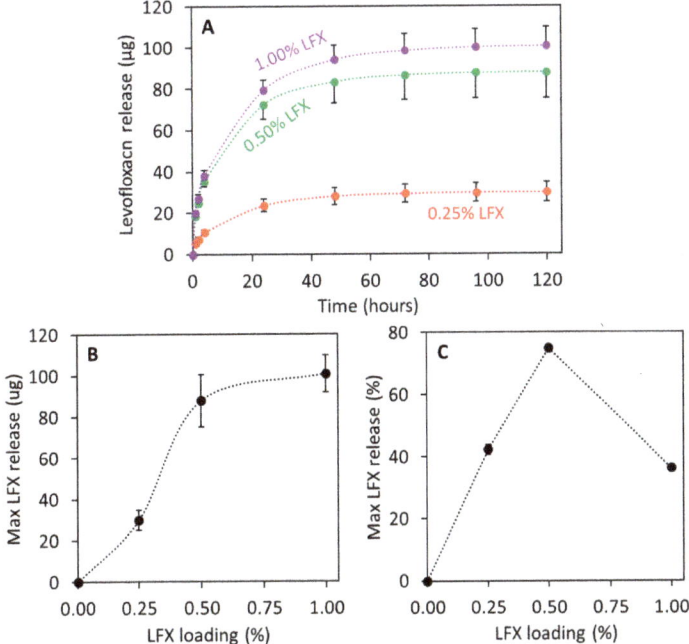

Figure 5. LFX release as a function of time for different LFX loaded 3D printed meshes (**A**). Maximum LFX release expressed in µg (**B**) and percentage (**C**) as a function of initial LFX drug loading.

3.4. Antimicrobial Properties of LFX Loaded 3D Printed Meshes

Printed meshes (1 cm × 1 cm × 0.1 cm) containing different LFX concentrations were tested for antimicrobial effect on a bacterial culture of S. aureus and E. coli in order to evaluate good examples of bacteria that are involved in a variety of community-and hospital-acquired infections. The results of the zone of inhibition are presented in the Figure 6. In this case, the zone of inhibition indicates that both used bacteria either at the surface of the meshes or even for an area extending outwards from the mesh's surface is inhibited. All the meshes containing LFX showed a clear zone of inhibition in both S. aureus and E. coli plates. As expected, the results showed no zone of inhibition in plates containing the control meshes without LFX.

The zones of inhibition in both S. aureus and E. coli plates were increased by increasing the amount of LFX. The diameter of the zone of inhibition in the S. aureus plates with TPU meshes containing LFX ranged from 25.5 ± 1.4 mm to 28.6 ± 0.8 mm, and from 25.2 ± 0.9 to 28.2 ± 0.8 in the E. coli plates. Statistical analysis showed that there were significant differences between the zones of inhibition caused by meshes containing 0.25% and 0.5% or 1% LFX ($p < 0.05$). This behaviour was observed for both cultures, S. aureus and E. coli. However, there were no significant differences in the zone of inhibition caused by meshes containing 0.5% and 1% LFX ($p > 0.05$). Once again, this trend was observed for both bacterial strains. These results are is in line with the obtained drug release profile for the meshes containing LFX (Figure 5A). In addition, when the zones of inhibition of E. coli and S. aureus were compared for the same concentration of LFX (0.25%, 0.5% and 1%), no significant differences were observed for any LFX concentration ($p > 0.05$). Therefore, it can be inferred that LFX had the same impact on both bacterial strains, which are the most frequent causes of many common bacterial infections.

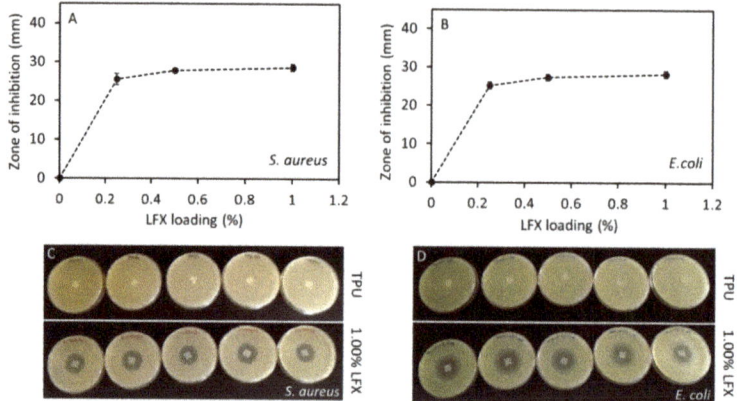

Figure 6. Correlation between the diameter of the zone of inhibition of *S. aureus* (**A**) and *E. coli* (**B**) and the concentration of LFX. Agar plates showing the zone of inhibition of meshes without LFX (TPU) and containing 1% of LFX for both bacterial strains, *S. aureus* (**C**) and *E. coli* (**D**).

4. Discussion

Historically, PP has been the choice material for pelvic floor repair since 1995 [13]. However, it has been shown that this material is not the ideal candidate for these applications due to the mechanical mismatch between the elastic paravaginal tissue and the strong and rigid PP [27]. Accordingly, the mechanical properties of PP mesh have generated multiple problems after mesh implantation. According to the US FDA, the use of PP mesh for pelvic floor repair can lead to serious complications associated with tissue erosion [28,29]. The ideal material for the production of pelvic floor repair mesh implants should possess elasticity and strength [12].

The present work describes the use of fused deposition modelling for the production of mesh implants for potential pelvic organ reconstructive surgery. TPU was selected as the ideal candidate for this purpose due to its elasticity and previously demonstrated biocompatibility [12,13,18]. This material has been used before for mesh implant manufacturing, showing superior capabilities than PP implants [12,13]. Additionally, TPU was combined with an antibiotic drug to prevent infection of this implantable material after surgery. Mesh-related infections are not common but when they occur they can compromise patients' well-being even leading to excision of the mesh implant or sepsis [30].

LFX was the antibiotic chosen for this application. In a previous work it was loaded in meshes prepared using electrospinning for hernia repair [26]. This antibiotic was combined with TPU using hot-melt extrusion to prepare filaments for further FDM applications. The materials displayed the homogeneous distribution of the drug. This was achieved using a single screw extruder coating the TPU pellets with LFX. This method has been previously used with successful results [14,19,31,32]. This is a quick way to obtain good mixtures between the drug and the polymer using a single screw extruder that is more accessible than a complicated and expensive twin-screw extruder. Figure 1A shows that the drug was properly dispersed within the material. FTIR results did not show any noticeable peak shift (Figure 1B). As mentioned before this can be due to the low drug loading. Similar behaviour was reported before for the combination of TPU and tetracycline or poly(urethane) and ciprofloxacin, a drug similar to LFX [14,33]. On the other hand, TGA results (Figure 1C) shows that there was interaction between LFX and TPU. Similar behaviour was reported when TPU was combined with tetracycline, ciprofloxacin or Schiff base additives [14,33,34]. It has been proposed that the C=O groups present in the TPU urethane groups can stablish non-covalent interactions with the drug.

The interaction of LFX with TPU can explain the behaviour obtained in the drug release profiles. In these experiments, meshes containing 1% of LFX showed a lower percentage of LFX released from the meshes than meshes containing 0.5% of LFX. The interactions between the polymer and the drug prevents a higher drug release. This has been observed previously for other drugs such as dipyridamole loaded into polyurethane [35]. Similarly, lower drug loadings (0.25% LFX) showed low release too. TPU is a non-degradable/hydrophobic polymer and, accordingly, the drug cargo located inside the material will not be released. Finally, the TPU meshes described in the present work are capable of providing releases of LFX for at least 3 days. A previously published work describing the use of electrospinning to prepare poly(caprolactone) surgical meshes loaded with LFX (0.5%) showed that this system was capable of providing drug release over 1 day. However, the nature of the mesh forming polymer was completely different.

This work was not only focused on the development of safer materials for mesh implant manufacturing but the use of techniques that allow clinicians to customize the mesh to patient's needs in a simple way. Therefore, FDM seems like an ideal technique for this purpose. TPU based meshes were successfully prepared using FDM (Figure 2). As expected, all the meshes had the same appearance and now noticeable drug aggregation was observed (Figure 2). Computed tomography was used to confirm drug distribution within the mesh matrix. Again, the results suggested that the drug was uniformly distributed within the mesh. In a previous study, computed tomography suggested that the combination of similar TPU with tetracycline showed some drug accumulation in certain parts of the material [14]. In this case, tetracycline was distributed all over the material, but some accumulation was observed using computed tomography.

The observed mechanical properties of the resulting meshes proved the initial approach: the resulting materials showed elastic behaviour unlike PP. The TPU-based meshes showed stiffness values ca. 0.4 N/mm while commercial PP meshes showed values ranging between 2 and 6 N/mm [25]. The design of the commercial meshes is different than the one proposed in the present paper but the testing conditions for these commercial meshes were similar. Some comparisons can be made. In order to compare the effect of the material in the mechanical properties, PP meshes were prepared using the same design used for the TPU based materials. Obviously, this PP is not exactly the same as the one used in conventional meshes, but it is a good example to compare the behaviour of both materials. The stiffness results obtained for PP (ca. 6 N/mm) were higher than those obtained for TPU meshes and the Force/displacement profile was completely different. Moreover, the stiffness values obtained for PP meshes were slightly higher than the previously reported results for commercial PP meshes (up to 5.3715 N/mm) [25]. However, the PP meshes tested in this work showed a different design than the commercial meshes. The mechanical characteristics of the material are important as it has been reported that materials with higher flexibility seem to adhere and conform to the tissues better than more rigid/stiffener meshes [36]. The design and size of the meshes can be hanged easily due to the versatility of FDM.

The 3D-printed meshes had a bacteriostatic activity on both *S. aureus* and *E. coli* cultures (Figure 6). This fact supports the premise that the extrusion and 3D printing processes did not affect the bacteriostatic activity of LFX. The risk of toxicity of these coated medical devices could be an important issue. Therefore, the possibility to print these medical devices using a small amount of the desired drug, and still have bacteriostatic activity, clearly minimizes the risk of toxicity in the patients. For instance, medical devices such as thermoplastic polyurethane (TPU) catheters were 3D-printed using up to 1% of tetracycline [14], thereby minimizing the risk of infection. Furthermore, Weisman et al. [31], in a different study, reported the possibility to print poly(lactic acid) (PLA) catheters using up to 2.5% of gentamicin. Additionally, it is also possible to print medical devices using higher percentages of drugs. Thus, for example, Genina et al. [37] 3D-printed drug-loaded intrauterine devices using different grades of ethylene vinyl acetate containing 5% and 15% of indomethacin.

PLA pellets coated with 1 wt % gentamicin were used to fabricate mesh prototypes for hernia repair [38]. In this study, they obtained a zone of inhibition of 1.1 ± 0.1 cm^2 for *E. coli* and 1.2 ± 0.1 cm^2 for *S aureus*. In a different work, polyvinyl alcohol (PVA) 3D meshes loaded with iodine were manufactured and these also showed a zone of inhibition against *E. coli* and *S. aureus* [39]. These results were far below to those found in our work. The diameter of the zone of inhibition in the *S. aureus* plates with TPU meshes of 0.25% LFX was 25.5 ± 1.4 mm and 28.6 ± 0.8 mm for meshes containing 1% LFX. As mentioned above, there were no significance differences between these results and the ones obtained in the *E coli* plates ($p > 0.05$). Therefore, it can be inferred that even the lower concentration (0.25%) of LFX had a significant zone of inhibition on both bacterial stains, which further minimises the risk of toxicity.

The use of medical devices such as transvaginal meshes, catheters or ventilators could be associated with the development of "nosocomial" or "health-care associated infections" (HCAIs) [40,41]. Although bacteria, viruses or fungal parasites can cause these infections, bacteria are the most common pathogens responsible for HCAI. Among these, bacterial species as *S. aureus* and *E. coli* have a major impact [42]. *S. aureus* is one of the most important pathogens responsible for nosocomial infections [43]. Moreover, *E. coli* is an emerging nosocomial pathogen, which is the leading cause of urinary tract infections (UTI) while, *S. aureus* is rarely found in these infections [43,44]. These infections may result in prolonged stays in the different health-care facilities, such as hospitals while increasing health-care costs [45]. Hence, the use of these 3D-printed meshes could decrease the rate of bacterial infections caused by the implant.

The majority of the FDM applications describing the combination of polymers with drugs are focused on the development of oral solid dosage forms [46,47]. We believe that this technology has the potential to be used for the manufacturing of medicated devices that can be produced on demand for a patient before a specific treatment/surgery. Previously we reported the use of FDM for dialysis catheter manufacturing [14,19] or antioxidant wound dressings. Some preliminary work has been done about the use of 3D printing for mesh implant manufacture. However, these works were not realistic as they propose the use of materials such as PLA or PCL that are biodegradable and do not present appropriate mechanical properties for this task [38,48,49]. Some of these works incorporated some antibiotics to the material. However, these works were not realistic due to material selection, but these studies worked as a proof of concept showing the potential of 3D printing for this purpose. Additionally, some recent work described the potential of using FDM as a tool for mesh implant manufacturing using PP [50]. The limitations of this material have been described previously. Moreover, these authors incorporated ciprofloxacin into the meshes by dip coating the implants. This is not ideal, as the manufacturing involves a two-step process. In the present work, the mesh is produced directly containing the drug within the device. Further research needs to be conducted about the in vivo biocompatibility of the meshes and shape optimization to adapt the mechanical properties of the mesh to patient's needs. The present work is a proof of concept that shows the potential of FDM technology to prepare elastic anti-infective materials. Finally, there are still regulatory aspects that should be addressed before 3D printing can be approved as a manufacturing technology for surgical devices. The US FDA has published some guidelines to manufactures about the appropriate use of this technology [51].

Author Contributions: Conceptualization, E.L. and D.A.L.; methodology, J.D.-R., C.M., E.M., I.G.-R., B.F.G. and E.L.; investigation and formal analysis, J.D.-R., C.M., E.L. and E.M.; data curation, J.D.-R., C.M. and E.L.; writing, J.D.-R., C.M., E.L. and D.A.L.; writing—review and editing, J.D.-R., C.M., E.M., I.G.-R., B.F.G., L.C., E.L. and D.A.L.; and supervision, E.L. and D.A.L. All authors have read and agreed to the published version of the manuscript.

Funding: This research received no external funding.

Conflicts of Interest: The authors declare no conflict of interest.

References

1. Wu, Y.M.; Welk, B. Revisiting current treatment options for stress urinary incontinence and pelvic organ prolapse: A contemporary literature review. *Res. Rep. Urol.* **2019**, *11*, 179–188. [CrossRef]
2. Mangir, N.; Chapple, C.R.; MacNeil, S. Synthetic Materials Used in the Surgical Treatment of Pelvic Organ Prolapse: Problems of Currently Used Material and Designing the Ideal Material. In *Pelvic Floor Disorders*; Rizvi, R., Ed.; InTechOpen: London, UK, 2018; Volume i, p. 13. ISBN 978-1-78-923245-5.
3. Vergeldt, T.F.M.; Weemhoff, M.; IntHout, J.; Kluivers, K.B. Risk factors for pelvic organ prolapse and its recurrence: A systematic review. *Int. Urogynecol. J.* **2015**, *26*, 1559–1573. [CrossRef]

4. Niaounakis, M. Medical, Dental, and Pharmaceutical Applications. In *Biopolymers: Applications and Trends*; Niaounakis, M., Ed.; Elsevier: Amsterdam, The Netherlands, 2015; pp. 291–405. ISBN 978-0-32-335399-1.
5. Mironska, E.; Chapple, C.; MacNeil, S. Recent advances in pelvic floor repair. *F1000Research* **2019**, *8*, 778. [CrossRef]
6. Rac, G.; Younger, A.; Clemens, J.Q.; Kobashi, K.; Khan, A.; Nitti, V.; Jacobs, I.; Lemack, G.E.; Brown, E.T.; Dmochowski, R.; et al. Stress urinary incontinence surgery trends in academic female pelvic medicine and reconstructive surgery urology practice in the setting of the food and drug administration public health notifications. *Neurourol. Urodyn.* **2017**, *36*, 1155–1160. [CrossRef]
7. The Food and Drug Administration. Obstetrical and Gynecological Devices; Reclassification of Surgical Mesh for Transvaginal Pelvic Organ Prolapse Repair; Final Order. *Fed. Regist.* **2016**, *81*, 353–361.
8. Mancuso, E.; Downey, C.; Doxford-Hook, E.; Bryant, M.G.; Culmer, P. The use of polymeric meshes for pelvic organ prolapse: Current concepts, challenges, and future perspectives. *J. Biomed. Mater. Res. Part B Appl. Biomater.* **2019**. [CrossRef]
9. FitzGerald, J.; Kumar, A. Biologic versus Synthetic Mesh Reinforcement: What are the Pros and Cons? *Clin. Colon Rectal Surg.* **2014**, *27*, 140–148.
10. Hympánová, L.; Rynkevic, R.; Román, S.; Mori da Cunha, M.G.M.C.; Mazza, E.; Zündel, M.; Urbánková, I.; Gallego, M.R.; Vange, J.; Callewaert, G.; et al. Assessment of Electrospun and Ultra-lightweight Polypropylene Meshes in the Sheep Model for Vaginal Surgery. *Eur. Urol. Focus* **2018**. [CrossRef]
11. De Tayrac, R.; Chentouf, S.; Garreau, H.; Braud, C.; Guiraud, I.; Boudeville, P.; Vert, M. In vitro degradation and in vivo biocompatibility of poly(lactic acid) mesh for soft tissue reinforcement in vaginal surgery. *J. Biomed. Mater. Res. Part B Appl. Biomater.* **2008**, *85*, 529–536. [CrossRef]
12. Shafaat, S.; Mangir, N.; Regureos, S.R.; Chapple, C.R.; MacNeil, S. Demonstration of improved tissue integration and angiogenesis with an elastic, estradiol releasing polyurethane material designed for use in pelvic floor repair. *Neurourol. Urodyn.* **2018**, *37*, 716–725. [CrossRef]
13. Hillary, C.J.; Roman, S.; Bullock, A.J.; Green, N.H.; Chapple, C.R.; MacNeil, S. Developing Repair Materials for Stress Urinary Incontinence to Withstand Dynamic Distension. *PLoS ONE* **2016**, *11*, e0149971. [CrossRef]
14. Mathew, E.; Domínguez-Robles, J.; Stewart, S.; Mancuso, E.; O'Donnell, K.; Larraneta, E.; Lamprou, D.A. Fused Deposition Modelling as an Effective Tool for Anti-Infective Dialysis Catheter Fabrication. *ACS Biomater. Sci. Eng.* **2019**, *5*, 6300–6310. [CrossRef]
15. Mathew, E.; Domínguez-Robles, J.; Larrañeta, E.; Lamprou, D.A. Fused Deposition Modelling as a Potential Tool for Antimicrobial Dialysis Catheters Manufacturing: New Trends vs. Conventional Approaches. *Coatings* **2019**, *9*, 515. [CrossRef]
16. Liang, K.; Brambilla, D.; Leroux, J.-C. Is 3D Printing of Pharmaceuticals a Disruptor or Enabler? *Adv. Mater.* **2019**, *31*, 1805680. [CrossRef]
17. Trenfield, S.J.; Awad, A.; Madla, C.M.; Hatton, G.B.; Firth, J.; Goyanes, A.; Gaisford, S.; Basit, A.W. Shaping the future: Recent advances of 3D printing in drug delivery and healthcare. *Expert Opin. Drug Deliv.* **2019**, *16*, 1081–1094. [CrossRef]
18. Stewart, S.; Domínguez-Robles, J.; Donnelly, R.; Larrañeta, E. Implantable Polymeric Drug Delivery Devices: Classification, Manufacture, Materials, and Clinical Applications. *Polymers* **2018**, *10*, 1379. [CrossRef]
19. Domínguez-Robles, J.; Martin, N.; Fong, M.; Stewart, S.; Irwin, N.; Rial-Hermida, M.; Donnelly, R.; Larrañeta, E. Antioxidant PLA Composites Containing Lignin for 3D Printing Applications: A Potential Material for Healthcare Applications. *Pharmaceutics* **2019**, *11*, 165. [CrossRef]
20. Turner, B.N.; Strong, R.; Gold, S.A. A review of melt extrusion additive manufacturing processes: I. Process design and modeling. *Rapid Prototyp. J.* **2014**, *20*, 192–204. [CrossRef]
21. Matos, B.D.M.; Rocha, V.; da Silva, E.J.; Moro, F.H.; Bottene, A.C.; Ribeiro, C.A.; dos Santos Dias, D.; Antonio, S.G.; do Amaral, A.C.; Cruz, S.A.; et al. Evaluation of commercially available polylactic acid (PLA) filaments for 3D printing applications. *J. Therm. Anal. Calorim.* **2019**, *137*, 555–562. [CrossRef]
22. Domínguez-Robles, J.; Larrañeta, E.; Fong, M.L.; Martin, N.K.; Irwin, N.J.; Mutjé, P.; Tarrés, Q.; Delgado-Aguilar, M. Lignin/poly(butylene succinate) composites with antioxidant and antibacterial properties for potential biomedical applications. *Int. J. Biol. Macromol.* **2020**, *145*, 92–99. [CrossRef]
23. Muwaffak, Z.; Goyanes, A.; Clark, V.; Basit, A.W.; Hilton, S.T.; Gaisford, S. Patient-specific 3D scanned and 3D printed antimicrobial polycaprolactone wound dressings. *Int. J. Pharm.* **2017**, *527*, 161–170. [CrossRef] [PubMed]

24. Hou, X.; Zheng, W.; Kodur, V.; Sun, H. Effect of temperature on mechanical properties of prestressing bars. *Constr. Build. Mater.* **2014**, *61*, 24–32. [CrossRef]
25. Afonso, J.S.; Martins, P.A.L.S.; Girao, M.J.B.C.; Natal Jorge, R.M.; Ferreira, A.J.M.; Mascarenhas, T.; Fernandes, A.A.; Bernardes, J.; Baracat, E.C.; Rodrigues de Lima, G.; et al. Mechanical properties of polypropylene mesh used in pelvic floor repair. *Int. Urogynecol. J.* **2008**, *19*, 375–380. [CrossRef]
26. Hall Barrientos, I.J.; Paladino, E.; Brozio, S.; Passarelli, M.K.; Moug, S.; Black, R.A.; Wilson, C.G.; Lamprou, D.A. Fabrication and characterisation of drug-loaded electrospun polymeric nanofibers for controlled release in hernia repair. *Int. J. Pharm.* **2017**, *517*, 329–337. [CrossRef]
27. Li, X.; Kruger, J.A.; Jor, J.W.Y.; Wong, V.; Dietz, H.P.; Nash, M.P.; Nielsen, P.M.F. Characterizing the ex vivo mechanical properties of synthetic polypropylene surgical mesh. *J. Mech. Behav. Biomed. Mater.* **2014**, *37*, 48–55. [CrossRef]
28. Bako, A.; Dhar, R. Review of synthetic mesh-related complications in pelvic floor reconstructive surgery. *Int. Urogynecol. J.* **2009**, *20*, 103–111. [CrossRef]
29. *Urogynecologic Surgical Mesh: Update on the Safety and Effectiveness of Transvaginal Placement for Pelvic Organ Prolapse*; The Food and Drug Administration (FDA): Hampton, VA, USA, 2011.
30. Mangir, N.; Roman, S.; Chapple, C.R.; MacNeil, S. Complications related to use of mesh implants in surgical treatment of stress urinary incontinence and pelvic organ prolapse: Infection or inflammation? *World J. Urol.* **2019**. [CrossRef]
31. Weisman, J.A.; Nicholson, J.C.; Tappa, K.; Jammalamadaka, U.; Wilson, C.G.; Mills, D.K. Antibiotic and chemotherapeutic enhanced three-dimensional printer filaments and constructs for biomedical applications. *Int. J. Nanomed.* **2015**, *10*, 357–370.
32. Tappa, K.; Jammalamadaka, U.; Weisman, J.; Ballard, D.; Wolford, D.; Pascual-Garrido, C.; Wolford, L.; Woodard, P.; Mills, D. 3D Printing Custom Bioactive and Absorbable Surgical Screws, Pins, and Bone Plates for Localized Drug Delivery. *J. Funct. Biomater.* **2019**, *10*, 17. [CrossRef]
33. Choi, Y.; Nirmala, R.; Lee, J.Y.; Rahman, M.; Hong, S.-T.; Kim, H.Y. Antibacterial ciprofloxacin HCl incorporated polyurethane composite nanofibers via electrospinning for biomedical applications. *Ceram. Int.* **2013**, *39*, 4937–4944. [CrossRef]
34. Naik, A.D.; Fontaine, G.; Bellayer, S.; Bourbigot, S. Salen based Schiff bases to flame retard thermoplastic polyurethane mimicking operational strategies of thermosetting resin. *RSC Adv.* **2015**, *5*, 48224–48235. [CrossRef]
35. Punnakitikashem, P.; Truong, D.; Menon, J.U.; Nguyen, K.T.; Hong, Y. Electrospun biodegradable elastic polyurethane scaffolds with dipyridamole release for small diameter vascular grafts. *Acta Biomater.* **2014**, *10*, 4618–4628. [CrossRef] [PubMed]
36. Siegel, A.L. Vaginal mesh extrusion associated with use of Mentor transobturator sling. *Urology* **2005**, *66*, 995–999. [CrossRef]
37. Genina, N.; Holländer, J.; Jukarainen, H.; Mäkilä, E.; Salonen, J.; Sandler, N. Ethylene vinyl acetate (EVA) as a new drug carrier for 3D printed medical drug delivery devices. *Eur. J. Pharm. Sci.* **2016**, *90*, 53–63. [CrossRef] [PubMed]
38. Ballard, D.H.; Weisman, J.A.; Jammalamadaka, U.; Tappa, K.; Alexander, J.S.; Griffen, F.D. Three-dimensional printing of bioactive hernia meshes: In vitro proof of principle. *Surgery* **2017**, *161*, 1479–1481. [CrossRef]
39. Boyer, C.J.; Ballard, D.H.; Weisman, J.A.; Hurst, S.; McGee, D.J.; Mills, D.K.; Woerner, J.E.; Jammalamadaka, U.; Tappa, K.; Alexander, J.S. Three-Dimensional Printing Antimicrobial and Radiopaque Constructs. *3D Print. Addit. Manuf.* **2018**, *5*, 29–36. [CrossRef] [PubMed]
40. CDC. Types of Healthcare-Associated Infections. Healthcare-Associated Infections (HAIs). Available online: https://www.cdc.gov/HAI/infectionTypes.html (accessed on 10 March 2019).
41. Khan, H.A.; Baig, F.K.; Mehboob, R. Nosocomial infections: Epidemiology, prevention, control and surveillance. *Asian Pac. J. Trop. Biomed.* **2017**, *7*, 478–482. [CrossRef]
42. Horan, T.C.; Andrus, M.; Dudeck, M.A. CDC/NHSN surveillance definition of health care–associated infection and criteria for specific types of infections in the acute care setting. *Am. J. Infect. Control* **2008**, *36*, 309–332. [CrossRef]
43. Khan, H.A.; Ahmad, A.; Mehboob, R. Nosocomial infections and their control strategies. *Asian Pac. J. Trop. Biomed.* **2015**, *5*, 509–514. [CrossRef]

44. Lausch, K.R.; Fuursted, K.; Larsen, C.S.; Storgaard, M. Colonisation with multi-resistant Enterobacteriaceae in hospitalised Danish patients with a history of recent travel: A cross-sectional study. *Travel Med. Infect. Dis.* **2013**, *11*, 320–323. [CrossRef]
45. Hall, C.W.; Mah, T.-F. Molecular mechanisms of biofilm-based antibiotic resistance and tolerance in pathogenic bacteria. *FEMS Microbiol. Rev.* **2017**, *41*, 276–301. [CrossRef] [PubMed]
46. Kollamaram, G.; Croker, D.M.; Walker, G.M.; Goyanes, A.; Basit, A.W.; Gaisford, S. Low temperature fused deposition modeling (FDM) 3D printing of thermolabile drugs. *Int. J. Pharm.* **2018**, *545*, 144–152. [CrossRef] [PubMed]
47. Goyanes, A.; Buanz, A.B.M.; Basit, A.W.; Gaisford, S. Fused-filament 3D printing (3DP) for fabrication of tablets. *Int. J. Pharm.* **2014**, *476*, 88–92. [CrossRef] [PubMed]
48. Ballard, D.H.; Jammalamadaka, U.; Tappa, K.; Weisman, J.A.; Boyer, C.J.; Alexander, J.S.; Woodard, P.K. 3D printing of surgical hernia meshes impregnated with contrast agents: In vitro proof of concept with imaging characteristics on computed tomography. *3D Print. Med.* **2018**, *4*, 13. [CrossRef]
49. Calero Castro, F.J.; Yuste, Y.; Pereira, S.; Garvín, M.D.; López García, M.Á.; Padillo, F.J.; Portilla, F. Proof of concept, design, and manufacture via 3-D printing of a mesh with bactericidal capacity: Behaviour in vitro and in vivo. *J. Tissue Eng. Regen. Med.* **2019**, *13*, 1955–1964. [CrossRef]
50. Qamar, N.; Abbas, N.; Irfan, M.; Hussain, A.; Arshad, M.S.; Latif, S.; Mehmood, F.; Ghori, M.U. Personalized 3D printed ciprofloxacin impregnated meshes for the management of hernia. *J. Drug Deliv. Sci. Technol.* **2019**, *53*, 101164. [CrossRef]
51. Statement by FDA Commissioner Scott Gottlieb, M.D., on FDA Ushering in New Era of 3D Printing of Medical Products; Provides Guidance to Manufacturers of Medical Devices. Available online: https://www.fda.gov/news-events/press-announcements/statement-fda-commissioner-scott-gottlieb-md-fda-ushering-new-era-3d-printing-medical-products (accessed on 15 March 2019).

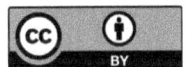

© 2020 by the authors. Licensee MDPI, Basel, Switzerland. This article is an open access article distributed under the terms and conditions of the Creative Commons Attribution (CC BY) license (http://creativecommons.org/licenses/by/4.0/).

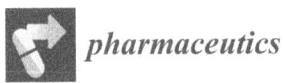

Article

Influence of High, Disperse API Load on Properties along the Fused-Layer Modeling Process Chain of Solid Dosage Forms

Marius Tidau [1,2,*], Arno Kwade [1,2] and Jan Henrik Finke [1,2]

[1] Institute for Particle Technology, TU Braunschweig, Volkmaroder Str. 5, 38104 Braunschweig, Germany; a.kwade@tu-braunschweig.de (A.K.); jfinke@tu-braunschweig.de (J.H.F.)
[2] Center of Pharmaceutical Engineering, TU Braunschweig, Franz-Liszt-Str. 35A, 38106 Braunschweig, Germany
* Correspondence: m.tidau@tu-braunschweig.de; Tel.: +49-531-391-65549

Received: 15 March 2019; Accepted: 16 April 2019; Published: 22 April 2019

Abstract: In order to cope with the increasing number of multimorbid patients due to demographic changes, individualized polypill solutions must be developed. One promising tool is fused layer modeling (FLM) of dosage forms with patient-specific dose combinations and release individualization. As there are few approaches reported that systematically investigate the influence of high disperse active pharmaceutical ingredient (API) loads in filaments needed for FLM, this was the focus for the present study. Different filaments based on polyethylene oxide and hypromellose (HPMC) with different loads of theophylline as model API (up to 50 wt.%) were extruded with a twin-screw extruder and printed to dosage forms. Along the process chain, the following parameters were investigated: particle size and shape of theophylline; mechanical properties, microstructure, mass and content uniformity of filaments as well as dosage forms and the theophylline release from selected dosage forms. Especially for HPMC, increasing theophylline load enhanced the flexural strength of filaments whilst the FLM accuracy decreased inducing defects in microstructure. Theophylline load had no significant effect on the dissolution profile of HPMC-based dosage forms. Therefore, a thorough analysis of particle-induced effects is necessary to correlate mechanical properties of filaments, printability, and the dosage-and-release profile adjustment.

Keywords: additive manufacturing; modified release; filament extrusion; fused layer modeling; theophylline; high API load

1. Introduction

Considering the demographic changes of society and the connected increase in multimorbid patients, new individualized therapies must be developed including the combination of highly dosed formulations in a single dosage form to improve patient compliance. To produce dosage forms with individual doses and release profiles, new production processes are necessary. As a promising tool for the production of individualized solid dosage forms, additive manufacturing techniques have emerged in pharmaceutical research in the past two decades [1,2]. With these techniques, three-dimensional objects are made without molds or tools by successive build-up of layers of source materials [3]. Depending on the source material, different physical principals are applicable, like powder-bed binding via laser sintering or binder fluid, extrusion freeforming, and stereo lithography [3]. All named techniques are also applicable for the production of solid dosage forms [2]. The first and only approved additively manufactured pharmaceutical, Spritam®, is produced by the ZipDose® technology where a powder bed of levetiracetam is selectively bound with a binder fluid to generate an ultra-rapidly disintegrating tablet [4]. However, as there are only few different doses approved and only one dissolution profile is available, Spritam® does not utilize all advantages of additive manufacturing to produce individual dosage forms on demand. Another technique, selective laser sintering, was used to produce orally disintegrating [5] or modified-release tablets [6]. Extrusion-based techniques include the selective deposition of hydrogels loaded with active pharmaceutical ingredients (API) [7,8] which after drying, were tested with up to five different drugs with each having a different excipient to obtain different release profiles [9]. Furthermore, fused layer modeling (FLM), where a polymer-API formulation is selectively deposited via a hot nozzle, also represents extrusion-based technologies and is currently the fastest evolving technique in pharmaceutical research [1].

Few approaches use direct melt extrusion of polymer-API powder blends [10,11]. However, most FLM machines use polymer wires, so-called filaments, as source material [1]. The first applications of FLM in pharmaceutics soaked commercially available polyvinyl alcohol filaments in API solutions to additively produce dosage forms [12,13]. More recent works use mostly hot melt extrusion (HME) to produce API-loaded filaments [1]. In general, HME of polymer-API blends is an advantageous process to improve solubility of BCS type-II and -IV APIs by intensively compounding the materials to gain solid dispersions and solutions [14]. For more soluble APIs, the compounding in polymeric excipients can be used to achieve modified and control release kinetics. To gain lower viscosities and therefore lower process temperatures in HME, plasticizers are frequently used [15]. However, it has to be considered that every substance in the process can have a plasticizing, viscosity decreasing, or even viscosity increasing effect. For example, absorbed water may plasticize polymers and alter the melting process [16], but can also cause polymer degradation [17] and physical instability of preliminary stable solid solutions [18]. Amorphous, molecularly dispersed APIs also have a plasticizing effect [19,20]. On the contrary, dispersely mixed APIs increase viscosity [21,22]. To produce filaments suitable for FLM machines adequate process parameters for HME and formulation are crucial. Thus, adequate mechanical stability, a consistent diameter, and a homogeneous API distribution are required [23]. There are different excipients of pharmaceutical grade that can be used as matrix polymer or plasticizer [24]. Depending on the excipient used, different release kinetics can be adjusted. It is also possible to mix different polymeric excipients to gain better applicability to FLM [24,25].

For the production of API-loaded filaments, different machinery was applied. For example, filaments were produced by the extrusion of powder blends with a single-screw extruder [23,26] with marginal shear and melt mixing or with a self-constructed ram-extruder [27] without any melt mixing. However, in most cases a co-rotating twin-screw extruder is applied [28–31] to obtain well-compounded, homogeneous filaments.

Different API-loaded filaments were, as mentioned before, successfully used in FLM to produce immediate [27] and controlled [23,25,28] release solid dosage forms. This includes first approaches with two formulations using a dual FLM machine to obtain delayed release and dosage forms with API combinations [32–34]. However, in most cases the used formulations include low API loads [23,33]; only few use API loads higher than 40 wt.% [31,35].

Especially for polypill applications, it is necessary to use source materials with high API loads to limit the dosage form size whilst increasing the maximum dose for each API. There are only few approaches to systematically investigate the influence of highly disperse API load on filament and additively produced dosage form properties. Therefore, the aim of the present work is to investigate the introduction of theophylline as model drug at different concentrations into different polymer matrices via HME. The obtained filaments and additively produced dosage forms were methodically characterized concerning parameters crucial over the whole process chain such as mechanical properties, content and mass uniformity, and drug release.

2. Materials and Methods

2.1. Materials

Hypromellose (HPMC) suited for HME (AFFINISOL™ HPMC HME 15lv), polyethylene glycole (PEG) with a molecular weight of 8000 g/mol (CARBOWAX™ PEG 8000), semi-crystalline polyethylene oxide (PEO) with a molecular weight of 100,000 (Sentry POLYOX™ WSR N-10–NF Grade;) and one (PEO-L) with a molecular weight of 2,000,000 (Sentry POLYOX™ WSR N-60K–NF Grade) were used as matrix polymers and were kindly donated by Dow (Bomlitz, Germany). As model API, theophylline (≥99%, anhydrous powder) was obtained from Sigma-Aldrich (Darmstadt, Germany). All solvents used were of analytical grade.

2.2. Methods

2.2.1. Analysis of Particle Size Distributions

The particle size distributions of raw material powders were measured using laser diffraction (Mastersizer 3000; Malvern Panalytical GmbH, Kassel, Germany) through a dry powder dispersing cell. The pressure of the dispersing air jet was set to 4 bar and the obtained data were evaluated applying Fraunhofer theory. For each material, the average of three measurements over 5 s was calculated and the volumetric distribution with the corresponding 10%, 50% and 90% cumulative undersize (d_{10}, d_{50}, d_{90}) was determined.

2.2.2. Preparation of Theophylline-Loaded Filaments

Filaments with a diameter of 2.85 mm ± 0.1 mm were produced applying a co-rotating twin-screw extruder (KETSE 12/36; Brabender® GmbH & Co. KG, Duisburg, Germany) with a die diameter of 2.7 mm (except for pure HPMC filament that was produced by applying a Pharma 11 HME (ThermoFischer ScientificTM, Karlsruhe, Germany) with a die diameter of 3 mm, obtained filament diameter was also 2.85 mm ± 0.1 mm through pull-off speed adjustment) in rotation speed-controlled mode at 100 rpm at temperatures adapted to formulations (Table 1). Pre-mixed powder blends (Table 1) were fed with a twin-screw gravimetric feeder (Brabender® GmbH & Co. KG, Duisburg, Germany). Filaments were pulled off by a conveyor belt (Brabender® GmbH & Co. KG, Duisburg, Germany) with constant velocity set to yield filament diameters of 2.85 ± 0.1 mm and cooled with compressed air if necessary to enable complete solidification over the belt length.

Table 1. Filament formulations and extrusion die temperatures.

Designation	Formulation in Fractions [wt.%]					Extrusion Temperatures [°C]
	HPMC	PEG	PEO	PEO-L	Theoph.	
HPMC *	95.00	5.00	-	-	-	150 *
HPMC15	81.53	4.08	-	-	14.38	160
HPMC35	62.95	3.15	-	-	33.90	160
HPMC50 **	48.78	2.44	-	-	48.78	170 **
PEO	-	-	100.00	-	-	120
PEO15	-	-	85.00	-	15.00	120
PEO15-P	-	4.08	81.53	-	14.38	120
PEO35	-	-	65.00	-	35.00	120
PEO35-PL	-	-	59.09	9.09	31.82	120

*: different extruder, **: different screw speed (200 rpm).

2.2.3. Content Uniformity (CU) of Filaments and 3D Prints

The theophylline distribution in filaments was proven by taking samples of about 100 mg every 10 cm from the filament—five of each end of every filament roll. The samples were dissolved in 0.1 N HCl and the theophylline concentrations were determined via UV/Vis spectrometry (Specocord

210plus, Analytic Jena, Jena, Germany). Polymers and additives did not influence the measurements. The content uniformity (CU) of 3D-printed full material cylinders was determined in the same way.

2.2.4. He-Pycnometry

Raw material densities and densities of filaments and 3D-printed tablets were measured by helium pycnometry (UltraPyc 1200e; Quantachrome GmbH & Co. KG, Duisburg, Germany). Five consecutive volume-measurements show a standard deviation less than 0.01 cm^3, up to ten measurements were averaged.

2.2.5. Differential Scanning Calorimetry (DSC) and Thermogravimetric Analysis (TGA)

All ingredients, filaments, and 3D-printed dosage forms were analyzed via dynamic differential scanning calorimetry (DSC) to investigate possible influences of the formulation and the process on the thermal behavior of the polymeric matrix. Therefore, each sample was tested in an aluminum crucible with a perforated lid over a heating/cooling/heating profile (HPMC-based: 20 °C/200 °C/0 °C/200 °C; PEO-based: 20 °C/160 °C/0 °C/160 °C) in a DSC apparatus (DSC 1, Mettler Toledo GmbH, Switzerland) with a heating rate of 10 K/min and a nitrogen flush of 150 mL/min inside and 50 mL/min outside of the cell.

Thermal stability of theophylline and the matrix materials was investigated via thermogravimetric analysis (TGA/DSC 1 sTAR^e; Mettler-Toledo GmbH, Greifensee, Switzerland) conducted from 30–950 °C in air with a heating rate of 10 K/min.

2.2.6. Additive Manufacturing of Solid Dosage Forms

A dual filament 3D printer (Ultimaker 3, Ultimaker, Geldermalsen, The Netherlands) operated via the Cura software (Version 2.7, Ultimaker, Geldermalsen, The Netherlands) was used for the production of samples. As only dosage forms of one material were produced in this study, only one of the printer's nozzles was used at a time. Every printable filament (iteratively determined material-specific printing parameters for reproducible, neat samples; aberrations from the printing profile of Cura for generic poly lactic acid (PLA) filament; in Table 2) was used to produce several compact samples of cylinders (8-mm diameter, 3-mm height), rings (10-mm outer diameter, 7.21-mm inner diameter, 4-mm height) and spheres (6.6-mm diameter) with the same volume of 150.8 mm^3 but different surface to volume ratios (sphere: 0.91-mm^{-1}; cylinder: 1.17-mm^{-1}; ring: 1.93-mm^{-1}) and (only for HPMC15) cylinders (8-mm diameter, 3-mm height) with different open porosity (20%, 50%, 80%). The mass uniformity (MU) of printed dosage forms was checked by weighing.

Table 2. Specific printing parameter deviating from Cura generic PLA profile for every filament.

Designation	Aberration from Standard Generic PLA Profile (Cura 2.7)
HPMC	Retraction distance: 8 mm; printing temperature: 220 °C
HPMC15	Retraction distance: 8 mm
HPMC35	Retraction distance: 8 mm; buildplate temperature: 70 °C
HPMC50	Retraction distance: 8 mm; buildplate temperature: 80 °C; printing temperature: 210 °C; print cooling: disabled
PEO/PEO15	Retraction distance: 8 mm; buildplate temperature: 55 °C; printing temperature: 110 °C; print cooling: 100% fanspeed at 1st layer; print speed: 40 mm/s
PEO15-P	
PEO35	Not printable
PEO35-PL	

2.2.7. Oscillatory Rheology

A rotary rheometer (MCR 302, Anton Paar GmbH, Graz, Austria) equipped with a heated parallel plate with a diameter of 25 mm was applied to determine the melt viscosity of extruded samples. After melting the sample, a gap of 1 mm was adjusted and measurements were conducted as temperature sweep with constant amplitude (0.36°) and frequency (1 Hz), both approved by amplitude and frequency sweep tests. Each sample was heated to the maximum of a material-specific temperature ramp (PEO-based: 40–120 °C; HPMC-based: 120–200 °C) then moderately cooled down while the rotor was already sweeping and afterwards reheated to the maximum temperature again. During reheating 16 data points were collected each over an integration time of 20 s and an aberration tolerance of 0.2%.

2.2.8. Mechanical Testing (Three-Point Bending and Brazilian Test)

Mechanical stability of the filaments and 3D-printed tablets was tested using a material tester (Z2.5, Zwick GmbH & Co. KG, Ulm, Germany). The flexural strength of the filaments was tested via three-point-bending with a span distance of 16 mm and a speed of 10 mm/min. The tablets' tensile strength was investigated with the Brazilian test (diametral breakage test) with a speed of 10 mm/min.

2.2.9. Microstructural Investigation via Micro-Computer Tomography (µCT) and SEM

Microstructure of dosage forms was investigated via µCT imaging using a micro-computer tomographic apparatus (MicroXCT-400 Xradia; Zeiss, Oberkochen, Germany). Furthermore, the surface of different dosage forms and filaments was recorded with a scanning electron microscope (SEM) (Helios G4 CX; FEI Deutschland GmbH, Dreieich, Germany) after being sputtered with 6-nm of platinum in a vacuum coater (EM ACE 600; Leica Microsysteme GmbH, Wetzlar, Germany).

2.2.10. Disintegration Behavior and Dissolution Testing of Dosage Forms

Disintegration of the full material cylinders was measured with an automatic apparatus (DT50, Sotax AG, Aesch, Switzerland) in 0.1 N HCl at 37 °C.

Theophylline release was investigated with an automated USP4 flow cell device (CE7 smart; Sotax AG, Aesch, Switzerland) including an UV/Vis spectrometer (Specord 200plus; Analytic Jena, Jena, Germany). All tests were conducted at 37 °C using 0.1 N HCl for the first two hours and then automatically switching to phosphate-buffered solution at pH = 6.8. The sample-specific flowrates can be obtained from Table 3.

Table 3. Sample-specific flow rates for dissolution testing in flow cell apparatus.

Flowrate [mL/min]	Samples
4	HPMC15 samples (including cylinders with open porosity)
	HPMC35 samples
8	HPMC50 samples
	PEO15 samples
16	PEO15-P samples

3. Results and Discussion

3.1. Filament Characteristics

3.1.1. Raw Material Particle Characteristics

All raw materials had relatively broad particle size distributions (Figure 1A). Except PEG, all materials had nearly the same median particle size of about 110 µm and PEO and theophylline nearly had the same size distribution. However, PEG with a median particle size of 169 µm is still in the same size range. Therefore, a segregation due to different particle sizes is unlikely. However, other properties like the materials' true densities or the particle morphology like the acicular shape of the theophylline particles (Figure 1B) might still affect segregation of particle mixtures.

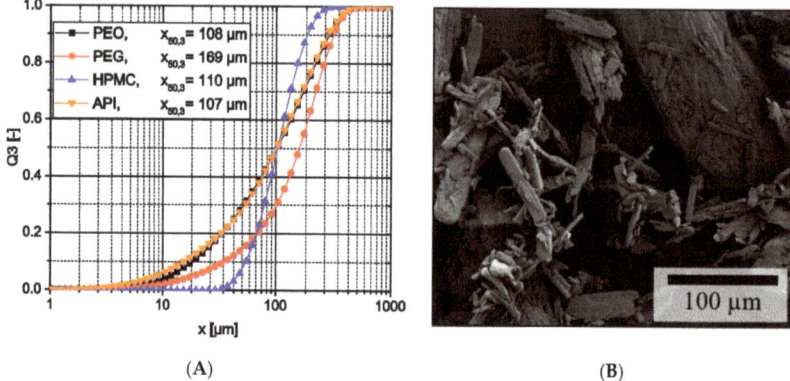

Figure 1. (A) Particle size distribution of raw materials; (B) SEM image of theophylline crystals.

3.1.2. Development of True Densities along the Process Chain

Filaments were successfully produced with a consistent diameter of 2.85 ± 0.05 mm. An increase of theophylline load resulted in a whitening of the light brown/yellowish HPMC and the yellowish/greenish PEO, depicting the increase in crystalline theophylline particles. Theoretical densities (Table 4) of all filaments were calculated using the formulation and the measured true densities of raw materials. As theophylline had a significantly higher true density, the density of the formulations increases with the theophylline load. The densities of all filaments and 3D-printed cylinders of all printable materials were determined and the deviation from the theoretical densities was calculated (Table 4). The negative difference of filament densities compared with theoretical densities allows an estimation of the closed pore volume within the filaments. As there is a trend towards higher densities along the process chain from filament to 3D print, these closed pores are opened and deaerated, respectively, during the tapering of the filament inside the 3D-printer's hot nozzle. The significant decrease of the density of HPMC and HPMC15 during the 3D print indicates enclosed air between the single layers. To the best of the authors' knowledge, the present work is the first to use the development of true densities along the process chain as a quality assurance tool in pharmaceutical research. However, as enclosed air, both in filaments and 3D prints, can alter the predefined properties like MU, CU, floatability, and dissolution behavior, porosity of filaments for 3D-printing of dosage forms should thoroughly be considered.

Table 4. Development of true densities along the process chain (He-pycnometer) with deviation from theoretical density of formulations.

Designation	Theoretical Density * [g/cm^3]	Filament Density [g/cm^3]	Density Deviation Filament [%]	3D-Print Density [g/cm^3]	Density Deviation 3D-Print [%]
HPMC	1.255	1.192	−5.29	1.182	−6.18
HPMC15	1.289	1.268	−1.66	1.237	−4.00
HPMC35	1.335	1.300	−2.63	1.309	−1.95
HPMC50	1.371	1.342	−2.12	1.356	−1.04
PEO	1.250	1.202	−3.99	1.207	−3.56
PEO15	1.286	1.251	−2.78	1.275	−0.90
PEO15-P	1.278	1.244	−2.63	1.256	−1.71
PEO35	1.335	1.277	−4.36	N/A	N/A
PEO35-PL	1.328	1.253	−5.67	N/A	N/A

* Raw material densities [g/cm^3]: PEO (1.25), PEO-L (1.26), PEG (1.081), HPMC (1.264), theophylline (1.492).

3.1.3. Microstructure of Filaments

Microstructural investigation of HPMC-based filaments via SEM depicted all the same visible effects of theophylline particles on both surface and fracture face which got more distinct with increasing theophylline load. On the filaments' surfaces crystalline structures occur (Figure 2A,C). As there are no comparable structures on HPMC filaments without theophylline (Figure 3A), these crystals can be identified as theophylline. In addition, defects on the crystals arise with increasing theophylline load (Figure 2C). Views of the fracture faces of theophylline-loaded HPMC filaments show the elongated theophylline crystals mainly in line with the extrusion direction of the filament (Figure 2B). In addition, some tooth-shaped structures appear on the fracture face at higher theophylline loads (Figure 2D) between the larger theophylline crystals which displays the higher amount of small theophylline particles, which are dispersed in the polymer matrix without orientation.

On the surfaces of theophylline-loaded filaments based on PEO, theophylline crystals were also visible (Figure 4A,B), which could not be observed on the surface of pure PEO filament (Figure 3B). Furthermore, the surfaces of all PEO-based filaments exhibited octagonal structuring (Figure 4A: magnified insert) depicting the crystalline part of the semi-crystalline polymer accordingly to the crystal structure of PEO [36]. However, as the polymer PEO also consists of an amorphous part with a glass transition temperature below 0 °C (cf. Figure 5B), significant plastic yielding can be observed at fracture faces (Figure 4D). Similar to HPMC-based, theophylline-loaded filaments, PEO filaments with theophylline show elongated particles mainly in line with the extrusion direction on the inside (Figure 4C). However, small theophylline crystals without orientation between the bigger ones, as they were observed in HPMC50 filaments (Figure 2D), could not be observed within PEO-based filaments. Therefore, these small crystals may be induced by the significantly higher melt viscosity of HPMC and the associated higher shear and dispersing during extrusion.

Due to the observations during microstructural investigation of filaments, particle-related effects on the FLM process can be expected. The theophylline crystals on the filament surface could get abraded during the tapering of the diameter inside of the hot nozzle where they could accumulate and degrade due to long exposure to heat. Furthermore, the aligned elongate particles can cause temporary blockage of the hot nozzle as it has been reported before by Kempin et al. [27].

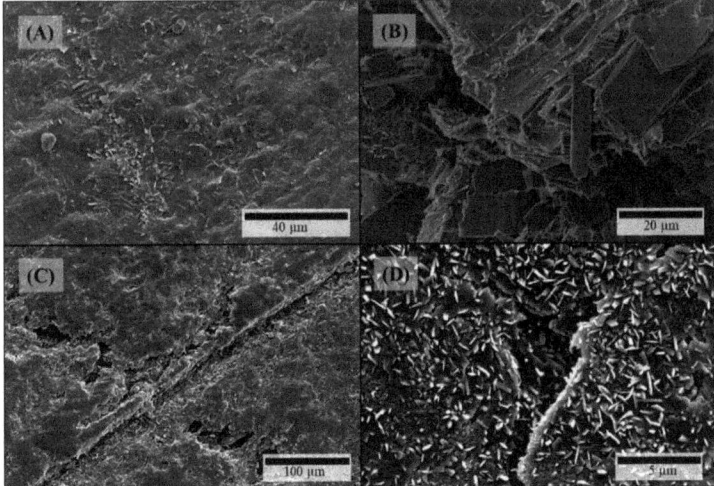

Figure 2. SEM pictures of HPMC-based filaments: (**A**) HPMC15 surface; (**B**) HPMC15 fracture face; (**C**) HPMC50 surface; (**D**) HPMC50 fracture face.

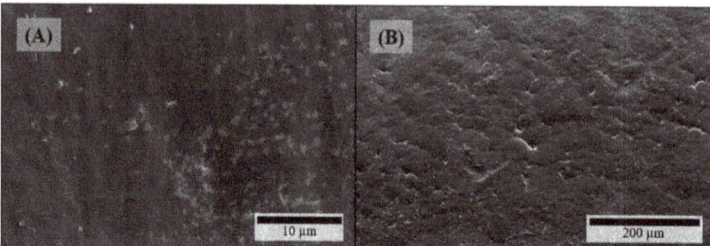

Figure 3. SEM pictures of filaments without any API: (**A**) HPMC surface; (**B**) PEO surface.

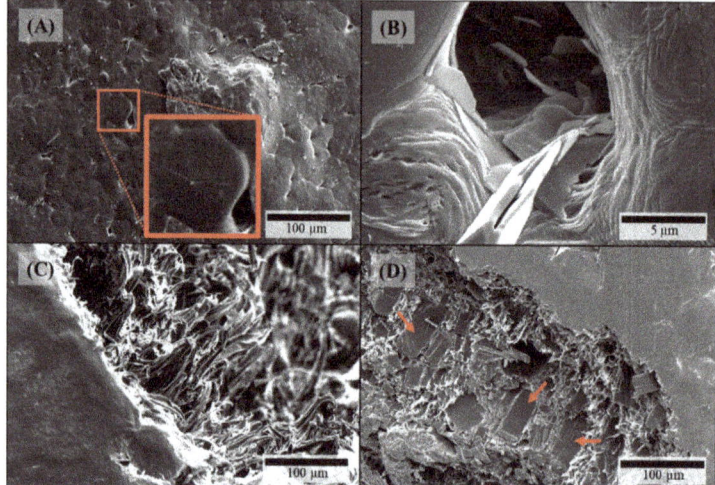

Figure 4. SEM pictures of PEO-based filaments: (**A**) PEO15-P surface, insert: magnification of octagonal structure; (**B**) PEO15-P surface close-up; (**C**) PEO15 fracture face; (**D**) PEO35 fracture face.

3.1.4. Thermal Analysis along the Process Chain

All raw materials show thermal stability within the temperature range of all processes (Figure 5A). Theophylline is the first of the used materials to degrade at above 200 °C [35], here approximately 230 °C. The slight mass decrease of HPMC around 100 °C indicates the loss of water bound during storage, which corresponds to the USP guideline [37]. This loss of water, around 1.5 wt.%, may induce inaccuracies in the theophylline load of filaments as the water evaporates after weighing during the extrusion through the venting hole of the extruder. Furthermore, the raw materials show different thermal events within the temperature range (Figure 5B). Theophylline does not show any event up to 200 °C. However, PEG and PEO show a significant melting at around 60 °C, depicting the crystalline part of the polymers. The amorphous HPMC has a glass transition temperature around 110 °C.

Each produced filament based on PEO and each 3D print made with these filaments only show one melting event within the temperature range around 60 °C (Figure 5C). The only remarkable observation is the decrease of the specific melting enthalpy for samples with increasing theophylline load which displays the higher load of nonmelting material.

During the first heating in the course of DSC measurements of filaments and 3D prints based on HPMC, two events could be detected (Figure 5D; dashed lines): The first endothermic event at around 60 °C presumably shows the melting of the PEG contained in the formulation; the second event is exothermic and occurs from 140–160 °C. This may indicate a recrystallization of amorphous theophylline. However, as during the second heating no significant events could be detected by other means and to the best of the authors' knowledge this behavior has not been described before, the effect is not safely attributed to these physical phenomena. In future work, this will be further investigated as an effect on printability and storage stability of filament and 3D-print.

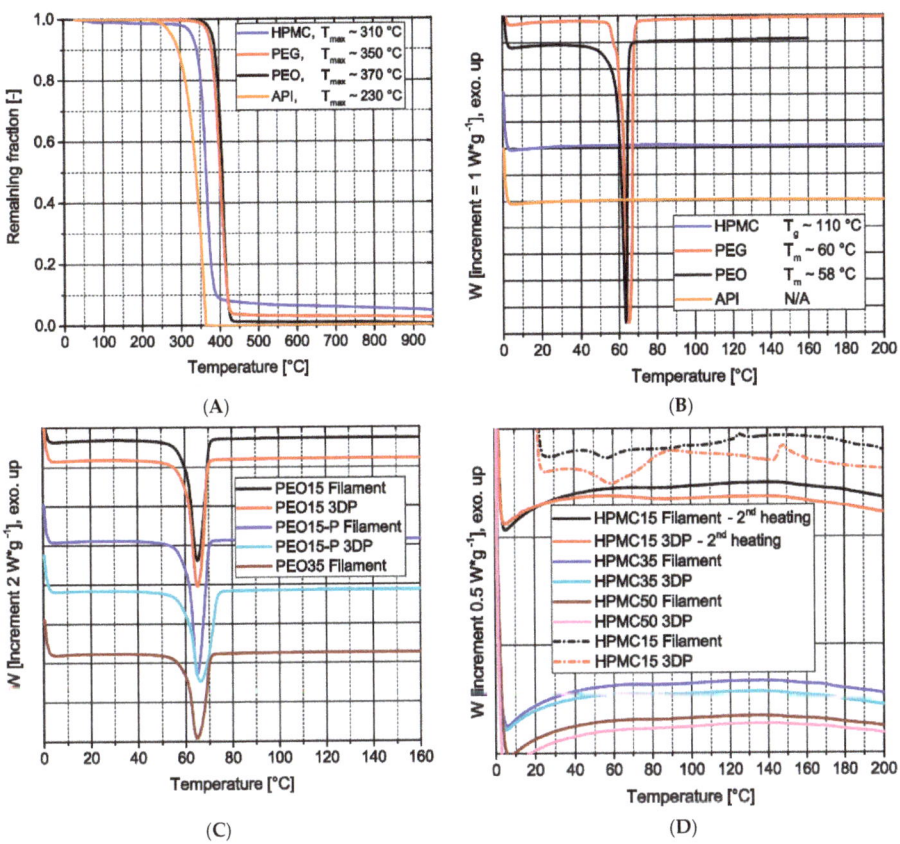

Figure 5. Thermal analysis: (**A**) TGA profiles of raw materials (under oxygen); (**B**) DSC profiles of raw materials (2nd heating); (**C**) DSC profiles of PEO-based materials (2nd heating); (**D**) DSC profiles of HPMC-based products (1st and 2nd heating).

3.1.5. Theophylline Content and Distribution in Filaments

The average theophylline content of all loaded filaments is near the adjusted loads through formulation (Table 5). The slightly higher theophylline contents of the HPMC-based filaments, especially of HPMC15, may be induced by evaporation of water absorbed on the HPMC powder, as described above. Except for PEO15-P and PEO35-PL, all filaments show a deviation of theophylline content along the spool length which may be induced by an instable process or segregation of the premixed powder blends. Especially the HPMC-based filaments show an increasing content deviation along the spool length with increasing matrix fraction. As described above, this may be a result of the significantly higher particle size of PEG.

The homogeneous theophylline distribution along the whole filament spool is crucial as one spool is several meters long but the amount which is needed for one tablet is only several millimeters of filament. Therefore, a thorough understanding of the production process of a filament is necessary to produce dosage forms with uniform theophylline content.

Table 5. Filament investigation for homogeneity of theophylline (in table API) distribution.

Designation	Theoretical API Content [wt.%]	API Content First End [wt.%]	API Content Second End [wt.%]	API Content Average [wt.%]
HPMC15	14.38	14.71 ± 0.28	16.54 ± 0.22	15.62 ± 0.95
HPMC35	33.90	33.09 ± 0.28	34.79 ± 0.33	33.94 ± 0.90
HPMC50	48.78	49.02 ± 0.53	49.70 ± 0.43	49.36 ± 0.59
PEO15	15.00	14.17 ± 0.17	16.03 ± 0.24	15.10 ± 0.95
PEO15-P	14.38	15.34 ± 0.15	15.76 ± 0.15	15.55 ± 0.26
PEO35 *	N/A *	N/A *	N/A *	N/A *
PEO35-PL	31.82	32.27 ± 0.42	32.76 ± 0.45	32.52 ± 0.50

*: Filament was too brittle; only small strands could be produced.

3.1.6. Influence of Polymer Matrix and Theophylline Load on Flexural Strength of Filaments

As intense stresses are applied to filaments during FLM, they need good mechanical stability. The flexural strength measured via three-point-bending combined with the relative flexural angle—which was derived by the bending angle of the filaments at flexural strength divided by the cross-sectional area—were taken as surrogates for the processability of filaments in FLM. In general, the results show that filaments made of HPMC have higher flexural strength than those made of PEO (Figure 6). Furthermore, an increase in flexural strength and a decrease in the relative bending angle were observed for HPMC-based filaments with increasing theophylline load. This shows that the needle-like theophylline crystals stiffen the HPMC matrix and shift the material behavior from elastic to more rigid and brittle. Filaments based on PEO first show an increase in flexural strength and decrease in bending angle as observed for HPMC. However, increasing the theophylline load from 15 wt.% to 35 wt.% weakens the filaments as a decrease in the flexural strength occurs. In both filaments an addition of PEG or PEO with different molecular weight leads to a slight increase in both flexural strength and relative bending angle.

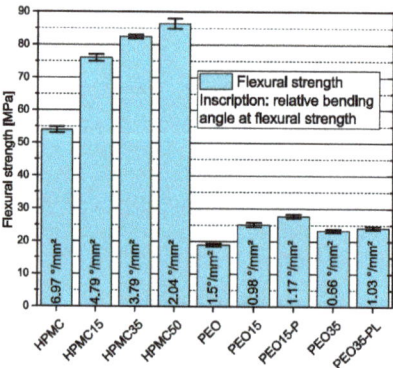

Figure 6. Flexural strength and relative bending angle of filaments measured via three-point-bending span = 16 mm; n = 6.

Zhang et al. reported that filaments should exhibit a minimum flexural strength of 28.85 MPa and a maximum bending angle of 9.15° to be suitable for FLM [28]. As they do not report the filament diameters, the relative flexural angle cannot be calculated and therefore not compared with our results. However, as the flexural strength should be independent of the filament diameter the minimum flexural strength reported should be adaptable to our results. The only two filaments that were not suitable for FLM due to extensive breakage during the forwarding of the filament inside the 3D-printer were PEO35 and PEO35-PL. This shows that the value reported by Zhang et al., which is significantly higher than the flexural strength of the other PEO filaments cannot be applied as a universal rule for

FLM filaments. Other characteristics like the tensile strength as reported before [31,38], or the abrasion resistance or the FLM machinery properties should also be considered to identify the suitability of filaments for FLM and will be analyzed in future work.

3.1.7. Influence of Theophylline Load on Melt Viscosity of Prepared Filament Formulations

In both the twin-screw extrusion of filaments and FLM, the melt viscosity of the applied formulation is a crucial parameter. To determine the influence of different theophylline loads on the melt viscosity of the used matrix polymers, the complex viscosity was determined via oscillatory viscosimetry at constant amplitude and frequency during the reheating of the sample in the temperature region of the extrusion and FLM processes. The measurements show that pure PEO has a higher melt viscosity than the formulations containing theophylline, which indicates a plasticizing effect (Figure 7). However, with increasing theophylline load from 15 wt.% towards 35 wt.% the melt viscosity again increases. Compared to the data of Van Renterghem et al. [21] the initial viscosity decrease may emanate from partly dissolved theophylline in the polymer matrix while the increasing amount of particulate theophylline at higher loads again increases the melt viscosity. The high temperatures needed to prepare HPMC-based samples for viscosimetry slowly induce degradation of the material visible by a brownish discoloration. Only the pure HPMC matrix and the sample with 15 wt.% theophylline melted sufficiently for rheological analysis before significant degradation. The measured viscosity curves (Figure 7) show higher viscosities for the theophylline-loaded material. Therefore, the plastifying effect of the dissolved theophylline, if there is any, cannot outweigh the thickening effect of non-dissolved theophylline particles.

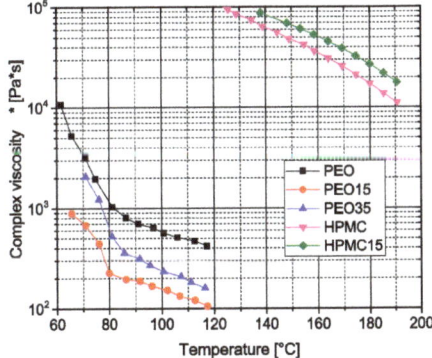

Figure 7. Oscillatory melt viscosity of different filament formulations (heating graph).

3.2. Characteristics of 3D-Printed Dosage Forms

3.2.1. Feasibility of the Additive Production of Dosage Forms and their Mass and Content Uniformity

Except for PEO35 and PEO35-PL, all filaments were successfully used in an FLM machine to produce different geometries with the same volume (Figure 8A). The formulation-specific printing parameters were established iteratively (data not shown). It could be determined that the nozzle temperature is the most important parameter with a narrow range; at too low temperatures the material has a too high viscosity, which can lead to a too-low extrusion and to damage of the filament in the feed unit; at too high temperatures the printed lines smear and the printed structures have an inhomogeneous surface and patterns cannot be reproducibly manufactured. During the production process of PEO-based materials, a thorough cooling was needed to gain neat structures due to the relatively low melt viscosity of PEO compared to the melting point of the crystalline fraction. Therefore, no complex structures like spheres could be produced from PEO-based filaments. FLM with HPMC-based filaments was hardly challenging. Only the temperature of the printhead nozzle and the build plate had to be raised with increasing theophylline load to gain smooth layers with good adhesion. This may be attributed to the higher amount of non-melting material as more particle-particle contacts occur with weaker interactions than the polymer parts that melt into each other. However, surprisingly, the HPMC filament without any theophylline needed the highest nozzle temperatures for good layer adhesion although the melt viscosity was lower than with theophylline load. This may be explained by the missing glass transition for HPMC containing theophylline, hinting at a plasticizing effect of dissolved theophylline molecules in the HPMC matrix. The higher viscosity induces lower interfacial forces between the printed layers as layers cannot be attached to each other smoothly. Another possible reason for the weaker layer adhesion could be the rougher surface of theophylline-loaded HPMC formulations as it can be observed in the SEM pictures (cf. Figures 2C, 3A and 8B). The amount of small visible theophylline crystals on the surface of 3D-printed objects is much higher than on filaments. This may indicate a post-process recrystallization on the 3D-print surface, which experienced high temperatures through direct nozzle contact.

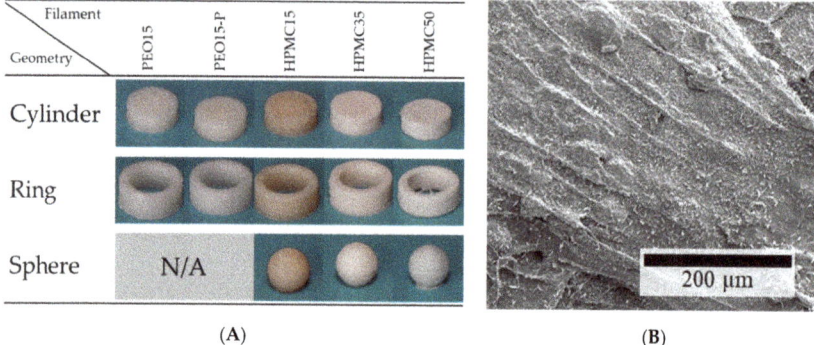

Figure 8. (**A**) Images of 3D-printed theophylline-loaded dosage forms with the same volume; (**B**) SEM image of the surface of a 3D-printed object made from HPMC15 filament.

Although every formulation based on HPMC was suitable for FLM, the accuracy decreased with increasing theophylline loads. The microstructural defects which were detected via µCT (Figure 9) were presumably, as discussed above, induced by temporary nozzle blockage which has already been reported elsewhere [27]. These structural defects can cause deviations in mass and content uniformity if the blockages are not detected during the process. Therefore, intensive studies are necessary for a better understanding of the relationship between the process, the formulation and the final properties, especially at high API loads.

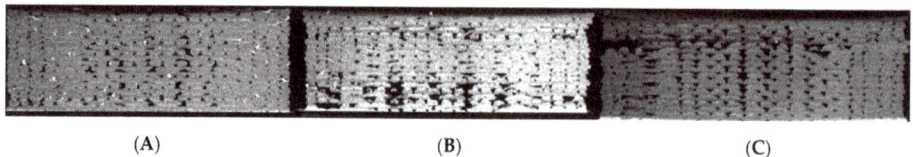

Figure 9. Microstructural cross section of 3D-printed HPMC cylinders via µCT (**A**) HPMC15, (**B**) HPMC35, (**C**) HPMC50.

With increasing theophylline loads for both HPMC and PEO-based printed cylinders and spheres, the adverse variances from the theoretical masses also increased (Table 6). The fact that some formulations show better results for the printed rings, for example HPMC15, is induced by printing parameters as the rings did not have an "infill" structure, which are printed with slightly different settings like faster print speed and acceleration. Furthermore, the theophylline content in the cylinders based on HPMC and PEO is near to the expected values. However, it has to be taken into account that the theoretical values are based on the measured weight. Therefore, the same effect of increasing adverse variance with increasing theophylline load could be detected by content determination.

Table 6. Theoretical and measured dosage form masses and theophylline CU of cylinders, n = 3–6.

Design	$m_{theor.}$ [mg]	$m_{cylinder}$ [mg]	m_{ring} [mg]	m_{sphere} [mg]	Cylinder Theophylline Content [mg]	
					Theoretic *	Measured
HPMC	189.18	175.37 ± 1.48	190.08 ± 0.37	183.23 ± 0.37	N/A	N/A
HPMC15	186.60	176.01 ± 1.56	183.47 ± 4.78	178.70 ± 1.18	27.89 ± 1.70	25.59 ± 0.51
HPMC35	197.44	180.14 ± 6.41	191.10 ± 0.85	174.87 ± 0.66	62.76 ± 3.72	63.53 ± 3.44
HPMC50	204.55	176.64 ± 6.50	172.33 ± 0.90	186.20 ± 1.85	88.83 ± 1.99	86.92 ± 2.61
PEO	188.50	162.97 ± 4.47	174.28 ± 1.61	N/A	N/A	N/A
PEO15	185.27	176.91 ± 1.46	188.37 ± 1.77	N/A	26.69 ± 1.69	29.10 ± 0.10
PEO15-P	192.22	171.52 ± 1.68	182.18 ± 3.16	N/A	27.15 ± 0.92	27.55 ± 0.78

*: Derived from measured tablet weights and average theophylline content of filaments including standard deviation.

3.2.2. Influence of Formulation and Production on the Tensile Strength of 3D-Printed Cylinders

Another influence of the previously described process-related microstructural defects in HPMC-based samples emerged from the investigation of the mechanical properties of printed full-material cylinders via Brazilian test. Instead of a material property, the diametric compression test yielded a value more dependent on layer adhesion. Neglecting the total values (Figure 10A), the significant increase in standard deviation with increasing theophylline load represents on one hand the increasing number of defects and their statistical occurrence. On the other hand, the matrix volume decreases with increasing theophylline load inducing more particle-particle contacts with weaker interfacial attraction. The significantly lower tensile strength of HPMC cylinders without theophylline confirms the above-discussed hypothesis that the theophylline particles enhance the layer adhesion and mechanical filament properties in some way.

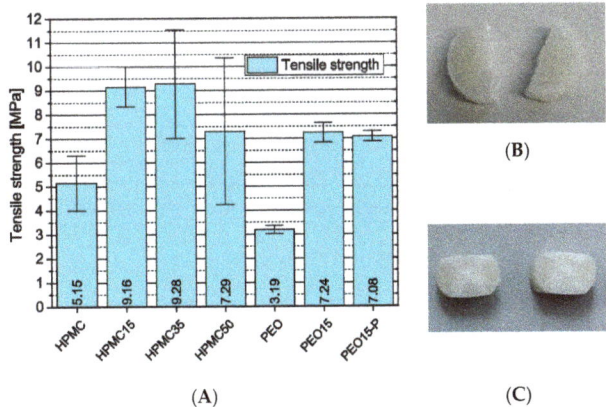

Figure 10. (A) Tensile strength of 3D-printed cylinders via Brazilian test, n = 6; (B) PEO cylinders after test; (C) PEO15 cylinders after test.

The PEO-based cylinders did not delaminate under diametric pressure. Instead, the pure PEO cylinders depicted nearly perfect diametric breakage as it can be observed with standard compressed tablets (Figure 10B). The cylinders containing theophylline, however, did not break but were compressed (Figure 10C). The difference is induced by dissolved theophylline molecules inside the PEO matrix plastifying the polymer and by the needle-like shape of the theophylline particles. The elongate particles are pulled out of the matrix during material failure and therefore induce a better adhesion between the fragments.

3.2.3. Influence of Formulation and Geometry on Dissolution Profiles and Release Kinetics

Dissolution testing of the 3D-printed cylindrical tablets and spheres made from HPMC formulations with different theophylline loads indicated that the theophylline load had no significant influence on the release profiles (Figure 11A). All cylinders and rings of the three formulations released nearly 60% of their theophylline content over six hours. During the first two hours, being characteristic for the passage through the stomach, all release curves follow a first-order kinetic up to a theophylline release of 30%. After changing the testing medium with a shift in pH from 1 to 6.8, all curves follow a zero-order kinetic. However, the dissolution testing of printed rings with a higher surface-area-to-volume ratio showed a drug release of nearly 95% over 6 h for all formulations (compared with approx. 60% for cylindrical tablets and spheres) and higher differences between different drug loads (higher flowrate for 50 wt.% formulation must be considered) due to lower diffusion lengths within the ring structure. Of course, the theophylline mass actually released from dosage forms made with different formulations differs due to the different theophylline contents (Figure 11B). However, the same trend towards higher theophylline release from rings can be observed. These observations show that with the used HPMC grade as matrix polymer which swells in water forming a diffusion barrier, extended release dosage forms can be produced which's release profiles are irrespective of the theophylline-content at low surface area to volume ratios and provide comparable relative release kinetics (spheres: 0.91 mm^{-1}, cylinders: 1.17 mm^{-1}, rings: 1.93 mm^{-1}).

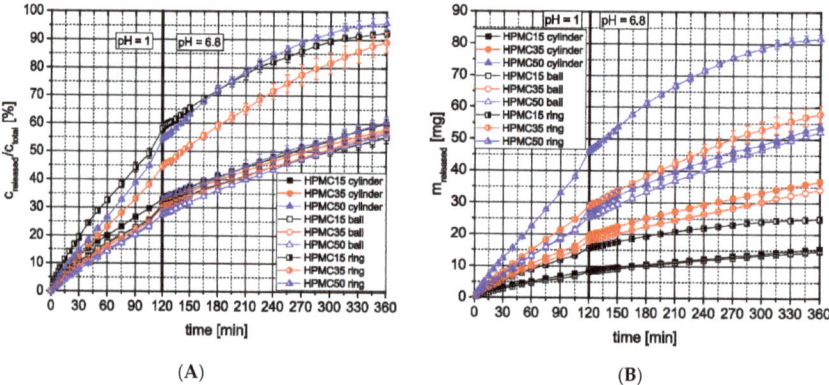

Figure 11. In vitro theophylline release from HPMC-based 3D-printed dosage forms using flow through apparatus; (**A**) relative release; (**B**) total release; $n = 3$.

3D-printed cylinders with open porosity controlled by the infill option of the printer's software consist of an outer full material ring filled with a structure whose density depends on the chosen infill value [%]. Therefore, the mass of a dosage form also depends on this value. During dissolution testing of cylinders with different open porosities based on HPMC15, different behavior of the dosage forms could be observed (Figure 12). The inner structure of the dosage form with only 20% infill was washed out after several minutes leaving a ring behind. Instead of being washed out, the inner structures of both dosage forms with 50% and 80% swelled, generating a cylindrical shape. Therefore, the relatively released theophylline increases with decreasing infill. In addition, dosage forms which generate a cylinder during dissolution testing release the theophylline after comparable but faster kinetic as a full material cylinder does.

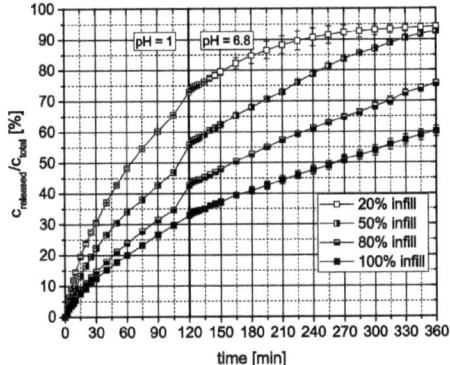

Figure 12. In vitro theophylline release from HPMC15 3D-printed cylinders with different open porosity defined via "infill" setting, $n = 3$.

Dissolution testing of dosage forms made from PEO (data shown in Supplementary Files) showed rapid theophylline release. Depending on the geometry and open porosity, 100% theophylline release was reached after 15–60 min. Therefore, PEO-based materials are suitable for fast releasing parts of polypill applications.

4. Conclusions

For individualization approaches of pharmaceuticals, combining different APIs into one dosage form by 3D-printing, a high API load in the respective intermediate products is needed. This makes the thorough evaluation of highly loaded filaments inevitable. However, by increasing disperse API content, properties of filaments for 3D-printing may be altered, modulating the performance along the process chain. Therefore, particle-induced effects on printability and product properties must be elucidated to finally enable the prediction of overall process performance based on formulation and API particle properties.

In general, particles inside the polymer matrix proved to particularly alter the mechanical properties of both filaments and 3D prints. The systematic adaption of specific FLM parameters can attenuate several challenges such as layer adhesion to a certain extent. However, as the influence of size and shape of particles and their behavior during multiple heating, such as in filament extrusion and FLM itself, and their interplay with dissolved API molecules in the melt are not fully understood, further investigations are required.

Additionally, higher API content can cause instabilities in the 3D-printing process, making prediction of dosage form mass and therefore content uniformity more challenging. For tested HPMC formulations, the release profile of geometries with low surface-area-to-volume ratio is independent of the API content, facilitating an independent adjustment of the dose-and-release profile as well as the application of highly loaded polymer formulations in polypill applications.

To conclude, all experimental data demonstrate the significance of the impact of the API load over the whole process chain of 3D-printing of tablets. This knowledge must be extended further to derive models that should be taken into consideration during product development of individualized medicines.

Supplementary Materials: The following are available online at http://www.mdpi.com/1999-4923/11/4/194/s1, Figure S1: In vitro theophylline release from PEO-based 3D-printed dosage forms, $n = 3$.

Author Contributions: Conceptualization, A.K. and J.H.F.; methodology, M.T. and J.H.F.; formal analysis, M.T.; investigation, M.T. and J.H.F.; resources, A.K. and J.H.F.; data curation, M.T.; writing—original draft preparation, M.T.; writing—review and editing, J.H.F. and A.K.; visualization, M.T.; supervision, A.K. and J.H.F.; project administration, J.H.F.

Funding: This research received no external funding.

Acknowledgments: The authors want to acknowledge Meinolf Brackhagen and Heiko Feldmann from DowDuPont Specialty Products (DuPont) Division for their support with material and their aid at filament extrusion. Further acknowledgements go to Manuela Handt from the Institute of Pharmaceutical Technology and Daniela Scholz and Alexander Diener both from the Institute for Particle Technology all from the TU Braunschweig for their great help with DSC, TGA and µCT measurements, respectively. Additionally, we acknowledge support by the German Research Foundation and the Open Access Publication Funds of the Technische Universität Braunschweig.

Conflicts of Interest: The authors declare no conflicts of interest.

References

1. Hsiao, W.-K.; Lorber, B.; Reitsamer, H.; Khinast, J. 3D printing of oral drugs: A new reality or hype? *Expert Opin. Drug Deliv.* **2018**, *15*, 1–4. [CrossRef]
2. Norman, J.; Madurawe, R.D.; Moore, C.M.V.; Khan, M.A.; Khairuzzaman, A. A new chapter in pharmaceutical manufacturing: 3D-printed drug products. *Adv. Drug Deliv. Rev.* **2017**, *108*, 39–50. [CrossRef] [PubMed]
3. Verein Deutscher Ingenieure. *Additive Fertigungsverfahren Grundlagen, Begriffe, Verfahrensbeschreibungen.* VDI 3405; ICS 25.020 (VDI 3405); Beuth Verlag GmbH: Berlin, Germany, 2014.
4. Spritam®. Available online: https://www.spritam.com (accessed on 10 November 2018).
5. Fina, F.; Madla, C.M.; Goyanes, A.; Zhang, J.; Gaisford, S.; Basit, A.W. Fabricating 3D printed orally disintegrating printlets using selective laser sintering. *Int. J. Pharm.* **2018**, *541*, 101–107. [CrossRef] [PubMed]
6. Fina, F.; Goyanes, A.; Madla, C.M.; Awad, A.; Trenfield, S.J.; Kuek, J.M.; Patel, P.; Gaisford, S.; Basit, A.W. 3D printing of drug-loaded gyroid lattices using selective laser sintering. *Int. J. Pharm.* **2018**, *547*, 44–52. [CrossRef]
7. Khaled, S.A.; Burley, J.C.; Alexander, M.R.; Roberts, C.J. Desktop 3D printing of controlled release pharmaceutical bilayer tablets. *Int. J. Pharm.* **2014**, *461*, 105–111. [CrossRef]
8. Khaled, S.A.; Burley, J.C.; Alexander, M.R.; Yang, J.; Roberts, C.J. 3D printing of tablets containing multiple drugs with defined release profiles. *Int. J. Pharm.* **2015**, *494*, 643–650. [CrossRef] [PubMed]
9. Khaled, S.A.; Burley, J.C.; Alexander, M.R.; Yang, J.; Roberts, C.J. 3D printing of five-in-one dose combination polypill with defined immediate and sustained release profiles. *J. Control. Release* **2015**, *217*, 308–314. [CrossRef]
10. Shor, L.; Güçeri, S.; Chang, R.; Gordon, J.; Kang, Q.; Hartsock, L.; An, Y.; Sun, W. Precision extruding deposition (PED) fabrication of polycaprolactone (PCL) scaffolds for bone tissue engineering. *Biofabrication* **2009**, *1*, 15003. [CrossRef] [PubMed]
11. Lee, S.-H.; Cho, Y.S.; Hong, M.W.; Lee, B.-K.; Park, Y.; Park, S.-H.; Kim, Y.Y.; Cho, Y.-S. Mechanical properties and cell-culture characteristics of a polycaprolactone kagome-structure scaffold fabricated by a precision extruding deposition system. *Biomed. Mater.* **2017**, *12*, 55003. [CrossRef]
12. Goyanes, A.; Buanz, A.B.M.; Basit, A.W.; Gaisford, S. Fused-filament 3D printing (3DP) for fabrication of tablets. *Int. J. Pharm.* **2014**, *476*, 88–92. [CrossRef]
13. Goyanes, A.; Buanz, A.B.M.; Hatton, G.B.; Gaisford, S.; Basit, A.W. 3D printing of modified-release aminosalicylate (4-ASA and 5-ASA) tablets. *Eur. J. Pharm. Biopharm.* **2015**, *89*, 157–162. [CrossRef] [PubMed]
14. Almeida, A.; Claeys, B.; Remon, J.P.; Vervaet, C. Hot-melt Extrusion Developments in the Pharmaceutical Industry. In *Hot-Melt Extrusion: Pharmaceutical Applications*; Douroumis, D., Ed.; Wiley: Chichester, UK; West Sussex, UK, 2012; pp. 43–70.
15. Crowley, M.M.; Zhang, F.; Repka, M.A.; Thumma, S.; Upadhye, S.B.; Battu, S.K.; McGinity, J.W.; Martin, C. Pharmaceutical applications of hot-melt extrusion: Part I. *Drug Dev. Ind. Pharm.* **2007**, *33*, 909–926. [CrossRef] [PubMed]
16. Pirayavaraporn, C.; Rades, T.; Tucker, I.G. Determination of moisture content in relation to thermal behaviour and plasticization of Eudragit RLPO. *Int. J. Pharm.* **2012**, *422*, 68–74. [CrossRef] [PubMed]
17. Crowley, M.M.; Zhang, F.; Koleng, J.J.; McGinity, J.W. Stability of polyethylene oxide in matrix tablets prepared by hot-melt extrusion. *Biomaterials* **2002**, *23*, 4241–4248. [CrossRef]
18. Zhang, Y.; Luo, R.; Chen, Y.; Ke, X.; Hu, D.; Han, M. Application of carrier and plasticizer to improve the dissolution and bioavailability of poorly water-soluble baicalein by hot melt extrusion. *AAPS Pharmscitech.* **2014**, *15*, 560–568. [CrossRef] [PubMed]

19. De Brabander, C.; van den Mooter, G.; Vervaet, C.; Remon, J.P. Characterization of ibuprofen as a nontraditional plasticizer of ethyl cellulose. *J. Pharm. Sci.* **2002**, *91*, 1678–1685. [CrossRef] [PubMed]
20. Wu, C. Non-traditional plasticization of polymeric films. *Int. J. Pharm.* **1999**, *177*, 15–27. [CrossRef]
21. Van Renterghem, J.; Vervaet, C.; de Beer, T. Rheological Characterization of Molten Polymer-Drug Dispersions as a Predictive Tool for Pharmaceutical Hot-Melt Extrusion Processability. *Pharm. Res.* **2017**, *34*, 2312–2321. [CrossRef]
22. Yang, M.; Wang, P.; Suwardie, H.; Gogos, C. Determination of acetaminophen's solubility in poly(ethylene oxide) by rheological, thermal and microscopic methods. *Int. J. Pharm.* **2011**, *403*, 83–89. [CrossRef]
23. Goyanes, A.; Chang, H.; Sedough, D.; Hatton, G.B.; Wang, J.; Buanz, A.; Gaisford, S.; Basit, A.W. Fabrication of controlled-release budesonide tablets via desktop (FDM) 3D printing. *Int. J. Pharm.* **2015**, *496*, 414–420. [CrossRef]
24. Melocchi, A.; Parietti, F.; Maroni, A.; Foppoli, A.; Gazzaniga, A.; Zema, L. Hot-melt extruded filaments based on pharmaceutical grade polymers for 3D printing by fused deposition modeling. *Int. J. Pharm.* **2016**, *509*, 255–263. [CrossRef] [PubMed]
25. Alhijjaj, M.; Belton, P.; Qi, S. An investigation into the use of polymer blends to improve the printability of and regulate drug release from pharmaceutical solid dispersions prepared via fused deposition modeling (FDM) 3D printing. *Eur. J. Pharm. Biopharm.* **2016**, *108*, 111–125. [CrossRef] [PubMed]
26. Goyanes, A.; Robles Martinez, P.; Buanz, A.; Basit, A.W.; Gaisford, S. Effect of geometry on drug release from 3D printed tablets. *Int. J. Pharm.* **2015**, *494*, 657–663. [CrossRef] [PubMed]
27. Kempin, W.; Domsta, V.; Grathoff, G.; Brecht, I.; Semmling, B.; Tillmann, S.; Weitschies, W.; Seidlitz, A. Immediate Release 3D-Printed Tablets Produced Via Fused Deposition Modeling of a Thermo-Sensitive Drug. *Pharm. Res.* **2018**, *35*, 124. [CrossRef] [PubMed]
28. Boetker, J.; Water, J.J.; Aho, J.; Arnfast, L.; Bohr, A.; Rantanen, J. Modifying release characteristics from 3D printed drug-eluting products. *Eur. J. Pharm. Sci.* **2016**, *90*, 47–52. [CrossRef]
29. Genina, N.; Holländer, J.; Jukarainen, H.; Mäkilä, E.; Salonen, J.; Sandler, N. Ethylene vinyl acetate (EVA) as a new drug carrier for 3D printed medical drug delivery devices. *Eur. J. Pharm. Sci.* **2016**, *90*, 53–63. [CrossRef]
30. Zhang, J.; Feng, X.; Patil, H.; Tiwari, R.V.; Repka, M.A. Coupling 3D printing with hot-melt extrusion to produce controlled-release tablets. *Int. J. Pharm.* **2017**, *519*, 186–197. [CrossRef] [PubMed]
31. Verstraete, G.; Samaro, A.; Grymonpré, W.; Vanhoorne, V.; van Snick, B.; Boone, M.N.; Hellemans, T.; van Hoorebeke, L.; Remon, J.P.; Vervaet, C. 3D printing of high drug loaded dosage forms using thermoplastic polyurethanes. *Int. J. Pharm.* **2018**, *536*, 318–325. [CrossRef]
32. Goyanes, A.; Wang, J.; Buanz, A.; Martínez-Pacheco, R.; Telford, R.; Gaisford, S.; Basit, A.W. 3D Printing of Medicines: Engineering Novel Oral Devices with Unique Design and Drug Release Characteristics. *Mol. Pharm.* **2015**, *12*, 4077–4084. [CrossRef]
33. Gioumouxouzis, C.I.; Katsamenis, O.L.; Bouropoulos, N.; Fatouros, D.G. 3D printed oral solid dosage forms containing hydrochlorothiazide for controlled drug delivery. *J. Drug Deliv. Sci. Technol.* **2017**, *40*, 164–171. [CrossRef]
34. Okwuosa, T.C.; Pereira, B.C.; Arafat, B.; Cieszynska, M.; Isreb, A.; Alhnan, M.A. Fabricating a Shell-Core Delayed Release Tablet Using Dual FDM 3D Printing for Patient-Centred Therapy. *Pharm. Res.* **2017**, *34*, 427–437. [CrossRef]
35. Pietrzak, K.; Isreb, A.; Alhnan, M.A. A flexible-dose dispenser for immediate and extended release 3D printed tablets. *Eur. J. Pharm. Biopharm.* **2015**, *96*, 380–387. [CrossRef]
36. Takahashi, Y.; Tadokoro, H. Structural Studies of Polyethers, (-(CH2)m-O-)n. X. Crystal Structure of Poly(ethylene oxide). *Macromolecules* **1973**, *6*, 672–675. [CrossRef]
37. The United States Pharmacopeial Convention. *Hypromellose*; The United States Pharmacopeial Convention: Rockville, MD, USA, 2015.
38. Korte, C.; Quodbach, J. Formulation development and process analysis of drug-loaded filaments manufactured via hot-melt extrusion for 3D-printing of medicines. *Pharm. Dev. Technol.* **2018**, *23*, 1117–1127. [CrossRef]

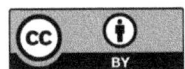

© 2019 by the authors. Licensee MDPI, Basel, Switzerland. This article is an open access article distributed under the terms and conditions of the Creative Commons Attribution (CC BY) license (http://creativecommons.org/licenses/by/4.0/).

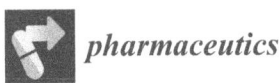

Article

Impact of Processing Parameters on the Quality of Pharmaceutical Solid Dosage Forms Produced by Fused Deposition Modeling (FDM)

Muqdad Alhijjaj [1,2,†], Jehad Nasereddin [1,†], Peter Belton [3] and Sheng Qi [1,*]

1. School of Pharmacy, University of East Anglia, Norwich, Norfolk NR4 7TJ, UK; muqdad.mousa@uobasrah.edu.iq (M.A.); J.Nasereddin@uea.ac.uk (J.N.)
2. College of Pharmacy, University of Basrah, Basrah 61004, Iraq
3. School of Chemistry, University of East Anglia, Norwich, Norfolk NR4 7TJ, UK; P.Belton@uea.ac.uk
* Correspondence: sheng.qi@uea.ac.uk; Fax: +44-1603592023
† These authors contributed equally to this work.

Received: 23 October 2019; Accepted: 25 November 2019; Published: 27 November 2019

Abstract: Fused deposition modeling (FDM) three-dimensional (3D) printing is being increasingly explored as a direct manufacturing method to product pharmaceutical solid dosage forms. Despite its many advantages as a pharmaceutical formulation tool, it remains restricted to proof-of-concept formulations. The optimization of the printing process in order to achieve adequate precision and printing quality remains to be investigated. Demonstrating a thorough understanding of the process parameters of FDM and their impact on the quality of printed dosage forms is undoubtedly necessary should FDM advance from a proof-of-concept stage to an adapted pharmaceutical manufacturing tool. This article describes the findings of an investigation into a number of critical process parameters of FDM and their impact on quantifiable, pharmaceutically-relevant measures of quality. Polycaprolactone, one of the few polymers which is both suitable for FDM and is a GRAS (generally regarded as safe) material, was used to print internally-exposed grids, allowing examination of both their macroscopic and microstructural reproducibility of FDM. Of the measured quality parameters, dimensional authenticity of the grids was found to poorly match the target dimensions. Weights of the grids were found to significantly vary upon altering printing speed. Printing temperature showed little effect on weight. Weight uniformity per batch was found to lie within acceptable pharmaceutical quality limits. Furthermore, we report observing a microstructural distortion relating to printing temperature which we dub The First Layer Effect (FLE). Principal Component Analysis (PCA) was used to study factor interactions and revealed, among others, the existence of an interaction between weight/dosing accuracy and dimensional authenticity dictating a compromise between the two quality parameters. The Summed Standard Deviation (SSD) is proposed as a method to extract the optimum printing parameters given all the perceived quality parameters and the necessary compromises among them.

Keywords: Fused Deposition Modeling 3D Printing; processing parameters; pharmaceutical quality control; hot-melt extrusion; solid dosage forms

1. Introduction

Three-dimensional (3D) printing continues to attract increasing attention in the pharmaceutical industry [1]. The flexibility and customisability potential offered by 3D printing promises to overcome some limitations of traditional pharmaceutical manufacturing techniques, particularly for personalised medicine [2]. The successful commercialisation of Spritam® 3D printed levetiracetam tablets, which are produced by powder-jetting 3D printing, further cemented the prospects of 3D printing as a realistic technique for pharmaceutical manufacturing [3]. Several variants of 3D printing exist. Khaled et al. demonstrated the use of semi-solid extrusion 3D printing to fabricate 5-in-1 polypills [4]. Awad et al. used selective laser sintering to 3D print ibuprofen-paracetamol bilayered pellets [5]. Robles-Martinez et al. used stereolithographic 3D printing to print stratified polypills containing six drugs [6]. Fused Deposition Modelling (FDM) is another type of 3D printing variant that has been increasingly investigation for pharmaceutical exploration [1,7]. FDM is an inexpensive and very widely available technique compared to other variants of 3D printing. The pairing of FDM with Hot-Melt Extrusion (HME) [8–10] extends the library of available materials for 3D printing to include many pharmaceutically-relevant polymers, allowing for material flexibility when formulating a pharmaceutical product. Furthermore, FDM is not liable to some of the limitations posed by other 3D printing variants. Objects produced by powder-based 3D printing and semi-solid extrusion are susceptible to mechanical weakness issues [7,11]. Stereolithography relies on ultraviolet curing to fabricate the object, which raises drug stability and safety concerns [7]. Because of those reasons, an increasing number of publications suggests that FDM may be a favourable 3D printing method for the fabrication of personalized medicines in the form of solid dosage forms [8,11–18]. It was demonstrated that even off-the-shelf FDM printers are capable of producing proof-of-concept formulations.

There is currently no FDM printer that has been specifically designed for pharmaceutical applications. Commercially available printers, such as the MakerBot® brand of printers, designed for fabricating plastic material-based prototype objects, have been frequently reported as the printers used when fabricating pharmaceutical dosage forms by FDM [1,8,9,14–16,18–20]. When characterizing the FDM printed objects, the non-pharmaceutical literature is largely concerned with the surface roughness and tensile strength of the fabricated objects [21–25]. In pharmaceutical applications, when the FDM printed objects are intended to be used as oral solid dosage forms, achieving precise and highly reproducible dimensions and weight is critical. However, to date, there is no debate on whether the fundamental design of these prototype-building FDM printers is suitable for pharmaceutical manufacturing. This study performed a detailed investigation of the influences of the processing parameters on the key quality attributes of the printed objects, including uniformity, reproducibility, and adherence to design specifications required for the pharmaceutical standards.

Although this study is limited to one particular printing machine it is intended to indicate the design parameters that must be considered when producing a 3D FDM printer for clinical pharmaceutical applications

In the FDM printing process, and any printing process, the quality of the printed object is the result of a complex interplay between the properties of the printing material and the settings of the machine (both adjustable and non-adjustable), the relevant parameters for FDM printing are shown in Figure 1. For the printer used in this work, the machine adjustable parameters are print speed, extrusion temperature, build plate temperature, and layer thickness. These represent the main variables in the FDM printing process. Temperature will necessarily affect the material properties, in particular, its rheological properties [26]. These, in turn, will determine the flow out of the printing head, often known as melt flow, which is one of the factors investigated in this study, and the spread on the build plate, which may then affect the reproducibility and dimensional precision of the printed object. Under some circumstances, high temperature may increase the fluidity of the printing material and cause unstable layer deposition. At the other extreme, low temperatures may cause reduced flow resulting in the print head, resulting in a blockage or a flow rate too small to print adequately at some printing speeds. Rheology may also affect flow after deposition on the build plate. In this work, we examine the interaction of the machine adjustable parameters and the print material rheological properties as indicated by the melt flow index and their effect on the reproducibility and adherence to design specification of the printed object. We note that some research suggests that computational factors such as slicing (the process by which the computer-generated 3D model is translated into movement instructions for the printer motors) algorithms could play a significant role in the overall quality of the printed object [27,28]. In this work, we restrict ourselves to exploring the relevant physical parameters, as other parameters cannot be manipulated without physically modifying the machine.

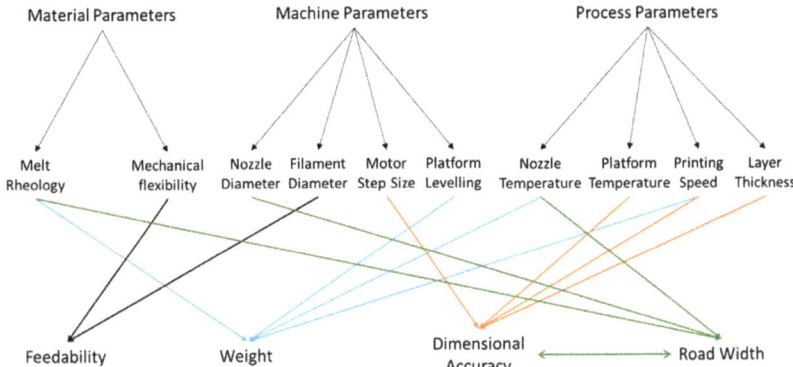

Figure 1. Summary of the interactions between the materials properties and the machine and process parameters in a fused deposition modeling (FDM) three-dimensional (3D) printing process.

In addition, prior to the printing process, the 'leveling' of the printer, which is to ensure that the distance between the printing head and the build plate is constant across the printing area, should be performed to ensure the reproducible quality of the printed objects. It has been reported [8] that, for a machine of the same make and model, the outcome of this process could be operator dependent, indicating that the printing outcome may be irreproducible between operators. We report below on our examination of this problem.

Polycaprolactone (PCL), being one of the very few polymers approved for pharmaceutical use that is also suitable for FDM without further formulation [9,19], was used as the model polymer to investigate the effect of material and process parameters on the quality of printing. In the course of the work, it was noted that the first deposited layer tended to have different morphology to the layers above. We have dubbed this phenomenon The First Layer Effect (FLE). Apart from the variables discussed above, it is possible that the surface properties of the build plate may affect the first layer so the printing behaviour on different surfaces was also investigated. This is expected to have great importance for selecting the best build plate lining that allows the most suitable adherence of the printing material to the build plate during the building process and provides the easy peel-off of the object after the complete production of the printed dosage forms.

2. Materials and Methods

2.1. Materials

PCL commercial filament was purchased from MakerBot Industries (MakerBot Industries LLC., New York, NY, United States). PCL pure powder (CAPA™, Grade 6506) was purchased from Perstorp Chemicals (Perstorp Chemicals GmbH, Arnsberg, Germany), acetylsalicylic acid (ASA) was purchased from Sigma Aldrich (Sigma Aldrich Ltd., Dorset, United Kingdom).

2.2. Methods

2.2.1. Preparation of Drug Loaded Filaments by HME

Three drug loaded PCL filaments containing 5%, 10%, and 15% ASA were prepared using HME. For each batch of the filament, the power mixes were accurately weighed then thoroughly mixed using a mortar and pestle. The powder mixes were fed into a Haake II minilab compounder

(Thermo Scientific, Karlsruhe, Germany) equipped with a co-rotating twin screw set and a circular die with a diameter of 1.75 mm. Extrusion was performed at 100 °C with a screw rotation speed of 100 revolutions per second (RPM). All formulations were cycled in the extruder for 5 min to ensure homogeneous mixing of ASA and PCL prior to being flushed out.

2.2.2. FDM 3D Printing of Commercial Filaments and Drug-Loaded Filaments

A MakerBot Replicator 2X twin nozzle desktop 3D printer (MakerBot Industries LLC, New York, NY, United States), equipped with nozzles of diameter 400 µm, was used for printing all filaments. The solid dosage form used in this study was a three-layered square film with 25 mm in length and width, and 0.6 mm in thickness (with 0.2 mm thickness per layer) (Figure 2). The film is comprised of 31 identical rods (rod dimensions: 0.4 mm wide, 0.2 mm thick, and 25 mm long). The design of the film is illustrated in Supplementary Materials Figure S1. The film was designed using Blender software and was then exported in stereolithography file format (STL file). The STL file was printed using MakerBot MakerWare™.

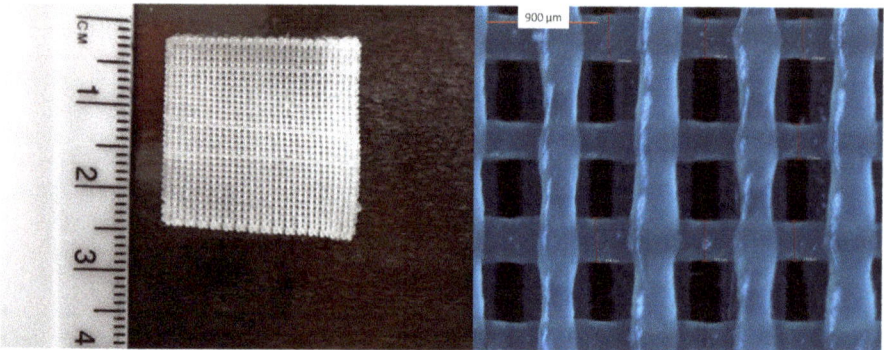

Figure 2. Macroscopic (left) and light microscopy image (right) of the 3D printed film.

Twelve sets of different printing experiments were conducted, each varying either one of three factors (nozzle temperature, build plate temperature, and printing speed), as seen in Table 1. Five films were printed using each set of printing parameters, the printed film was weighed and the dimensions of the films were then accurately measured using a digital calliper. Printing of the drug-loaded filaments was performed using the MakerBot Replicator 2X printer. The filaments were printed with a nozzle temperature of 100 °C, an unheated build plate and were printed at a speed of 90 mm/s.

Table 1. Experimental parameters used for printing the selected 3D object using MakerBot® Flexible filament.

Nozzle Temperature (°C)	Platform Temperature (°C)	Printing Speed (mm/s)
100	30	30
100	30	90
100	30	160
110	30	30
110	30	90
110	30	160
120	30	30
120	30	90
120	30	160
100	45	30
100	45	90
100	45	160

2.2.3. In Vitro Drug Release Studies

ASA release studies from the 5%, 10%, and 15% loaded 3D printed grid films were conducted using the United States Pharmacopoeia (USP) apparatus II (paddle) using a revolution rate of 50 RPM. The grids were placed in 750 mL of pH 1.2 simulated gastric fluid for 2 h, then transferred to 900 mL of pH 6.8 phosphate buffer saline. Determination of amount of ASA released was conducted using a Perkin Elmer Lambda 35 UV/Vis spectrophotometer (PerkinElmer, Inc., Waltham, MA, United States) at a wavelength of 265 nm [29].

2.2.4. Melt Flow Index Measurements

The melt flow index (MFI) of the filaments was measured using an adaptation of the ISO 1133-1 standard method [30]. The printing head of a MakerBot® Replicator 2X desktop FDM 3D printer (MakerBot Industries LLC. New York, NY, United States) was detached from its roller feeding zone and used to melt the filaments. A piston attached to a metal weight of 80 g was used to propel 2 cm slices of the filament through the nozzle (Supplementary Materials Figure S2). The filament melt flowing from the nozzle was collected at specified time intervals and weighed. The mass of the polymer (in milligrams) extruded per second was regarded as the MFI of the polymer. Using this adapted method maintains the gravimetric flow of the polymer melt that is characteristic of standard MFI measurements, but over the relevant capillary diameter of the printing nozzle. The MFI measurements for PCL were performed using a temperature range of 70 °C to 130 °C.

The quantity (in milligrams) of material deposited per second during an actual FDM printing process is defined in this study as the FDM-MFI. The FDM-MFI values of the PCL filaments were measured at three different printing speeds (30 mm/s, 90 mm/s, and 160 mm/s) over a range of processing temperatures (70–130 °C). For both MFI and FDM-MFI measurements, the rate of deposition of the objects was then expressed as weight deposited per unit time (mg/min).

2.2.5. Leveling of the Build Plate of the Printer

Two investigations of the platform leveling were performed. Inter-person calibration: the platform was leveled by two operators, then six square films were printed and their weights and dimensions quantified. Same person inter-day calibration: the platform was leveled by the same operator on two different days; then, a set of six squares were printed and their weights and dimensions were quantified. The object used for calibration was a simple square design with an edge length of 10 mm and a thickness of 1 mm printed using standard printer settings at 100 °C.

Leveling was conducted as per the standard printer leveling procedure outlined in the user manual of the printer [31]. The card supplied with the instrument was placed between the nozzle and the build plate at various positions around the build plate and the leveling screws were adjusted until the card can just slide between the build plate and the nozzle.

2.2.6. Printing on Different Surfaces

The FLE was further investigated by printing the PCL films on three different surfaces, Kapton® (polyimide) Tape, aluminum, and glass. Aluminum and glass were secured to the build plate using double adhesive tape, to ensure that there was no movement of the test surface during printing. All of these printing experiments were conducted using a nozzle temperature of 100 °C and a printing speed of 90 mm/s. The build plate was leveled following the protocol described in 2.2.4 before each printing attempt.

2.2.7. Characterization of Printed Solid Dosage Forms

Microscopic images were acquired using a Linkam Imaging Station, equipped with a Linkam MDS600 heating/cooling stage (Linkam Scientific Instruments, Tadworth, United Kingdom). Image analysis (dimensions measurements) was conducted using LINK software version 1.0.5.9

(Linkam Scientific Instruments, Tadworth, United Kingdom) to measure the road widths of the 3D printed objects.

Fourier-Transform Infrared (FTIR) spectroscopy was used to characterize all materials used in this study. Spectra were acquired using a Vertex 70 infrared spectrometer (Bruker Optics Ltd., Coventry, United Kingdom), equipped with Golden Gate, heat-enabled Attenuated Total Reflectance (ATR) accessory (Specac Ltd., Orpington, United Kingdom) fitted with a diamond internal reflection element. The spectra were acquired in absorbance mode, with a resolution of 2 cm^{-1}, and 32 scans per sample. Scanning range was set to 4000 cm^{-1}–600 cm^{-1}. Spectral analysis was conducted using OPUS software, version 7.8 (Bruker Optics Ltd., Coventry, United Kingdom).

Differential Scanning Calorimetry (DSC) was carried out using a TA Universal Q2500 Discovery series DSC (TA Instruments, Newcastle, DE, United States). DSC was used to characterize the pure materials (PCL commercial filament, PCL powder, and ASA powder), the physical mixes, and extruded filaments. PCL powder was characterized using a heat-cool-reheat method with a range from 20 °C to 120 °C, followed by cooling to −90 °C, then reheating to 120 °C. ASA powder and physical mixes of all three formulations were scanned using a heat-cool-reheat method; samples were tested over a range of 20 °C to 150 °C, then cooled to −90 °C, and then reheated to 150 °C. All extruded filaments were characterized using a heat-cool-reheat method using a temperature range of −90 °C to 150 °C. A heating/cooling rate of 10 °C/min was used for all experiments. All samples were equilibrated for 3 min at either 20 °C or −90 °C at the start of each experiment. All characterization experiments were carried out in triplicates.

2.2.8. Statistical Analysis

Independent sample T-tests were conducted using Microsoft Excel (version 2016) expanded with the statistical data analysis add-on.

Summed Standard Deviation (SSD) was calculated as follows: for each value of temperature (T) and speed (S) the normalised standard deviations (P') of the measured parameters weight (M), length (L), width (W), thickness (D), and road width (R), were calculated using the following equation:

$$P'_i = \left(\frac{\sigma_i^p}{P_i}\right)_{T,S} \qquad (1)$$

where P_i is the value of the measured parameter at a fixed value of S and T and σ_i^p is its standard deviation. These were summed up, as shown in Equation (2):

$$SSD = \sum_{\substack{S=n \\ T=n \\ S=0 \\ T=0}} [P'_M + P'_L + P'_W + P'_D + P'_R]_{T,S} \qquad (2)$$

Principal Component Analysis (PCA) was conducted on all the measured responses using IBM® SPSS statistics (version 25). Following the Kaiser criterion, only principal components with an eigenvalue ≥ 1 were extracted ($n = 2$), yielding a total explained variance of 82.15% (Principal Component 1: 57.77%. Principal Component 2: 24.38%). The unrotated components matrix showed no factor that could be explained solely by either principal component (coefficient < 0.4); therefore, Varimax rotation was conducted such that each factor is solely described by a single principal component. The loadings plot was used to extract variable scores for each of the two factors (printing temperature, and printing speed), the scores were imported into Microsoft Excel and used to generate a biplot [32,33].

3. Results and Discussion

3.1. Impacts of Build Plate Leveling

It has been previously reported in the literature that the leveling of the build plate of MakerBot® printers causes a significant difference in the weights of the 3D printed objects when conducted by different operators [8]. In an attempt to prevent this discrepancy from misattributing other findings of this work, calibration prints were conducted as described in Section 2.2.5. The weights and dimensions of the two sets were then compared via an Independent Sample T-Test. The results are shown below in Tables 2 and 3.

As seen in Table 2, the P-value for the T-tests for all of the parameters was >0.05, indicating no significant difference between the objects printed when the leveling was carried out by two different operators.

Table 3 shows the results of the calibration prints when the platform was leveled by the same operator on two different days. The P-value for width was the only T-Test parameter found >0.05, indicating no significant difference. P-values for length, thickness, and weight were all <0.05, indicating significant difference.

Table 2. Effect of leveling by different operators on the weight and dimensions of the printed objects. RSD: Relative standard deviation ($(Standard\ deviation/Mean) \times 100$).

	Operator I			
n	Thickness (mm)	Length (mm)	Width (mm)	Weight (mg)
1	1.09	9.92	10.01	110.6
2	1.04	10.03	10.10	114.6
3	1.07	10.00	10.16	113.4
4	1.05	10.00	10.09	111.0
5	1.10	9.91	10.02	109.8
6	1.05	9.99	10.20	111.0
RSD	2.25%	0.48%	0.74%	1.65%
	Operator II			
n	Thickness (mm)	Length (mm)	Width (mm)	Weight (mg)
1	1.03	10.05	10.16	107.7
2	1.08	10.05	10.23	112.6
3	1.04	10.06	10.13	111.1
4	1.06	10.05	10.20	112.5
5	1.04	9.96	10.18	108.7
6	1.06	9.94	10.10	110.1
RSD	1.71%	0.53%	0.46%	1.8%
	Independent Sample T-Test			
p-Value (Length)	p-Value (Width)	p-Value (Thickness)	p-Value (Weight)	
0.223	0.101	0.127	0.137	

Table 3. Inter-day variation in leveling on the weight and dimensions of the printed objects. RSD: Relative standard deviation (($Standard\ deviation/Mean$) × 100).

		Day 1		
n	Thickness (mm)	Length (mm)	Width (mm)	Weight (mg)
1	1.09	9.92	10.01	110.6
2	1.04	10.03	10.10	114.6
3	1.07	10.00	10.16	113.4
4	1.05	10.00	10.09	111.0
5	1.10	9.91	10.02	109.8
6	1.05	9.99	10.20	111.0
RSD	2.25%	0.48%	0.74%	1.65%
		Day 2		
n	Thickness (mm)	Length (mm)	Width (mm)	Weight (mg)
1	1.02	10.08	10.11	108.7
2	1.04	10.09	10.12	108.4
3	1.07	10.03	10.14	105.2
4	1.03	10.06	10.11	107.9
5	1.02	10.03	10.08	104.5
6	1.04	10.06	10.14	109.7
RSD	1.83%	0.25%	0.23%	1.93%
		Independent Sample T-Test		
p-Value (Length)	p-Value (Width)	p-Value (Thickness)	p-Value (Weight)	
0.004	0.213	0.04	0.006	

A study conducted by Melocchi et al. using the same model of the FDM printer [8] previously reported a significant difference when the build plate was leveled by different operators. We acknowledge that the results reported herein contradict with those findings. However, as shown in Table 3, we observed a significant difference (most importantly in weights of the printed objects) when the printer was leveled by the same operator on two different days. Both our findings and what was reported by Melocchi et al. serve to highlight the operator dependence of the calibration of this model of printer which can be a potential problem in this design of the printer if it is used for printing pharmaceutical standard products. The current method employed by the printer to level the build plate is very subjective, relying on what the operator's judgment as 'suitable friction' between the nozzle tip and leveling card. While this may be adequate for printing large commercial prototype objects, it is unlikely to be a suitable 'calibration' method for pharmaceutical printing of oral solid dosage forms where high printing precision is required. Therefore, we believe that the leveling process of any printer to be used for manufacturing pharmaceutical standard solid dosage forms needs to be modified to a more robust procedure.

3.2. Impacts of Melt Flow of the Printed Materials

The Melt Flow Index (MFI), is defined by the ISO standard 1133-1 as "the mass of the molten polymer, in grams, that flows through a capillary of a specific diameter in 10 min" [30]. The MFI of a filament is often cited as one of the key factors defining the success of an FDM printing process [9,19,34]. The MFI is highly associated with the thermal viscosity of the filament materials at a certain printing temperature [26]. Therefore, MFI measurements (which describe the amount of PCL deposited due to its melt flow) were compared to the amount deposited during FDM printing (referred to as FDM-MFI in Figure 3b). Despite the temperature dependence of rheology seen in the MFI experiments (Figure 3a), there was a very weak temperature dependence of deposition rates when printed using FDM (Figure 3b). This implies that over the range of relevant printing temperatures, the change in the melt flow of the filament is not too great to significantly impact the amount of material being deposited by the print head. The only effect was seen at 70 °C, where printing was only possible at a printing speed of

30 mm/s. This leads to the hypothesis that, provided that the operating speed is sufficient to allow free flow of the polymer melt, the contribution of operating temperature to the printability of the material is not of prime importance.

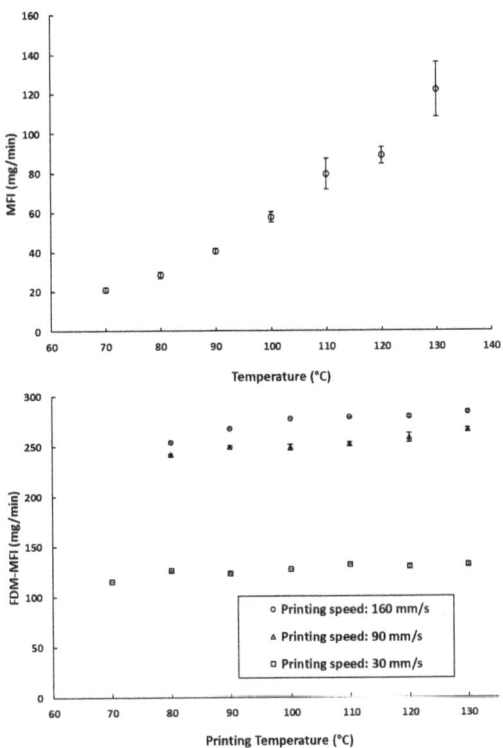

Figure 3. (a) The measured MFI values of the PCL filaments at different temperatures (the arrow indicates the manufacturer recommended printing temperature); (b) FDM-MFI of the PCL filaments measured at different printing speeds across different printing temperature. *: printing at 90 mm/s and 160 mm/s was not possible at this speed.

3.3. Impact of Processing Conditions on Weight Uniformity

MFI measurements showed that PCL has measurable melt flow index at a temperature of 70 °C; however, printing of PCL was only possible at this temperature at the lowest speed of 30 mm/s. In addition, objects printed at 80 °C and either 90 mm/s or 160 mm/s were much distorted, with very poor printing quality and erratic melt deposition. Therefore, samples printed at 70 °C and 80 °C were disregarded. This suggests that there is a lower limit to the melt flow index, below which good quality printing is not possible.

Despite that, on average, the impact of the printing temperature on melt deposition rate was not as significant as printing speed (Figure 3b). It appears that it may impact the reproducibility of the weights of the printed objects. As can be seen in Figure 4a, at a fixed printing speed, increasing the printing temperature resulted in an increase in the weights of the printed objects. This is to be expected, as melt flow of PCL increases with temperature. The standard deviations of weights do not seem to follow any trends either with temperature or printing speed. The largest recorded standard deviation was ±3.2 mg at 90 mm/s and 120 °C. The second largest being ±3.0 mg at 30 mm/s and 70 °C, and the third largest being ±2.4 mg at 30 mm/s and 110 °C. Notably, fixing the printing speed at 160 mm/s yields the narrowest standard deviations, with the smallest standard deviation at that speed being

±0.1 mg at 100 °C, and the largest being ±0.9 mg, seen at both 120 °C and 130 °C. Even though all the reported standard deviations fall well within acceptable limits for weight uniformity specified in the pharmacopoeias, it is worth noting that changing the printing conditions was seen to substantially impact weights of the printed objects, by as much as 31.3 mg. The lightest printed object weighed 169.1 mg (±0.5 mg, printed at 70 °C, and 160 mm/s), and the heaviest printed object weighing 200.3 mg (±1.5 mg, printed at 130 °C, and 30 mm/s). These results indicate that if FDM is to be utilized in personalized medicine, careful screening of the printing parameters, and choosing the appropriate conditions to match the target dose is of utmost importance [2].

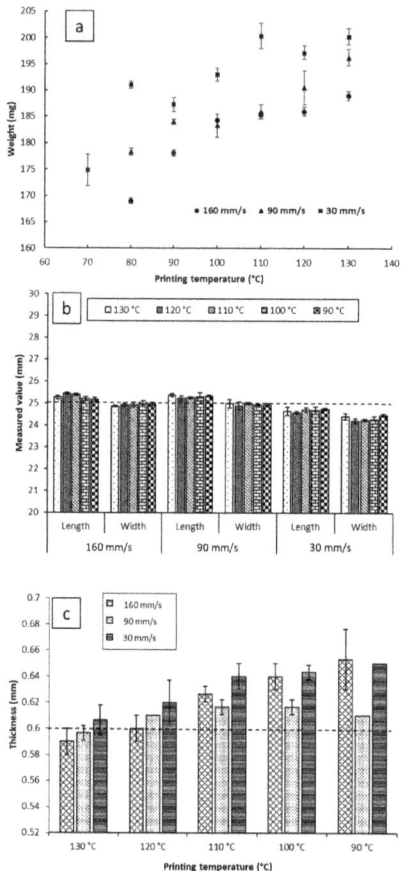

Figure 4. (a) The weight; (b) the length and width; and (c) the thickness of the films printed at a range of speed and temperature. The dotted lines at 25 mm in (b) and 0.6 mm in (c) indicate the theoretical targeted values of the dimensions.

3.4. Impact of Processing Conditions on Dimensional Authenticity

For the commercial printers, the pre-set (target) object parameters are dimensions instead of weight. Therefore, it is important to understand the effect of the process parameters by comparing the measured printed object dimensions to the target values pre-set by the STL file. Despite the source STL file being designed as a square in this study, all the objects printed displayed a difference between length and width. To avoid ambiguity, length was defined as the dimension parallel to the roads of the first layer, and width as the dimension perpendicular to the roads of the first layer. The impacts of the printing temperature on the dimensions (width, length, and thickness) of the objects are illustrated in Figure 4b,c. For each printing condition, the length of the objects was found to be larger than the width of the objects. The printing temperature shows no significant effect on the reproducibility of the length and width of the printed films at a fixed printing speed.

Reducing the printing temperature increases the thickness of the films for both 30 and 160 mm/s printing speeds but there is no significant effect at the printing speed of 90 mm/s. Microscopic imaging of the printed films (Table S1) revealed that the road width of the first layer is much larger than that of the subsequent layers, and the width of the first layer appears to be correlated with the nozzle temperature. This correlation between first layer road width and the reduction of object thickness with increasing temperature suggests that when the first layer is deposited on the build plate, the fluid melt spreads sideways, increasing in width and decreasing in thickness, resulting in the observed effect on road width and thickness. We have chosen to dub this phenomenon the First Layer Effect (FLE), which is discussed in a further section.

Printing at 90 mm/s and 160 mm/s yielded objects that possessed greater length and lower width than the target (25.29 mm ± 0.06 mm × 24.95 mm ± 0.04 mm for 90 mm/s, and 25.29 mm ± 0.11 mm × 24.93 mm ± 0.04 mm for 160 mm/s), showing no significant difference in dimensions between the two conditions. However, printing at 30 mm/s yielded objects that were smaller than the target geometry of 25 mm × 25 mm (with the films being 24.68 mm ± 0.06 mm × 24.33 mm ± 0.11 mm). At this speed, no changes in length and width relative to changing the temperature were observed. In terms of reproducibility of lengths and widths, none of the three printing speeds showed remarkably different results, with no significant differences between the standard deviations of dimensions between the three printed conditions.

As can be seen in Figure 4c, the thickness of the 3D printed objects tends to decrease with increasing temperature for both 160 mm/s and 30 mm/s, going from 0.65 mm ± 0.00 mm at 90 °C to 0.61 mm ± 0.01 mm at 130 °C when printed at 30 mm/s, and from 0.65 mm ± 0.02 mm to 0.59 ± 0.01 mm when printing at 160 mm/s. Objects printed at 90 mm/s had, on average, consistent thickness, independent of printing temperature. Furthermore, printing at 90 mm/s appears to have the most reproducible object thicknesses, with the narrowest recorded standard deviation at said speed being ± 0.00 mm, and the widest being ± 0.01 mm (within the limits of detection of the digital caliper used).

3.5. The First Layer Effect (FLE)

Figure 5a shows the average road width of each layer under different printing conditions. The top layer is the closest to the nozzle. The platform layer is the bottommost layer resting on the build plate of the printer. No significant difference was seen between the top and middle layers of the objects, regardless of printing conditions. The average road width for the top layer was 347.0 μm ± 12.00 μm at 30 mm/s, 345.0 μm ± 15.37 μm at 90 mm/s, and 323.5 μm ± 25.62 μm at 160 mm/s. The average road width for the middle layer was 341.3 μm ± 18.46 μm at 30 mm/s, 310.4 μm ± 13.56 μm at 90 mm/s, 316.8 μm ± 27.45 μm at 160 mm/s. The platform layer displayed a larger road width than the corresponding top and middle layers at every printing condition, with the average road width of the platform layer being 438.8 μm ± 51.79 μm at 30 mm/s, 425.8 μm ± 34.56 μm at 90 mm/s, 436.1 μm ± 68.63 μm at 160 mm/s.

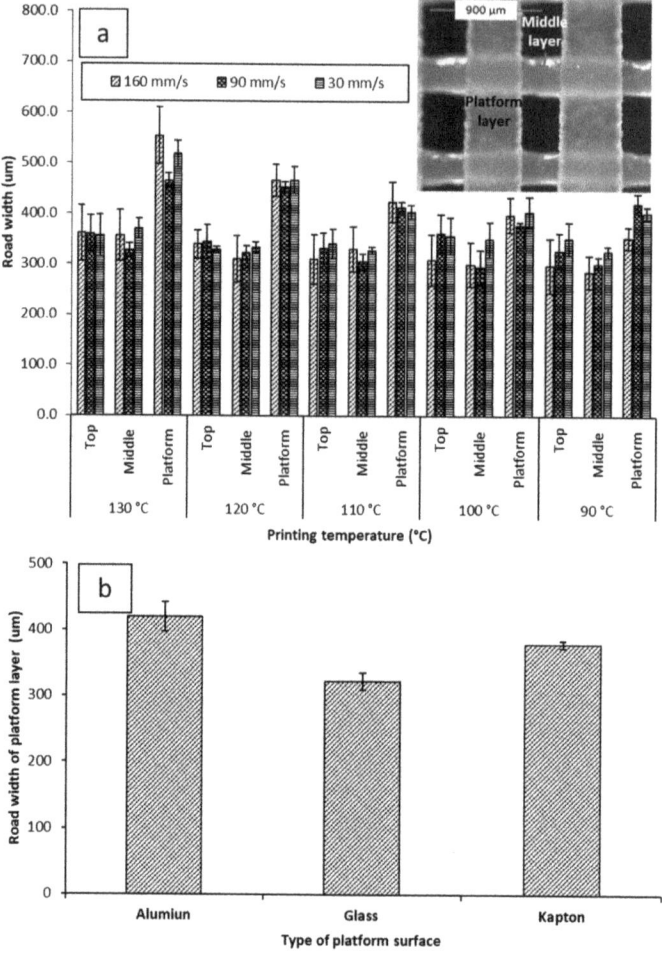

Figure 5. (a) Impacts of printing temperature and printing speed on the road width measurements of the platform (the first layer deposited on the build plate), middle, and top layer (with inserted microscopic image illustrating the platform and mid layers); (b) impact of different printing surfaces on the road width of the platform layer when printed at 90 mm/s and 100 °C. Microscopic images of printed films can be seen in supplementary materials Table S1.

The road width of the platform layer was also observed to vary inversely with printing temperature. There was a notable decrease in the average road width of the first layer at different printing temperatures; at 30 mm/s, the road width increased from 402.1 µm ± 12.9 µm at 90 °C to 517.5 µm ± 26.0 µm at 130 °C. At 90 mm/s, the road width increased from 420.5 µm ± 19.1 µm at 90 °C to 465.2 µm ± 14.9 µm. At 160 mm/s, the road width increased from 422.0 µm ± 35.7 µm at 90 °C to 554.0 µm ± 55.9 µm at 130 °C. Due to the platform layer being the first layer constructed during the fabrication of the object, this phenomenon has been dubbed The First Layer Effect (FLE). This spreading effect is assumed to be caused by the nature of the interaction of PCL with the surface of the Kapton® tape. Therefore, printing was attempted on different surfaces. Printing on different surfaces yielded different spreading amounts (Figure 5b). Building on glass was found to yield the narrowest average road width (322.3 µm ± 13.03 µm). Building on aluminum was found to yield the widest road width

(419.8 µm ± 22.00 µm). The increased spreading with temperature when printing on Kapton® is likely due to decreased viscosity of PCL at higher temperatures allowing it to flow more prior to solidifying.

When printed at higher temperatures (>110 °C), PCL was found to bind strongly to the Kapton® tape. When printed at lower temperatures (i.e., 80 °C–100 °C), the PCL films were easily removed. However, no sticking to aluminum or glass was observed. The temperature-dependent spreading, and the sticking of the objects to the Kapton® tape at elevated temperatures is probably due to the formation of PCL-polyimide interactions at elevated temperatures, yielding greater wetting and adhesion to the surface.

3.6. Impact of Drug Incorporation

Drug incorporation can often cause changes to the printability of polymeric filaments, in most cases due to the plasticisation effect of the drug when a molecular dispersion is formed between the drug and the polymer. Three levels of drug loading were used to create filaments that were either true molecular dispersions or supersaturated with the crystalline drug in the filaments. DSC and ATR-FTIR spectroscopy were used to characterize the physical state of the ASA in the filaments prepared by HME (Figure S3 and Figure 6). The results indicate the formation of a molecular dispersion of ASA in PCL at 5% drug loading, whereas both the 10% and 15% formulation contain a crystalline fraction of ASA. The shifted peaks of the C–O and C–OH groups indicate the molecular interaction of ASA and PCL via hydrogen bonding at the carboxyl groups, as seen in Figure 6. The detailed analysis of the formulation characterisation data can be found in the Supplementary Materials Section S1.1.

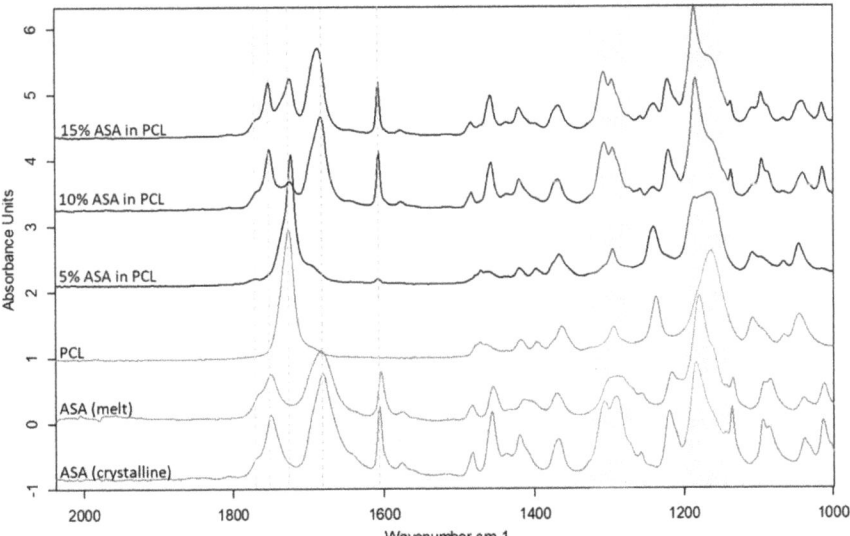

Figure 6. ATR-FTIR spectra of drug loaded PCL filaments in comparison to the raw material and the placebo filament. Shifted C-O stretching peak regions at ~1160 cm^{-1} and ~1290 cm^{-1} are highlighted in blue.

It would be expected that a drug-polymer molten solution would exhibit different spreading behaviour when printed on the surface since the incorporation of the drug would be expected to alter the physical properties of the mix [35]. This was investigated by printing ASA-loaded PCL filaments at a median condition of 100 °C and 90 mm/s. Followed by determination of the average road width per layer. The results can be seen in Figure 7 against a placebo filament printed at the same conditions. No significant difference was seen in the nozzle and middle layer between the three drug-loaded filaments and the placebo filament. However, there is a significant increase in the average road width of the first layer that was brought about by incorporation of ASA in PCL; printing at 90 mm/s and 100 °C showed an increase in the first layer road width from ≈390 µm to >600 µm. This is likely due to the presence of ASA in the PCL matrix decreasing the viscosity of the melt, allowing for a greater extent of spreading before the road completely solidifies. No significant difference was seen between the three drug-loaded formulations, this could be attributed to the ASA-PCL melt reaching the maximum possible wettability it can achieve on Kapton® before it solidifies, regardless of drug loading. Notably, the drug-loaded objects exhibited greater sticking to the platform than their placebo counterparts, requiring very careful peeling off the platform with a razor blade to avoid severely deforming the object printed.

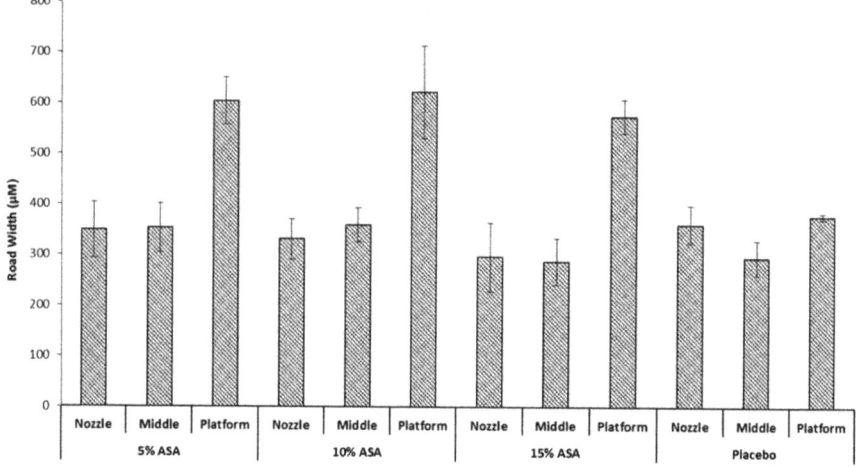

Figure 7. Impact of drug loading on the road width of the printed films.

3.7. In Vitro Drug Release Studies

Figure 8 shows the in vitro drug release rates for the 5%, 10%, and 15% ASA-loaded formulations in PCL. A significant difference in the release rate of the 5% formulation compared to its higher loading counterparts was observed. Both the 10% and 15% formulation achieved ~100% release in under 300 min. The 5% drug-loaded formulation, however, had released only ~30% of the drug after 8 h. As previously discussed, the 5% drug-loaded formulation was the only formulation in which the ASA was molecularly dispersed within the matrix of PCL, while both 10% and 15% drug-loaded contained phase separated crystalline ASA. This is further evidenced by the aforementioned differences in release rate. PCL is a biodegradable polymer that is commonly used for implantable, long-term release formulations [36]. It is insoluble in aqueous media, and only degrades over time via hydrolysis of its ester linkages in physiological conditions. In the 5% drug-loaded formulation, the ASA is molecularly dispersed within the polymer, thus the drug release relies on the slow diffusion of ASA molecules from the PCL matrices and the polymer degradation. On the other hand, the 10% and 15% drug-loaded formulations contain phase–separated crystalline ASA which can dissolve much faster. No visible disintegration of the FDM printed films was observed over the 8 h dissolution tests.

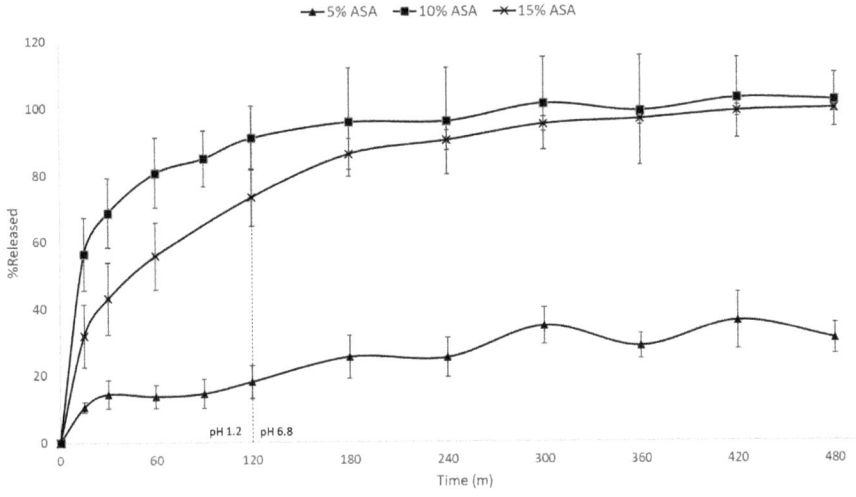

Figure 8. In vitro drug release profiles of FDM printed PCL films containing 5%, 10%, and 15% ASA.

3.8. Statistical Analysis

The data above demonstrated the quality of the printed dosage form is a result of the complex interplay between different processing and materials factors. These factors also often interact such that varying the level of factors concurrently has a greater impact over a perceived measure of goodness than varying either parameter individually. Furthermore, while one can measure particular properties of the 3D printed object (such as weight, dimensions, road width, etc.) to be utilized as measures of goodness for parameter selection, this remains a non-straightforward process. Mainly because processing conditions that appear to produce a more favoured object when observing one measure of goodness fail when another measure of goodness is considered (i.e., weight versus dimensional authenticity). Therefore, it is clear that there exists a need for an overarching method for selecting the optimum printing conditions that will produce the objects with the greatest overall quality. For this purpose, we propose basing this method on a measure of goodness to determine the printing conditions which will produce objects with the highest overall printing reproducibility. Said conditions are those that will yield the minimum Summed Standard Deviation (SSD) score. This proposed SSD can be calculated by summing the standard deviations of each measured value at each condition.

The SSD scores for all printing conditions can be seen in Figure 9. The processing parameters 120 °C and 90 mm/s yielded the lowest SSD while 130 °C and 160 mm/s yielded the highest SSD. Objects printed at 90 mm/s notably had lower SSD scores for every single temperature than their counterparts printed at 30 mm/s and 160 mm/s. The SSD scores represent a figure of merit, which can be used to select a set of printing conditions which will give minimal overall variability.

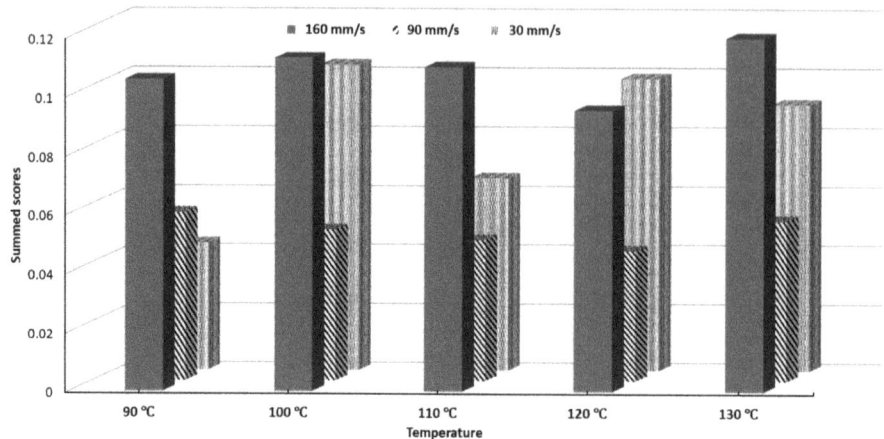

Figure 9. Summed Standard Deviation (SSD) scores of printability of all tested conditions.

While the SSD provides a quick method to determine the optimum printing conditions for a given filament, further statistical analysis techniques can be used to extract more information about the process parameters and how they interact to influence the process. Therefore, PCA was conducted as an exploratory data analysis tool to investigate the interplay between the different perceived quality parameters.

Figure 10 shows the loadings plot of the measured responses in rotated space. Principal Component 1 (PC1) was found to describe object mass, road width, length, width, and the printer deposition index, corresponding to 57.77% of the total variance. Principal Component 2 (PC2) was found to describe object thickness, and first layer width, corresponding to 24.38% of the total variance.

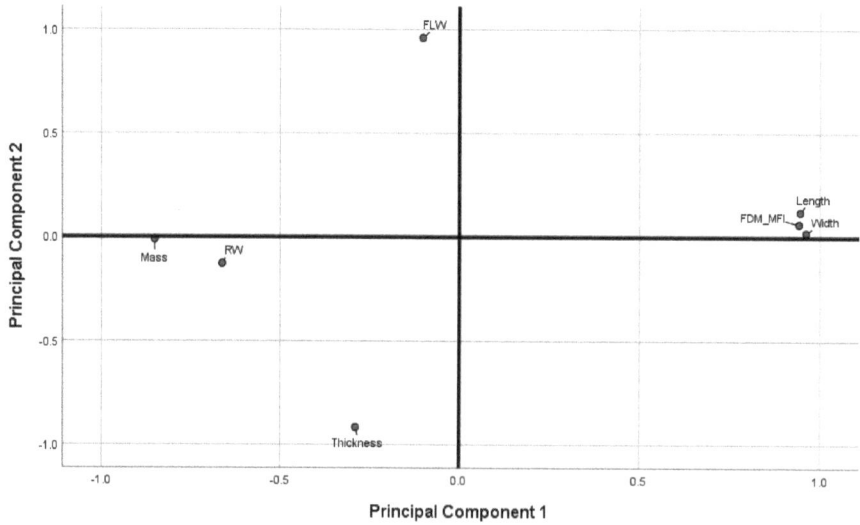

Figure 10. Loadings plot in rotated space. (FLW: first layer width. RW: road width).

As discussed in previous sections, object thickness and the first layer effect were found to correlate more strongly with printing temperature than with printing speed (Figures 4c and 5a), while object mass, length and width, and the FDM-MFI were found to vary more significantly in response to change in printing speed rather than printing temperature. Therefore, one may extrapolate that PC1 may be redubbed the speed axis, as it describes variance introduced due to change in printing speed. Similarly, PC2 may be named the temperature axis as the variables it describes are those that alter more significantly in response to changes in printing temperature. Since PC1 accounts for the majority of the total explained variance (57.77%), one may deduce that printing speed a more significant contributor to the perceived quality parameters of FDM printed objects than printing temperature.

Observing the measured variables as described by the loadings plot allows for a more overarching look at how printing speed and temperature both influence perceived quality attributes, as well as how the quality attributes relate to one another. Object thickness and first layer width load opposite to each other on the temperature axis, suggesting the two are anti-correlated. This suggests that the spreading of the first layer not only increases its road width, but also decreases road height in the Z-axis. Furthermore, first layer width loads positively, while thickness loads negatively on the axis, indicating that wider road widths are brought about by higher temperatures, while greater object thickness is a result of lower printing temperature. Therefore, a conclusion can be drawn that printing at higher temperatures leads to a more drastic FLE, while printing at lower temperatures leads to thicker objects.

Length, width, mass, FDM-MFI, and road width were all described by the speed axis. Length, width, and FDM-MFI being anti-correlated to mass and road width, with the former three loading positively, and the latter negatively, indicating that length, width, and the FDM-MFI are directly correlated to printing speed, while mass and road width are inversely correlated. The length/width versus road width correlation is an interesting one as it gives insight into the operation of the feeding motors, as well as printer accuracy; the anti-correlation between road width and printing speed suggests that at higher printing speeds, the printer is not feeding sufficient material to keep up with the demands of the higher printing speed, leading to the road being deposited to be tugged as the print head is moving, stretching it thinner (leading to a decrease in road width) and longer (leading to an increase in length/width). This argument relating printing speed and feeding speed suggests that, at higher print speeds, the printer is not providing enough material feed to faithfully replicate a print at lower speeds. Therefore, objects printed at higher speeds should have less mass than their lower speed counterparts. This was found to be true as mass loaded negatively on the speed axis, and was found to be anti-correlated to length, width, and FDM-MFI. The latter, which was found to increase relative to speed (Figure 3b) was, unsurprisingly, found to load positively on the speed axis.

Figure 11 shows the biplot obtained when case scores were projected onto the loadings plot shown in Figure 10. The X-axis, denoting the scores of the cases against PC 1, unsurprisingly separates the cases into three clusters relative to printing speed, with three clusters showing clear separation between the 30 mm/s set, followed by 90 mm/s, and followed by 160 mm/s. The clustering pattern fits the argument presented prior relating printing speed to object mass and dimensions, as the leftmost cluster, falling on the "largest mass" quadrant of the biplot belonged to the 30 mm/s, then 90 mm/s, which was then followed by 160 mm/s, the "widest dimensions" set. Notably, there is less separation between the latter two sets than between 30 mm/s and 90 mm/s, which strongly mirrors the FDM-MFI results displayed in Figure 3b.

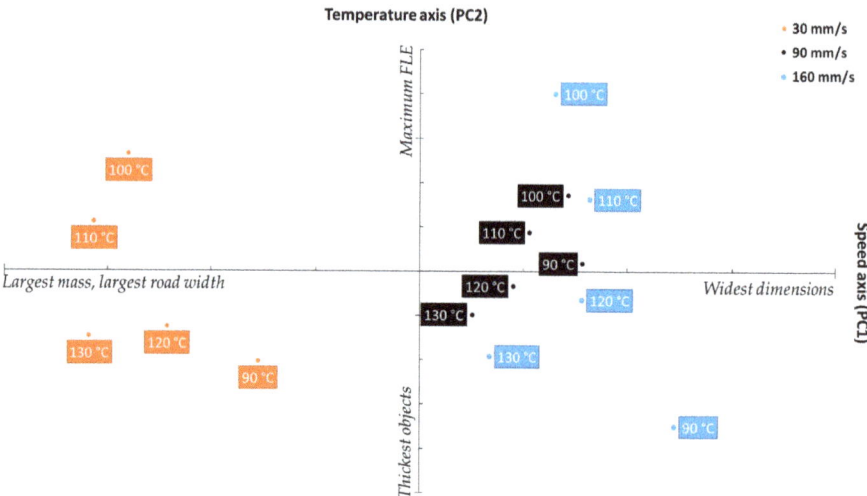

Figure 11. Biplot projecting the scores of the studied cases onto the response loadings.

The Y-axis, which shows the scores loadings relative to PC2 (the temperature axis) describes quality parameters which are influenced by printing temperature (object thickness, and the FLE). While the clusters do not appear to offer any meaningful metric towards either parameter at first glance, closer observation reveals that both object thickness and FLE are not described within each cluster, but rather between the clusters. With respect to object thickness, looking at objects printed at the same temperature (i.e., 90 °C), the one printed at 160 mm/s was the thickest, followed by the object printed at 30 mm/s, with 90 mm/s coming in third. Similarly with respect to FLE, of the objects printed at 100 °C, the one printed at 160 mm/s had the largest FLE, followed by the one printed at 30 mm/s, followed by the one printed at 90 mm/s. This inter-cluster pattern was found to apply to all the observed cases. This data pattern suggests that there may be either a more complex physical phenomenon, or a speed–temperature interaction that skews what is perceived as the impact printing temperature has on the quality parameters.

Of the three clusters, the 90 mm/s group appears to show the least variance relative to change in printing temperature. This indicates that that printing speed further minimizes the significance of printing temperature. Furthermore, the 90 mm/s cluster was the most centered cluster with respect to the four quadrants of the biplot, indicating that 90 mm/s offers the best compromise between the opposing quality parameters. This sits in agreement with the result obtained from the SSD displayed in Figure 9, in which printing at a speed of 90 mm/s yielded the lowest SSD, regardless of printing temperature, indicating that higher reproducibility is achieved when printing at 90 mm/s. Therefore, one may extrapolate that, for the PCL filament used herein, printing at 90 mm/s offers the most predictable and reproducible results, making it the optimum printing speed for this filament.

4. Conclusions

The results of this study demonstrated the significant impact processing parameters have on some of the perceived quality attributes of 3D printed dosage forms (weight, dimensional authenticity, road width, and overall print reproducibility). For the printer used in the study, printing speed exhibited a more profound impact on the weight uniformity and dimension authenticity of the printed dosage forms than printing temperature. Printing temperature and the build plate surfaces were found to contribute significantly to the FLE.

The repeatability and consistency of the calibration of the print was examined using the statistic variation observed in build plate leveling. The results confirmed that the build plate leveling is a source of significant operator-dependent error. This finding indicates the needs to redesign the build plate leveling mechanism to allow more consistent and operator-independent calibration of the printer.

The use of summed standard deviations (SSD) enables the calculation of a figure of merit indicating the most reproducible set of printing conditions, and by extension, the optimal printing parameters.

PCA was used as factor exploration method to further investigate the impact of processing parameters on the quality attributed measured herein, and possibly explore some factor interplay that may not necessarily be obvious by looking at the impact processing parameters may have on a single quality parameter outside the context of the entire set of quality attributes.

By using PCA, printing speed was found to explain more data variance than printing temperature. Factoring in that printing was not possible at a printing temperature of 70 °C and printing speed ≥90 mm/s, we can conclude that, provided that the temperature is sufficient to overcome polymer viscosity, printing speed will have a greater contribution to the perceived quality parameters of the printed object.

Printing speed was found to be negatively correlated with object road width, and more notably with object mass. Control of the latter being critical for accurate dosing in a pharmaceutical manufacturing context. Which leads us to deduce that increasing printing speed does not equal increased printing throughput, and is not a valid method for the scaling-up of a pharmaceutical FDM printing process.

The use of PCA did prove to be an effective chemometric method to determine the optimum printing conditions for the filament studied herein, as it revealed the processing parameters that produce objects that offer the best compromise between the extremes of all the perceived quality parameters. Said processing conditions were deemed to be the optimum because they offer the most reproducible and predictable prints, and not because they match a desired target value.

For pharmaceutical applications, the control of such impacts should be thoroughly understood as it can affect the performance of the printed formulation. These results brought to the conclusion of that careful engineering for a pharmaceutically suitable FDM 3D printer should be treated as a priority for making the shift of FDM 3D printing from proof-of-concept to industrial application.

Supplementary Materials: The following are available online at http://www.mdpi.com/1999-4923/11/12/633/s1, Figure S1. Computer-generated image of the STL file design for the porous film. Figure S2. Illustration for the method adapted for measuring the melt flow index for different materials. Figure S3. DSC thermograms of (A) Raw materials. (B) ASA-PCL powder mixtures (first heating cycle). (C) ASA-PCL powder mixtures (second heating cycle). (D) HME fabricated filaments. Table S1. Microscopic images depicting road width measurements. N.B. images may be resized for viewing the full details of the measurements.

Author Contributions: Conceptualization, J.N., M.A.; Data curation, J.N.; Formal analysis: J.N.; Investigation, J.N., M.A.; Methodology, J.N., M.A.; Supervision: P.B., S.Q.; Validation, J.N., P.B., and S.Q.; Visualization: J.N.; Writing—original draft, J.N.; Writing—review and editing, J.N., P.B., and S.Q.

Funding: This research received funding from the Interreg 2 Seas program 2014–2020 co-funded by the European Regional Development Fund under subsidy contract 2S01-059_IMODE.

Acknowledgments: The authors would like to thank Laszlo Fabian of the University of East Anglia for his help in proof-reading sections of this manuscript.

Conflicts of Interest: The authors declare no conflict of interest.

References

1. Hsiao, W.-K.; Lorber, B.; Reitsamer, H.; Khinast, J. 3D printing of oral drugs: A new reality or hype? *Expert Opin. Drug Deliv.* **2017**, *15*, 1–4. [CrossRef] [PubMed]
2. Wening, K.; Breitkreutz, J. Oral drug delivery in personalized medicine: Unmet needs and novel approaches. *Int. J. Pharm.* **2011**, *404*, 1–9. [CrossRef] [PubMed]
3. Joo, Y.; Shin, I.; Ham, G.; Abuzar, S.M.; Hyun, S.-M.; Hwang, S.-J. The advent of a novel manufacturing technology in pharmaceutics: Superiority of fused deposition modeling 3D printer. *J. Pharm. Investig.* **2019**. [CrossRef]

4. Khaled, S.A.; Burley, J.C.; Alexander, M.R.; Yang, J.; Roberts, C.J. 3D printing of five-in-one dose combination polypill with defined immediate and sustained release profiles. *J. Control. Release* **2015**, *217*, 308–314. [CrossRef]
5. Awad, A.; Fina, F.; Trenfield, S.; Patel, P.; Goyanes, A.; Gaisford, S.; Basit, A. 3D Printed Pellets (Miniprintlets): A Novel, Multi-Drug, Controlled Release Platform Technology. *Pharmaceutics* **2019**, *11*, 148. [CrossRef]
6. Robles-Martinez, P.; Xu, X.; Trenfield, S.J.; Awad, A.; Goyanes, A.; Telford, R.; Basit, A.W.; Gaisford, S. 3D printing of a multi-layered polypill containing six drugs using a novel stereolithographic method. *Pharmaceutics* **2019**, *11*, 274. [CrossRef] [PubMed]
7. Alhnan, M.A.; Okwuosa, T.C.; Sadia, M.; Wan, K.W.; Ahmed, W.; Arafat, B. Emergence of 3D Printed Dosage Forms: Opportunities and Challenges. *Pharm. Res.* **2016**, *33*, 1817–1832. [CrossRef] [PubMed]
8. Melocchi, A.; Parietti, F.; Maroni, A.; Foppoli, A.; Gazzaniga, A.; Zema, L. Hot-melt extruded filaments based on pharmaceutical grade polymers for 3D printing by fused deposition modeling. *Int. J. Pharm.* **2016**, *509*, 255–263. [CrossRef] [PubMed]
9. Alhijjaj, M.; Belton, P.; Qi, S. An investigation into the use of polymer blends to improve the printability of and regulate drug release from pharmaceutical solid dispersions prepared via fused deposition modeling (FDM) 3D printing. *Eur. J. Pharm. Biopharm.* **2016**, *108*, 111–125. [CrossRef]
10. Prasad, E.; Islam, M.T.; Goodwin, D.J.; Megarry, A.J.; Halbert, G.W.; Florence, A.J.; Robertson, J. Development of a hot-melt extrusion (HME) process to produce drug loaded Affinisol^{TM} 15LV filaments for fused filament fabrication (FFF) 3D printing. *Addit. Manuf.* **2019**, *29*, 100776. [CrossRef]
11. Norman, J.; Madurawe, R.D.; Moore, C.M.V.; Khan, M.A.; Khairuzzaman, A. A new chapter in pharmaceutical manufacturing: 3D-printed drug products. *Adv. Drug Deliv. Rev.* **2017**, *108*, 39–50. [CrossRef] [PubMed]
12. Katstra, W.E.; Rowe, C.W.; Palazzolo, R.D.; Giritlioglu, B.; Teung, P.; Cima, M.J.; Katstra, W.E.; Palazzolo, R.D.; Giritlioglu, B.; Teung, P.; et al. Oral dosage forms fabricated by Three Dimensional Printing. *J. Control. Release* **2000**, *66*, 11–17. [CrossRef]
13. Pietrzak, K.; Isreb, A.; Alhnan, M.A. A flexible-dose dispenser for immediate and extended release 3D printed tablets. *Eur. J. Pharm. Biopharm.* **2015**, *96*, 380–387. [CrossRef] [PubMed]
14. Goyanes, A.; Robles Martinez, P.; Buanz, A.; Basit, A.W.; Gaisford, S. Effect of geometry on drug release from 3D printed tablets. *Int. J. Pharm.* **2015**, *494*, 657–663. [CrossRef] [PubMed]
15. Goyanes, A.; Buanz, A.B.M.M.; Hatton, G.B.; Gaisford, S.; Basit, A.W. 3D printing of modified-release aminosalicylate (4-ASA and 5-ASA) tablets. *Eur. J. Pharm. Biopharm.* **2015**, *89*, 157–162. [CrossRef]
16. Goyanes, A.; Buanz, A.B.M.; Basit, A.W.; Gaisford, S. Fused-filament 3D printing (3DP) for fabrication of tablets. *Int. J. Pharm.* **2014**, *476*, 88–92. [CrossRef]
17. Korte, C.; Quodbach, J. Formulation development and process analysis of drug-loaded filaments manufactured via hot-melt extrusion for 3D-printing of medicines. *Pharm. Dev. Technol.* **2018**, *23*, 1117–1127. [CrossRef]
18. Skowyra, J.; Pietrzak, K.; Alhnan, M.A. Fabrication of extended-release patient-tailored prednisolone tablets via fused deposition modelling (FDM) 3D printing. *Eur. J. Pharm. Sci.* **2015**, *68*, 11–17. [CrossRef]
19. Nasereddin, J.M.; Wellner, N.; Alhijjaj, M.; Belton, P.; Qi, S. Development of a Simple Mechanical Screening Method for Predicting the Feedability of a Pharmaceutical FDM 3D Printing Filament. *Pharm. Res.* **2018**, *35*, 151. [CrossRef]
20. Lim, S.H.; Kathuria, H.; Tan, J.J.Y.; Kang, L. 3D printed drug delivery and testing systems—A passing fad or the future? *Adv. Drug Deliv. Rev.* **2018**. [CrossRef]
21. Peng, A.; Xiao, X.; Yue, R. Process parameter optimization for fused deposition modeling using response surface methodology combined with fuzzy inference system. *Int. J. Adv. Manuf. Technol.* **2014**, *73*, 87–100. [CrossRef]
22. Bakar, N.S.A.; Alkahari, M.R.; Boejang, H. Analysis on Fused Deposition Modelling Performance. *J. Zhejiang Univ. Sci. A* **2010**, *11*, 972–977. [CrossRef]
23. Ziemian, S.; Okwara, M.; Ziemian, C.W. Tensile and fatigue behavior of layered acrylonitrile butadiene styrene. *Rapid Prototyp. J.* **2015**, *21*, 270–278. [CrossRef]
24. Weeren, R.V.; Agarwala, M.; Jamalabad, V.R.; Bandyophadyay, A.; Vaidyanathan, R.; Langrana, N.; Ballard, C. Quality of Parts Processed by Fused Deposition. In Proceedings of the 1995 International Solid Freeform Fabrication Symposium, Austin, TX, USA, 1995; The University of Texas at Austin: Austin, TX, USA, 1995; pp. 314–321.

25. Bharath Vasudevarao, B.; Dharma Prakash Natarajan, D.P.; Henderson, M.M.; Vasudevarao, B.; Natarajan, D.P.; Henderson, M.M. Sensitivitiy of RP Surface Finish to Process Parameter Variation. *Solid Free. Fabr. Proc.* **2000**, 251–258.
26. Dawson, P.C. Flow Properties of Molten Polymers. In *Mechanical Properties and Testing of Polymers*; Springer: Dordrecht, The Netherlands, 1999; pp. 88–95.
27. Lu, L.; Chen, B.; Sharf, A.; Zhao, H.; Wei, Y.; Fan, Q.; Chen, X.; Savoye, Y.; Tu, C.; Cohen-Or, D. Build-to-last: Strength to Weight 3D Printed Objects. *ACM Trans. Graph.* **2014**, *33*, 1–10. [CrossRef]
28. Gokstorp, D. Prototyping a Custom 3D Printing Slicer Implementation of a Prototype Modular Infill, Tool Path and Gcode Generator in Houdini. Master's Thesis, Bournemouth University, Poole, UK, 2016.
29. Wang, Y.; Xu, P.P.; Li, X.X.; Nie, K.; Tuo, M.F.; Kong, B.; Chen, J. Monitoring the hydrolyzation of aspirin during the dissolution testing for aspirin delayed-release tablets with a fiber-optic dissolution system. *J. Pharm. Anal.* **2012**, *2*, 386–389. [CrossRef]
30. International Organization for Standardization. ISO 1133-1:2011–Plastics—Determination of the Melt Mass-Flow Rate (MFR) and Melt Volume-Flow Rate (MVR) of Thermoplastics—Part 1: Standard Method. Available online: https://www.iso.org/standard/44273.html (accessed on 21 July 2018).
31. Makerbot LLC. (n.d.). User Manual|Replicator®2X Dual Extrusion Experimental 3D Printer. Available online: http://downloads.makerbot.com/replicator2x/MakerBot_Replicator_2X_User_Manual.pdf (accessed on 4 October 2017).
32. Ringnér, M. What is principal component analysis? *Nat. Biotechnol.* **2008**, *26*. [CrossRef]
33. Williams, L.J. Principal Component Analysis. *Wiley Interdiscip. Rev. Comput. Stat.* **2010**, *2*, 433–470.
34. Sadia, M.; Isreb, A.; Abbadi, I.; Isreb, M.; Aziz, D.; Selo, A.; Timmins, P.; Alhnan, M.A. From 'fixed dose combinations' to 'a dynamic dose combiner': 3D printed bi-layer antihypertensive tablets. *Eur. J. Pharm. Sci.* **2018**, *123*, 484–494. [CrossRef]
35. Tian, Y.; Booth, J.; Meehan, E.; Jones, D.S.; Li, S.; Andrews, G.P. Construction of drug-polymer thermodynamic phase diagrams using flory-huggins interaction theory: Identifying the relevance of temperature and drug weight fraction to phase separation within solid dispersions. *Mol. Pharm.* **2013**, *10*, 236–248. [CrossRef]
36. Rowe, R.; Sheskey, P.; Quinn, M. *Handbook of Pharmaceutical Excipients*, 6th ed.; Pharmaceutical Press: London, UK, 2009.

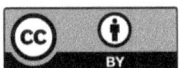

© 2019 by the authors. Licensee MDPI, Basel, Switzerland. This article is an open access article distributed under the terms and conditions of the Creative Commons Attribution (CC BY) license (http://creativecommons.org/licenses/by/4.0/).

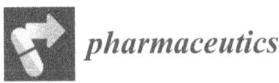

Article

A 3D Bioprinted Pseudo-Bone Drug Delivery Scaffold for Bone Tissue Engineering

Pariksha Jolene Kondiah, Pierre P. D. Kondiah, Yahya E. Choonara, Thashree Marimuthu and Viness Pillay *

Wits Advanced Drug Delivery Platform Research Unit, Department of Pharmacy and Pharmacology, School of Therapeutic Sciences, Faculty of Health Sciences, University of the Witwatersrand, Johannesburg, 7 York Road, Parktown 2193, South Africa; parikshakondiah@gmail.com (P.J.K.); pierre.kondiah@wits.ac.za (P.P.D.K.); yahya.choonara@wits.ac.za (Y.E.C.); Thashree.marimuthu@wits.ac.za (T.M.)
* Correspondence: viness.pillay@wits.ac.za; Tel.: +27-11-717-2274

Received: 31 December 2019; Accepted: 6 February 2020; Published: 17 February 2020

Abstract: A 3D bioprinted pseudo-bone drug delivery scaffold was fabricated to display matrix strength, matrix resilience, as well as porous morphology of healthy human bone. Computer-aided design (CAD) software was employed for developing the 3D bioprinted scaffold. Further optimization of the scaffold was undertaken using MATLAB® software and artificial neural networks (ANN). Polymers employed for formulating the 3D scaffold comprised of polypropylene fumarate (PPF), free radical polymerized polyethylene glycol- polycaprolactone (PEG-PCL-PEG), and pluronic (PF127). Simvastatin was incorporated into the 3D bioprinted scaffolds to further promote bone healing and repair properties. The 3D bioprinted scaffold was characterized for its chemical, morphological, mechanical, and in vitro release kinetics for evaluation of its behavior for application as an implantable scaffold at the site of bone fracture. The ANN-optimized 3D bioprinted scaffold displayed significant properties as a controlled release platform, demonstrating drug release over 20 days. The 3D bioprinted scaffold further displayed formation as a pseudo-bone matrix, using a human clavicle bone model, induced with a butterfly fracture. The strength of the pseudo-bone matrix, evaluated for its matrix hardness (MH) and matrix resilience (MR), was evaluated to be as strong as original bone, having a 99% MH and 98% MR property, to healthy human clavicle bones.

Keywords: 3D bioprinting; polymeric ink; optimization; pseudo-bone; implantable scaffold; computer-aided design (CAD) design; drug delivery

---

1. Introduction

3D bioprinting is currently the most explored field of research in mechanical microenvironment tissue-engineered systems [1]. The most common impairments employing 3D bioprinting research significantly focus on therapeutics designed to treat bone fractures as well as bone defects [2]. Consequently, bone-related costs and therapy are escalating [3]. Typical treatment for these impairments includes bone grafts or metal prosthetic implants. However, this form of therapy is restricted in many incidents due to significant tissue loss resulting from surgery, long recovery periods, and donor site morbidity [4]. Nonetheless, the limitations related to these forms of therapy have opened doors to the evolution of 3D bioprinting technology, employing cutting edge design and execution of drug delivery engineered platforms [5]. Bone tissue repair and regeneration employing noninvasive procedures have become a significant focus due to the implementation of 3D bioprinting technology [6–8].

3D bioprinted scaffolds employed for bone tissue repair and healing, using computer-aided design (CAD) software, has numerous benefits such as intensive care patient-specific dose designs, customized geometrical site-specific drug delivery applications, as well as controlled drug release implantable platforms employing internal architecture modification designs [9,10]. To date, 3D printing has gained superior recognition in the industrial market, ranging from medical devices, engineering components to pharmaceutical drug technologies [11–14]. Previous studies conducted in 3D printing and bone tissue engineering have employed polymers of similar nature, designed to strengthen scaffold conformation designs, as well as obtain suitable bioinks/ polymeric inks, for a variety of printing architecture. Studies have reported hydrogel formulations for bone support (injectable hydrogels), bone regeneration using natural (chitin and alginate derivatives) and synthetic polymers (silicone and inorganic complexes), various 3D inkjet bio-fabrications, as well as incorporation of growth factors within porous scaffold designs [10–17]. Biomineralization, osteogenesis, and hard tissue promoting therapeutics have also been an area of significant focus due to exponential cases of accident-related bone fractures and osteoporotic pathologies. However, an essential component of such research should provide a means of improving the cost-effectiveness of products, thereby causing minimum wastage and time efficiency over the synthetic process. Nevertheless, this will also require highly accurate batches when undertaking 3D bioprinting, so as to achieve reproducible therapeutic delivery systems [15–18].

In this study, we synthesized a pseudo-bone drug delivery scaffold, possessing properties of comparable matrix hardness and resilience to healthy bone tissue, following in situ analysis. This study follows as a trajectory from previous pre-formulation studies undertaken [19], with further optimization employing 3D bioprinting for advanced drug delivery. The 3D bioprinted pseudo-bone scaffold formulations were designed using polymer-variable concentration optimization, employing MATLAB® software (MathWorks®, Natick, MA, USA) and artificial neural networks. The 3D bioprinted scaffold was designed using Inventor® (Autodesk®, San Rafael, CA, USA) auto CAD, fabricating a strategic cylindrical-shaped drug delivery scaffold, with uniform bioprinted filaments and pore size geometrical configuration. The pseudo-bone 3D bioprinted scaffold was designed to mimic the morphology, matrix strength, and matrix resilience of healthy human bone. This was evaluated using healthy human clavicles in which butterfly fractures were induced. Ethical clearance waiver was granted from the Department of Human Anatomy, University of the Witwatersrand, for undertaking this study (ethics clearance number: W-CJ-140604-1; granted date: 3 July 2018).

This drug delivery system was optimized as a controlled release platform incorporating the drug simvastatin. The polymeric ink was designed to gradually degrade and release its loaded contents in a sustained manner, allowing contact adhesion between fractured/damaged bone and formation of a pseudo-bone matrix within these sites. Polymers employed for formulating the polymeric ink of the pseudo-bone scaffold consisted of polypropylene fumarate (PPF), free radical polymerized polyethylene glycol-polycaprolactone (PEG-PCL-PEG), and Pluronic (PF127). The 3D bioprinted scaffold was characterized for its chemical, morphological, mechanical, and in vitro release properties and optimization design using MATLAB® software and artificial neural networks.

The analysis of a designed multilayered network, using a feed-forward backpropagation, with multiple inputs, outputs, as well as varied hidden layers, was designed. This system comprised of multilayer nonlinear networks. In the design, a back-propagation relationship using large input and output datasets, determining network mapping, thereby not requiring a definite mathematical equation to undertake the modeling, was achieved. This model, employing a gradient descent algorithm using backpropagation, was classified as the Widrow–Hoff learning rule, using multiple-layer networks, with various degrees of optimization to the algorithm.

In this study, the 3D bioprinted scaffolds, designed and evaluated as 39 formulations using MATLAB® software, comprised of variables of PPF (8% w/v–20% w/v) and PF127 (14% w/v–16% w/v). Results presented from these design scaffold formulations were studied in response to duration of release of simvastatin and the degree of thermogelation of the polymeric ink formulation. Analysis was undertaken determining the formulation compositions and response factor from each design, using a 3D Simulink design graph. The release analysis of further evaluating the relationship between the hydrophobic chain regions of PPF encapsulating simvastatin was undertaken, correlating the duration of drug release from the 3D bioprinted scaffold over time.

2. Materials and Methods

2.1. Materials

PEG (Mw 4000), stannous octoate, 92.5%; Pluronic F-127; poly(ethylene glycol) diacrylate; epsilon-caprolactone, 99%; petroleum ether, 90%; and simvastatin (molecular weight: 418.57), 97% purity, were procured from Sigma-Aldrich (St. Louis, MO, USA). Methanol, 99%; diethyl fumarate, 98%; dichloromethane, diethyl ether (anhydrous); hydroquinone, 99% purity; methylene chloride; propylene glycol (1,2-propandiol); hydrochloric acid, 1.85% v/v; sodium sulphate; and zinc chloride were purchased from Merck (Pty) Ltd. (Modderfontein, South Africa). All software employed in this study was procured from EnvisionTEC® GmbH (Gladbeck, Germany). All other reagents were of analytical grade and were employed as received. All reactions were undertaken under inert conditions.

2.2. Synthesis of the Polymeric Ink Formulation

A strategically designed copolymeric blend of polymers, polypropylene fumarate (PPF), PEG-PCL-PEG, and pluronic PF 127, was optimized for 3D bioprinting and loaded with simvastatin drug. Free radical polymerization was undertaken for preparation of copolymer PEG-PCL-PEG using PEG (Mw 4000) as the macroinitiator and catalyst stannous octoate (Sn(Oct)$_2$). Briefly, 0.007 M of PEG 4000 and 0.098 M of ε-caprolactone was reacted in a round bottom flask, purged with nitrogen, at a temperature of 125 °C, under constant magnetic stirring (3500 rpm). The catalyst (100 μL) was then added to the reaction and left for 6 h under nitrogen purging. PPF (8% w/v–20% w/v) and PF 127 (14% w/v–16% w/v) were then added to the reaction mixture, specifying the concentrations as obtained by the designed formulations using MATLAB® software. The reaction temperature was then increased to 140 °C and left for 6 h under constant magnetic stirring of 3000 rpm. The reaction mixture was then allowed to cool to room temperature, with further addition to Dichloromethane (DCM), and washing thrice with deionized water. The organic solvent was then removed using rotary evaporation and stored at 10 °C for further use. Details of the above synthesis have previously been reported by authors [19]. Simvastatin was then loaded into the copolymer, with a therapeutic dose calculated at 10 mg per scaffold. The dose for loading was calculated according to the material required for bioprinting, dependent on parameters employed, according to the optimization of fabrication procedures on the bioprinted scaffold, as discussed in Section 2.4. The polymeric ink paste was then fabricated by formulating a ratio of 6:3:1 of the copolymer: methanol: deionized water, respectively. The copolymer then underwent microwave-assisted heating using a specific laboratory designed MAS-II Plus Microwave Synthesis Workstation (Sineo, China) at 50 °C for 10 min, at 600 W. Distilled water was added to the polymeric ink (polymeric ink: water ratio; 6.5:3.5) for its application of drug loading and release analysis. Ten milligrams of drug was loaded in the polymeric ink at a temperature of 10 °C for 6 h. Thereafter, the loaded polymeric ink was incubated at 25 °C for 2 h to ensure maximum drug loading occurred during the gelling phase. The loading of drug was back-calculated according to sample volume in each printing cartridge such that 10 mg of simvastatin was present in a total of 7 layers of the 3D printed scaffold.

2.3. Artificial Neural Network Design and Optimization of the 3D Bioprinted Scaffold

Artificial neural networks (ANN) can be used to determine linear and nonlinear sophisticated relationships between dependent and independent variables in a study [20]. The fundamental benefit of using ANN is the capacity for the neural network to learn directly from an informal dataset that has not been associated directly with a mathematical equation. In this study, MATLAB Simulink® R2016a edition (The MathWorks, Inc.) was employed to undertake neural networking.

Formulations were derived using variables of 14% w/v–16% w/v of PF 127 and 8% w/v–20% w/v of PPF. Formulations were obtained using MATLAB®, determining combination integer matrices, in 1% w/v concentration increments within the variable range of PPF and PF 127. The concentrations of PEG-PCL-PEG polymer and all other reagents were kept constant during the design of the study.

A total of 39 formulations were derived and synthesized using this software, as noted in Table 1. All formulations were evaluated for parameters of the temperature of gelation before bioprinting and the duration of drug release after bioprinting. This was then analyzed as a factor (Equation (1)), with the highest factor representing the optimized formulation matrix.

Table 1. Design specifications of the 3D bioprinted scaffold formulations using MATLAB Simulink®.

Formulation Number	PPF (% w/v)	PF-127 (% w/v)
1	8	14
2	9	14
3	10	14
4	11	14
5	12	14
6	13	14
7	14	14
8	15	14
9	16	14
10	17	14
11	18	14
12	19	14
13	20	14
14	8	15
15	9	15
16	10	15
17	11	15
18	12	15
19	13	15
20	14	15
21	15	15
22	16	15
23	17	15
24	18	15
25	19	15
26	20	15
27	8	16
28	9	16
29	10	16
30	11	16
31	12	16
32	13	16
33	14	16
34	15	16
35	16	16
36	17	16
37	18	16
38	19	16
39	20	16

$$Factor = \frac{tg}{bt} \times Rd \quad (1)$$

where tg represents the thermogelation temperature of the synthesized copolymer, bt represents body temperature, and Rd represents the drug release duration. Performance training of the neural network was evaluated by the mean square error and regression analysis [20].

A designed network, using a multilayer feed forward-back propagation, containing an input, output, as well as a variety of hidden layers, refers to a system architecture where the gradient is computed for multilayer nonlinear networks. This backpropagation relationship thus uses large input and output datasets to determine a network mapping, thereby not requiring a definite mathematical equation to undertake the modeling. This gradient descent algorithm using backpropagation is classified as the Widrow–Hoff learning rule, using multiple-layer networks, with various degrees of optimization to the algorithm.

For the neural network to display training algorithms on the basis of lowest mean square error and highest accuracy correlations, a training percentage value of 70% was selected in the network. Validation of 15% was undertaken, measuring the network generalization, thereby terminating training when generalization of the network stops improving. A testing percentage of 15% was selected, resulting in no effect on training parameters and providing an indication of an independent measure of performance during and after training of the network. Thus, this complies with 100% evaluation split into 3 categories of network priority. The algorithm employed in a study depends on the complexity of variables and desired strategic outcome of modeling. In this study, we used 3 types of algorithms, such as Levenberg–Marquardt, Scaled Conjugate Gradient, and Bayesian Regularization. The algorithm that obtained the best training results was employed for the ANN study [20].

In terms of expressing data in the form of equation variables, the input to hidden layer U was expressed by:

$$(U) = (W)(I) \tag{2}$$

W, representing the weight, and I the input. Each term of the hidden layer matrix can be explained as follows:

$$Uj = \sum_{i=1}^{n} W i I i - \Theta \tag{3}$$

Θ, representing the associated bias. Optimization in the hidden layer using transfer functions was conducted. Nonlinear functions {log-sigmoid (logsig), hyperbolic tangent sigmoid function (tansig)}, and linear function (purelin) were undertaken to investigate the ability to achieve optimum results. Equations (4)–(6) were employed to understand the sequencing of optimization of the network:

$$f(U) = u \tag{4}$$

$$f(U) = \frac{1}{\left[1 + e^{(-u)}\right]} \tag{5}$$

$$f(U) = \frac{2}{\left[1 + e^{(-2u)}\right] - 1} \tag{6}$$

As a means of determining the effectiveness of the models, the determination coefficient (R^2) and the mean square error (MSE) were employed as follows:

$$MSE = \frac{1}{n} = \sum_{i=1}^{n} (Y\ response\ predicted - Y\ response\ experimental)^2 \tag{7}$$

$$R^2 = 1 - \frac{\sum_{i=1}^{n} (Y\ response\ predicted - Y\ response\ experimental)^2}{\sum_{i=1}^{n} (Y\ response\ experimental - Y\ response\ mean)^2} \tag{8}$$

The adaptation learning function employed was the gradient descent, with momentum weight and bias learning function. Optimization of the learning function also varied with the number of neurons, resulting in observational learning with greater percentage validity. Parameters of the number of epochs, minimum gradient, and Mu employed were evaluated at 10^2, 1^{-10}, and 0.01, respectively.

Thermogelation analysis on the 39 polymeric ink design formulations, as seen in Table 1, were undertaken using a Modular Advanced Rheometer (ThermoHaake MARS Modular Advanced Rheometer, Thermo Electron, Karlsruhe, Germany), comprising a C 35/1° Ti sensor. A temperature range of 10–40 °C was conducted, using a cone and plate inertia of 1.721 × 10^{-6} kg m^2, analyzing 5 mL of sample. The sample was analyzed in the range of 0–1.0 Hz, in the region of the shear independent plateau of the strain amplitude sweep stress (11). G', representing the effects of elastic energy (storage modulus), and G", representing the effects of viscous energy (loss modulus), were evaluated. The point of thermogelation occurred when the fluid nature of the gel (G") transitioned to a semi-solid composition (G'), being subjected to an increase in temperature, over constant sinusoidal oscillation.

2.4. 3D Design of the Bioprinted Pseudo-Bone Drug Delivery Scaffold

The 3D bioprinted scaffold was designed using Autodesk Inventor®, 3D computer-aided design (CAD), for precise fabrication prototyping of the polymer-based biomaterial. The scaffold was designed as a cylindrical implant, with dimensions comprising 16 mm radius and a height of 4.2 mm. After generating a Stereolithography (STL) file on Inventor®, this file was imported to EnvisionTEC Visual Machines software, thereby converting to a Borland Package Library (BPL) file for bioprinting processing. Design of internal features and uniform slicing of the design was then undertaken on this software, printing a strand diameter of 600 µm and creating an inner structure pattern between layers at 30°. The inner structural printing pattern of 30° was not designed in the CAD model, instead, it was implemented in the EnvisionTEC Visual Machines software as per the desired printing conformation. A needle tip of 0.8 mm diameter was used for printing the scaffold, which was set at an optimum 80% offset. This resulted in an average height of 0.6 mm printing diameter, with a deviation of +/−60 µm per given strand. The deviation was due to drying of each strand between layers, which resulted minimally in the designed size. The designed scaffold, with a total number of 7 layers, is depicted in Figure 1.

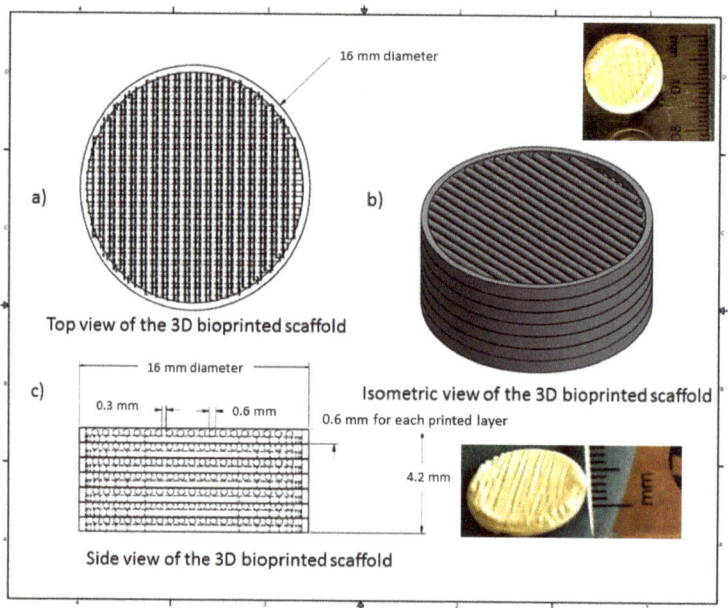

Figure 1. Computer-aided design (CAD) specification of the optimized 3D bioprinted scaffold.

A 3D Bioplotter® (EnvisionTEC GmbH, Gladbeck, Germany) was employed, using a pressure and temperature regulated syringe, with parameters optimized at 1.0 bar of pressure, speed at 1 mm/s, and syringe temperature regulated at 20 °C. The temperature of the printing platform was maintained at 40 °C. The transfer height and needle offset were set at 5 mm and 0.5 mm, respectively. Pre-flow delay, post-flow delay, and time between layers were set as 0, 0, and 120 s, respectively. The low pressure and speed of printing provided sufficient time for the structure to solidify, thereby promoting accuracy and scaffold platform building to occur. This technology allows the development of any object to be printed, provided the appropriate uniform viscosity is maintained throughout. Figure 1 illustrates the CAD design of the 3D bioprinted scaffold model.

2.5. Chemical and Thermal Evaluation of the 3D Bioprinted Pseudo-Bone Scaffold

Nuclear magnetic resonance (NMR) was undertaken on the 3D printed scaffold using a Bruker AVANCE II 500 MHz (Bruker Avance Biospin, Germany) instrument. Deuterated chloroform (DCl_3) was used to dissolve the scaffold, evaluating the sample at 25 °C.

Thermogravimetric analysis was undertaken using a TGA 4000 thermogravimetric analyzer (PerkinElmer Inc, Massachusetts, USA) over a temperature range of 30–900 °C. This was undertaken at a ramping rate of 10 °C/min, under inert conditions, with a purge rate of 20 mL/min of nitrogen. A sample weight of 10 mg was used, evaluating the percentage degradation of the 3D bioprinted scaffold. The 1st derivative was obtained after analysis of the thermogram, detecting the point of inflection for analysis. This peak indicates the point of the greatest rate of change of the 3D bioprinted scaffold, with most significant weight loss observed.

2.6. Morphological Analysis of the 3D Bioprinted Pseudo-Bone Scaffold and Rheological Evaluation of the Polymeric Ink

Scanning electron microscopy (SEM) analysis was undertaken to confirm the pore architecture of the 3D bioprinted scaffold as well as to determine the accuracy of bioprinting parameters in relation to morphological characteristics between all 7 layers of the 3D scaffold. The 3D bioprinted scaffold sample was prepared by sputter coating on an aluminium spud, employing an EPI sputter coater (SPI Module TM sputter-coater and control unit, West Chester, PA, USA). The sample was then analyzed using an FEI ESEM Quanta 400 F (FEITM, Hillsboro, OR, USA) electron microscope, with an electron acceleration charge of 20 kV, producing high-resolution images of the 3D bioprinted scaffold.

The viscoelastic behavior of the polymeric ink was evaluated using a Modular Advanced Rheometer (ThermoHaake MARS Modular Advanced Rheometer, Thermo Electron, Karlsruhe, Germany) comprising of a C 35/1° Ti sensor. Rheological measurements were evaluated at 10–40 °C, using a cone and plate inertia of 1.721×10^{-6} kg.m². 0.5 mL of the sample was examined over a range of 0–1.0 Hz, falling within the shear independent plateau of the strain amplitude sweep stress [12]. The effects of elastic energy (storage modulus or G′) and viscous energy (loss modulus or G″) were observed after subjecting the sample to sinusoidal oscillation.

2.7. In Vitro Drug Release Evaluation on the Designed 3D Bioprinted Pseudo-Bone Drug Delivery Scaffolds.

All 39 bioprinted scaffolds (n = 3) were evaluated, employing a dialysis membrane (MWCO: 1.2 kDa) immersed in phosphate buffer solution (PBS, pH 6.8). Samples were evaluated in an orbital shaker incubator (LM-530-2, MRC Laboratory Instruments Ltd., Hahistadrut, Holon, Israel) at 37.5 °C, 50 rpm. One milliliter of sample was removed at each time point from the buffer and replaced equally with new buffer, which was conducted over a period of 30 days. Release samples were then analyzed for simvastatin concentration using a UV spectrophotometer at wavelength 238 nm (IMPLEN Nanophotometer[TM], Implen GmbH, München Germany). This was undertaken using a 10 times dilution factor of path-length 0.1 mm [21].

2.8. Textural Analysis of the Human Clavicle Bone and 3D Bioprinted Pseudo-Bone Scaffold

Matrix hardness (MH) and matrix resilience (MR) analysis, employing a textual analyzer (TA.XTplus, Stable Microsystems, Surrey, UK) under parameters of temperature at 37.5 °C and pressure of 1 atm, were undertaken on a healthy human clavicle bone (obtained with ethical waiver clearance) and thereafter on the area of the bone that was fractured and treated with the 3D bioprinted scaffold. A steel flat tip probe of 2 mm diameter was used for MH determination, and a steel cylindrical probe of 50 mm diameter was employed for MR evaluation. The clavicles were induced with a 4 mm diameter fracture in the region between the cervical fascia and the area below the conoid tubercle [22]. This was undertaken using a 4mm punch and dye apparatus, with a hydraulic pressure of 0.6 MPa. The fracture-induced human clavicle bone was then tested after incubation at 37.5 °C for 2 h, following hydration of the scaffold with 2 mL of PBS at the fracture site, with evaluation of the properties of matrix hardness and resilience on the bone thereafter.

3. Results and Discussion

3.1. Design and Optimization of the 3D Bioprinted Pseudo-Bone Drug Delivery Scaffold Employing Artificial Neural Networks

The 3D bioprinted scaffolds, evaluated as 39 design formulations using MATLAB® software, comprised of variables of PPF (8% w/v–20% w/v) and PF127 (14% w/v–16% w/v), as presented in Table 1. These design scaffold formulations were studied in response to duration of release of simvastatin and the degree of thermogelation of the polymeric ink formulation. Figure 2 reflects the formulation compositions and response factor from each design, using a 3D Simulink design graph. It was observed that with incremental increases in the concentration of PPF at constant PF127 levels, a comparatively greater concentration of simvastatin was released for the formulations. This can be attributed to the increasing incompatibility created by the hydrophobic chain regions of PPF encapsulating simvastatin, a biopharmaceutics classification system (BCS) class 2 drug, at higher concentrations. It was also observed that, as the PF127 variable increased, the scaffolds biodegraded over an extended duration due to stronger gelation of the scaffold with increased PF127 concentration, further controlling the release rate of the loaded drug. This slower sustained release effect of PF127 in the formulation is desirable for implantable systems [23]. Furthermore, the formulations also demonstrated a decrease in gelation temperature as the concentration of PF127 was increased, as observed in Figure 4.

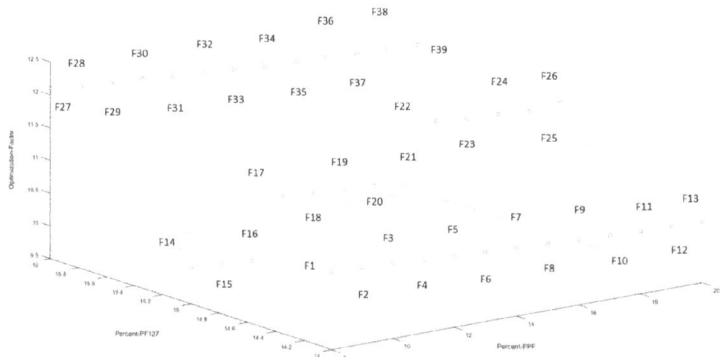

Figure 2. 3D representation of the artificial neural networks (ANN) design formulations, reflecting the percentage of PPF and PF127, with the optimization factor for each formulation.

Providing these inputs in the software, Equation (1) was employed in determining the variable concentrations for the optimized formulation, thereafter training these inputs using ANN. The 546 number data set involved in the study was undertaken by varying the number of neurons in the hidden layer, using the sigmoid symmetric transfer function and using 3 different training functions for developing the model. The optimum network was derived using performance indicators of error function and R^2 values. A variation in the number of neurons in the hidden layer is an essential component in ANN. The network thus becomes underperforming or highly entangled to sort, when the number of neurons is too high or low. Thus, a region between 6 and 16 neurons was investigated and considered an efficient model for optimum results. The optimum number of neurons after testing was found to be 10, thus producing the lowest mean square error and highest regression values for various training models.

For training of the network, the feed-forward backpropagation method was employed. Using the Levenberg–Marquardt, Bayesian Regularization, and Scaled conjugate gradient training networks, the training network that resulted in the lowest error functions (Equation (7)) and the highest regression value (Equation (8)) was evaluated. After much training and evaluation of input data, the Levenberg–Marquardt training function was observed to be the most effective algorithm employed using the sigmoid (tansig) function. Table 2 reflects the results obtained from the training algorithm and parameter performance observed.

Table 2. Training functions undertaken for optimization of the design formulations.

Training Algorithm	Mean Square Error (MSE)	Regression Function (R^2)
Levenberg-Marquardt	≤0.1	9.99
Bayesian Regularization	≤0.1	9.82
Scaled conjugate gradient	0.7	9.14

Figure 3 reflects a 3D cubic function of optimization parameters using a surface computed plot. The optimized formulation with the greatest factor, representing an optimum ratio of release duration and polymeric ink thermogelation, was found to be 14% *w/v* of PPF and 16% *w/v* of PF 127. This optimized formulation composition was thus selected as the superior formulation specification. Figure 4 represents the thermogelation temperature of the 39 polymeric ink formulations, highlighting a decrease in gelation temperature as the concentration of PF127 was increased due to the characteristic nature of the polymer.

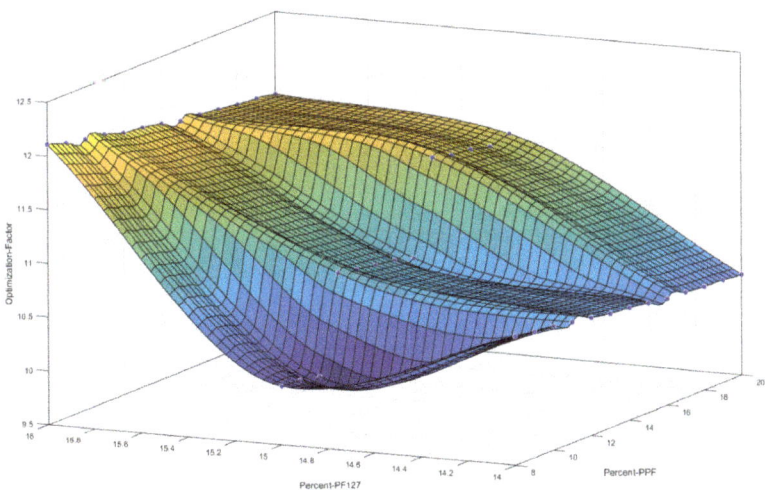

Figure 3. 3D representation of the designed polymeric ink formulations using a cubic function surface plot, with the highest point on the surface plot representing the optimum polymer concentrations.

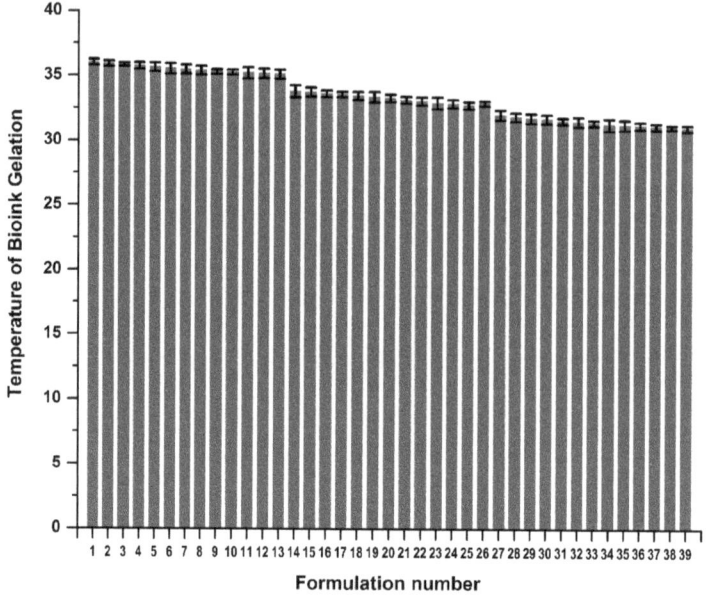

Figure 4. Gelation temperature of the 39 polymeric ink design formulations prior to 3D printing.

3.2. Chemical and Thermogravimetric Analysis of the Optimized 3D Bioprinted Pseudo-Bone Scaffold

NMR analysis was undertaken on the 3D bioprinted scaffold, evaluating each chemical component in the formulation. As visualized in Figure 5, the broad signal peaks in the region of 3.5 ppm and 3.65 ppm represent the $-(CH_2)-$ functional groups present in PEG, with PCL functionalities of $-OCCH_2-$ and $-CH_2OOC-$ in the regions of 1.6 ppm and 2.2 ppm, respectively. Evaluating peaks responsible for PPF, it was evident that the defining functionalities of $-HC=CH-$ in the region of 6.75 ppm remained intact in the PPF backbone structure. The $-CH_3-$ functionality of PF127 was identified in the region of 1.1 ppm, with further evaluation reflecting no chemical shifting of this functionality of protons in the backbone of PEG-PCL. The peaks observed in regions 1–1.3 ppm can thus be attributed to the $-CH_3-$ groups present in PPF and PF 127, respectively, responsible for chemical shifts from the parent compounds. Peaks for PF 127 were also identified in the region of 3.4 ppm, reflecting protons of individual functional groups. Minor peaks of PPF, not evident in the 3D bioprinted scaffold, was suggestive of successful copolymeric blending interaction, with the end groups of the PPF polymeric chain implicated in the interaction [24–26].

The thermogravimetric analysis was undertaken to determine the temperature range, resulting in the greatest weight loss experienced in the 3D bioprinted scaffold, after being exposed to temperatures of 30–900 °C. Figure 6a represents polymer PEG-PCL-PEG, producing a double point of inflection, with the maximum degradation for PEG and PCL chains observed in the region of 387 °C and 448 °C, respectively. An initial percentage of degradation below 100 °C was attributed to the release of moisture in the sample, due to the hygroscopic nature of the polymer. PF 127 demonstrated significant biodegradation in the range of 412 °C, with PPF reflecting substantial weight loss at 379 °C, as seen in Figure 6b,c, respectively. Figure 6d depicts the 3D bioprinted pseudo-bone scaffold. As observed, the higher point of inflection at 448 °C indicated that the scaffold possessed greater thermal stability compared to individual polymers, possibly due to properties of increasing interfacial adhesion in the scaffold matrix.

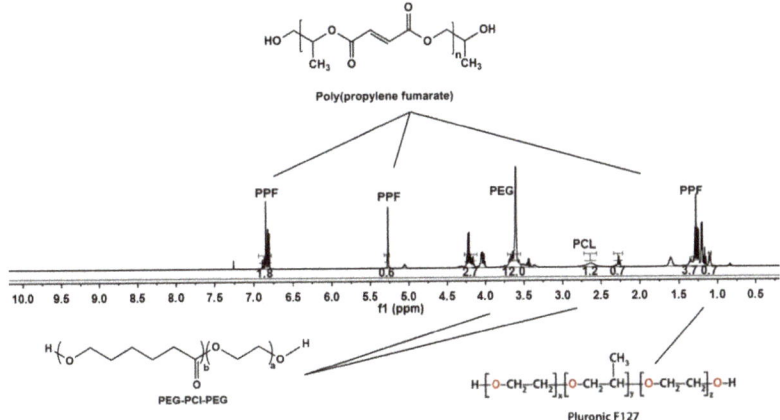

Figure 5. NMR analysis of the 3D bioprinted pseudo-bone scaffold, reflecting chemical shifts and copolymeric composition.

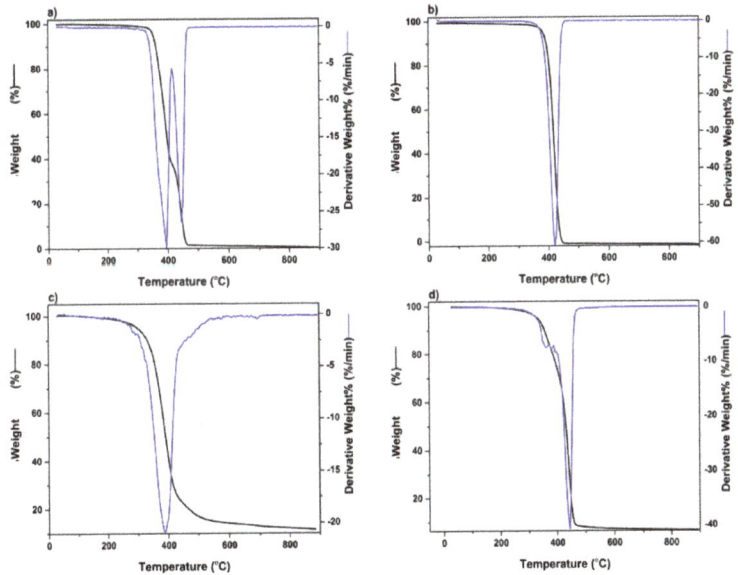

Figure 6. TGA analysis undertaken in the region of 30 °C to 900 °C for (**a**) PEG-PCL-PEG, (**b**) PF127, (**c**) PPF, and (**d**) 3D bioprinted scaffold.

3.3. Morphological Analysis Undertaken on the 3D Bioprinted Pseudo-Bone Scaffold

Scanning electron microscopy was undertaken on the 3D bioprinted scaffold for determining the microarchitectural design according to the CAD bioprinting parameters. The morphology was investigated employing electron microscopy at an average of 3500 times magnification. As seen in Figure 7, each layer of the scaffold reflected a similar porosity configuration, with uniform intercalated threads of fibrous 3D printing, bioengineered for cell growth within the porous network. This configuration further allows easy diffusion of tissue medium through the scaffold matrix. Printing under low-pressure and low-speed parameters, thus, allows for maximum consistency and uniformity in the microarchitectural design of the 3D scaffold. As observed in Figure 7, the intercalated "rope-like" nature with porous network architecture can be identified with multiple sites of scaffold printing, bonding between each designed layer. Macrostructural analysis undertaken after 3D printing confirmed a 600 μm strand diameter, with a deviation of +/− 60 μm per given strand. This can be attributed to air pressure accumulation during 3D printing, as well as, drying rates between each layer, once printed. A slight change in temperature could also affect the drying rate of each layer, thus contributing to the slight deviation of strand diameter thickness.

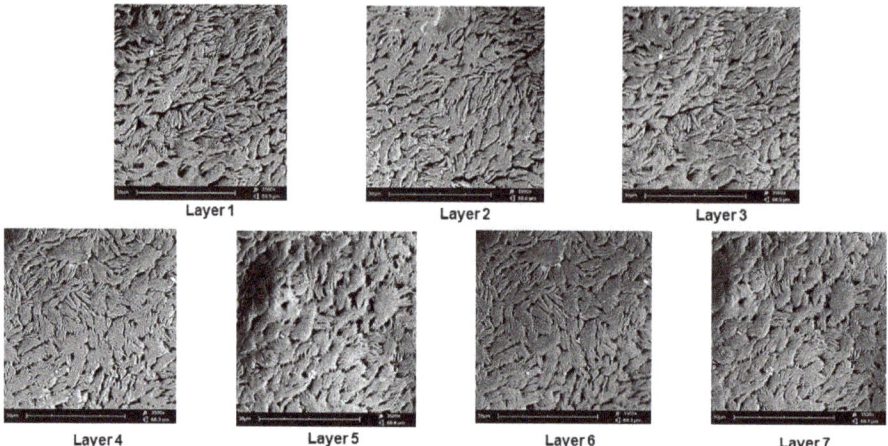

Figure 7. SEM analysis of the 3D bioprinted scaffold at 3500 times magnification, demonstrating the microarchitecture and inner porous nature of the 7 layers of the designed 3D scaffold matrix.

The polymeric ink was evaluated with respect to change in temperature at a constant applied force, evaluating the change in temperature, as seen in Figure 8. G' is described as the measure of deformation energy, referring to the elastic, solid properties of the polymeric ink that would adhere to the fracture of the bone. In contrast, G" is the measure of the viscous and deformation energy used and lost in the polymeric ink over a given temperature range. As seen in Figure 8, G' begins at 23 °C, starting to form a semi-solid gelling property, and thereafter at 32 °C, completely switches to the elastic phase property, remaining above G" throughout the evaluation of the sample. It was observed that the viscosity of the sample gradually increases above room temperature, ± 25 °C, maintaining a higher elastic phase property than the liquid state at body temperature conditions.

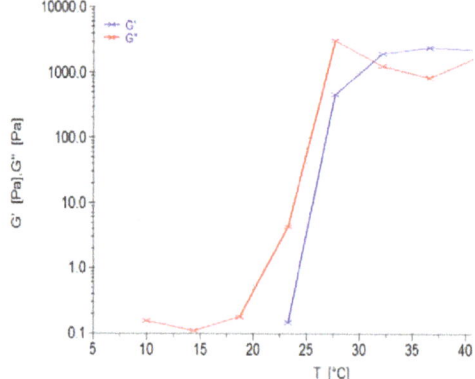

Figure 8. Rheological evaluation of the polymeric ink in relation to change in temperature.

Thus, we can determine that the polymeric ink has substantial thermo-responsive properties, with a significant change in modulus due to temperature variations. At controlled storage temperature of 10–20 °C, only viscous modulus is present in the range of 0.1–0.3 Pa, allowing ideal 3D printing to occur. When the higher temperature is reached, the polymeric ink increases strength by 45,000 times, allowing swelling and adhesion to occur (from 0.1 Pa to 4500 Pa). As body temperature is reached by the polymeric ink, the gel forms a solid, semi-elastic substance, thereby gradually releasing drug in a controlled, sustainable manner.

3.4. In Vitro Analysis of the Designed 3D Bioprinted Drug Delivery Scaffolds

The 39 designed 3D scaffold formulations were analyzed for their simvastatin release behavior. It was observed that as PPF polymer (8% *w/v*–20% *w/v*) was increased in percentage in the formulation, greater release of simvastatin from the scaffold over 24 h was observed. This can be attributed to the ester linkage of PPF, accounting for hydrolysis of the polymer into biocompatible and excretable degradation products of fumaric acid and propylene glycol, with associated release of the drug from the matrix [27].

PF 127 was incorporated at concentrations 14% *w/v* to 16% *w/v* in the formulations. It was observed that as the concentration of PF 127 was increased in the 3D scaffold, release of the loaded drug from the formulation was gradually slowed. This could possibly be explained in terms of increasing the amphiphilic nature of the 3D scaffold, resulting in an improved controlled release profile. The thermogelling capabilities of the system also contribute to the controlled release potential of the system by preventing particle aggregation, balancing hydrophilicity, surface roughness, and surface charge [23]. As observed in Figure 9, formulations 1–16 released drug up to 13 days, formulations 17–26 up to 16 days, formulations 27–32 up to 19 days, and formulation 33–39 up to 20 days. All formulations demonstrated near zero-order release kinetics. The optimized 3D bioprinted scaffold formulation, resulting in the highest factor of response (most sustained drug release), was thus synthesized incorporating 14% *w/v* PPF and 16% *w/v* PF127. The optimized 3D bioprinted scaffold displayed a controlled release of simvastatin over a 20-day duration, as seen in Figure 10, with significant correlation to the predicted release kinetics ascertained using ANN. It can be further emphasized that the morphological configuration in terms of the specialized shape and internal architecture significantly influenced the release kinetics and biodegradation of the 3D bioprinted drug delivery scaffold. It can be concluded that the optimized 3D bioprinted scaffold possessing highly specific design features of microarchitectural pores and uniform bioprinted filaments of specific dimensional properties has favorable controlled release kinetics in vitro, which demonstrated good correlation to the release predicted by the ANN model.

An advantage of employing 3D printing over these parameters holds premise for the incorporation of cellular/biological materials to be integrated for future studies. Another advantage of this delivery system is attributed to the hydrophobic chain regions of PPF encapsulating a class of BCS 2 drugs, at higher concentrations. As PF 127 concentration increased, the scaffolds biodegraded over an extended duration of time, resulting in stronger gelation of the scaffold with increased PF 127 concentration. This can also be seen in Figure 9, as further controlling the release rate of the loaded drug was observed. Thus, a major advantage in the design was the slower sustained release effect of PF 127 in the formulation, being desirable for implantable systems.

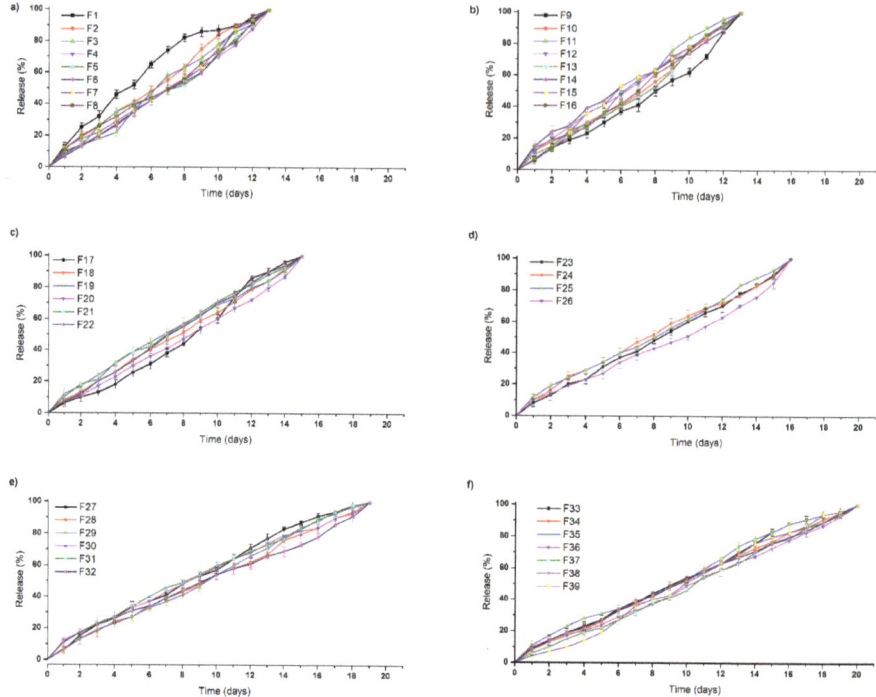

Figure 9. In vitro simvastatin release analysis of the designed 3D bioprinted drug delivery scaffolds. (**a**,**b**) formulations 1–16, released drug up to 13 days; (**c**,**d**) formulations 17–26, released up to 16 days; (**e**) formulations 27–32, released up to 19 days; and (**f**) formulation 33–39, released over a duration of 20 days.

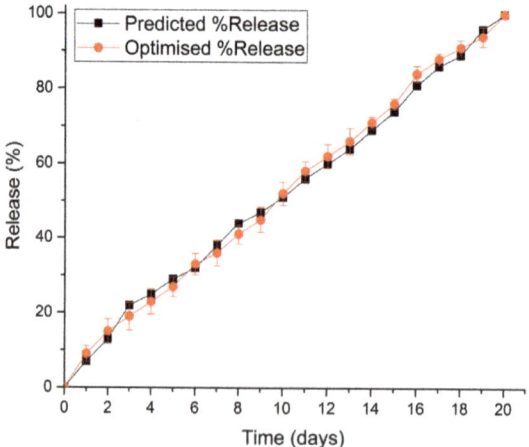

Figure 10. Correlation of in vitro simvastatin release analysis of the optimized 3D bioprinted scaffold with predicted release kinetics using ANN modeling.

3.5. Matrix Analysis of the 3D Bioprinted Scaffold in Fracture-Induced Human Clavicle Bones

Mechanical properties of 3D scaffolds are essential in relation to their site-specific application [28,29]. The butterfly fracture was induced using a 4 mm punch and dye apparatus, using a hydraulic pressure of 0.6 MPa, under standard conditions (temperature of 25 °C and pressure of 1atm). A steel flat tip probe of 2 mm diameter was used to determine the MH and a steel cylindrical probe of 50 mm diameter used for determination of MR. The MH and MR were evaluated employing a texture analyzer resulting in values of 18.61 N/mm^2 and 9.48%, respectively, for the human clavicle before fracture. Figure 11a–c depicts an X-ray image of the human clavicle bone before fracture, after fracture, and after treatment with the 3D bioprinted scaffold, respectively [29–31]. Following fracture, the missing bone mass was observed in the X-ray image (Figure 11b), as well as in Figure 11e, which is circled in red. After inducing the fracture, the 3D scaffold was applied at the site of defect, with immersion in PBS, and incubated at 37 °C for 20 days. The bone was then evaluated for MH and MR. It was found that a MH of 18.45 N/mm^2 and MR of 9.33% were observed at the site of the fracture, thus possessing similar results to the non-fractured bone. Figure 11d represents a light microscope image at 24 times magnification of the 3D bioprinted scaffold immersed in PBS. After incubation of the scaffold in PBS at 37.5 °C for 2 h at the fracture site, microscopic visualization revealed significant filling of the fracture site, as observed in Figure 11f (depicting the architecture of the bone and the scaffold sealed sites). These values of MH and MR further exemplifies the unique properties of the 3D bioprinted pseudo-bone scaffold to fill in fracture sites in bones, thus promoting greater adhesion of bone and restoration of damaged bone to its intended mechanical integrity.

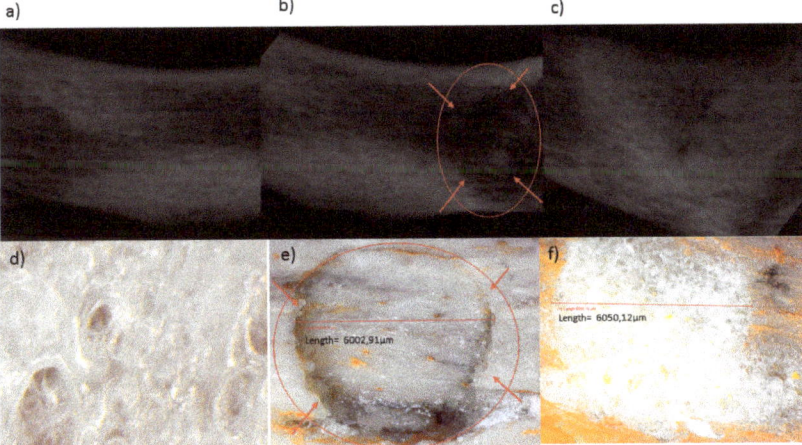

Figure 11. X-ray images of the human clavicle bone (**a**) before fracture, (**b**) after fracture, and (**c**) after treatment with the 3D bioprinted scaffold, respectively. (**d**) Light microscope image at 24 times magnification of the 3D bioprinted scaffold immersed in phosphate buffer solution, (**e**) human clavicle bone induced with a fracture, representing missing bone fragments, (**f**) human clavicle bone tested after incubation at 37.5 °C for 2 h, demonstrating sealing of the induced fracture site, with properties of matrix hardness and resilience comparable to original bone properties.

4. Conclusions

A 3D bioprinted pseudo-bone drug delivery scaffold was designed to mimic the morphology, matrix strength, and matrix resilience of healthy human bone. The 3D bioprinted scaffold was developed using computer-aided design (CAD) software, with further optimization of the design formulations employing MATLAB® software and artificial neural networks. Polymers employed for formulating the 3D bioprinted scaffold consisted of polypropylene fumarate (PPF), free radical polymerized polyethylene glycol- polycaprolactone (PEG-PCL-PEG), and pluronic (PF 127). Simvastatin was incorporated into the 3D bioprinted scaffolds to further promote bone healing and repair properties. The 3D bioprinted scaffold was characterized for its chemical, morphological, mechanical, and in vitro release properties for evaluation of its behavior for application as an implantable scaffold at the site of fracture. The ANN-optimized 3D bioprinted scaffold demonstrated favorable properties as a controlled release platform, displaying sustained drug release over 20 days. The 3D bioprinted scaffold thus promoted contact adhesion between fractured/damaged bone using a human clavicle bone model, promoting the formation of a pseudo-bone matrix within the fractured site. Future investigations to be reported include in vitro cell culture studies, with biocompatibility evaluation on the 3D bioprinted scaffold, with completion following in vivo analysis. In in vivo studies in New Zealand, Albino rabbit model is being undertaken to confirm the degree of bone repair and regeneration promoted by the 3D bioprinted scaffold. It can thus be concluded that the significant research undertaken will demonstrate promising results for future research endeavors in bone healing and repair.

Author Contributions: Conceptualization, methodology, software, and validation of this research was undertaken by P.J.K. Formal analysis, investigation, resources, and data curation was undertaken by all authors, including P.J.K., P.P.D.K., Y.E.C., T.M., and V.P. Authorship has thus been limited to those who have contributed substantially to the work reported. All authors have read and agreed to the published version of the manuscript.

Funding: This research was funded by the National Research Foundation (N.R.F) of South Africa (SARCI 191219497422).

Acknowledgments: We would like to acknowledge the N.R.F for supporting this research project.

Conflicts of Interest: The authors declare no conflict of interest.

References

1. Ferracini, R.; Martínez Herreros, I.; Russo, A.; Casalini, T.; Rossi, F.; Perale, G. Scaffolds As Structural Tools For Bone-Targeted Drug Delivery. *Pharmaceutics* **2018**, *10*, 122. [CrossRef] [PubMed]
2. Özcan, İ.; Bouchemal, K.; Segura-Sánchez, F.; Özer, Ö.; Güneri, T.; Ponchel, G. Synthesis And Characterization Of Surface-Modified PBLG Nanoparticles For Bone Targeting: In Vitro And In Vivo Evaluations. *J. Pharm. Sci.* **2011**, *100*, 4877–4887. [CrossRef] [PubMed]
3. Caetano, G.; Violante, R.; Sant'Ana, A.; Murashima, A.; Domingos, M.; Gibson, A.; Bártolo, P.; Frade, M. Cellularized Versus Decellularized Scaffolds For Bone Regeneration. *Mater. Lett.* **2016**, *182*, 318–322. [CrossRef]
4. Bosco, A.; Faleiros, P.; Carmona, L.; Garcia, V.; Theodoro, L.; de Araujo, N.; Nagata, M.; de Almeida, J. Effects Of Low-Level Laser Therapy On Bone Healing Of Critical-Size Defects Treated With Bovine Bone Graft. *J. Photochem. Photobiol. B Biol.* **2016**, *163*, 303–310. [CrossRef]
5. Bujoli, B.; Scimeca, J.; Verron, E. Fibrin As A Multipurpose Physiological Platform For Bone Tissue Engineering And Targeted Delivery Of Bioactive Compounds. *Pharmaceutics* **2019**, *11*, 556. [CrossRef]
6. Tsai, S.; Yu, W.; Hwang, P.; Huang, S.; Lin, H.; Hsu, Y.; Hsu, F. Fabrication And Characterization of Strontium-Substituted Hydroxyapatite-Cao-Caco3 Nanofibers with a Mesoporous Structure as Drug Delivery Carriers. *Pharmaceutics* **2018**, *10*, 179. [CrossRef]
7. Heintz, K.; Bregenzer, M.; Mantle, J.; Lee, K.; West, J.; Slater, J. Biomimetic Microfluidic Networks: Fabrication Of 3D Biomimetic Microfluidic Networks In Hydrogels (Adv. Healthcare Mater. 17/2016). *Adv. Healthc. Mater.* **2016**, *5*, 2152. [CrossRef]
8. Li, J.; He, L.; Zhou, C.; Zhou, Y.; Bai, Y.; Lee, F.; Mao, J. 3D Printing For Regenerative Medicine: From Bench To Bedside. *Mrs Bull.* **2015**, *40*, 145–154. [CrossRef]
9. Lee, J.; Hong, J.; Jung, J.; Shim, J.; Oh, J.; Cho, D. 3D Printing Of Composite Tissue With Complex Shape Applied To Ear Regeneration. *Biofabrication* **2014**, *6*, 024103. [CrossRef]
10. Huang, G.; Wang, L.; Wang, S.; Han, Y.; Wu, J.; Zhang, Q.; Xu, F.; Lu, T. Engineering Three-Dimensional Cell Mechanical Microenvironment With Hydrogels. *Biofabrication* **2012**, *4*, 042001. [CrossRef]
11. del Castillo-Santaella, T.; Ortega-Oller, I.; Padial-Molina, M.; O'Valle, F.; Galindo-Moreno, P.; Jódar-Reyes, A.; Peula-García, J. Formulation, Colloidal Characterization, And In Vitro Biological Effect Of BMP-2 Loaded PLGA Nanoparticles For Bone Regeneration. *Pharmaceutics* **2019**, *11*, 388. [CrossRef]

12. Gioffredi, E.; Boffito, M.; Calzone, S.; Giannitelli, S.; Rainer, A.; Trombetta, M.; Mozetic, P.; Chiono, V. Pluronic F127 Hydrogel Characterization And Biofabrication In Cellularized Constructs For Tissue Engineering Applications. *Procedia Cirp* **2016**, *49*, 125–132. [CrossRef]
13. Kang, K.; Hockaday, L.; Butcher, J. Quantitative Optimization Of Solid Freeform Deposition Of Aqueous Hydrogels. *Biofabrication* **2013**, *5*, 035001. [CrossRef] [PubMed]
14. Wang, C.; Tang, Z.; Zhao, Y.; Yao, R.; Li, L.; Sun, W. Three-Dimensional In Vitro Cancer Models: A Short Review. *Biofabrication* **2014**, *6*, 022001. [CrossRef] [PubMed]
15. Arai, K.; Iwanaga, S.; Toda, H.; Genci, C.; Nishiyama, Y.; Nakamura, M. Three-Dimensional Inkjet Biofabrication Based On Designed Images. *Biofabrication* **2011**, *3*, 034113. [CrossRef] [PubMed]
16. Choonara, Y.; du Toit, L.; Kumar, P.; Kondiah, P.; Pillay, V. 3D-Printing And The Effect On Medical Costs: A New Era? *Expert Rev. Pharm. Outcomes Res.* **2016**, *16*, 23–32. [CrossRef]
17. Shirosaki, Y.; Furuse, M.; Asano, T.; Kinoshita, Y.; Kuroiwa, T. Skull Bone Regeneration Using Chitosan–Siloxane Porous Hybrids—Long-Term Implantation. *Pharmaceutics* **2018**, *10*, 70. [CrossRef]
18. Götz, W.; Tobiasch, E.; Witzleben, S.; Schulze, M. Effects Of Silicon Compounds On Biomineralization, Osteogenesis, And Hard Tissue Formation. *Pharmaceutics* **2019**, *11*, 117. [CrossRef]
19. Kondiah, P.; Choonara, Y.; Kondiah, P.; Kumar, P.; Marimuthu, T.; du Toit, L.; Pillay, V. Development Of An Injectable Pseudo-Bone Thermo-Gel For Application In Small Bone Fractures. *Int. J. Pharm.* **2017**, *520*, 39–48. [CrossRef]
20. Agami, N.; Atiya, A.; Saleh, M.; El-Shishiny, H. A Neural Network Based Dynamic Forecasting Model For Trend Impact Analysis. *Technol. Forecast. Soc. Chang.* **2009**, *76*, 952–962. [CrossRef]
21. Liu, C.; Zeng, Y.; Kankala, R.; Zhang, S.; Chen, A.; Wang, S. Characterization And Preliminary Biological Evaluation Of 3D-Printed Porous Scaffolds For Engineering Bone Tissues. *Materials* **2018**, *11*, 1832. [CrossRef] [PubMed]
22. Sanchez-Molina, D.; Velazquez-Ameijide, J.; Quintana, V.; Arregui-Dalmases, C.; Crandall, J.; Subit, D.; Kerrigan, J. Fractal Dimension And Mechanical Properties Of Human Cortical Bone. *Med Eng. Phys.* **2013**, *35*, 576–582. [CrossRef] [PubMed]
23. Raval, A.; Pillai, S.; Bahadur, A.; Bahadur, P. Systematic Characterization Of Pluronic ®Micelles And Their Application For Solubilization And In Vitro Release Of Some Hydrophobic Anticancer Drugs. *J. Mol. Liq.* **2017**, *230*, 473–481. [CrossRef]
24. Zhou, Q.; Zhang, Z.; Chen, T.; Guo, X.; Zhou, S. Preparation And Characterization Of Thermosensitive Pluronic F127-B-Poly(ε-Caprolactone) Mixed Micelles. *Colloids Surf. B Biointerfaces* **2011**, *86*, 45–57. [CrossRef] [PubMed]
25. Behravesh, E.; Shung, A.; Jo, S.; Mikos, A. Synthesis And Characterization Of Triblock Copolymers Of Methoxy Poly(Ethylene Glycol) And Poly(Propylene Fumarate). *Biomacromolecules* **2002**, *3*, 153–158. [CrossRef] [PubMed]
26. Jo, S.; Engel, P.; Mikos, A. Synthesis Of Poly(Ethylene Glycol)-Tethered Poly(Propylene Fumarate) And Its Modification With GRGD Peptide. *Polymer* **2000**, *41*, 7595–7604. [CrossRef]
27. Salarian, M.; Xu, W.; Biesinger, M.; Charpentier, P. Synthesis And Characterization Of Novel Tio2-Poly(Propylene Fumarate) Nanocomposites For Bone Cementation. *J. Mater. Chem. B* **2014**, *2*, 5145–5156. [CrossRef]
28. Buj-Corral, I.; Bagheri, A.; Petit-Rojo, O. 3D Printing Of Porous Scaffolds With Controlled Porosity And Pore Size Values. *Materials* **2018**, *11*, 1532. [CrossRef]
29. Xu, T.; Binder, K.; Albanna, M.; Dice, D.; Zhao, W.; Yoo, J.; Atala, A. Hybrid printing of mechanically and biologically improved constructs for cartilage tissue engineering applications. *Biofabrication* **2012**, *5*, 015001. [CrossRef]
30. Iannolo, M.; Werner, F.; Sutton, L.; Serell, S.; VanValkenburg, S. Forces Across The Middle Of The Intact Clavicle During Shoulder Motion. *J. Shoulder Elb. Surg.* **2010**, *19*, 1013–1017. [CrossRef]
31. Schramm, G. *A Practical Approach to Rheology and Rheometry. Thermo Electron (Karlsruhe)*; GmbH: Karlsruhe, Germany, 2004; Volume 2.

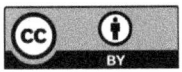

© 2020 by the authors. Licensee MDPI, Basel, Switzerland. This article is an open access article distributed under the terms and conditions of the Creative Commons Attribution (CC BY) license (http://creativecommons.org/licenses/by/4.0/).

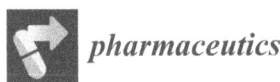

Article

Development of Bio-Active Patches Based on Pectin for the Treatment of Ulcers and Wounds Using 3D-Bioprinting Technology

Eleftherios G. Andriotis *, Georgios K. Eleftheriadis, Christina Karavasili and Dimitrios G. Fatouros

Department of Pharmaceutical Technology, School of Pharmacy, Aristotle University of Thessaloniki, GR-54124 Thessaloniki, Greece; gkelefth@pharm.auth.gr (G.K.E.); karavasc@pharm.auth.gr (C.K.); dfatouro@pharm.auth.gr (D.G.F.)
* Correspondence: andrioti@pharm.auth.gr; Tel.: +30-6948-469-406

Received: 17 December 2019; Accepted: 7 January 2020; Published: 9 January 2020

Abstract: Biodegradable 3D-printable inks based on pectin have been developed as a system for direct and indirect wound-dressing applications, suitable for 3D printing technologies. The 3D-printable inks formed free-standing transparent films upon drying, with the latter exhibiting fast disintegration upon contact with aqueous media. The antimicrobial and wound-healing activities of the inks have been successfully enhanced by the addition of particles, comprised of chitosan and cyclodextrin inclusion complexes with propolis extract. Response Surface Methodology (RSM) was applied for the optimization of the inks (extrusion-printing pressure, shrinkage minimization over-drying, increased water uptake and minimization of the disintegration of the dry patches upon contact with aqueous media). Particles comprised of chitosan and cyclodextrin/propolis extract inclusion complexes (CCP), bearing antimicrobial properties, were optimized and integrated with the produced inks. The bioprinted patches were assessed for their cytocompatibility, antimicrobial activity and in vitro wound-healing properties. These studies were complemented with ex vivo skin adhesion measurements, a relative surface hydrophobicity and opacity measurement, mechanical properties, visualization, and spectroscopic techniques. The in vitro wound-healing studies revealed that the 3D-bioprinted patches enhanced the in vitro wound-healing process, while the incorporation of CCP further enhanced wound-healing, as well as the antimicrobial activity of the patches.

Keywords: wound-healing; 3D bio-printing; pectin; propolis; cyclodextrin; 3D bio-inks

---

1. Introduction

There is a vast number of materials available for wound dressing, currently under investigation for different types of wounds and different treatment approaches [1–4]. The type, depth, and location of a wound, in addition to the extent of damage, the amount of wound exudates and the presence of an infection in the wound site, are key factors in the selection of dressing type. The application of traditional dressings, like cotton bandages or gauzes, absorb the moisture contained by the wound, leading to dehydration of the wound surface, and subsequently decreasing the healing rate. Alternative dressings, fabricated by polymers in the form of films, foams or gels, have already been developed and extensively applied for wound management, as they provide the optimum conditions for wound-healing by maintaining the moisture of the wound and at the same time providing a sense of relief to the patient [3,4]. To this end, the aim of this study was the development of a wound-dressing system that could provide an adequate moisture environment under occlusive conditions, and the capability to protect the wound from infection and contamination [5], based on natural, non-toxic materials, like pectin, honey, and propolis.

Pectin belongs to a wider class of materials applied for the fabrication of hydrocolloid dressings, that are well-known to promote wound-healing by maintaining a proper, moist environment 5]. These types of dressing can form a gel upon direct contact with wound exudates, leading to high fluid absorption [6], and at the same time provide an adequate protective barrier against bacterial infection [7]. Pectin serves as a hydrophilic agent that reacts with the wound fluid towards the formation of a soft gel over the wound bed that helps to remove or control exudates. The acidity of the resulting pectin solution enhances the bacterial or viral barrier properties of the system. These wound dressings are well known and extensively studied systems for loading and releasing APIs like antibiotics, analgesics, growth factors and others [7,8].

Pectin has also been studied in combination with honey towards the development of wound dressings [8]. Honey possesses multiple bioactivities related to the wound-healing process and exhibits a broad-spectrum antibacterial activity with variation in potency between different types. Despite the fact that many honey varieties have been studied for their beneficial effects on the wound site, the majority of the research is focused on Manuka honey. The main difference between Manuka honey and other honey varieties is methylglyoxal (MGO), which enhances its antibacterial properties [9]. This honey variety can be diluted by wound exudates (up to 7-fold) and still maintain its inhibition activity against bacteria [10], while its acidity increases the release of oxygen from hemoglobin, creating a less favorable environment for destructive proteases. Additionally, the high osmolarity of honey draws fluid out of the wound bed, creating an outflow of lymph similar to negative pressure wound therapy [10].

Another natural material used in this study is propolis. More than 300 different compounds have been identified in propolis, including aliphatic acids, esters, aromatic acids, fatty acids, carbohydrates, aldehydes, amino acids, ketones, chalcones, dihydrochalcones, terpenoids, vitamins, and inorganic substances, with flavonoids being the most widely studied [11,12]. The positive therapeutic effects of propolis are well established and mostly attributed to the antioxidant activity of polyphenols [11]. It is also well-documented that propolis contains active compounds, like caffeic acid, caffeic phenyl ester, artepillin C, quercetin, resveratrol, galangin, and genistein, that promote cell proliferation [11]. Propolis, in general, is studied for its antiseptic, antibacterial, antimycotic, astringent, spasmolytic, anti-inflammatory, anesthetic, antioxidant, antifungal, antiulcer, anticancer, and immunomodulatory effects. The acceleration of burned tissue repair by propolis is also supported by the literature, and a connection between the ability of flavonoid compounds to reduce lipid peroxidation and prevent necrosis of cells has been suggested [11,13].

Pectin, propolis and Manuka honey could be combined towards the fabrication of wound-healing patches using 3D printing technology. 3D printing is a significant platform that can be used for the production of films and patches in complex geometries, in a controlled manner. 3D printers could be an asset for the development of personalized wound-healing patches to meet the specific needs of individual patients and treatments [14,15]. The fact that 3D bioprinting is a prominent platform for combining cells, growth factors, bio-molecules, and bio-polymers in a controlled manner, makes the use of this technology advantageous compared to traditional techniques for the production of patches, like the solvent-casting method.

In this study, free-standing wound patches that disintegrate in aqueous media were fabricated using a 3D bioprinter. The 3D bioinks were a combination of high methoxylated pectin with Manuka honey, designed either for direct application to the wound site or as free-standing patches after drying. The antimicrobial and wound-healing properties of the fabricated films were enhanced by the addition of propolis inclusion complexes with beta-cyclodextrin. The inclusion complexes were prepared by adding an ethanolic extract of propolis to beta-cyclodextrin. The propolis complexes were further combined with chitosan in order to enhance their adhesion to pectin, by exploiting the ionic bonds formed between the two polymers [16].

2. Materials and Methods

2.1. Materials

All reagents used were of standard analytical grade. HM pectin from apple (HMP, Degree of esterification = 70–75%, Sigma-Aldrich, Darmstadt, Germany) was used as received. Manuka Honey (MGO 550+, Manuka Health, Auckland, New Zealand) and crude propolis (Propolis from Taygetus Mountain, Green Family-Ellinikon, Thessaloniki, Greece) were kept in the dark at 4 °C and warmed to room temperature prior to use. Beta cyclodextrin (kleptose®, Roquette, Zaventem, Belgium) was used as received.

2.2. Preparation of 3D Printed Patches

The preparation of 3D-printable pectin inks was realized by the addition of predetermined amounts of apple pectin in 10 mL sterile, double-distilled water, pH 8, to prevent early gelation of pectin. The mixture was left at room temperature for 24 h, under constant magnetic stirring, to ensure wetting and swelling of pectin powder. Subsequently, the temperature of the system was raised to 80 °C under continuous mixing, until a homogeneous viscous mixture was formed (pectin dissolution). Afterward, the pH value of the mixture was lowered (pH 2.6 ± 0.2), by the addition of 20 mg Citric Acid (16.7% *w/v* in double distilled H_2O), to form a non-freely flowing gel. The gel was cooled to room temperature under continuous mixing, and predetermined amounts of Manuka honey were added. The addition of Manuka honey leads to the formation of harder gels, with a gum-like texture. The prepared 3D-printable pectin inks were loaded to a 3D Bioprinter (CELLINK®Inkredible, Gothenburg, Sweden) and films of various geometries were printed, depending on the needs of experiments. Film thickness was determined using a 0–25 mm (±0.01 mm) handheld caliper at five random positions on each film to obtain an average value.

2.3. Design of Experiments

Central Composite Design of Experiments (CCDE) was applied with using the Minitab 17.1.0 software (Minitab® 17.1.0, Minitab Inc., State College, PA, USA), for the construction of the design matrixes. In order to quantitatively elucidate the effects of the variables, the responses were subjected to regression analysis, and mathematical models were obtained. Contour plots were constructed based on those models and the preferred experimental conditions were chosen accordingly. The validity of the models is assessed by confirmation experiments contacted in triplicateat the preferred conditions.

2.4. Preparation of Propolis Ethanolic Extract (EEP)

The extract was prepared according to a published method [12]. In summary, propolis was cut into small pieces (≈2–3 mm) and mixed with 99% ethanol, at a ratio of 1:10 (propolis:ethanol). The mixture was magnetically stirred for 48 h, in dark at room temperature. The extract was filtered to clarification, and ethanol was removed under reduced pressure. EEP was dissolved in 99% ethanol at a final concentration of 56% *w/v* and stored at 4 °C in an amber vial.

2.5. Preparation of Chitosan and β-Cyclodextrin/Propolis Extract Inclusion Complexes (CCP)

Chitosan and β-cyclodextrin/propolis extract inclusion complexes (CCP) were prepared according to literature, with minormodification [13]. Briefly, chitosan (CS) stock solution (1% *w/v*) was prepared in aqueous acetic acid solution (2% *v/v*) and mixed with an aqueous solution of β-CD (5% *w/v*), at predetermined ratios. EEP solution was added dropwise, and the final mixture was sonicated using a probe sonicator (SONICS, vibracell™, Newtown, CT, USA), in an ice bath, to prevent thermal decomposition of EEP. Ethanol was removed under reduced pressure and CCP particles were collected after freeze-drying. Freeze-dried CCP was grounded using a mortar and a pestle, and passed through a

125 µm mesh. The fine powder was gradually added to the 3D-printable pectin ink, under continuous mixing, until a homogeneous ink was formed.

2.6. Determination of Total Polyphenol Content

The total polyphenol content of CCP particles was determined according to the Folin–Chiocaltau method [17]. Briefly, CCP samples (10 mg) were suspended in 200 µL ethanol and placed in a rotary mixer for 1 h, in the dark and at room temperature. After the extraction of propolis from CCP, the mixture was centrifuged at 4500 rpm, and 50µL of the supernatant was added to a solution containing 50 µL of theFolin–Chiocaltau reagent, 700 µL H_2O and 200 µL of 10% *w/v* sodium carbonate solution. The solution was placed for 1 h at room temperature and color development was measured at 650 nm. The color development intensities of the sample extracts were expressed as Gallic Acid Equivalent per mg of sample (mg GAE/mg).

2.7. Dynamic Light Scattering and ζ-Potential Measurements

Dynamic light scattering (DLS) and ζ-potential measurements were performed using a Malvern Nanosizer ZS, Malvern Instruments (UK). The droplet size, polydispersity index (PDI), and z-potential values were recorded in triplicate and evaluated.

2.8. Film Swelling Studies

Rectangular patches (1 × 1 cm) were printed and left to dry at 75 °C until at a constant weight. The patches were weighted and placed in 50 mL PBS for 60 s, under mild agitation. Subsequently, the swollen patches were withdrawn, gently blotted with filter paper and weighted. The swelling properties were expressed as the percentage weight gain over the initial dry weight. The patches were then left to dry at 75 °C until the weight variations were stabilized, and reweighed to calculate the mass loss during the swelling test.

2.9. 3D Printing Shape Fidelity Assessment

The shape fidelity of the 3D-printed patches was quantified based on the variance between the theoretical and experimental dimensions of the 3D printed patches, after drying. Briefly, 3D-printed patches (2 × 2 cm) were fabricated and left to dry until a constant weight was achieved at 75 °C. The dimensions of the dry patches were compared to a computer-designed control frame (2 × 2 cm), using a conventional desktop 2D scanner (HP DesckJet 2630, Hewlett-Packard, Palo Alto, CA, USA) (Figure 1) and an image analysis software (ImageJ public domain software, NIH, Bethesda, MD, USA). The deviation from the expected shape is expressed as Equation (1),

$$F(\%) = 100 \times (Ac - As)/Ac \qquad (1)$$

where Ac and As are the projection areas (in pixels) of the control frame and the 3D-printed patch, respectively.

2.10. Determination of Film Opacity

Film opacity was determined according to previously reported studies. Rectangular strips of 3D-printed Pectin films (3d Pec), containing various amounts of CCP, were printed according to the geometry of a UV–Vis cuvette. The 3D printed patches were then placed in contact with the inner wall of the cuvette, and the absorption spectrum of the patches was obtained from 400–700 nm in a UV-Visible spectrophotometer (Shimadzu 1601, Kyoto, Japan). Film opacity was defined as the area under the curve, divided by the film thickness and expressed as Absorbance Units × nanometers/millimeters (AU × nm/mm). All measurements were conducted in triplicate.

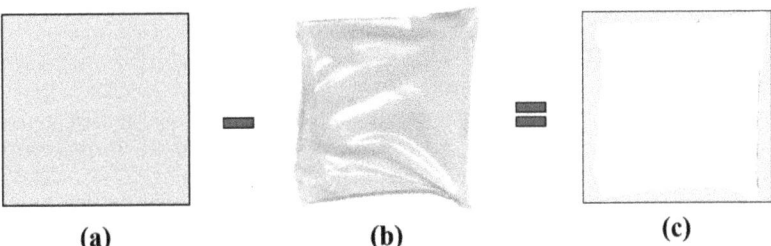

Figure 1. Theoretical dimentions of the patches (**a**), experimental dimensions of the 3D-printed patches after drying (**b**), and their difference (**c**), as it is calculated by Equation (1).

2.11. Optical Microscopy

All 3D-printed patches were observed under an optical microscope (Celestron MicroDirect 1080p HD Handheld Digital Microscope, Celestron, Torrance, CA, USA) at a magnification of 220×.

2.12. Determination of Relative Surface Hydrophobicity

The relative surface hydrophobicity of the films was estimated by the sessile drop method, based on the optical contact angle method [18,19]. A 2 µL droplet of ethylene–glycol was deposited onto the patch surface. Contact angle measurements were carried out using a digital microscope (CelestronMicroDirect 1080p HD Handheld Digital Microscope). The digital camera of the microscope was placed horizontally to capture the droplet image. Image analysis software (ImageJ public v1.52a, NIH, Bethesda, MD, USA) was used to measure the angle between the patch surface and the tangent to the drop of liquid, at the point of contact with the film surface. Seven parallel measurements were performed for each film at 25 °C.

2.13. Mechanical Tests

The tensile properties of the formulated films were investigated using a TA-XT2i instrument (Stable Micro Systems, Godalming, Surrey, UK) ($n = 3$). To achieve this, dumbbell-shaped films with 50 × 10 × 0.2 mm dimensions were 3D-printed. Thickness was measured using a caliper, and an average value of five points was obtained. The fabricated films were fixed onto the clamps of the instrument, and tensile tests were performed under a speed of 0.5 mm/s, to determine the tensile strength and the elongation at break [20].

2.14. Biodhesion Studies

The bioadhesion performance of the films was examined using a TA-XT2i instrument (Stable Micro Systems, Godalming, Surrey, UK) ($n = 3$). Freshly excised porcine skin was supplied by a local slaughterhouse. Porcine skin was used as anex vivomodel for bioadhesion studies [21]. The skin was attached onto PET films with cyano-acrylate glue, to avoid the extensive deposition of glue residues on the instrumentation, and subsequently fixed onto the platform of the device with double adhesive tape. The films were mounted onto the probe using double-adhesive tape. The performance of the films was assessed under dry conditions, to simulate the direct use of the films on a dry wound. Alternatively, 100 µL of PBS or liquid 3D pectin ink were instilled onto the skin, to simulate the application of the films onto a wet wound surface or the indirect utilization of the films as a support dressing on wounds, covered with the 3D pectin ink. A force of 1 N was applied, to maintain contact of the formulations with the skin for 60 s, and the probe was withdrawn at a speed of 1 mm/s [22]. The maximum force (F_{max}) of detachment was recorded, whereas the work of adhesion (W_{ad}) was determined from the area under the curve of the force-versus-distance plot.

2.15. Determination of Antimicrobial Properties

A medium pouring method was used to determine the antimicrobial activity of the 3D-printed patches containing CCP against two bacterial strains (*Staphylococcus aureus* and *Escherichia coli*) [23]. Three-dimensional-printed patches (discs with diameter 1 cm, height 0.15 mm and weight 40 mg) were sterilized by UV light (30 W, 1.0 m) for 30 min. The sterile patches were added to 15 mL polypropylene tubes, containing 1 mL 10^7 CFU/mL bacterial suspension, diluted in 9 mL sterile saline solution. After the complete dissolution of the patches, the solution was cultivated in sterile plates. All the plates were incubated at 37 °C for 24 h, and the colony number was measured. Bacteriostasis was calculated by Equation (2),

$$Q(\%) = 100 \times (A - B)/A \qquad (2)$$

where Q, A, and B represent the growth inhibition, the mean colony count (CFU/mL) of the control group and the mean colony count (CFU/mL) of the sample group, respectively.

2.16. Film Disintegration Test

An ERWEKA Disintegration Tester (ERWEKA GmbH, Langen, Germany) was used to measure the disintegration time of the 3D-printed films, modifying the USP30<701> Disintegration procedure, using 900 mL of distilled water at 37 °C. Disks of 1 cm diameter and 0.12 mm average thickness were printed and placed into individual tubes of the basket-rack assembly. Time was recorded until complete erosion of the films.

2.17. Scanning Electron Microscopy

The morphological features of the 3D-printed patches were assessed using a Zeiss SUPRA 35VP SEM microscope (Zeiss GmbH, Oberkochen, Germany). Samples were placed on aluminum stubs and coated with 15 nm gold, using an Emitech K550X DC sputter coater (Emitech Ltd. Ashford, Kent, UK) apparatus, prior to imaging.

2.18. Fourier-Transform Infra-Red (FTIR).

The chemical structure of the 3D printed patches was confirmed by recording the FTIR spectra (IR Prestige-21, Shimadzu, Japan). The resolution of the spectrum was set at 4 cm^{-1}. The recorded wavenumber range was 800–4000 cm^{-1}, and 64 spectra were averaged. The commercially available software IR Solutions (Shimadzu, Japan) was used to process the spectral data.

2.19. Cell Culture

Dermal human fibroblast cells (HDFa, ATCC® PCS-201-012™) were cultured in 96-well plates containing high-glucose DMEM with 10% v/v heat-inactivated fetal bovine serum (FBS) and 1% (v/v) antibiotic antimycotic at 37 °C in a humidified atmosphere of 5% CO_2 [24].

2.20. Cell Viability—MTT Assay

The viability of HDFa cells was evaluated using the MTT assay based on the ability of viable cells to convert thiazolyl blue tetrazolium bromide solution to purple formazan crystals in their mitochondria [25,26]. The HDFa cells were seeded into 96-well plates and incubated with three different concentrations of dissolved patches containing different concentrations of CCP (0.1, 1 and 5 mg/mL 3DPect of 0, 2.5, 5, 10, 20 and 30% CCP w/w of dry film, respectively) for 24 and 48 h. The culture medium was then removed, and the cells were rinsed three times with PBS. The MTT agent (5 mg/mL in PBS) was added into the wells and the plates were incubated at 37 °C for 3 h. Sequentially, formazan crystals were dissolved in DMSO and the absorbance of each well was measured at 540 nm. Cell viability was calculated using Equation (3),

$$\text{Cell Viability (\%)} = 100 \times (A_S - A_B)/(A_C - A_B) \qquad (3)$$

where A_S, A_C, and A_B are the absorbance values of the sample well, control well and blank well, respectively.

2.21. Cell Scratch Assay (In Vitro Wound Healing)

The cell scratch assay was proposed for the assessment of the wound-healing properties of the 3D-printed patches, as a facile and low-cost in vitro method to evaluate the migration ability of cells [24]. Briefly, HDFa cells were seeded into 6-well plates, at an initial density of 2×10^5 cells/well and incubated at 37 °C for 72 h (in high glucose DMEM with 10% v/v FBS). Two perpendicular scratches were generated in each well, via a sterile tip of a pipette (200 μL), as well as an intersection at a point close to the center of the well. The cross-shaped scratch was used as a location marker. After rinsing with PBS, the cells were incubated with three different concentrations of dissolved 3D-printed patches (0.1, 1 and 5 mg/mL 3DPect) and serum-free medium. The distribution and quantity of cells in the scratch area in each well were monitored under a microscope, and images were recorded at 0, 24 and 72 h, respectively. Wound width and wound closure were calculated according to Equations (4) and (5),

$$\text{Relative Wound Width (\%)} = 100 \times W_f/W_i \quad (4)$$

where, W_i and W_f are the initial and final wound width, respectively.

$$\text{Relative Wound Closure (\%)} = 100 \times (A_i - A_f)/A_i \quad (5)$$

where, A_i and A_f are the initial and final cell-free area of the simulated wound, respectively.

Wound width was calculated as the average distance between the edges of the scratch. Manual quantification was carried out and the initial and final wound width was calculated as the average of 50 width measurements across the scratch. The wound area was calculated based on the cell-free area in captured images using the ImageJ public domain software (NIH, Bethesda, MD, USA).

2.22. Statistical Analysis

All experiments are reported in triplicate, and statistical analysis was performed for data derived from different samples. All results are expressed as mean ± standard deviation and checked by normality tests. OriginLab v9.0.0software (Originlab Corporation, Wellesley Hills, MA, USA) was used for statistical analysis. Student's paired t-test was performed to compare the data of paired samples. A value of $P < 0.05$ indicated statistical significance.

3. Results and Discussion

3.1. Process Optimization

3.1.1. Optimization of 3D Printable Pectin Inks

CCDE was performed, based on Manuka honey/pectin ratio and pectin concentration. The design matrix and the corresponding responses are listed in Table 1. Six centerpoints have been selected (runs 1, 3, 7, 10, 13, and 14) and the corresponding responses are listed in Table 1. The differences between the values of the response for the centerpoints are indicative of the system variability, caused mainly by the addition of undiluted Manuka honey. The direct use of viscous materials like honey induces experimental variations, mainly due to the intense gelation of pectin at honey-rich regions of the mixture. These variations are surpassed by the continuous mixing of the system until homogeneity is reached. These alterations have an impact on the measured responses and they are taken under consideration by the Response Surface Methodology process. The following equations (Equations (6)–(9)) were obtained by regression analysis (using the full quadratic model) of the swelling properties of the patches (S), the mass loss of the patches after swelling (D), the shape fidelity of the patches (F) and the maximum pressure needed for the ink to be extruded through the printer nozzle (P), relating X_1 and X_2 (Manuka honey/pectin ratio and pectin concentration, respectively):

$$P \text{ (kPa)} = 27.5 - 697 \times (X_2) + 302 \times (X_1) + 5781 \times (X_2)^2 - 5162 \times (X_1)^2 + 3400 \times (X_2) \times (X_1), (R^2 = 0.894) \quad (6)$$

$$F \text{ (\%)} = 30.98 - 119 \times (X_2) - 46 \times (X_1) + 429 \times (X_2)^2 + 1817 \times (X_1)^2 - 1357 \times (X_2) \times (X_1), (R^2 = 0.679) \quad (7)$$

$$S \text{ (\%)} = 662 - 5000 \times (X_2) - 6289 \times (X_1) + 14{,}032 \times (X_2)^2 + 15{,}158 \times (X_1)^2 + 34{,}733 \times (X_2) \times (X_1), (R^2 = 0.421) \quad (8)$$

$$D \text{ (\%)} = 82.2 - 1119 \times (X_2) + 149 \times (X_1) + 3968 \times (X_2)^2 - 1679 \times (X_1)^2 + 174 \times (X_2) \times (X_1), (R^2 = 0.709) \quad (9)$$

Table 1. Central-composite design matrix defining conditions for printing patches by using 3D pectin inks, together with the experimental values of the respective responses.

Run	Variables in Uncoded Unit		P (kPa)	F (%)	S (%)	D (%)
	Manuka honey/pectin (w/v)	Pectin (w/v)				
1	0.05	0.10	32	5.8	230	4.0
2	0.00	0.15	40	21.2	180	8.8
3	0.05	0.10	33	19.1	200	11.3
4	0.00	0.05	10	28.3	600	31.8
5	0.10	0.15	73	16.4	180	4.4
6	0.10	0.05	9	37.1	250	25.6
7	0.05	0.10	32	15.4	240	9.1
8	0.12	0.10	20	25.1	170	11.4
9	0.05	0.03	10	23.9	120	65.1
10	0.05	0.10	30	28.8	240	13.0
11	0.00	0.10	25	23.3	200	7.6
12	0.05	0.18	134	14.5	340	10.4
13	0.05	0.10	20	16.9	190	4.4
14	0.05	0.10	60	17.5	180	6.5

Contour plots have been constructed in order to visualize the aforementioned models (Equations (6)–(9)). Figure 2a shows a distinct area of moderate working extrusion pressure (20–120 kPa), that is considered ideal for the printing process. Figure 2b shows a distinct minimum shape-deviation from the theoretical dimensions of patches, for a pectin concentration 0.125–0.18 w/v of ink, and Manuka honey/pectin ratio over 0.05 w/w. Figure 2c shows two maxima of film-swelling for a pectin concentration less than 0.075 w/v of ink and more than 0.15 w/v of ink and for a Manuka honey/pectin ratio less than 0.025 w/w and more than 0.1 w/w. Both of these maxima are located to extreme areas that are not preferred due to intense ink gelation (high Manuka honey concentration) or insufficient ink gelation (low Manuka honey concentration). Finally, Figure 2d shows a minimum film weight loss for a pectin concentration over 0.1 w/v of ink, depending almost exclusively on pectin concentration. Based on the visualization of the trends of the responses, as they are depicted by the above contour plots, the selected value for pectin concentration was 0.13 w/v of ink, and the value for Manuka honey/pectin ratio was 0.08 w/w. The model describing the swelling properties of the films failed to fit the data properly, and it was not taken into consideration for the final selection.

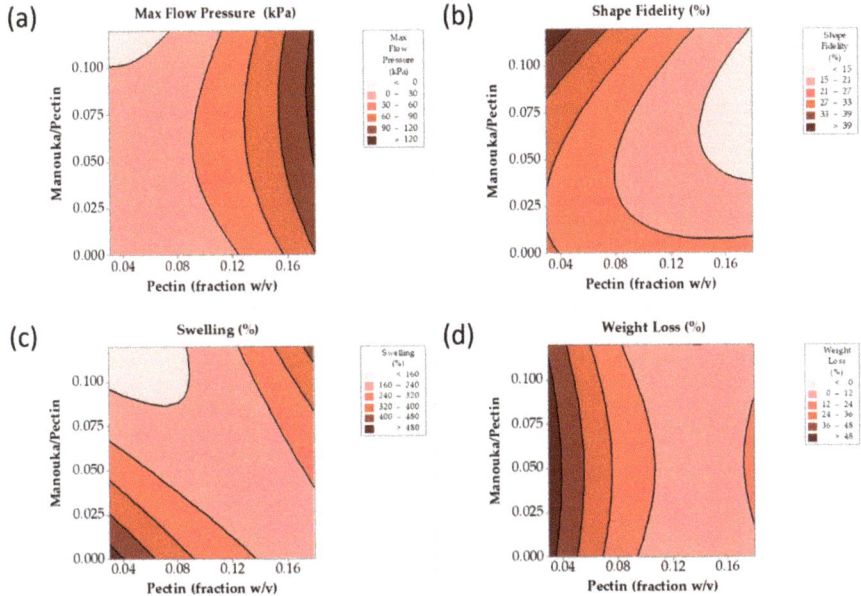

Figure 2. Maximum flow pressure (**a**), shape fidelity (**b**), film swelling (**c**) and film weight loss (**d**) contour lines against pectin concentration and Manuka honey/pectin ratio.

3.1.2. Optimization of Chitosan and Cyclodextrin/Propolis Extract Inclusion Complexes

Table 2 summarizes the design matrix and the corresponding responses. The responses were subjected to regression analysis (using full quadratic model) and the following equations (Equations (10)–(13)) were obtained for particle size (d_{nm}), zeta potential (ζ), PDI and EEP-loading, based on Gallic acid equivalent, as determined by the Folin–Chiocaltau method (GAE), relating X_1 and X_2 (EEP and chitosan concentration, respectively):

$$d_{nm}(nm) = 880 - 1 \times (X1) - 115 \times (X2) - 14.6 \times (X1)^2 + 601 \times (X2)^2 - 8 \times (X1) \times (X2), (R^2 = 0.608) \quad (10)$$

$$\zeta\ (mV) = -40.6 + 27.3 \times (X1) + 201.2 \times (X2) - 1.89 \times (X1)^2 - 100.5 \times (X2)^2 - 23.41 \times (X1) \times (X2), (R^2 = 0.859) \quad (11)$$

$$PDI = 0.350 + 0.0407 \times (X1) - 0.097 \times (X2) + 0.0006 \times (X1)^2 + 0.200 \times (X2)^2 - 0.0837 \times (X1) \times (X2), (R^2 = 0.367) \quad (12)$$

$$GAE\ (\mu g/mg) = -13.6 + 18.0 \times (X1) + 42.7 \times (X2) - 3.37 \times (X1)^2 - 45.3 \times (X2)^2 - 0.5 \times (X1) \times (X2), (R^2 = 0.147) \quad (13)$$

Contour plots have been constructed to visualize the aforementioned models (Equations (10)–(13)). Figure 3a shows a distinct minimum of particle size for an EEP concentration more than 3.8% *v/v* and a chitosan concentration less than 0.45% *w/v*. A broad range of chitosan and EEP concentrations exhibited zeta potential values greater than 40 mV (Figure 3b). The PDI (Figure 3c) was less than 0.4 (narrow distribution) for a broad range of chitosan and EEP concentrations. Finally, Figure 3d shows a distinct maximum of GAE for EEP concentration in the range of 1.5–4.5% *v/v* and chitosan concentration in the range 0.2–0.8% *w/v*. Based on the visualization of the trends in the responses, as they are depicted by the above contour plots, the selected value for EEP concentration was 4.5% *v/v* and the value for chitosan concentration was 0.6% *w/v*. The models describing the PDI and GAE for the EEP concentration of the CCP failed to fit the data properly and they were not taken into consideration for the final selection.

Table 2. Central-composite design matrix defining conditions for the production of CCP, together with the experimental values of the respective responses.

Run	Variables in Uncoded Unit		d (nm)	ζ (mV)	PDI	GAE (μg/mg)
	EEP (%)	Chitosan (%)				
1	1	0	760	−26.8	0.35	2.57
2	2.5	0.5	1080	61.1	0.29	3.82
3	0.4	0.5	1140	59.8	0.41	0.23
4	4.5	0.5	720	60	0.42	5.07
5	2.5	0.5	780	59.5	0.42	5.00
6	4	1	1080	55.4	0.26	2.67
7	2.5	0	1130	44.1	0.62	4.41
8	4	0	510	32.7	0.44	7.77
9	2.5	0.5	850	55.6	0.37	3.35
10	1	1	1250	54.6	0.38	0.52
11	2.5	1	1360	55.2	0.41	1.51
12	2.5	0.5	650	59.6	0.25	5.09
13	2.5	0.5	750	61.2	0.31	8.8
14	1	0	760	−26.8	0.35	2.57

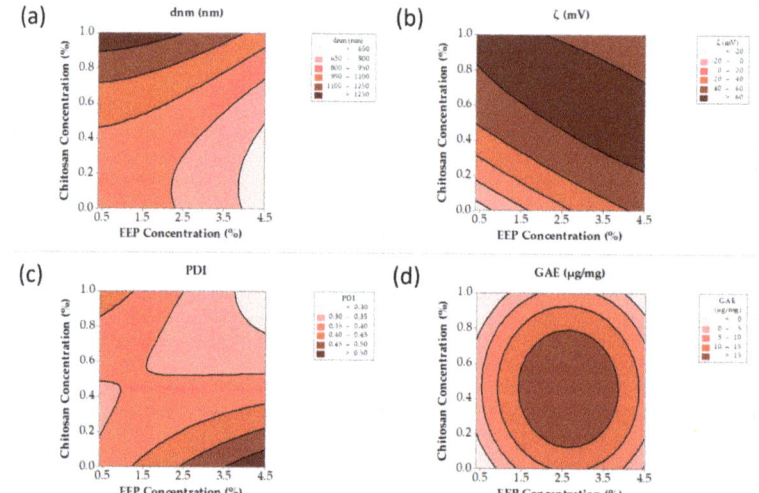

Figure 3. Particle size (**a**), zeta potential (**b**), polydispersity index (PDI) (**c**) and Gallic acid equivalent (**d**), contour lines versus propolis ethanoic extract (EEP) and chitosan concentration.

3.1.3. Confirmation Experiments

Response Surface Methodology was chosen as a statistical tool to screen experimental conditions through the visualization of the trend of the responses. The obtained models from the regression analysis were used for the construction of the contour plots and subsequently for the selection of the formulation, according to the depicted trends. Models that do not fit the experimental data (low R^2 values), were not taken into account for the selection of the final experimental conditions. The selection of the experimental conditions was performed by setting the desirable limits of the final responses based on the contour plots. In order to confirm the validity of the selected experimental conditions, additional experiments were carried out. The maximum flow pressure, shape fidelity, film swelling, and film weight loss for the printed patches, along with the particle size, ζ-potential, PDI and Gallic acid equivalent for the CCP particles, were obtained for the selected conditions, as listed in Tables 3 and 4, respectively. The desirable limits (Target Limits), along with the theoretical and experimental values of the responses, are listed in Tables 3 and 4. The reproducibility of the results for the selected conditions within the desirable limits validates that the RSM was a useful approach for screening and selecting the experimental conditions.

Table 3. Confirmation experiments executed for the selected conditions for 3D pectin inks.

EEP (%)	Chitosan (%)	Parameter	d (nm)	ζ (mV)	PDI	GAE (µg/mg)
4.5	0.6	Target Limit	650–800	>60	0.30–0.35	5–10
		Theoretical Value	715	65	0.33	7.9
		Experimental Value	715 ± 8	62 ± 1.8	0.4 ± 0.11	5.1 ± 0.2

Table 4. Confirmation experiments executed for the selected conditions for CCP particles.

Manuka Honey/Pectin	Pectin	Parameter	P (kPa)	F (%)	S (%)	D (%)
0.08	0.13	Target Limit	30–60	15–21	160–240	0–12
		Theoretical Value	62	17	204	7
		Experimental Value	35 ± 4	14 ± 5	220 ± 16	12 ± 8

3.2. Evaluation of 3D Pectin Patches Containing CCP

The optimum ink formulation was mixed with the optimally prepared CCP, under various final CCP concentrations (0%, 2.5%, 5%, 10%, 20% and 30% *w/w* CCP based on the amount of dry pectin). The prepared inks were loaded to the bioprinter, and the resulting patches were dried at room temperature to achieve a constant weight of the formulations. The free-standing films were stored in a desiccator, at room temperature.

3.2.1. Film Opacity

The 3D pectin patches with different amounts of CCP were assessed for their opacity. Transparent wound dressings permit the inspection of a wound without the need for dressing removal, and thus they are recommended for application on superficial and shallow wounds with low exudates [4]. The opacity quantitative analysis of the patches is shown in Figure 4a, while the actual patches are shown in Figure 5 (optical microscopy with 220× magnification). Patches, comprised of 0%, 2.5% and 5% *w/w* of CCP, are considered transparent (Figure 5a–c) with an increasing opacity correlated to higher concentrations of CCP. CCP-free patches were visually transparent, while the presence of CCP in the films resulted in a darker and more yellow appearance. As shown in Figures 4a and 5, the film opacity of the 3D-printed pectin films was relatively low, exhibiting an increase in relation to CCP incorporation. The notably higher opacity of the CCP-containing films, compared to the control, is attributed to their extensive light scattering, due to the inhomogeneous film structure, originating from CCP, which aggregates, expanding over the continuous pectin-rich phase. A key factor that influences the extent of dispersion of CCP in the film matrix, and consequently the opacity of the films, is the interaction between pectin and chitosan (present in CCP). The different charges of pectin and chitosan lead to the formation of ionic bonds that directly result in the topical cross-linking of pectin around CCP [14], thus inhibiting extended dispersion of the later. This topical cross-linking can elucidate the presence of the larger coagulants that were visible in the films.

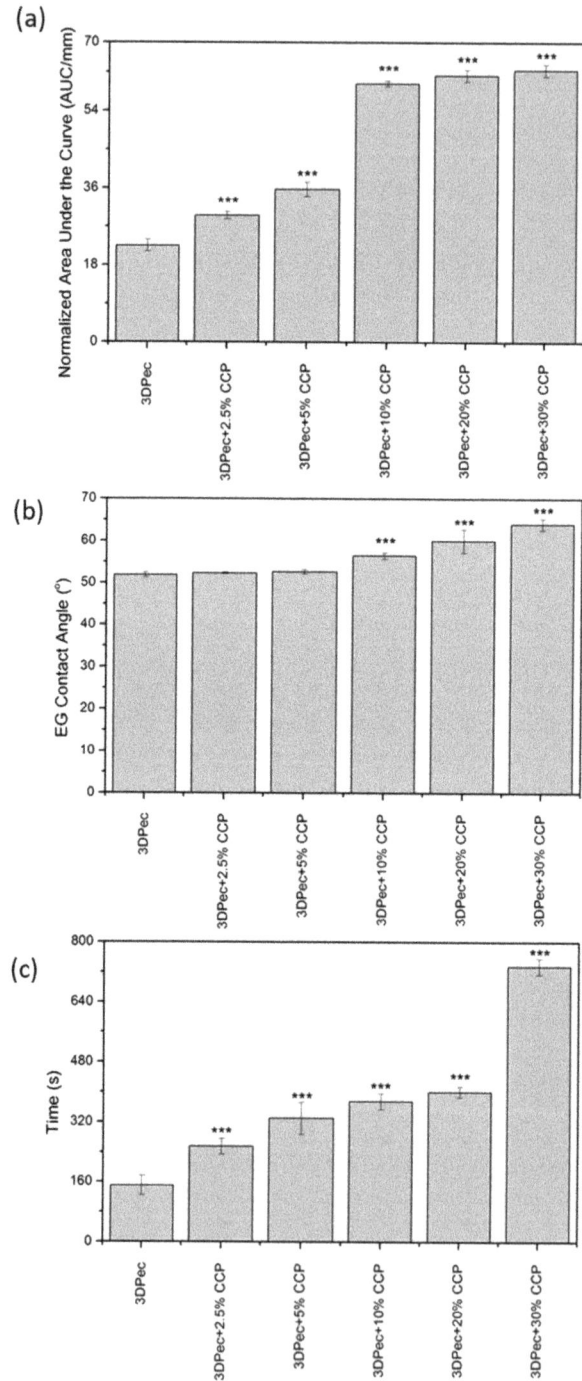

Figure 4. Data of (**a**) film opacity, (**b**) relative surface hydrophobicity, and (**c**) film disintegration time, obtained for patches with different concentrations of CCP. *** $P < 0.05$ vs. control.

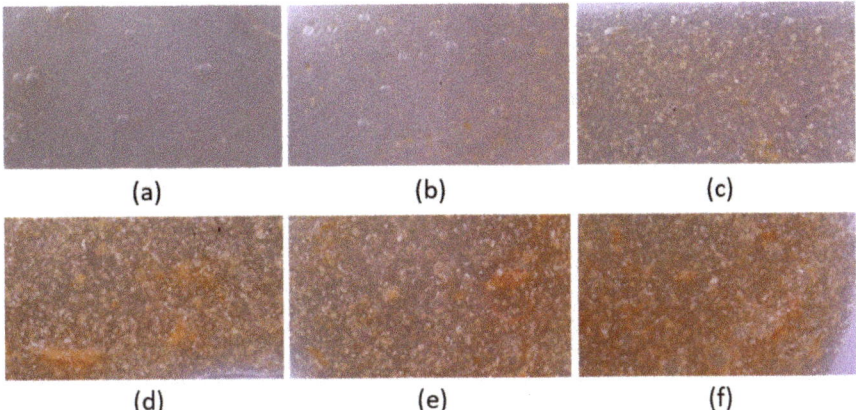

Figure 5. Optical microscopy images of 3D-printed pectin films with: (**a**) 0%, (**b**) 2.5%, 5%, (**c**) 10%, (**d**) 20% and (**e**,**f**) 30% w/w CCP.

3.2.2. Relative Surface Hydrophobicity

Low contact angles, less than 90°, measured for CCP-free and composite films, are typical of hydrophilic materials, like pectin films. CCP incorporation up to 5% w/w into the pectin films does not influence the hydrophilic characteristics of the resulting film surface ($P > 0.05$), as was deduced from the data for contact angles presented in Figure 4b. On the other hand, CCP incorporation higher than 5% w/w into the pectin films affected the hydrophilic character of the film surface ($P < 0.05$). Despite the statistical significance of this effect, the film surface was still considered hydrophilic, with contact angles less than 65°. These negligible alterations to the hydrophobicity of the patches suggest that hydrophobicity is preferentially influenced by the changes in surface roughness following CCP incorporation, rather than by chemical or compositional changes to the surface. In conclusion, the increase in the hydrophobicity of the film surface is considered artifactual, as the ethylene–glycol droplet used for the contact angle measurements is considered to exclusively contact the pectin matrix.

3.2.3. Film Disintegration Test

A disintegration test of the 3D-printed patches is shown in Figure 4c. The incorporation of CCP into the films is suggested to influence the disintegration time of the patches ($P < 0.05$), compared to the control film. The disintegration time presented an increasing trend, proportional to the addition of CCP, with a six-fold increase in the case of films comprising 30% w/w CCP, compared to the control group. This increase is solely attributed to cross-linked pectin moieties, due to the formation of ionic bonds with the incorporated chitosan molecules.

3.2.4. Film Surface Observation

The films' surface was observed by optical microscopy and SEM (Figures 5 and 6). Both techniques revealed the presence of printing-related defects on the surface of the control film. These defects are characterized by the presence of voids, formed during the printing process, which gradually decreased in size and resulted in a bubble-like formation. The inhomogeneity of the composite films, as is depicted in Figure 5b–f, is attributed to the presence of CCP coagulants, with increasing intensity as the concentration of CCP is increased. The transparency and the color of the films are clearly depicted in Figure 5, where films with more than 5% w/w CCP appear to be opaque with a distinct, dark yellow color, due to propolis. Finally, the CCP micrograph shows the structure of propolis-containing particles that are smaller than those incorporated in the films, indicating the presence of intense coagulation due to topical cross-linking.

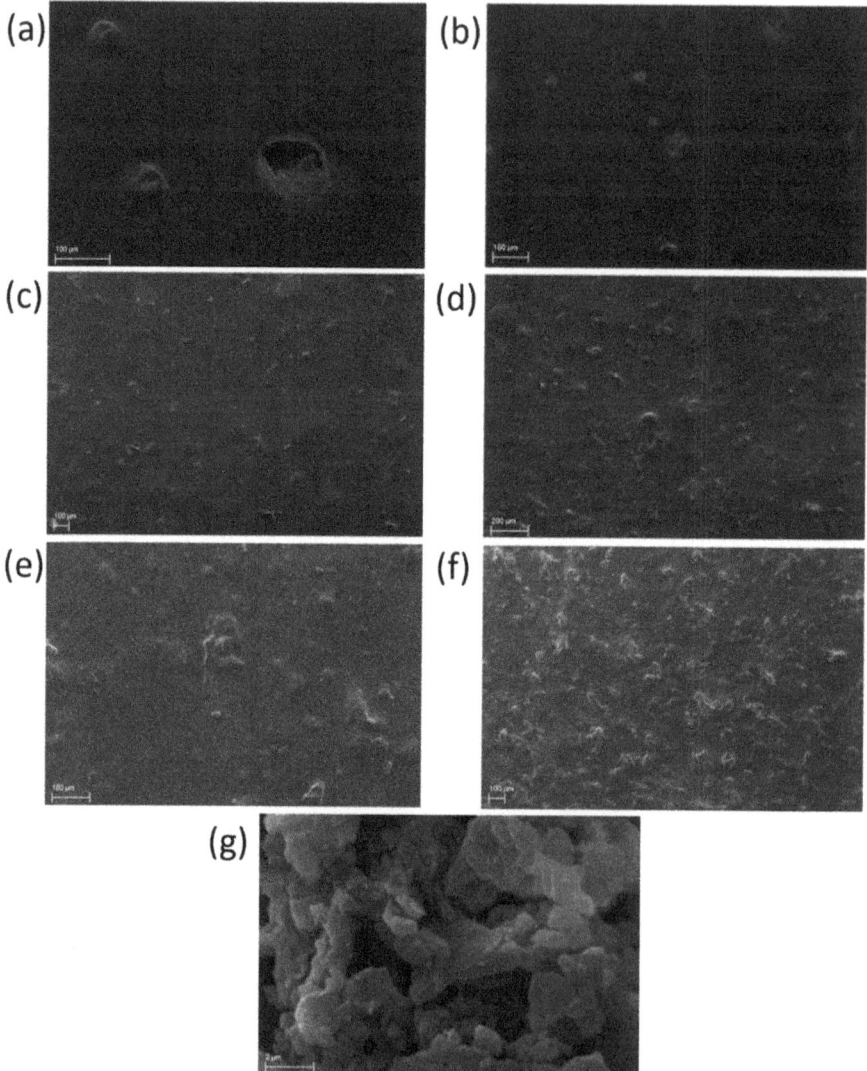

Figure 6. SEM images of 3D-printed pectin films with: (**a**) 0%, (**b**) 2.5%, 5%, (**c**) 10%, (**d**) 20% and (**e**,**f**) 30% w/w propolis extract inclusion complexes (CCP); and (**g**) CCP powder.

3.2.5. Fourier-Transform Infra-Red (FTIR)

The chemical structure of the surface of the 3D-printed patches was confirmed by recording their ATR-FTIR spectra. Figure 4, summarizes the ATR-FTIR spectra of the patches, the spectra of their composites with CCP, and the spectra of CCP. The spectra in Figure 7 revealed a broad band around 3700–3000 cm^{-1} for all films and for CCP, typical for polysaccharides, attributed to the O–H stretching vibration (OH), while peaks around 3000–2800 cm^{-1} were attributed to C–H stretching vibrations (vCH) [14]. Regarding the spectrum of pectin films, two bands were detected between 1800–1500 cm^{-1}, which were attributed to the stretching vibrations of the carbonyl group (vC=O) [14]. The band located at 1733 cm^{-1} corresponds to the vC=O of the methyl ester group (COOCH$_3$) and to the non-dissociated carboxyl group (COOH), while the band located at 1624 cm^{-1} is assigned to the asymmetric stretching vibration of the carbonyl group of the carboxyl ion (COO−) [14]. The CCP spectrum revealed a band centered at 1647 cm^{-1}, attributed to the νC=O of the amide group (also known as Amide I band) of the acetylated units of chitosan, present in the CCP. The almost identical spectra of the control 3D-printed pectin films and the composite films with CCP are indicative of the surface composition of the films that are mainly composed of a pectin matrix, while CCP particles are coated with pectin to such an extent that the presence of free CCP on the surface is considered negligible.

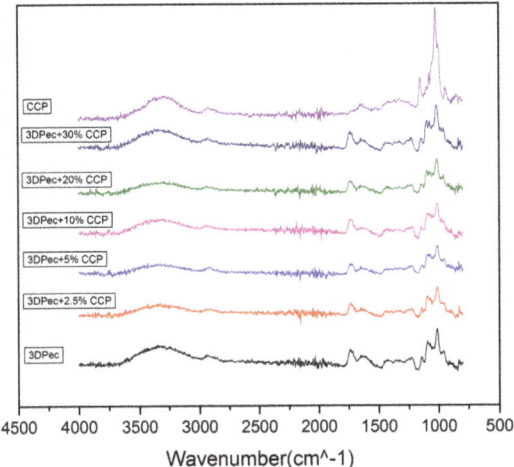

Figure 7. ATR-FTIR Spectra of 3D-printed pectin films with: 0%, 2.5%, 5%, 10%, 20% and 30% *w/w* CCP; and CCP powder.

3.2.6. Mechanical Tests

The tensile properties of the prepared films are presented in Table 5. It has been reported that the mechanical properties of wound dressings are key to the optimal applicability of the formulations on the skin and the avoidance of mechanical abrasion [27,28]. The incorporation of propolis-based microparticles resulted in significant alterations in the tensile strength of the specimens ($P < 0.05$). The maximum tensile performance was recorded in the case of the formulation with 2.5% *w/w* CCP, presenting values of tensile strength and elongation of approximately 50 N/mm^2 and 2.7% *w/w*, respectively. Formulations with a higher content of CCP reduced tensile properties, due to the simultaneous incorporation of chitosan, as it has been documented that chitosan-based films exhibit poor mechanical properties [29]. Furthermore, it was hypothesized that large amounts of the particles in the ink induced the formation of low-homogeneity structures, as was previously discussed, thus affecting the mechanical properties of the films. The results for the Young Modulus of the fabricated pectin films show an increase, following the incorporation of CCP, from 7.76 to 9.1 N × mm^{-2} ($P < 0.05$). Films with 2.5%, 5%, and 10% *w/w* CCP have similar Young Modulus values, in contrast with the films with 20% and 30% *w/w* CCP, which are stiffer. The loss of elasticity, due to CCP incorporation, is also attributed to the cross-linking that takes place between pectin and chitosan moieties of the CCP.

Table 5. Data obtained from the mechanical tests for the tensile strength, elongation at break, and Young Modulus of the fabricated 3D-printed pectin films with different amounts of CCP.

Formulation	Tensile Strength (N × mm^{-2})	Elongation (%)	Young Modulus (N × mm^{-2})
3DPec	29.68 ± 3.05	1.91 ± 0.08	7.76 ± 0.47
3DPec + 2.5% CCP	49.62 ± 1.71	2.72 ± 0.22	9.14 ± 0.43
3DPec + 5% CCP	43.65 ± 2.23	2.35 ± 0.03	9.28 ± 0.36
3DPec + 10% CCP	36.96 ± 2.79	1.91 ± 0.06	9.67 ± 0.43
3DPec + 20% CCP	35.62 ± 1.62	1.63 ± 0.13	10.95 ± 0.38
3DPec + 30% CCP	36.31 ± 3.22	1.59 ± 0.11	11.41 ± 0.22

3.2.7. Bioadhesion Studies

The bioadhesive performances of the formulated films, under dry and wet conditions, are reported in Table 6. Negligible adhesion was observed under dry conditions, in all cases. The instillation of PBS onto the porcine skin induced a significantly higher adhesion performance ($P < 0.05$). Further studies were conducted with the incorporation of liquid pectin ink onto the porcine skin. The experiments revealed greater F_{max} and W_{ad} values for all specimens, compared to PBS.

Table 6. Data obtained from the bioadhesion studies of the fabricated 3D printed pectin films with different amounts of CCP, for direct contact with the tissue (dry), after wetting the tissue with double distilled H$_2$O (wet) and after wetting the tissue with 3D-printable pectin ink (ink).

Formulation	Conditions	F_{max} (N)	Wad × 10 (N × mm)
3DPec	Dry	0.05 ± 0.03	0.07 ± 0.04
	Wet	0.48 ± 0.10	0.68 ± 0.13
	Ink	1.29 ± 0.11	3.44 ± 0.21
3DPec + 2.5% CCP	Dry	0.06 ± 0.02	0.13 ± 0.03
	Wet	0.85 ± 0.15	1.48 ± 0.34
	Ink	1.39 ± 0.08	5.38 ± 0.42
3DPec + 5% CCP	Dry	0.14 ± 0.07	0.52 ± 0.11
	Wet	1.59 ± 0.11	5.67 ± 0.37
	Ink		
3DPec + 10% CCP	Dry	0.17 ± 0.04	0.64 ± 0.14
	Wet	1.04 ± 0.09	2.28 ± 0.24
	Ink	1.47 ± 0.09	5.27 ± 0.32
3DPec + 20% CCP	Dry	0.26 ± 0.03	0.99 ± 0.16
	Wet	2.88 ± 0.14	6.43 ± 0.28
	Ink	3.66 ± 0.15	8.79 ± 0.35
3DPec + 30% CCP	Dry	0.17 ± 0.12	0.32 ± 0.19
	Wet	1.38 ± 0.25	2.76 ± 0.54
	Ink	2.04 ± 0.33	6.16 ± 0.98

Regarding the content of microparticles in the films, alterations in the bioadhesion parameters were further recorded, due to the simultaneous incorporation of the bioadhesive chitosan [30,31]. Up to a certain amount of CCP, a significant enhancement in the bioadhesive performance of the specimens was evidenced ($P < 0.05$), as the formulation comprising 20% w/w CCP exhibited F_{max} and W_{ad} values of approximately 6.4 and 8.8 N × mm, respectively. In line with the tensile tests, however, the higher content of CCP reversely affected the bioadhesive performance of formulation, with 30% w/w CCP, suggesting the limited homogeneity of the films.

3.2.8. Determination of Antimicrobial Properties

The antimicrobial properties of the 3D-printed films, comprised of pectin and Manuka honey, and their composites with CCP, were evaluated using the medium-pouring method. Figure 8 shows the percentage of microbial viability in the presence of dissolved patches. The results show that 3D-printed pectin films exhibit insufficient antimicrobial activity, despite the presence of manuka honey. This was an expected outcome, as the amount of honey in contact with the bacteria is highly diluted (more than 10-fold). On the other hand, CCP incorporation of up to 10% w/w CCP is followed by an intense increase of more than 95% in the antimicrobial activity of the films. Notably, the antimicrobial activity decreased for 20% and 30% w/w of CCP, presenting a minimum for CCP concentrations of 10% w/w. It was evidenced that the presence of insoluble CCP clusters, which were formed by the topical cross-linking of pectin with chitosan, affect the extent of the contact area between the propolis-containing particles and the bacteria incorporated into the aqueous media.

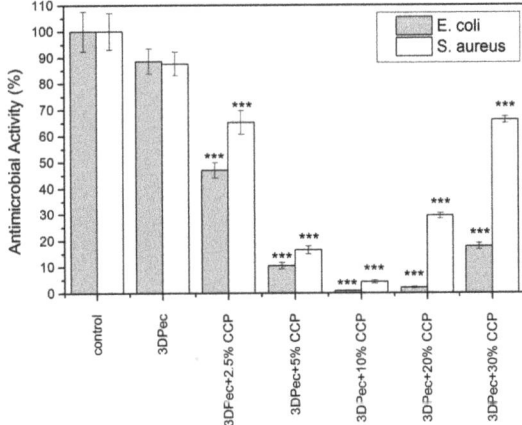

Figure 8. Antimicrobial activity of 3D-printed pectin films with: 0%, 2.5%, 5%, 10%, 20% and 30% w/w CCP, against two bacterial strains of interest. *** $P < 0.05$ vs. control.

3.2.9. Cell Viability Assay

The viability results of HDFa cells, treated with 3D-printed patches that contain different amounts of CCP, as well as for three different concentrations of the dissolved patches in the cell culture medium, are summarized in Figure 9. For the low concentration of dissolved patches in the cell culture medium (0.1 mg/mL), cell viability was not significantly affected for the first 24 h; however, decreased viability was evidenced at 48 h, estimated at 50% of the control culture. Additionally, cell viability was slightly reduced with increasing the CCP concentration in the films. This behavior was attributed to the addition of pectin films that resulted in a possible decrease in the pH of the medium, combined with an increase in the medium viscosity that is believed to affect cell proliferation. Another key factor that affects cell viability is the presence of insoluble material (especially for films containing higher amounts of CCP) that are capable of physically obstructing the cells, by either covering or immobilizing them. This phenomenon was more intense for higher concentrations of dissolved patches in the cell culture medium (1 and 5 mg/mL), where the decrease in cell viability was higher for the first 24 h, followed by the lack of a distinct pattern correlating CCP concentration with cell viability. The absence of a distinct pattern of cell viability for concentrations of 1 and 5 mg/mL of dissolved films in the cell culture medium is attributed to the inhomogeneous character of the films containing CCP, due to the presence of the topical cross-linking of pectin with chitosan. This immediately resulted in the presence of more insoluble material in the cell culture medium, and subsequently a more intense inhibition of cell growth.

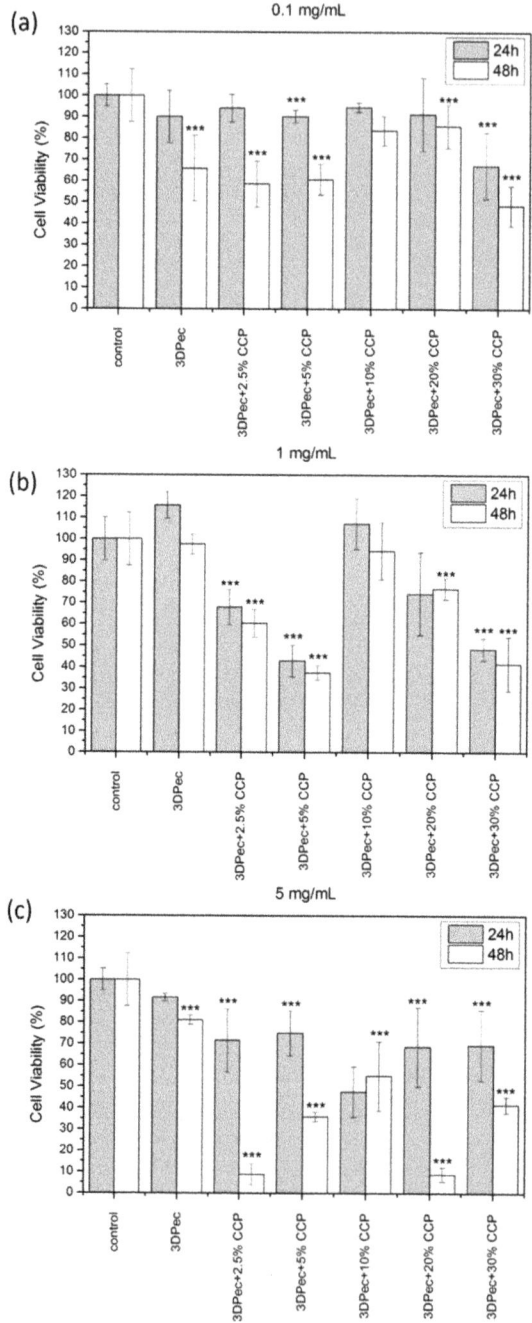

Figure 9. Cell viability assay of the 3D-printed pectin films with: 0%, 2.5%, 5%, 10%, 20% and 30% w/w CCP, for (**a**) 0.1 mg/mL, (**b**) 1 mg/mL and (**c**) 5 mg/mL of dissolved patches in the cell culture medium. *** $P < 0.05$ vs. control.

3.2.10. Cell Scratch Assay (In Vitro Wound Healing)

The cell scratch assay was applied for assessment of the wound-healing potential of the 3D-printed patches. The scratch assay was applied to different amounts of CCP and for three different concentrations of the dissolved patches in the cell culture medium (0.1, 1 and 5 mg/mL). HDFa cells were cultured, and a cross-shaped scratch was generated on the cell monolayer, simulating a wound. The wound closure in the presence of 3D-printed pectin patches containing CCP was monitored for 72 h. Figure 10a,b shows the relative wound width and the relative wound area, respectively. Figure 11 shows the time-lapse of the actual wound healing process. The results of the in vitro wound-healing assay revealed that the 3D-printed pectin patches exhibit strong wound-healing properties in vitro. This behavior is further enhanced by the addition of CCP (up to 5% w/w), where full closure (Relative Wound Width = 0% and Relative Wound Area = 0%) of the simulated wound was evidenced. In all cases, elongated cell formations with multiple infusions were observed, typical of migrating cells, along with changes in their spatial conformation. For CCP concentrations higher than 10% w/w, the presence of an insoluble film material exhibited an inhibitory effect on cell migration, despite the migration of individual cells towards the empty scratched area. The higher concentrations of dissolved patches in the cell culture medium presented a similar behavior to the samples containing 0.1 mg/mL of patches (with 20% and 30% w/w CCP), and thus they are not presented. It is suggested that the discrimination efficacy of the assay was compromised by higher amounts of insoluble film debridement, and thus the deduction of a safe conclusion was arbitrary.

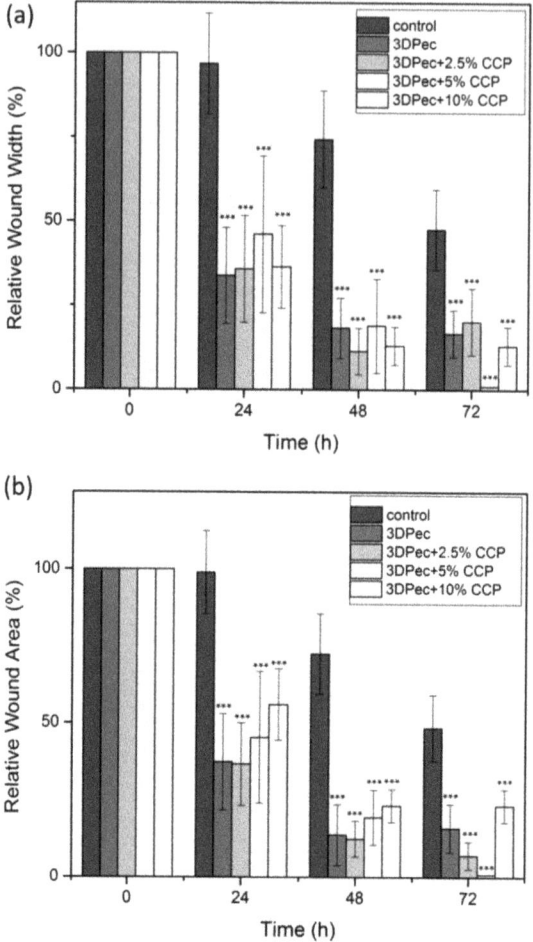

Figure 10. (a) Relative Wound Width and (b) Relative Wound Area calculated by the in vitro wound-healing assay for 3D-printed pectin films with: 0%, 2.5%, 5%, 10%, 20% and 30% w/w CCP, for 0.1 mg/mL of dissolved patches in the cell culture medium. *** $P < 0.05$ vs. control.

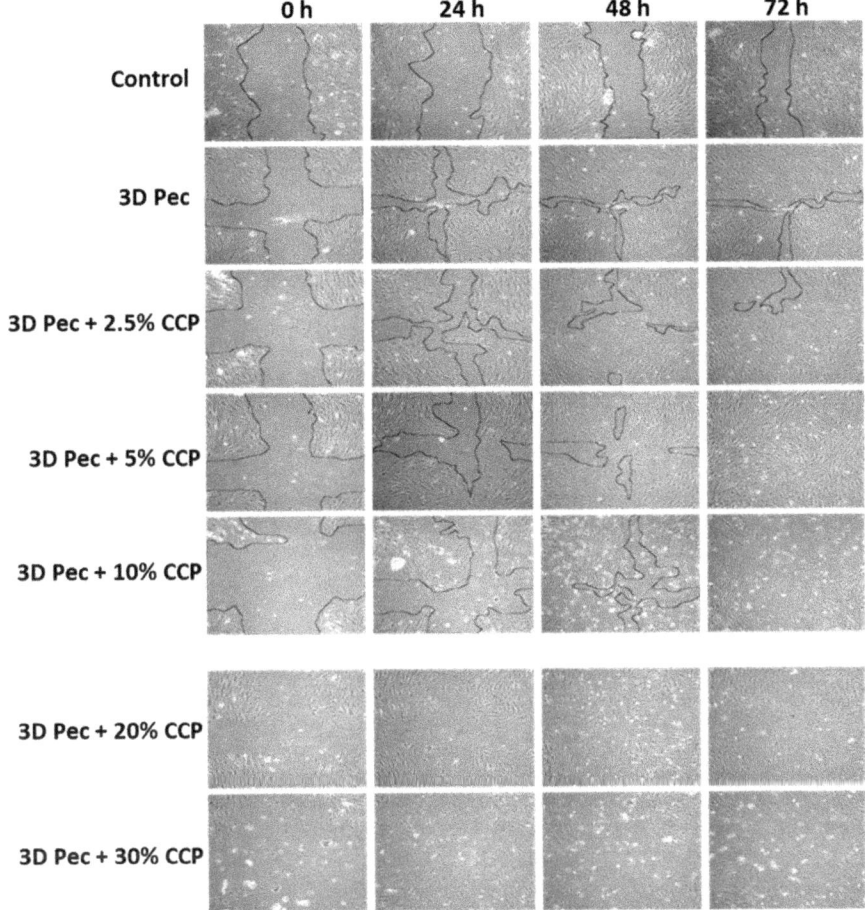

Figure 11. Time-lapse of in vitro wound healing process for 0.1 mg/mL of the dissolved patches in the cell culture medium (100× magnification).

4. Conclusions

Biodegradable, pectin-based 3D-printable inks have been developed as an efficient treatment approach for direct and indirect wound-dressing applications. The evaluation methodology followed in the current study rendered the inks suitable for 3D-printing applications. Free-standing transparent films that disintegrate upon contact with aqueous media were developed via 3D-bioprinting. The antimicrobial and wound-healing activities of the fabricated dressings were investigated and effectually enhanced by the incorporation of particles comprised of chitosan and cyclodextrin inclusion complexes with propolis extract.

Author Contributions: Conceptualization, E.G.A., G.K.E., C.K., and D.G.F.; methodology, E.G.A.; validation, E.G.A.; formal analysis, E.G.A.; investigation, E.G.A., G.K.E., C.K., and D.G.F.; resources, D.G.F.; writing—original draft preparation, E.G.A., and G.K.E.; writing—review and editing, E.G.A., G.K.E., C.K., and D.G.F.; visualization, E.G.A.; supervision, E.G.A., and D.G.F.; project administration, E.G.A., and D.G.F.; funding acquisition, D.G.F. All authors have read and agreed to the published version of the manuscript.

Funding: This research is carried out/funded in the context of the project "Development of bioactive patches for the treatment of acute and chronic ulcers and wounds using 3D printing technology" (MIS 5004712, '95347') under the call for proposals "Supporting researchers with emphasis on new researchers" (EDULLL 34). The project is co-financed by Greece and the European Union (European Social Fund-ESF) by the Operational Programme Human Resources Development, Education and Lifelong Learning 2014–2020.

Acknowledgments: The authors of this paper would like to express their gratitude to the Laboratory of Biochemistry, of the Department of Chemistry of the Aristotle University of Thessaloniki, for providing insights, expertise and assistance of great importance for the implementation of the antimicrobial assays and the cell studies.

Conflicts of Interest: The authors declare no conflict of interest.

References

1. Jantrawut, P.; Bunrueangtha, J.; Suerthong, J.; Kantrong, N. Fabrication and Characterization of Low Methoxyl Pectin/Gelatin/Carboxymethyl Cellulose Absorbent Hydrogel Film for Wound Dressing Applications. *Materials* **2019**, *12*, 1628. [CrossRef] [PubMed]
2. Paul, W.; Sharma, C.P. *Advances in Wound Healing Materials: Science and Skin Engineering*; Smithers Rapra Technology Ltd.: Shawbury, UK, 2015; ISBN 978-1-909030-36-7.
3. Rezvani Ghomi, E.; Khalili, S.; Nouri Khorasani, S.; Esmaeely Neisiany, R.; Ramakrishna, S. Wound dressings: Current advances and future directions. *J. Appl. Polym. Sci.* **2019**, *136*, 47738. [CrossRef]
4. Dhivya, S.; Padma, V.V.; Santhini, E. Wound dressings-a review. *BioMed* **2015**, *5*, 22. [CrossRef] [PubMed]
5. Kannon, G.A.; Garrett, A.B. Moist Wound Healing with Occlusive Dressings: A Clinical Review. *Dermatol. Surg.* **1995**, *21*, 583–590. [CrossRef]
6. Lanel, B.; Barthesbiesel, D.; Regnier, C.; Chauve, T. Swelling of hydrocolloid dressings. *Biorheology* **1997**, *34*, 139–153. [CrossRef]
7. Munarin, F.; Tanzi, M.C.; Petrini, P. Advances in biomedical applications of pectin gels. *Int. J. Biol. Macromol.* **2012**, *51*, 681–689. [CrossRef]
8. Giusto, G.; Vercelli, C.; Comino, F.; Caramello, V.; Tursi, M.; Gandini, M. A new, easy-to-make pectin-honey hydrogel enhances wound healing in rats. *BMC Complement. Altern. Med.* **2017**, *17*, 266. [CrossRef]
9. Minden-Birkenmaier, B.; Bowlin, G. Honey-Based Templates in Wound Healing and Tissue Engineering. *Bioengineering* **2018**, *5*, 46. [CrossRef]
10. Molan, P.; Rhodes, T. Honey: A Biologic Wound Dressing. *Wounds* **2015**, *27*, 141–151.
11. Martinotti, S.; Ranzato, E. Propolis: A new frontier for wound healing? *Burn. Trauma* **2015**, *3*, 9. [CrossRef]
12. Sameni, H.R.; Ramhormozi, P.; Bandegi, A.R.; Taherian, A.A.; Mirmohammadkhani, M.; Safari, M. Effects of ethanol extract of propolis on histopathological changes and anti-oxidant defense of kidney in a rat model for type 1 diabetes mellitus. *J. Diabetes Investig.* **2016**, *7*, 506–513. [CrossRef] [PubMed]
13. Sharaf, S.; El-Naggar, M.E. Wound dressing properties of cationized cotton fabric treated with carrageenan/cyclodextrin hydrogel loaded with honey bee propolis extract. *Int. J. Biol. Macromol.* **2019**, *133*, 583–591. [CrossRef] [PubMed]
14. Khaled, S.A.; Alexander, M.R.; Irvine, D.J.; Wildman, R.D.; Wallace, M.J.; Sharpe, S.; Yoo, J.; Roberts, C.J. Extrusion 3D Printing of Paracetamol Tablets from a Single Formulation with Tunable Release Profiles Through Control of Tablet Geometry. *AAPS PharmSciTech* **2018**, *19*, 3403–3413. [CrossRef] [PubMed]
15. Eleftheriadis, G.K.; Katsiotis, C.S.; Bouropoulos, N.; Koutsopoulos, S.; Fatouros, D.G. FDM printed pH-responsive capsules for the oral delivery of a model macromolecular dye. *Pharm. Dev. Technol.* **2020**, 1–23. [CrossRef]
16. Coimbra, P.; Ferreira, P.; de Sousa, H.C.; Batista, P.; Rodrigues, M.A.; Correia, I.J.; Gil, M.H. Preparation and chemical and biological characterization of a pectin/chitosan polyelectrolyte complex scaffold for possible bone tissue engineering applications. *Int. J. Biol. Macromol.* **2011**, *48*, 112–118. [CrossRef] [PubMed]
17. Katsube, T.; Tabata, H.; Ohta, Y.; Yamasaki, Y.; Anuurad, E.; Shiwaku, K.; Yamane, Y. Screening for Antioxidant Activity in Edible Plant Products: Comparison of Low-Density Lipoprotein Oxidation Assay, DPPH Radical Scavenging Assay, and Folin-Ciocalteu Assay. *J. Agric. Food Chem.* **2004**, *52*, 2391–2396. [CrossRef]
18. Matsakidou, A.; Biliaderis, C.G.; Kiosseoglou, V. Preparation and characterization of composite sodium caseinate edible films incorporating naturally emulsified oil bodies. *Food Hydrocoll.* **2013**, *30*, 232–240. [CrossRef]

19. Choi, W.S.; Han, J.H. Film-forming Mechanism and Heat Denaturation Effects on the Physical and Chemical Properties of Pea-Protein-Isolate Edible Films. *J. Food Sci.* **2002**, *67*, 1399–1406. [CrossRef]
20. Sezer, A.D.; Hatipoglu, F.; Cevher, E.; Oğurtan, Z.; Bas, A.L.; Akbuğa, J. Chitosan film containing fucoidan as a wound dressing for dermal burn healing: Preparation and in vitro/in vivo evaluation. *AAPS PharmSciTech* **2007**, *8*, E94–E101. [CrossRef]
21. Liu, L.; Kuffel, K.; Scott, D.K.; Constantinescu, G.; Chung, H.-J.; Rieger, J. Silicone-based adhesives for long-term skin application: Cleaning protocols and their effect on peel strength. *Biomed. Phys. Eng. Express* **2017**, *4*, 015004. [CrossRef]
22. Boateng, J.S.; Pawar, H.V.; Tetteh, J. Polyox and carrageenan based composite film dressing containing anti-microbial and anti-inflammatory drugs for effective wound healing. *Int. J. Pharm.* **2013**, *441*, 181–191. [CrossRef] [PubMed]
23. Zhang, Z.; Zhang, S.; Su, R.; Xiong, D.; Feng, W.; Chen, J. Controlled Release Mechanism and Antibacterial Effect of Layer-By-Layer Self-Assembly Thyme Oil Microcapsule. *J. Food Sci.* **2019**, *84*, 1427–1438. [CrossRef] [PubMed]
24. Zhang, C.; Li, Y.; Hu, Y.; Peng, Y.; Ahmad, Z.; Li, J.-S.; Chang, M.-W. Porous Yolk-Shell Particle Engineering via Nonsolvent-Assisted Trineedle Coaxial Electrospraying for Burn-Related Wound Healing. *ACS Appl. Mater. Interfaces* **2019**, *11*, 7823–7835. [CrossRef] [PubMed]
25. Mosmann, T. Rapid colorimetric assay for cellular growth and survival: Application to proliferation and cytotoxicity assays. *J. Immunol. Methods* **1983**, *65*, 55–63. [CrossRef]
26. Spanakis, M.; Bouropoulos, N.; Theodoropoulos, D.; Sygellou, L.; Ewart, S.; Moschovi, A.M.; Siokou, A.; Niopas, I.; Kachrimanis, K.; Nikolakis, V.; et al. Controlled release of 5-fluorouracil from microporous zeolites. *Nanomed. Nanotechnol. Biol. Med.* **2014**, *10*, 197–205. [CrossRef]
27. Boateng, J.S.; Matthews, K.H.; Stevens, H.N.E.; Eccleston, G.M. Wound Healing Dressings and Drug Delivery Systems: A Review. *J. Pharm. Sci.* **2008**, *97*, 2892–2923. [CrossRef]
28. Mohamad, N.; Mohd Amin, M.C.I.; Pandey, M.; Ahmad, N.; Rajab, N.F. Bacterial cellulose/acrylic acid hydrogel synthesized via electron beam irradiation: Accelerated burn wound healing in an animal model. *Carbohydr. Polym.* **2014**, *114*, 312–320. [CrossRef]
29. Prateepchanachai, S.; Thakhiew, W.; Devahastin, S.; Soponronnarit, S. Mechanical properties improvement of chitosan films via the use of plasticizer, charge modifying agent and film solution homogenization. *Carbohydr. Polym.* **2017**, *174*, 253–261. [CrossRef]
30. Mengoni, T.; Adrian, M.; Pereira, S.; Santos-Carballal, B.; Kaiser, M.; Goycoolea, F. A Chitosan—Based Liposome Formulation Enhances the In Vitro Wound Healing Efficacy of Substance P Neuropeptide. *Pharmaceutics* **2017**, *9*, 56. [CrossRef]
31. Eleftheriadis, G.K.; Ritzoulis, C.; Bouropoulos, N.; Tzetzis, D.; Andreadis, D.A.; Boetker, J.; Rantanen, J.; Fatouros, D.G. Unidirectional drug release from 3D printed mucoadhesive buccal films using FDM technology: In vitro and ex vivo evaluation. *Eur. J. Pharm. Biopharm.* **2019**, *144*, 180–192. [CrossRef]

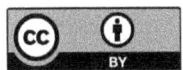

© 2020 by the authors. Licensee MDPI, Basel, Switzerland. This article is an open access article distributed under the terms and conditions of the Creative Commons Attribution (CC BY) license (http://creativecommons.org/licenses/by/4.0/).

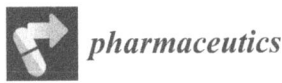

Article

Additive Manufacturing of Personalized Pharmaceutical Dosage Forms via Stereolithography

Andrew V. Healy [1], Evert Fuenmayor [1], Patrick Doran [2], Luke M. Geever [1], Clement L. Higginbotham [1] and John G. Lyons [3,*]

1. Materials Research Institute, Athlone Institute of Technology, Dublin Road, Athlone, Co., Westmeath N37 HD68, Ireland; andrewhealy@research.ait.ie (A.V.H.); e.fuenmayor@research.ait.ie (E.F.); lgeever@ait.ie (L.M.G.); chigginbotham@ait.ie (C.L.H.)
2. Applied Polymer Technologies Gateway, Athlone Institute of Technology, Dublin Road, Athlone, Co., Westmeath N37 HD68, Ireland; patrickdoran@ait.ie
3. Faculty of Engineering and Informatics, Athlone Institute of Technology, Dublin Road, Athlone, Co., Westmeath N37 HD68, Ireland
* Correspondence: slyons@ait.ie; Tel.: +353-(0)90-64-68150

Received: 18 October 2019; Accepted: 28 November 2019; Published: 3 December 2019

Abstract: The introduction of three-dimensional printing (3DP) has created exciting possibilities for the fabrication of dosage forms, paving the way for personalized medicine. In this study, oral dosage forms of two drug concentrations, namely 2.50% and 5.00%, were fabricated via stereolithography (SLA) using a novel photopolymerizable resin formulation based on a monomer mixture that, to date, has not been reported in the literature, with paracetamol and aspirin selected as model drugs. In order to produce the dosage forms, the ratio of poly(ethylene glycol) diacrylate (PEGDA) to poly(caprolactone) triol was varied with diphenyl(2,4,6-trimethylbenzoyl)phosphine oxide (Irgacure TPO) utilized as the photoinitiator. The fabrication of 28 dosages in one print process was possible and the printed dosage forms were characterized for their drug release properties. It was established that both drugs displayed a sustained release over a 24-h period. The physical properties were also investigated, illustrating that SLA affords accurate printing of dosages with some statistically significant differences observed from the targeted dimensional range, indicating an area for future process improvement. The work presented in this paper demonstrates that SLA has the ability to produce small, individualized batches which may be tailored to meet patients' specific needs or provide for the localized production of pharmaceutical dosage forms.

Keywords: stereolithography; three-dimensional printing; additive manufacturing; personalized medicine; 3D printed oral dosage forms; drug delivery; sustained drug release tablets; photopolymerization; paracetamol (acetaminophen); aspirin (acetylsalicylic acid)

1. Introduction

Three-dimensional printing (3DP) is an additive manufacturing (AM) process which involves the fabrication of an object or structure from a digital form by the deposition or binding of materials layer-by-layer [1–4]. Over the last few decades, 3DP has received extraordinary attention, particularly for its use within both the biomedical and pharmaceutical sectors. The introduction of 3DP has led to a potential shift in the way in which drug dosage forms may be manufactured. Further, with an ever-ageing population and the growing understanding of pharmacogenomics, there is an increased requirement for personalized medicine to be optimized. 3DP can facilitate the fabrication of dosage forms of complex geometries [5–7] with immediate [8–12] or modified [8,9,11,12] drug release profiles, some of which may contain multiple drugs [9,13–15]. These characteristics allow greater flexibility in the manufacturing of dosage forms, which would not otherwise be possible utilizing conventional manufacturing technologies [16,17], thus permitting the change from the current "one size fits all" approach [18]. This may revolutionize the production of personalized medicines [19,20] which will be of particular benefit in the treatment of patients who are known to have a pharmacogenetic polymorphism or are currently being treated with drugs which have narrow therapeutic indices [21].

Currently, there are numerous AM technologies available on the market, such as stereolithography (SLA), fused filament fabrication (FFF), and selective laser sintering (SLS) among others, many of which have been explored as potential fabrication approaches for drug delivery. For example, SLA has been investigated by Martinez and researchers [22] who examined the ability SLA offers in the fabrication of controlled release dosage forms and found that by modifying the water content in the formulation it was possible to alter the rate at which the drug was released. In a follow up study, Martinez et al. [6] explored the effect of geometry on drug release from dosage forms with their results indicating that out of all the geometric parameters examined the surface area to volume ratio had the greatest impact regarding drug release kinetics. Meanwhile, Fuenmayor and co-workers [23] evaluated the considerations that material choice plays in the FFF of dosage forms. Further to this, they compared FFF to direct compression (DC) and found that the manufacturing method utilized determined the drug release properties with FFF dosage forms taking considerably longer to release the active drug than that of DC, demonstrating the potential FFF has to offer for extended/modified release applications. In addition to this, Fuenmayor et al. [12] further compared FFF to two alternative manufacturing techniques, DC and injection molding, to conclude that through the manipulation of the printing parameters it was possible to alter the drug release characteristics, which would not be possible in the other two techniques they explored. Furthermore, Fina et al. [8] conducted a study to evaluate if the alternative AM technique SLS could potentially be exploited in the fabrication of oral dosage forms using pharmaceutical grade excipients. From their study, the authors [8] deduced that SLS has the capacity to yield personalized dosage forms and with careful selection of excipients it is possible to fabricate dosage forms of either immediate-release or modified-release. In addition to this study, Fina and researchers [10] built on their knowledge of the SLS process by fabricating orally disintegrating dosage forms that had increased drug release properties which were dictated by an adjustment of the printing parameters with accelerated release observed in a faster laser scanning speed, illustrating that the manipulation of printing parameters is not just limited to the FFF technique. All of the aforementioned studies and AM techniques employed highlight the current possibilities available to be exploited in both the area of drug delivery and personalized medicine.

However, the most remarkable use of 3DP in drug delivery to date is the first U.S. Food and Drug Administration (FDA) approved 3D printed medicine, Spritam® (levetiracetam), which is a rapidly disintegrating oral medicine [3,24]. The innovative technology employees a powder-based method of 3DP allowing dosage forms to be fabricated in various strengths, namely 250, 500, 750, and 1000 mg, [25] illustrating the potential benefits that it offers in terms of drug delivery with the possibility of manufacturing bespoke drug formulations which may be dependent on the patient's specific needs, further proving that it may offer the flexibility to prepare small batch sizes of personalized dosage forms [15,26,27].

The purpose of this study was to evaluate the possibility of fabricating drug dosage forms utilizing the AM technique of stereolithography. The stereolithography process was successful in the fabrication of the tablets with the tablets being characterized by a variety of testing procedures. Fourier transform infrared (FTIR) spectroscopic analysis was used to determine the chemical structure of the printed dosages and also evaluate the extent of the reaction, while thermal characterization assessed if the active drug was dissolved within the photopolymer solution. Furthermore, the tablets were analyzed for their dimensional accuracy, weight variation, and drug release kinetics with paracetamol and aspirin being selected as the model drugs for the study. Scanning electron microscopy (SEM) was also utilized to investigate the structure of the tablets.

2. Materials and Methods

2.1. Materials

Poly(ethylene glycol) diacrylate (PEGDA, average M_w 700, Batch number: MKBW9043V), paracetamol (acetaminophen, Batch number: MKCD6375), aspirin (acetylsalicylic acid, Batch number: SLBV2290), methanol and 2-propanol were purchased from Sigma Aldrich, Wicklow, Ireland). Poly(caprolactone) Triol, (PCL Triol), Capa™ 3031 (average M_w 300, Lot number: WBY 000428) was received as a gift from Perstorp UK Ltd., Cheshire, UK. Diphenyl(2,4,6-trimethylbenzoyl)phosphine oxide (Irgacure TPO, Batch number: 50019766) was also received as a gift from BASF, (Ludwigshafen, Germany). All salts required in the preparation of the dissolution media were also procured from Sigma Aldrich (Wicklow, Ireland). All materials were used as received unless otherwise stated.

2.2. Stereolithography

2.2.1. Preparation of Photopolymer Formulations

The photopolymer formulations were prepared as outlined in Table 1. The PEGDA and PCL Triol were added together and mixed for a duration of 2 h, after which the photoinitiator, Irgacure TPO, was added at a concentration of 1.00% (w/w). The solution was mixed thoroughly for a duration of 8 h to ensure that the photoinitiator had completely dissolved. Paracetamol or aspirin was then added to the solution at a concentration of 2.50% (w/w) or 5.00% (w/w) as shown in Table 1 with the solution constantly mixed until complete dissolution of the drug. All mixing of solutions was carried out using a magnetic stirrer and mixed at room temperature. In addition to this, all formulations were protected from light at all stages of production, mixing, and storage by the use of amber Duran bottles. Prior to printing, the prepared respective photopolymer solution was loaded into the printing tray.

Table 1. Composition of SLA formulations prepared.

SLA Formulation [1]	PEGDA [2]	PCL Triol [3]	Irgacure TPO [4]	Paracetamol	Aspirin
	% (w/w)				
2.50% Para	19.30	77.20	1.00	2.50	-
5.00% Para	18.80	75.20	1.00	5.00	-
2.50% Asp	19.30	77.20	1.00	-	2.50
5.00% Asp	18.80	75.20	1.00	-	5.00

[1] Stereolithography, [2] Poly(ethylene glycol) diacrylate, [3] Poly(caprolactone) Triol, [4] Diphenyl(2,4,6-trimethylbenzoyl)phosphine oxide.

2.2.2. Stereolithographic Printing

All stereolithographic printing was conducted by utilization of a Formlabs Form 2 SLA 3D printer (Formlabs Inc., Somerville, MA, USA) which is equipped with 405 nm wavelength light source. The SLA printer has the capabilities of fabricating objects with a resolution that allows for a layer thickness of 25, 50, or 100 μm. The design for the 3D printed oral dosage form Figure 1 was designed in SolidWorks 2017 (Dassault Systèmes, Waltham, MA, USA) and exported as a stereolithography file (STL) to the 3D printer software (PreForm Software version 2.15.1). In order to print using the formulated photopolymer resin, "Open Mode" was enabled on the printer, which deactivates the dispensing of resin and the resin heating and wiping capabilities.

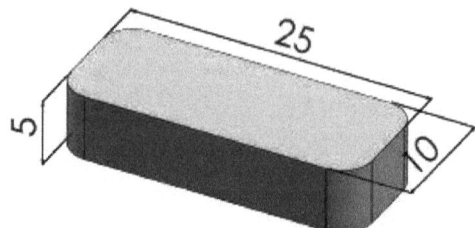

Figure 1. Computer-aided design (CAD) of the printed oral dosage form (length 25.00 mm, width 10.00 mm, height 5.00 mm).

2.3. Spectroscopic Analysis of Photoinitiator

2.3.1. UV/Vis Spectrophotometry

The UV/Vis spectra of the photoinitiator, Irgacure TPO was measured on a UV/Vis spectrophotometer (Shimadzu UV-1280, Milton Keynes, UK). The spectra were recorded for three different concentrations of the photoinitiator, 0.10%, 0.50%, and 1.00%, in two different solvents, methanol and 2-propanol, by conducting a wavelength scan ranging from 450–325 nm with the spectrophotometer being blanked with the respective solvent prior to the analysis being conducted.

2.3.2. Fourier Transform Infrared Spectrometry

Fourier transform infrared (FTIR) spectroscopy was carried out by the utilization of a Spectrum One FTIR spectrometer (Perkin Elmer, Dublin, Ireland) which incorporates a universal Attenuated Total Reflectance (ATR) sampling accessory. All data was recorded at ambient temperature, in the spectral range 4000–650 cm^{-1}, utilizing 16 scans per cycle at 4 cm^{-1} resolution and a fixed compression force of 80 N. Subsequent analysis was carried out on the Spectrum software.

2.4. Thermal Characterization

The printed dosage forms were characterized by the utilization of differential scanning calorimetry (DSC), DSC 2920 Differential Scanning Calorimeter (TA Instruments). Samples of between 6.0–8.0 mg were weighed out using a Sartorius analytical balance with a resolution of 1×10^{-5} g and placed in non-hermetic aluminum pans, which were crimped prior to testing with an empty crimped aluminum pan being used as the reference pan. Calorimetry scans were carried out by heating each sample at a rate of 10 °C/min from −20 °C to 200 °C.

However, for the thermal characterization of paracetamol, the second heating cycle was also evaluated in order to ascertain what polymorph the paracetamol existed in.

All DSC scans were carried out under a 30 mL/min flow of nitrogen. Prior to conducting the characterization, the DSC was calibrated using indium as standard.

2.5. Tablet Characterization

In order to evaluate the dimensional accuracy that the SLA printing process affords printed dosage forms ($n = 10$) were measured for their length, width and height using digital calipers with Figure 1 showing the anticipated measurements that should be obtained from the printed dosage form. A two-way ANOVA was used to analyze the variance between tablet dimensions with the Dunnett's multiple comparisons test used determine the significant difference between expected dimensions and printed dosage forms with differences being considered significant when $p \leq 0.05$. Furthermore, the printed dosage forms were analyzed for their uniformity of weight to evaluate the consistency of the printing process with ten tablets taken and measured on a Sartorius analytical balance with a resolution of 1×10^{-5} g.

2.6. Dissolution Analysis

Drug dissolution profiles for the printed dosage forms were obtained by utilization of a Distek dissolution system 2100B with a Distek temperature control system TCS 0200B (Distek Inc., North Brunswick, NJ, USA) according to USP dissolution apparatus I. The dosage forms were investigated in 0.2 M hydrochloric acid, pH 1.2 with 900 mL of media used per vessel. All testing was conducted at 37 ± 0.5 °C with the stir rate being 50 RPM. At pre-determined time intervals, 5 mL was withdrawn from each vessel and replaced with pre-heated dissolution media. The withdrawn samples were filtered through 0.45 µm filters with drug release being determined at 243.2 nm for paracetamol and 233.2 nm for aspirin by performing UV spectroscopy on a Shimadzu UV-1280 UV-VIS spectrophotometer (Shimadzu, Milton Keynes, UK). Drug dissolution studies were conducted in sextuplicate with the average percentage of drug release as a function of time being determined. A two-way ANOVA with multiple comparisons among subgroups was performed using a Bonferroni post-hoc test to differentiate drug release curves with differences being considered significant when $p \leq 0.05$.

2.7. Scanning Electron Microscopy

Surface and cross-section images at a range of magnifications of the printed dosage forms were taken by with a Mira SEM (Tescan, Oxford Instruments, Cambridge, UK). The samples were placed on aluminum stubs using double-sided conductive carbon tape which were then sputter-coated with gold using an SCD 005 sputter coater (Bal-Tec, Balzers, Liechtenstein) for 110 s at 0.1 mBar vacuum prior to observation. All images were generated using an accelerating voltage of 20 kV and were recorded at magnifications of 300, 500 and 1000×.

2.8. Statistical Analysis

Data handling and analysis were performed using GraphPad Prism (GraphPad Prism version 8.0.1 for Windows, GraphPad Software, San Diego, CA, USA). All test data was inputted into the software with the mean and standard deviations calculated for the replicate data sets. All data were assessed for normality of distribution after which the relevant statistical analysis was performed with differences being considered significant when $p \leq 0.05$. All data in figures are presented as mean with error bars representing standard deviation unless otherwise stated.

3. Results and Discussion

3.1. Stereolithographic Printing Process

The dosage forms in this study were fabricated utilizing the AM technique of SLA. SLA is a method in which objects may be fabricated or produced by using focused ultraviolet (UV) light and photocurable materials to produce solid 3D forms due to a photopolymerization reaction occurring. Photopolymerization is the use of light in order to initiate a polymerization reaction, thus resulting in the conversion of a liquid monomer to a solid polymer through a chemical reaction taking place [28]. The polymerization reaction is initiated by the addition of light-sensitive compounds called photoinitiators, which become active under the appropriate wavelengths, creating free radicals due to the conversion of the absorbed light energy [29]. These free radicals are then consumed in the reaction converting the liquid monomer into a solid-state, which may be referred to as a crosslinked hydrogel [28,29]. The photoinitiator used within this study is Irgacure TPO, a Norrish Type 1, photoinitiator which is a single-molecule and undergoes photocleavage into radical fragments when exposed to light from an appropriate wavelength as illustrated in Figure 2 [30,31].

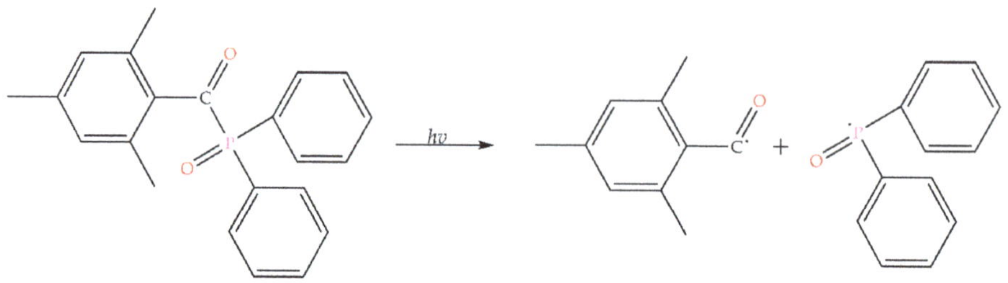

Figure 2. Norrish Type 1 photocleavage of Irgacure TPO.

In order to fabricate the drug dosage forms, it was necessary to prepare the photopolymer solutions to be loaded into the SLA 3D printer which was carried out by altering the ratio of PCL Triol to PEGDA in the formulation with the ratios being chosen based on previous experimentation work in our lab and on the rheological profiling of existing formulations.

PCL Triol is a biodegradable, semi-crystalline, aliphatic polyester, with low molecular weight and melting point which has been investigated to a great extent as a biomaterial as well as in drug delivery applications [32–34]. One reason for this is the degradation products of PCL being naturally occurring metabolites in the human body with sutures composed of PCL being approved by the US Food and Drug Administration (FDA) [35]. Further to this, low molecular weight PCL Triols have been investigated for their potential to act as plasticizers [33,36,37] with Kanis et al. [34] indicating that it is the three hydroxyl groups present which allow it to act as a plasticizer. Furthermore, PCL Triols due to their nature do not possess photopolymerizable terminal groups and therefore cannot crosslink on their own which is why PCL derivatives have been developed [38–40]. Like PCL Triol, poly(ethylene glycol) (PEG) itself cannot crosslink [41] and has also been investigated for use as a plasticizer [42,43] and in drug delivery applications [11,44–46]. Martinez et al. [22] conducted a study in which they added PEG 300 to the resin formulation and due to its inability to crosslink it would allow for a reduction in the intermolecular forces between the polymer chains, resulting in greater drug release.

Poly(ethylene glycol) (PEG) is a well-established synthetic polymeric material with PEG based hydrogels being well documented within the literature [29,47–50] owing to the exceptional properties they afford, such as being nontoxic, biocompatible, and having notable tunability, in addition to being approved by the FDA for use in a variety clinical uses [51,52]. PEGDA has been shown to be a beneficial polymer in drug delivery applications and was investigated by McAvoy et al. [53] to evaluate its potential to fabricate implants via UV polymerization in the release of both small and large drug molecules with the former being released at a greater rate than that of the latter. This indicates that by the careful selection of drugs it may be feasible to manipulate and control the rate at which they are released from the fabricated dosage form.

The model drugs, paracetamol and aspirin, were found to easily dissolve in their respective photopolymer solutions with the colors of both solutions being clear and the 3DP dosage forms displaying the same color as in Figure 3a,b. Although the concentrations of the model drugs were low the authors selected these concentrations based on previously published contributions with Goyanes et al. [20] fabricating topical drug delivery systems with the incorporation of 2.00% w/w salicylic acid the primary metabolite of aspirin. In addition to this, Wang et al. [41] and Martinez et al. [6] both fabricated dosage forms with the loading of paracetamol being 5.90% w/w and 4.00% w/w respectively. While the concentrations utilized do not have immediate clinical relevance, the formulations are intended to demonstrate the capability of the AM technique for bespoke batch production within a clinical setting. Despite this, the authors do believe that drug concentration could be increased, with Martinez et al. [54] incorporating 10.00% w/w of both model drugs used in this study, in addition to four other model drugs, to fabricate a multi-layered polypill via SLA. However, the effect on the increased drug concentration and thus decreased polymer concentration would need to be tested in order to identify how it would affect the printing process, curing process and drug release mechanism. Paracetamol and aspirin were identified as model drugs for this work, in part because of the difference in pKa values, 9.5 and 3.5 respectively [55,56], of the two active ingredients. A rectangular shape was selected as the geometry to be printed, as shown in Figure 3. However, 3DP has the capabilities of fabricating dosage forms of varied and complex shapes which has been demonstrated by Martinez et al. [6] who evaluated the role that geometry plays in drug release from printed dosage forms.

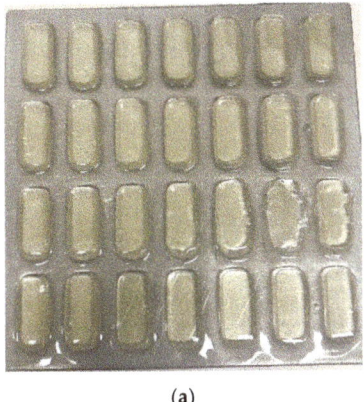
(a)

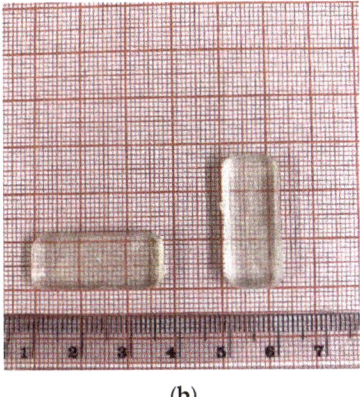
(b)

Figure 3. (a) Complete batch of printed dosage forms fabricated via SLA 3D printing ($n = 28$) (b) single dosage form.

As can be observed in Figure 3a, it was possible to fabricate 28 tablets in one single print illustrating the potential the 3DP affords in the area of personalized medicine specifically if the patient requires one dosage per day meaning that it is possible to fabricate a month's supply in one print. This finding has the possibility to revolutionize how pharmaceuticals are fabricated, and in particular when developing drug delivery methods for the treatment of rare diseases, as there is little to no waste from the printing process. Furthermore, through the manipulation of the dimensional design parameters of the dosage form, it may also be feasible to fabricate an amount greater than what was achieved in this study, 28 dosage forms, which would be advantageous if the patient was required to take more than one dose per day.

3.2. Spectroscopic Analysis of Photoinitiator

This study utilized Irgacure TPO which is a highly efficient photoinitiator that is used in the initiation of free radical polymerization [57] with McDermott et al. [58] reporting that it absorbs radiation in the region of 420–340 nm, making it ideal for use in the SLA process as the wavelength utilized by the SLA printer is 405 nm, as reported by Dizon et al. [59]. The UV/Vis spectra of the photoinitiator Irgacure TPO was measured at three different concentrations, namely 0.10%, 0.50%, and 1.00%, and in two different solvents, 2-propanol and methanol, to establish if the photoinitiator has the capabilities of absorbing in the operating range of the SLA printer. As can be observed in the spectra, as shown in Figure 4a,b, all three concentrations in both solvents absorb in the desired range, 405 nm. In both solvents, the TPO at a concentration of 0.10% showed a rather low absorption at 405 nm when compared to the other two concentrations, 0.50% and 1.00%. Furthermore, Arikawa et al. [60] evaluated a number of photoinitiators and light curing units and concluded that both TPO and the violet-LED light was the most optimum in the polymerization of a mixture of bisphenol A-glycidyl methacrylate (Bis-GMA) and triethylene glycol dimethacrylate (TEGDMA).

Despite only a slight variance being apparent in the absorbance value between the concentrations, 0.50% and 1.00%, the latter concentration was selected for the study conducted. The rationale for selecting this concentration, 1.00%, is owing to the fact that if there is insufficient photoinitiator incorporated in the formulation this may result in surface cure problems. However, on the other hand, if too high a concentration is selected, high levels of surface crosslinking may occur which will prevent the UV light used in the printing process from effectively penetrating to the lower layers which may result in inadequate curing. Although the loading of 1.00% may seem high there are a number of publications in the literature utilizing higher concentrations. In a publication by Steyrer and researchers [61], they illustrated the possibility of using a concentration loading of 1.18 wt% of Omnirad TPO-L (Ethyl (2,4,6-trimethylbenzoyl) phenylphosphinate) in the fabrication of 3D printed part on a 405 nm Digital Light Processing (DLP) printer, and although it may not be the same process used in this study it does, however, rely on a similar technology using UV light to cure the photopolymer. In addition to this, a concentration in excess of what is proposed in this study was utilized by Asikainen et al. [62] in which they assessed lidocaine drug release from photo-crosslinkable PCL scaffolds fabricated by SLA technology.

However, the photoinitiator used in the studies by Steyrer and co-workers [61] and Asikainen and researchers [62] was an acylphosphine oxide derivative similar to that of Irgacure TPO used in this study. Furthermore, Bausch & Lomb Incorporated. filed a patent in 2010 utilizing a 1.50 wt.% of Lucirin TPO, now called Irgacure TPO, in the formulation of contact lenses [63]. In addition to this, Martinez et al. [6] also carried out a study, to explore the role that geometry plays in the release of drugs from printed tablets, using the same photoinitiator that is to be used within this study at a concentration of 2.00% *w/w*. Additionally, both the photoinitiator, Irgacure TPO, and SLA printer, Formlabs Form 2, used in this study were also exploited in a study by Duan et al. [64], albeit that the concentration of photoinitiator was higher in their study.

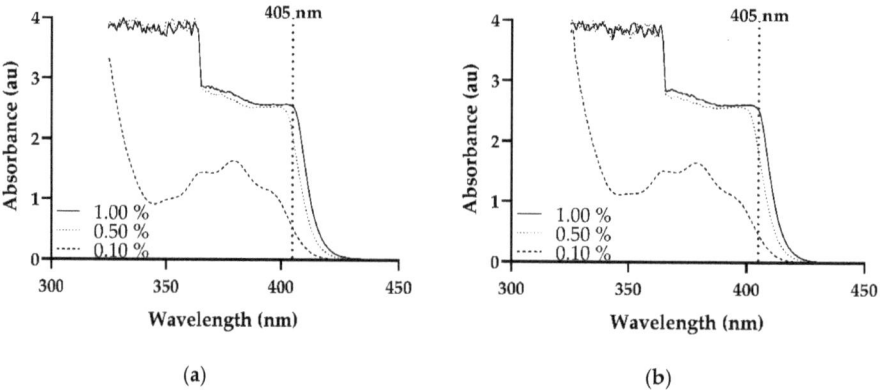

Figure 4. Absorbance spectra of photoinitiator at varying concentrations in (**a**) 2-propanol and (**b**) methanol.

3.3. Fourier Transform Infrared Spectroscopy

The printed dosage forms were characterized in order to evaluate the efficiency of the SLA printing process as the IR spectral changes that occurred during the photopolymerization process could be evaluated. This evaluation is possible as the alterations, peak shifts, which occur in the spectra are indicative that bonding has occurred between the individual constituents present in the photopolymer solution, therefore suggesting that crosslinking has occurred within the samples [57].

The double bond acrylate groups present at the end of the PEG chain in the PEGDA molecule is what gives rise for the polymer to undergo free radical polymerization in the presence of the TPO photoinitiator resulting in the fabrication of the dosage form. The UV light of the SLA printer activates the TPO, resulting in the TPO decomposing to generate two radicals, as previously shown in Figure 2. The free radicals are then available to react with the PEGDA monomer in the photopolymer solution resulting in the opening of the C=C bond present in the PEGDA monomer thus allowing a polymer network to be formed [65]. From conducting FTIR analysis of PEGDA (data not shown) the acrylate groups, C-H bending of the CH_2=CH–C=O and C–O–C stretching at 811 cm^{-1} and 1189 cm^{-1} respectively were identified with similar findings being reported elsewhere [66–68].

Figure 5a shows the results obtained from FTIR analysis of the paracetamol loaded dosage forms with the spectra for the aspirin samples being displayed in Figure 5b. The FTIR spectra of all printed samples, paracetamol and aspirin, were similar to one another, however, due to the higher ratio of PCL Triol present within the composition, there was over-saturation of the notable peaks of PCL Triol (data not shown) found in printed samples.

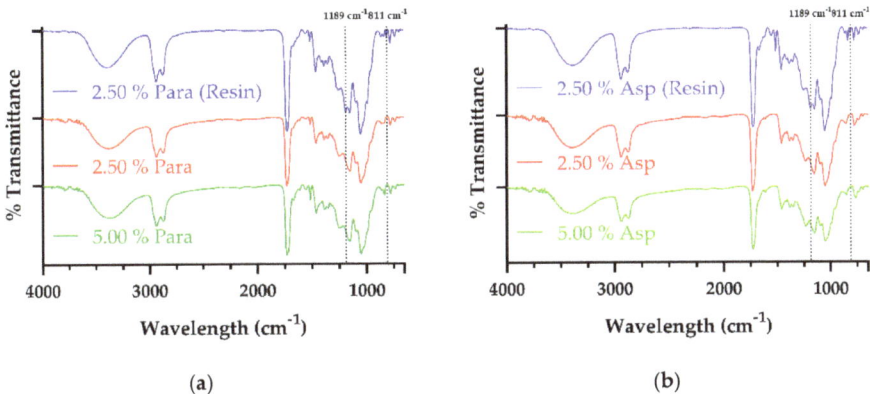

Figure 5. FTIR spectra of (a) 2.50% Para (Resin), 2.50% Para dosage form and 5.00% Para dosage form (b) 2.50% Asp (Resin), 2.50% Asp dosage form and 5.00% Asp dosage form.

As already stated, the higher ratio of PCL Triol within the photopolymer solution resulted in the spectra predominantly appearing as PCL Triol, with the broad peak ranging from 3394.19 to 3369.64 cm^{-1} in the samples being indicative of the free hydroxyl group (–OH) of the PCL Triol while the strong peak ranging from 1729.63 to 1726.05 cm^{-1} is characteristic of the stretching carbonyl (C=O) group of the molecule. It can also be observed that when both the 2.50% Para Resin and 2.50% Asp Resin is compared to their respective printed dosages there is the disappearance of peaks at 811 cm^{-1}, and 1189 cm^{-1} with similar findings being reported by Killion et al. [69] and Burke et al. [66,67] reporting that polymerization of a PEGDA derivative, PEGDMA, had occurred upon disappearance of the aforementioned peaks. This finding indicates that the SLA process undertaken within this study may be beneficial within the area of personalized medicine owing to its ability to cure the photopolymer solution and produce dosage forms of not only different active ingredients but also at different drug loading concentrations.

3.4. Thermal Characterization

The study of the thermal properties of the stereolithographic printed tablets and materials used in the fabrication of such tablets was evaluated by the utilization of DSC. Figure 6 shows the DSC thermograms of the materials used in the fabrication of the printed dosage forms. It can be observed that the photoinitiator, TPO, demonstrates a peak a melting peak around 92 °C, which corresponds to the melting point that is found in the materials technical data sheet [70]. The DSC of PEGDA displays an endotherm which is clearly identifiable at 14 °C, which is similar to what Martinez and researchers [22] found, establishing the melting point of PEGDA to be ca. 10 °C from the research that they conducted.

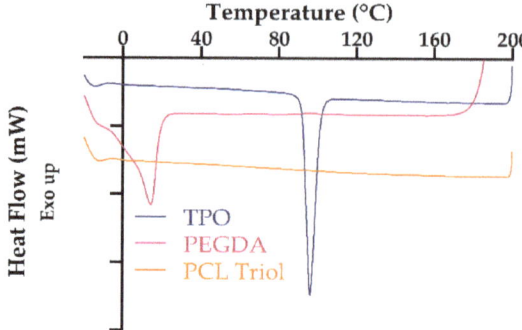

Figure 6. Overlaid DSC thermograms of starting materials.

Figure 7 displays the DSC thermograms for paracetamol (first and second heat cycles) and the two printed dosage forms which contain paracetamol. The DSC for paracetamol, (a) first heat cycle, shows a sharp endothermic peak at 169 °C with this melting point being in agreement with that which is found in the literature [5,71]. Furthermore, this melting point is indicative of paracetamol existing in its most stable form, that being the commercially marketed version, Form I (monoclinic) [72,73]. This is further confirmed upon observing the second heat cycle (b) as the melting point has shifted to a lower temperature of 159 °C with Sacchetti [72] noting similar results. Also, when the two heat cycles are compared, there is no cold crystallization peak noted in the first heat cycle, thus indicating that the paracetamol is present in its 100% crystalline form. However, upon observing the second heat cycle, it is apparent that the drug is 100% amorphous (Form II) with a glass transition temperature at 24 °C, with this finding been consistent with that of the literature [73,74]. Furthermore, the broad exothermal peak between 75 and 100 °C, with peak maxima around 80 °C, is typical of cold crystallization occurring with Rengarajan and Beiner [73] reporting results to support this. In addition to this, Rengarajan and Beiner [73] also indicate that the Form II crystals melt at 157 °C with the results of this study finding the onset to be at 155 °C with a maximum melt peak at 159 °C, which according to the literature the melting temperature ranges from 154 to 160 °C which is characteristic of Form II, orthorhombic paracetamol [71].

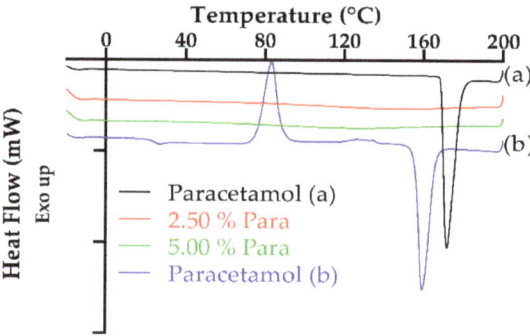

Figure 7. Overlaid DSC thermograms of paracetamol and printed paracetamol dosage forms. (**a**) first heat cycle, (**b**) second heat cycle.

The overlaid DSC thermograms of aspirin and printed dosage forms containing aspirin can be observed in Figure 8. The DSC for aspirin shows two melt peaks with the first endothermic peak being sharp and present at 144 °C (onset temperature 137 °C) with similar results being reported in the literature [75–77]. However, the second endotherm was noted at 179 °C (onset temperature 177 °C) may be attributed to the degradation of aspirin. There are various publications within the literature, [78–80], indicating that thermal degradation/decomposition of aspirin occurs in two processes with the first process ranging from 160 to 260 °C. Furthermore, thermogravimetric analysis (TGA) studies conducted by Al-Maydama et al. [81] and de A. Silva et al. [82] deduced that the temperature of maximum degradation (T_{DTG}) of aspirin occurred around 181 °C with further DSC studies conducted by de A. Silva et al. [82] confirming this result.

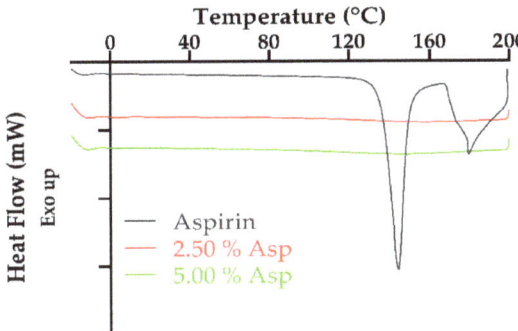

Figure 8. Overlaid DSC thermograms of aspirin and printed aspirin dosage forms.

As can be observed in both Figures 7 and 8, there was no endotherm observed for the dosages which contained either drug, paracetamol or aspirin, and either concentration, 2.50% or 5.00%, which is indicative of the active drug being entirely dissolved within the photopolymer solution. Similar results illustrating drug dissolution in the SLA photopolymer solution have been established with a number of publications [20,22,62] citing comparable findings.

3.5. Tablet Characterization

In order to evaluate the effectiveness of SLA as a suitable means of fabricating tablets to be utilized in the area of personalized medicine, both the dimensional accuracy of the printing process and uniformity of tablet weight were evaluated. The tablets were fabricated with a high degree of repeatability with respect to their physical dimensions and this was apparent due to the paracetamol and aspirin printed dosage forms producing results close to target dimensions: Length 25.00 mm, width 10.00 mm, and height 5.00 mm, as shown in Figure 9 and Table 2. However, some statistically significant differences were observed when the printed tablets were compared to that of their target dimensions. It was found that the 2.50% Para dosage forms displayed significant differences ($p < 0.05$) in both their length and width when compared to that of their target dimensions. In addition to this, significant differences ($p < 0.0001$) in both length and width were also observed for both the 2.50% Asp and 5.00% Asp dosage forms. Furthermore, there were no significant differences ($p > 0.05$) noted for the 5.00% Para dosage forms in their length and width when compared to that of the target dimension as well as no significant differences ($p > 0.05$) observed for any of the printed dosage forms irrespective of drug or drug loading in regard to the height of the fabricated dosage forms when compared to the expected dimension. The findings presented here are representative of what has previously been outlined in the literature. In two separate studies by Martinez et al. [22,54], the authors assessed the dimensional accuracy of SLA printing as a means of fabricating dosage forms for drug delivery and concluded it was achievable to produce prints with good uniformity in physical dimensions.

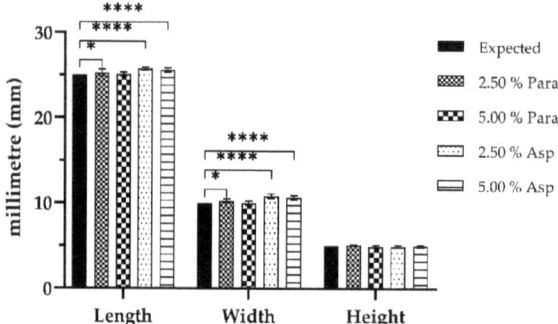

Figure 9. Dimensional analyses values of the paracetamol and aspirin printed dosage forms ($n = 10$, expected values; length 25.00 mm, width 10.00 mm, height 5.00 mm, * = $p < 0.05$, **** = $p < 0.0001$).

Table 2. Measured parameters of paracetamol and aspirin dosage forms ($n = 10$, expected values; length 25.00 mm, width 10.00 mm, height 5.00 mm).

SLA Formulation	Length (mm)	Width (mm)	Height (mm)
2.50% Para	25.26 ± 0.40	10.27 ± 0.20	5.12 ± 0.10
5.00% Para	25.05 ± 0.26	10.00 ± 0.27	4.96 ± 0.15
2.50% Asp	25.72 ± 0.18	10.85 ± 0.26	4.97 ± 0.11
5.00% Asp	25.58 ± 0.26	10.64 ± 0.25	5.00 ± 0.12

Further to the dimensional analysis being conducted, weight uniformity among the printed tablets was also evaluated with the results presented in Figure 10. Although the absolute weights of the two paracetamol formulations vary slightly from one another, all printed tablet weights ranged from 1324 to 1467 mg with no statistically significant difference ($p > 0.05$) between the two formulations regarding tablet weight observed. However, it was found that the absolute weights of the two aspirin formulations did exhibit some variation, with the printed tablet weights ranging from 1566 to 1918 mg and the differences in tablet weight being significant ($p < 0.002$).

In addition to comparing the printed dosage forms containing the same drugs, the tablets containing the same drug loadings, 2.50% or 5.00%, were also evaluated with respect to uniformity of weight. The printed dosage forms which contained a drug loading of 2.50% showed a significant difference in weight ($p < 0.0001$). Similarly, when the drug loading was 5.00% in the printed tablets they also showed a significant difference ($p < 0.0001$).

Overall, the weight uniformity of all the printed tablets, paracetamol and aspirin, ranges from a lower range of 1324 mg (paracetamol) to an upper range of 1918 mg (aspirin) with significant differences between some tablets being shown as previously outlined with the exception of significant differences between 2.50% Para and 5.00% Para.

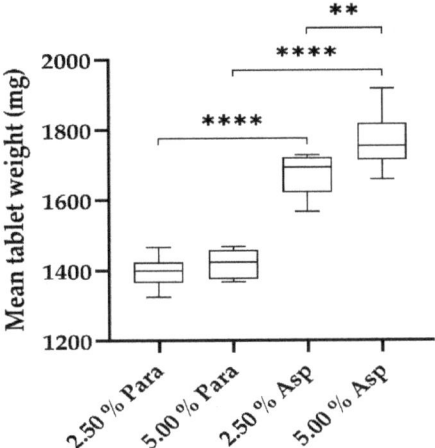

Figure 10. Weight uniformity of paracetamol and aspirin dosage forms ($n = 10$, ** $= p < 0.002$, **** $= p < 0.0001$).

These findings reported here of dimensional accuracy and weight uniformity as well as the observations reported in the literature [22,45,54,83–86] illustrate that AM and in particular the SLA process has the potential to be exploited in the fabrication of dosage forms for a variety of medical conditions. This is evident in the ability to print dosage forms comprised of various monomer(s)/photoinitiator(s)/drug concentrations and/or combinations of each which show excellent consistency in their dimensions with reference to the STL file that was imported into the software of the printer. Furthermore, the results obtained in this study indicate that it was feasible to fabricate a large batch of tablets in a single print, Figure 3a, with 28 dosage forms being produced. In addition to this finding, it should also be noted that a greater number of tablets could be attained through manipulation of the software which would be advantageous when treatment is required more than once per day.

3.6. Dissolution Analysis

Drug release studies were conducted for all of the printed dosage forms with the results shown in Figure 11. As can be observed both the paracetamol and aspirin loaded dosage forms exhibited sustained drug release which was maintained for the duration of the study, 24 h.

Looking at Figure 11, it can be observed that the printed paracetamol dosage forms displayed sustained release of the active drug over the 24 h testing period. It was found that the 2.50% Para exhibited a maximum release of 84.11% with the 5.00% loading achieving a release of 88.16% for the test duration. Over the test period it was found that upon comparison of the two different drug loadings there was statistical significance ($p < 0.0001$) up to the two hour time point after which no statistical significance ($p > 0.05$) was noted until the last and final time point, 24 h, ($p < 0.002$).

As with the paracetamol dosage forms, the aspirin dosage forms also exhibited a sustained rate of release from the 3DP matrices. However, there was a difference in the maximum release after 24 h with the 2.50% Asp having a maximum release rate of 95.85% after the 24 h period with the higher loading, 5.00% Asp, achieving a higher maximum release rate of 113.30% after the same time. However, although the 5.00% Asp dosage form released a greater amount of drug after 24 h, this is believed to have been due to the higher loading of the drug, and therefore less polymer within the polymer matrix. Furthermore, the rate at which aspirin was released from the printed dosage forms was not statistically significant ($p > 0.05$) for time points up to 4 h.

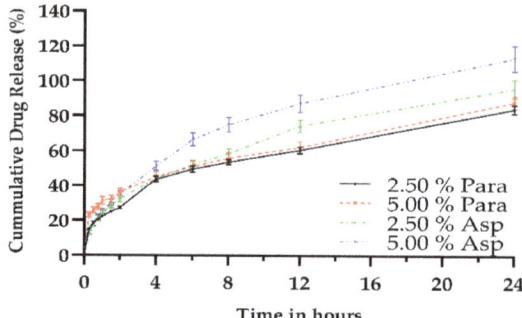

Figure 11. Drug release profiles of both paracetamol and aspirin printed dosage forms over a 24 h period in pH 1.2 ($n = 6$).

The results presented in this study differ from that reported by Wang and researchers [41] who describe that by altering the ratio of PEGDA to PEG it was possible to modulate drug release, of paracetamol and 4-amino salicylic acid, from the printed dosages with a low percentage of PEGDA (35%) showing faster release rates from that of their higher counterparts. The percentage of PEGDA which was utilized in this study was lower than what was used in the study by Wang et al. [41] with slower release rates been observed with a lower PEGDA content. It was found in the study by Wang and researchers [41] that at the 8 h (480 min) time point that close to 95% of paracetamol was released while at the same point in this study there was only 53% and 56% released from the 2.50% and 5.00% respective paracetamol loaded dosage forms. However, one explanation for this is the incorporation of PEG in the matrix of the dosage form as due to its hydrophilic nature and its inability to crosslink would allow for a reduction in the intermolecular forces between the polymer chains resulting in greater drug release [22]. Additionally, the results also conflict with what was presented by Vehse et al. [87] who incorporated various concentrations of aspirin into PEGDA matrices via a similar technology albeit a different wavelength, and found that more than 95% of aspirin was released within the first 3 h regardless of the drug loading concentration.

The lower release rates established in this study may be attributed to the higher PCL Triol content of the resin composition used in the formulation, with the PCL Triol influencing drug release due to the hydrophobic nature it affords. Asikainen et al. [62] noted that an increase in hydrophobic networks will result in slower drug release. Furthermore, the addition of low molecular weight molecules added to polymer matrices have been reported to have the ability to modulate drug release due to a reduction in the polymer-polymer interactions as a result of the plasticization effect [32,36,37]. Kanis et al. [34] conducted a study evaluating the effect of PCL Triol content imparted on drug release from a poly(ethylene-co-methyl acrylate) matrix and found that by increasing the amount of PCL Triol resulted in a lower amount of drug being released from the matrix. Therefore, it could be possible to control and manipulate the rate at which drug is released from the dosage form by adjusting the ratio of PCL Triol to PEGDA in the formulation, which would be advantageous if immediate release was a requirement of the dosage form.

3.7. Scanning Electron Microscopy

Scanning electron microscopy (SEM) images of selected paracetamol and aspirin printed dosage forms are presented in Figure 12a–d.

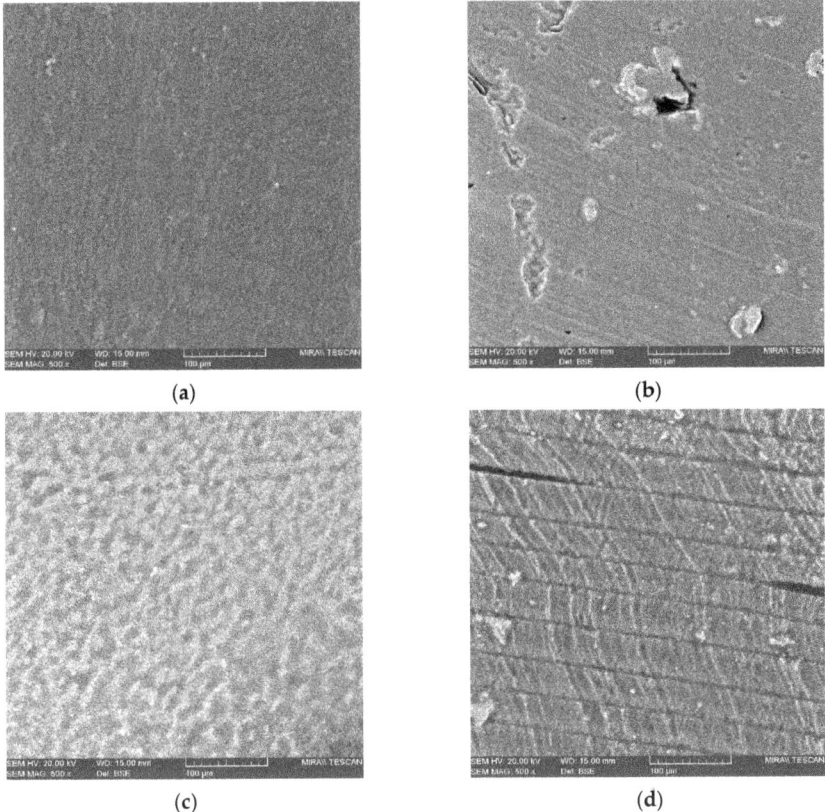

Figure 12. Scanning electron microscopy image of (**a**) 2.50% Para surface (**b**) 2.50% Para cross-section (**c**) 2.50% Asp surface and (**d**) 2.50% Asp cross-section all at 500× magnification.

From observing the images on the surface of the paracetamol loaded dosage forms, Figure 12a, it can be seen that there are no visible voids present indicative of the photopolymer resin curing to a high degree which was further confirmed via FTIR analysis, with the disappearance of the peaks at 811 cm^{-1} and 1189 cm^{-1} associated with polymerization occurring [67]. However, in the images displaying the cross-section of the 2.50% Para dosage form, Figure 12b, it appears that there are notable crystals present which may be TPO and/or paracetamol, suggesting that some of the crystals may not have dissolved in their entirety in the photopolymer solution.

The images obtained for the aspirin dosage forms however, Figure 12c,d, appear different to those of the paracetamol dosage forms. The image showing the surface of the 2.50% Asp dosage form, Figure 12c, the surface appears coarse in comparison to that of the paracetamol dosage form which may be as a result of undissolved TPO and/or aspirin settling on the surface of the print with further analysis that is beyond the scope of this work being required to ascertain this finding. In the cross-sectional images of the 2.50% Asp dosage forms, Figure 12d, the layering of the printing process/laser pass can be observed which demonstrates that polymerization of resin occurred with the binding of the resin in a layer-by-layer fashion as would be expected in the SLA process. However, in addition to this, in the 2.50% Asp dosage form there is evidence of voids present, indicating that incomplete curing may have occurred in these areas. Furthermore, there was also particles observed in the 2.50% Asp dosage form which may be present as a result of the TPO and/or aspirin not fully dissolving into the photopolymer solution.

The results found from conducting SEM demonstrate that SLA has the potential to fabricate dosage forms from photocurable resins, with little to no voids being observed on the surface of the dosage forms being indicative of a high level of curing. However, upon closer inspection and viewing the cross-sectional images of the dosage forms, it was found that there may have been incomplete dissolution or agglomeration occurring due to the inhomogeneous distribution of either drug and/or photoinitiator within the resin as crystals were noted. This may be a potential drawback to SLA as an AM technique for drug delivery applications with these findings requiring further investigation in order to elucidate if the observed particles are that of drug and/or photoinitiator.

4. Conclusions

The results which are laid out in this paper, like many others in the area of 3DP, illustrate the promising potential the technology offers with respect to dosage form production. The present study harnessed the polymerization of photocurable polymers to fabricate 28 drug dosage forms in one single print cycle, exploiting the additive manufacturing technique of stereolithography for bulk manufacture. The study also highlighted that the incorporation of the different drugs, paracetamol and aspirin, may have had an impact on the overall dimensions of the printed dosage forms, with statistically significant differences observed from their target dimensions. This finding indicates that this is an area which can be further investigated and improved upon in future work to advance the AM technique of SLA in relation to fabrication of personalized dosage forms. In addition to this, significant differences were noted in the mean tablet weight between the paracetamol and aspirin dosage forms, with the aspirin based device having a greater tablet weight which correlated with greater drug release than that of the paracetamol dosage forms. Additionally, as the drug loading was increased, there was also a greater release of active, paracetamol or aspirin, noted indicating that with specific drug loadings it may be possible to formulate patient-specific dosage forms, and that with fine-tuning it may be possible to further modulate drug release. The results presented here demonstrate that 3DP for drug delivery can provide opportunities for bespoke treatment of patients coupled to batch manufacturing. Future work to progress the SLA tablet printing approach must focus on elucidating the differences between traditional tableting, commercially available tablets based on additive manufacturing, and the photocurable polymer formulations described herein. Particular focus is needed on tablet physical properties such as hardness and friability, toxicity related to residual unreacted monomers or solvents, and the stability/shelf-life of photocurable formulations prior to printing.

Author Contributions: Conceptualization, A.V.H. and J.G.L.; Methodology, A.V.H., E.F. and J.G.L.; Validation, A.V.H.; Formal analysis, A.V.H.; Investigation, A.V.H.; Resources, A.V.H., P.D. and J.G.L.; Data curation, A.V.H.; Writing—original draft preparation, A.V.H.; Writing—review and editing, A.V.H. and J.G.L.; Visualization A.V.H. and J.G.L.; Supervision, P.D., L.M.G., C.L.H. and J.G.L.; Project administration P.D. and J.G.L.; Funding acquisition, L.M.G., C.L.H. and J.G.L.

Funding: This publication has emanated from research conducted with the financial support of Athlone Institute of Technology under the Presidents Seed Fund, Enterprise Ireland funding under the Technology Gateway program, grant number TG-2017-0114 and Science Foundation Ireland (SFI) under Grant Number 16/RC/3918.

Conflicts of Interest: The authors declare no conflict of interest.

References

1. Conner, B.P.; Manogharan, G.P.; Martof, A.N.; Rodomsky, L.M.; Rodomsky, C.M.; Jordan, D.C.; Limperos, J.W. Making sense of 3-D printing: Creating a map of additive manufacturing products and services. *Addit. Manuf.* **2014**, *1–4*, 64–76. [CrossRef]
2. Gross, B.C.; Erkal, J.L.; Lockwood, S.Y.; Chen, C.; Spence, D.M. Evaluation of 3D Printing and Its Potential Impact on Biotechnology and the Chemical Sciences. *Anal. Chem.* **2014**, *86*, 3240–3253. [CrossRef] [PubMed]
3. Prasad, L.K.; Smyth, H. 3D Printing technologies for drug delivery: A review. *Drug Dev. Ind. Pharm.* **2016**, *42*, 1019–1031. [CrossRef] [PubMed]

4. Pollack, S.; Venkatesh, C.; Neff, M.; Healy, A.V.; Hu, G.; Fuenmayor, E.A.; Lyons, J.G.; Major, I.; Devine, D.M. Polymer-Based Additive Manufacturing: Historical Developments, Process Types and Material Considerations. In *Polymer-Based Additive Manufacturing*; Devine, D.M., Ed.; Springer International Publishing: Cham, Switzerland, 2019; pp. 1–22.
5. Goyanes, A.; Robles Martinez, P.; Buanz, A.; Basit, A.W.; Gaisford, S. Effect of geometry on drug release from 3D printed tablets. *Int. J. Pharm.* **2015**, *494*, 657–663. [CrossRef]
6. Martinez, P.R.; Goyanes, A.; Basit, A.W.; Gaisford, S. Influence of Geometry on the Drug Release Profiles of Stereolithographic (SLA) 3D-Printed Tablets. *AAPS PharmSciTech* **2018**, *19*, 3355–3361. [CrossRef]
7. Fuenmayor, E.A.; Healy, A.V.; Dalton, M.; Major, I. Customised Interventions Utilising Additive Manufacturing. In *Polymer-Based Additive Manufacturing*; Devine, D.M., Ed.; Springer International Publishing: Cham, Switzerland, 2019; pp. 143–160.
8. Fina, F.; Goyanes, A.; Gaisford, S.; Basit, A.W. Selective laser sintering (SLS) 3D printing of medicines. *Int. J. Pharm.* **2017**, *529*, 285–293. [CrossRef]
9. Khaled, S.A.; Burley, J.C.; Alexander, M.R.; Yang, J.; Roberts, C.J. 3D printing of five-in-one dose combination polypill with defined immediate and sustained release profiles. *J. Control. Release* **2015**, *217*, 308–314. [CrossRef]
10. Fina, F.; Madla, C.M.; Goyanes, A.; Zhang, J.; Gaisford, S.; Basit, A.W. Fabricating 3D printed orally disintegrating printlets using selective laser sintering. *Int. J. Pharm.* **2018**, *541*, 101–107. [CrossRef]
11. Khaled, S.A.; Burley, J.C.; Alexander, M.R.; Yang, J.; Roberts, C.J. 3D printing of tablets containing multiple drugs with defined release profiles. *Int. J. Pharm.* **2015**, *494*, 643–650. [CrossRef]
12. Fuenmayor, E.; Forde, M.; Healy, A.V.; Devine, D.M.; Lyons, J.G.; McConville, C.; Major, I. Comparison of fused-filament fabrication to direct compression and injection molding in the manufacture of oral tablets. *Int. J. Pharm.* **2019**, *558*, 328–340. [CrossRef]
13. Goyanes, A.; Buanz, A.B.M.; Basit, A.W.; Gaisford, S. Fused-filament 3D printing (3DP) for fabrication of tablets. *Int. J. Pharm.* **2014**, *476*, 88–92. [CrossRef] [PubMed]
14. Gioumouxouzis, C.I.; Katsamenis, O.L.; Bouropoulos, N.; Fatouros, D.G. 3D printed oral solid dosage forms containing hydrochlorothiazide for controlled drug delivery. *J. Drug Deliv. Sci. Technol.* **2017**, *40*, 164–171. [CrossRef]
15. Khaled, S.A.; Burley, J.C.; Alexander, M.R.; Roberts, C.J.; Yang, J. Desktop 3D printing of controlled release pharmaceutical bilayer tablets. *Int. J. Pharm.* **2014**, *461*, 105–111. [CrossRef] [PubMed]
16. Goyanes, A.; Wang, J.; Buanz, A.; Martínez-Pacheco, R.; Telford, R.; Gaisford, S.; Basit, A.W. 3D Printing of Medicines: Engineering Novel Oral Devices with Unique Design and Drug Release Characteristics. *Mol. Pharm.* **2015**, *12*, 4077–4084. [CrossRef]
17. Norman, J.; Madurawe, R.D.; Moore, C.M.V.; Khan, M.A.; Khairuzzaman, A. A new chapter in pharmaceutical manufacturing: 3D-printed drug products. *Adv. Drug Deliv. Rev.* **2017**, *108*, 39–50. [CrossRef]
18. Trenfield, S.J.; Awad, A.; Goyanes, A.; Gaisford, S.; Basit, A.W. 3D Printing Pharmaceuticals: Drug Development to Frontline Care. *Trends Pharmacol. Sci.* **2018**, 1–12. [CrossRef]
19. Verstraete, G.; Samaro, A.; Grymonpré, W.; Vanhoorne, V.; Van Snick, B.; Boone, M.N.; Hellemans, T.; Van Hoorebeke, L.; Remon, J.P.; Vervaet, C. 3D printing of high drug loaded dosage forms using thermoplastic polyurethanes. *Int. J. Pharm.* **2018**, *536*, 318–325. [CrossRef]
20. Goyanes, A.; Det-Amornrat, U.; Wang, J.; Basit, A.W.; Gaisford, S. 3D scanning and 3D printing as innovative technologies for fabricating personalized topical drug delivery systems. *J. Control. Release* **2016**, *234*, 41–48. [CrossRef]
21. Afsana; Jain, V.; Haider, N.; Jain, K. 3D Printing in Personalized Drug Delivery. *Curr. Pharm. Des.* **2019**, *24*, 5062–5071. [CrossRef]
22. Martinez, P.R.; Goyanes, A.; Basit, A.W.; Gaisford, S. Fabrication of drug-loaded hydrogels with stereolithographic 3D printing. *Int. J. Pharm.* **2017**, *532*, 313–317. [CrossRef]
23. Fuenmayor, E.; Forde, M.; Healy, A.; Devine, D.; Lyons, J.; McConville, C.; Major, I. Material Considerations for Fused-Filament Fabrication of Solid Dosage Forms. *Pharmaceutics* **2018**, *10*, 44. [CrossRef] [PubMed]
24. Boetker, J.; Water, J.J.; Aho, J.; Arnfast, L.; Bohr, A.; Rantanen, J. Modifying release characteristics from 3D printed drug-eluting products. *Eur. J. Pharm. Sci.* **2016**, *90*, 47–52. [CrossRef]
25. Goole, J.; Amighi, K. 3D printing in pharmaceutics: A new tool for designing customized drug delivery systems. *Int. J. Pharm.* **2016**, *499*, 376–394. [CrossRef] [PubMed]

26. Zema, L.; Melocchi, A.; Maroni, A.; Gazzaniga, A. *Three-Dimensional Printing of Medicinal Products and the Challenge of Personalized Therapy*; Elsevier Inc.: Amsterdam, The Netherlands, 2017; Volume 106, ISBN 3902503246.
27. Preis, M.; Öblom, H. 3D-Printed Drugs for Children—Are We Ready Yet? *AAPS PharmSciTech* **2017**, *18*, 303–308. [CrossRef] [PubMed]
28. McDermott, S.; Walsh, J.E.; Howard, R.G. A novel application of UV-LEDs in the contact lens manufacturing process. In Proceedings of the Opto-Ireland 2005: Optical Sensing and Spectroscopy, Dublin, Ireland, 3 June 2005; Volume 5826, p. 119.
29. Geever, T.; Killion, J.; Grehan, L.; Geever, L.M.; Chadwick, E.; Higginbotham, C. Effect of Photoinitiator Concentration on the Properties of Polyethylene Glycol Based Hydrogels for Potential Regenerative Medicine Applications. *Adv. Environ. Biol. Adv. Environ. Biol* **2014**, *8*, 7–17.
30. Bernauer, U.; Chaudhry, Q.; Coenraads, P.; Degen, G.; Dusinska, M.; Gawkrodger, D.; Lilienblum, W.; Luch, A.; Nielsen, E.; Platzek, T.; et al. *Scientific Committee on Consumer Safety Trimethylbenzoyl Diphenylphosphine Oxide (TPO)*; European Commission: Luxembourg, 2014.
31. Ligon, S.C.; Liska, R.; Stampfl, J.; Gurr, M.; Mülhaupt, R. Polymers for 3D Printing and Customized Additive Manufacturing. *Chem. Rev.* **2017**, *117*, 10212–10290. [CrossRef]
32. Meier, M.M.; Kanis, L.A.; de Lima, J.C.; Pires, A.T.N.; Soldi, V. Poly(caprolactone triol) as plasticizer agent for cellulose acetate films: Influence of the preparation procedure and plasticizer content on the physico-chemical properties. *Polym. Adv. Technol.* **2004**, *15*, 593–600. [CrossRef]
33. Wessler, K.; Nishida, M.H.; Da Silva, J.; Pezzin, A.P.T.; Pezzin, S.H. Thermal properties and morphology of poly(3-hydroxybutyrate-co-3- hydroxyvalerate) with poly(caprolactone triol) mixtures. *Macromol. Symp.* **2006**, *245–246*, 161–165. [CrossRef]
34. Kanis, L.A.; Soldi, V. Poly(ethylene-co-methyl acrylate)/poly(caprolactone) triol blends for drug delivery systems: Characterization and drug release. *Quim. Nova* **2012**, *35*, 297–300. [CrossRef]
35. Li, Z.; Li, J. Control of hyperbranched structure of polycaprolactone/ poly(ethylene glycol) polyurethane block copolymers by glycerol and their hydrogels for potential cell delivery. *J. Phys. Chem. B* **2013**, *117*, 14763–14774. [CrossRef]
36. Duarte, M.A.T.; de Rezende Duek, E.A.; Motta, A.C. In vitro degradation of poly (L-co-D,L lactic acid) containing PCL-T. *Polímeros Ciência e Tecnol.* **2014**, *24*, 1–8. [CrossRef]
37. Meier, M.M.; Kanis, L.A.; Soldi, V. Characterization and drug-permeation profiles of microporous and dense cellulose acetate membranes: Influence of plasticizer and pore forming agent. *Int. J. Pharm.* **2004**, *278*, 99–110. [CrossRef] [PubMed]
38. Elomaa, L.; Teixeira, S.; Hakala, R.; Korhonen, H.; Grijpma, D.W.; Seppälä, J.V. Preparation of poly(ε-caprolactone)-based tissue engineering scaffolds by stereolithography. *Acta Biomater.* **2011**, *7*, 3850–3856. [CrossRef] [PubMed]
39. Chung, I.; Xie, D.; Puckett, A.D.; Mays, J.W. Syntheses and evaluation of biodegradable multifunctional polymer networks. *Eur. Polym. J.* **2003**, *39*, 1817–1822. [CrossRef]
40. La Gatta, A.; De Rosa, A.; Laurienzo, P.; Malinconico, M.; De Rosa, M.; Schiraldi, C. A novel injectable poly(ε-caprolactone)/calcium sulfate system for bone regeneration: Synthesis and characterization. *Macromol. Biosci.* **2005**, *5*, 1108–1117. [CrossRef]
41. Wang, J.; Goyanes, A.; Gaisford, S.; Basit, A.W. Stereolithographic (SLA) 3D Printing of Oral Modified-Release Dosage Forms. *Int. J. Pharm.* **2016**, *503*, 207–212. [CrossRef]
42. Pivsa-Art, W.; Fujii, K.; Nomura, K.; Aso, Y.; Ohara, H.; Yamane, H. The effect of poly(ethylene glycol) as plasticizer in blends of poly(lactic acid) and poly(butylene succinate). *J. Appl. Polym. Sci.* **2016**, *133*, 1–10. [CrossRef]
43. Li, D.; Jiang, Y.; Lv, S.; Liu, X.; Gu, J.; Chen, Q.; Zhang, Y. Preparation of plasticized poly (lactic acid) and its influence on the properties of composite materials. *PLoS ONE* **2018**, *13*, 1–15. [CrossRef]
44. Serra, T.; Ortiz-Hernandez, M.; Engel, E.; Planell, J.A.; Navarro, M. Relevance of PEG in PLA-based blends for tissue engineering 3D-printed scaffolds. *Mater. Sci. Eng. C* **2014**, *38*, 55–62. [CrossRef]
45. Kollamaram, G.; Croker, D.M.; Walker, G.M.; Goyanes, A.; Basit, A.W.; Gaisford, S. Low temperature fused deposition modeling (FDM) 3D printing of thermolabile drugs. *Int. J. Pharm.* **2018**, *545*, 144–152. [CrossRef]

46. Melocchi, A.; Parietti, F.; Loreti, G.; Maroni, A.; Gazzaniga, A.; Zema, L. 3D printing by fused deposition modeling (FDM) of a swellable/erodible capsular device for oral pulsatile release of drugs. *J. Drug Deliv. Sci. Technol.* **2015**, *30*, 360–367. [CrossRef]
47. Clark, E.A.; Alexander, M.R.; Irvine, D.J.; Roberts, C.J.; Wallace, M.J.; Sharpe, S.; Yoo, J.; Hague, R.J.M.; Tuck, C.J.; Wildman, R.D. 3D printing of tablets using inkjet with UV photoinitiation. *Int. J. Pharm.* **2017**, *529*, 523–530. [CrossRef]
48. Morris, V.B.; Nimbalkar, S.; Younesi, M.; McClellan, P.; Akkus, O. Mechanical Properties, Cytocompatibility and Manufacturability of Chitosan:PEGDA Hybrid-Gel Scaffolds by Stereolithography. *Ann. Biomed. Eng.* **2017**, *45*, 1–11. [CrossRef]
49. Killion, J.A.; Geever, L.M.; Devine, D.M.; Grehan, L.; Kennedy, J.E.; Higginbotham, C.L. Modulating the mechanical properties of photopolymerised polyethylene glycol–polypropylene glycol hydrogels for bone regeneration. *J. Mater. Sci.* **2012**, *47*, 6577–6585. [CrossRef]
50. Killion, J.A.; Kehoe, S.; Geever, L.M.; Devine, D.M.; Sheehan, E.; Boyd, D.; Higginbotham, C.L. Hydrogel/bioactive glass composites for bone regeneration applications: Synthesis and characterisation. *Mater. Sci. Eng. C* **2013**, *33*, 4203–4212. [CrossRef]
51. Browning, M.B.; Cereceres, S.N.; Luong, P.T.; Cosgriff-Hernandez, E.M. Determination of the in vivo degradation mechanism of PEGDA hydrogels. *J. Biomed. Mater. Res. Part A* **2014**, *102*, 4244–4251.
52. Zhong, C.; Wu, J.; Reinhart-King, C.A.; Chu, C.C. Synthesis, characterization and cytotoxicity of photo-crosslinked maleic chitosan-polyethylene glycol diacrylate hybrid hydrogels. *Acta Biomater.* **2010**, *6*, 3908–3918. [CrossRef]
53. McAvoy, K.; Jones, D.; Thakur, R.R.S. Synthesis and Characterisation of Photocrosslinked poly(ethylene glycol) diacrylate Implants for Sustained Ocular Drug Delivery. *Pharm. Res.* **2018**, *35*, 36. [CrossRef]
54. Robles-Martinez, P.; Xu, X.; Trenfield, S.J.; Awad, A.; Goyanes, A.; Telford, R.; Basit, A.W.; Gaisford, S. 3D Printing of a Multi-Layered Polypill Containing Six Drugs Using a Novel Stereolithographic Method. *Pharmaceutics* **2019**, *11*, 274. [CrossRef]
55. de Martino, M.; Chiarugi, A. Recent Advances in Pediatric Use of Oral Paracetamol in Fever and Pain Management. *Pain Ther.* **2015**, *4*, 149–168. [CrossRef]
56. Kanani, K.; Gatoulis, S.C.; Voelker, M. Influence of differing analgesic formulations of aspirin on pharmacokinetic parameters. *Pharmaceutics* **2015**, *7*, 188–198 [CrossRef]
57. McElroy, D.M.; Geever, L.M.; Higginbotham, C.L.; Devery, S.M. The Effect of Photoinitiator Concentration on the Physicochemical Properties of Hydrogel Contact Lenses. *Appl. Mech. Mater.* **2014**, *679*, 118–127. [CrossRef]
58. McDermott, S.L.; Walsh, J.E.; Howard, R.G. A comparison of the emission characteristics of UV-LEDs and fluorescent lamps for polymerisation applications. *Opt. Laser Technol.* **2008**, *40*, 487–493. [CrossRef]
59. Dizon, J.R.C.; Chen, Q.; Valino, A.D.; Advincula, R.C. Thermo-mechanical and swelling properties of three-dimensional-printed poly (ethylene glycol) diacrylate/silica nanocomposites. *MRS Commun.* **2018**, 1–9. [CrossRef]
60. Arikawa, H.; Takahashi, H.; Kanie, T.; Ban, S. Effect of various visible light photoinitiators on the polymerization and color of light-activated resins. *Dent. Mater. J.* **2009**, *28*, 454–460. [CrossRef]
61. Steyrer, B.; Neubauer, P.; Liska, R.; Stampfl, J. Visible Light Photoinitiator for 3D-Printing of Tough Methacrylate Resins. *Materials* **2017**, *10*, 1445. [CrossRef]
62. Asikainen, S.; van Bochove, B.; Seppälä, J.V. Drug-releasing biopolymeric structures manufactured via stereolithography. *Biomed. Phys. Eng. Express* **2019**, *5*, 025008. [CrossRef]
63. Meng, R.F.; Mao, S.; Chapoy, L. Contact Lens. U.S. Patent 8461226, 11 June 2013.
64. Duan, A.; Li, Y.; Li, B.; Zhu, P. 3D-printable thermochromic acrylic resin with excellent mechanical performance. *J. Appl. Polym. Sci.* **2019**, *137*, 48277. [CrossRef]
65. Yang, W.; Yu, H.; Liang, W.; Wang, Y.; Liu, L. Rapid fabrication of hydrogel microstructures using UV-induced projection printing. *Micromachines* **2015**, *6*, 1903–1913. [CrossRef]
66. Burke, G.; Cao, Z.; Devine, D.M.; Major, I. Preparation of Biodegradable Polyethylene Glycol Dimethacrylate Hydrogels via Thiol-ene Chemistry. *Polymers* **2019**, *11*, 1339. [CrossRef]
67. Burke, G.; Barron, V.; Geever, T.; Geever, L.; Devine, D.M.; Higginbotham, C.L. Evaluation of the materials properties, stability and cell response of a range of PEGDMA hydrogels for tissue engineering applications. *J. Mech. Behav. Biomed. Mater.* **2019**, *99*, 1–10. [CrossRef]

68. Wu, Y.H.; Park, H.B.; Kai, T.; Freeman, B.D.; Kalika, D.S. Water uptake, transport and structure characterization in poly(ethylene glycol) diacrylate hydrogels. *J. Memb. Sci.* **2010**, *347*, 197–208. [CrossRef]
69. Killion, J.A.; Geever, L.M.; Devine, D.M.; Kennedy, J.E.; Higginbotham, C.L. Mechanical properties and thermal behaviour of PEGDMA hydrogels for potential bone regeneration application. *J. Mech. Behav. Biomed. Mater.* **2011**, *4*, 1219–1227. [CrossRef] [PubMed]
70. BASF. *Irgacure®TPO-Technical Data Sheet*; BASF SE: Ludwigshafen, Germany, 2015.
71. Burger, A.; Ramberger, R. On the polymorphism of pharmaceuticals and other molecular crystals. I. *Mikrochim. Acta* **1979**, *72*, 259–271. [CrossRef]
72. Sacchetti, M. Thermodynamic Analysis of DSC Data for Acetaminophen Polymorphs. *J. Therm. Anal. Calorim.* **2001**, *63*, 345–350. [CrossRef]
73. Trichy Rengarajan, G.; Beiner, M. Relaxation Behavior and Crystallization Kinetics of Amorphous Acetaminophen. *Lett. Drug Des. Discov.* **2006**, *3*, 723–730. [CrossRef]
74. Rengarajan, G.T.; Enke, D.; Beiner, M. Crystallization Behavior of Acetaminophen in Nanopores. *Open Phys. Chem. J.* **2007**, *1*, 18–24. [CrossRef]
75. Jain, H.; Khomane, K.S.; Bansal, A.K. Implication of microstructure on the mechanical behaviour of an aspirin–paracetamol eutectic mixture. *CrystEngComm* **2014**, *16*, 8471–8478. [CrossRef]
76. Kundu, S.P.; Amjad, F.M.; Sultana, S.; Sultan, Z. Study of Differential Scanning Calorimetry of complex of Magnesium Sulfate with Aspirin, Paracetamol and Naproxen. *Banladesh Pharm. J.* **2012**, *15*, 7–12.
77. Semalty, A.; Semalty, M.; Singh, D.; Rawat, M.S.M. Development and Characterization of Aspirin-Phospholipid Complex for Improved Drug Delivery. *J. Pharm. Sci.* **2010**, *3*, 940–947.
78. Tita, B.; Fulias, A.; Rusu, G.; Tita, D. Thermal Behaviour of Acetylsalicylic Acid-active Substance and Tablets Kinetic Study under Non-isothermal Conditions. *Rev. Chim.* **2009**, *60*, 419–423.
79. Tita, D.; Jurca, T.; Fulias, A.; Marian, E.; Tita, B. Compatibility study of the acetylsalicylic acid with different solid dosage forms excipients. *J. Therm. Anal. Calorim.* **2013**, *112*, 407–419. [CrossRef]
80. Campanella, L.; Micieli, V.; Tomassetti, M.; Vecchio, S. Kinetic investigation and predictive model for the isothermal degradation time in two commercial acetylsalicylic acid-based pharmaceutical tablet formulations. *Thermochim. Acta* **2011**, *526*, 151–156. [CrossRef]
81. Al-Maydama, H.M.; Abduljabbar, A.A.; Al-Maqtari, M.A.; Naji, K.M. Study of temperature and irradiation influence on the physicochemical properties of Aspirin. *J. Mol. Struct.* **2018**, *1157*, 364–373. [CrossRef]
82. de A. Silva, E.M.; de A. Melo, D.M.; de F. V. de Moura, M.; de Farias, R.F. An investigation about the solid state thermal degradation of acetylsalicylic acid: Polymer formation. *Thermochim. Acta* **2004**, *414*, 101–104. [CrossRef]
83. Goyanes, A.; Kobayashi, M.; Martínez-Pacheco, R.; Gaisford, S.; Basit, A.W. Fused-filament 3D printing of drug products: Microstructure analysis and drug release characteristics of PVA-based caplets. *Int. J. Pharm.* **2016**, *514*, 290–295. [CrossRef]
84. Beck, R.C.R.; Chaves, P.S.; Goyanes, A.; Vukosavljevic, B.; Buanz, A.; Windbergs, M.; Basit, A.W.; Gaisford, S. 3D printed tablets loaded with polymeric nanocapsules: An innovative approach to produce customized drug delivery systems. *Int. J. Pharm.* **2017**, *528*, 268–279. [CrossRef]
85. Zhang, J.; Yang, W.; Vo, A.Q.; Feng, X.; Ye, X.; Kim, D.W.; Repka, M.A. Hydroxypropyl methylcellulose-based controlled release dosage by melt extrusion and 3D printing: Structure and drug release correlation. *Carbohydr. Polym.* **2017**, *177*, 49–57. [CrossRef]
86. Goyanes, A.; Allahham, N.; Trenfield, S.J.; Stoyanov, E.; Gaisford, S.; Basit, A.W. Direct powder extrusion 3D printing: Fabrication of drug products using a novel single-step process. *Int. J. Pharm.* **2019**, *567*, 118471. [CrossRef]
87. Vehse, M.; Petersen, S.; Sternberg, K.; Schmitz, K.-P.; Seitz, H. Drug Delivery From Poly(ethylene glycol) Diacrylate Scaffolds Produced by DLC Based Micro-Stereolithography. *Macromol. Symp.* **2014**, *346*, 43–47. [CrossRef]

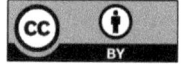

© 2019 by the authors. Licensee MDPI, Basel, Switzerland. This article is an open access article distributed under the terms and conditions of the Creative Commons Attribution (CC BY) license (http://creativecommons.org/licenses/by/4.0/).

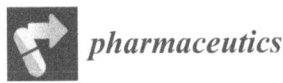

Article

3D Printing of a Multi-Layered Polypill Containing Six Drugs Using a Novel Stereolithographic Method

Pamela Robles-Martinez [1], Xiaoyan Xu [1], Sarah J. Trenfield [1], Atheer Awad [1], Alvaro Goyanes [2,3], Richard Telford [4], Abdul W. Basit [1,2,*] and Simon Gaisford [1,2,*]

1. Department of Pharmaceutics, UCL School of Pharmacy, University College London, 29–39 Brunswick Square, London WC1N 1AX, UK; pamela.martinez.13@ucl.ac.uk (P.R.-M.); xiaoyan.xu.13@ucl.ac.uk (X.X.); sarah.trenfield.16@ucl.ac.uk (S.J.T.); atheer.awad.15@ucl.ac.uk (A.A.)
2. FabRx Ltd., 3 Romney Road, Ashford TN24 0RW, UK; a.goyanes@fabrx.co.uk
3. Departamento de Farmacología, Farmacia y Tecnología Farmacéutica, R + D Pharma Group (GI-1645), Universidade de Santiago de Compostela, 15782 Santiago de Compostela, Spain
4. School of Chemistry and Forensic Sciences, University of Bradford, Richmond Road, Bradford BD7 1DP, UK; R.Telford@bradford.ac.uk
* Correspondence: a.basit@ucl.ac.uk (A.W.B.); s.gaisford@ucl.ac.uk (S.G.)

Received: 7 May 2019; Accepted: 3 June 2019; Published: 11 June 2019

Abstract: Three-dimensional printing (3DP) has demonstrated great potential for multi-material fabrication because of its capability for printing bespoke and spatially separated material conformations. Such a concept could revolutionise the pharmaceutical industry, enabling the production of personalised, multi-layered drug products on demand. Here, we developed a novel stereolithographic (SLA) 3D printing method that, for the first time, can be used to fabricate multi-layer constructs (polypills) with variable drug content and/or shape. Using this technique, six drugs, including paracetamol, caffeine, naproxen, chloramphenicol, prednisolone and aspirin, were printed with different geometries and material compositions. Drug distribution was visualised using Raman microscopy, which showed that whilst separate layers were successfully printed, several of the drugs diffused across the layers depending on their amorphous or crystalline phase. The printed constructs demonstrated excellent physical properties and the different material inclusions enabled distinct drug release profiles of the six actives within dissolution tests. For the first time, this paper demonstrates the feasibility of SLA printing as an innovative platform for multi-drug therapy production, facilitating a new era of personalised polypills.

Keywords: three-dimensional printing; fixed-dose combinations; additive manufacturing; 3D printed drug products; printlets; tablets; personalized medicines; multiple-layer dosage forms; stereolithography; vat polymerisation

1. Introduction

Multiple drug therapies have gained increasing attention in healthcare because of improved treatment outcomes for diseases with complex pathologies, such as HIV-1 infection, hypertension, tuberculosis and type II diabetes mellitus [1–4]. Despite this, polypharmacy (involving the administration of five or more medicines) is arguably the most pressing prescribing issue, linked to increasing rates of non-adherence and patient confusion due to the high pill burden and complex administration requirements [5]. Such challenges can be overcome by utilising fixed-dose combinations (FDCs) or polypills, whereby more than one drug is incorporated into the same drug product [6–8]. Indeed, the commercially available polypill (Polycap™), which contains enteric-coated aspirin, ramipril, simvastatin, atenolol, and hydrochlorothiazide, has been shown to be effective in reducing multiple cardiovascular risk factors [9,10].

The main barrier to the widespread introduction of FDCs, however, lies in their manufacturing and lack of flexibility in dosing. Conventional powder compaction typically produces homogeneous tablets containing fixed strengths on a large commercial scale, an approach that is wholly unsuitable for therapies that require flexibility in dosing or drug combination(s). For example, if a patient requires a change in dose and/or drug whilst maintained on a FDC, often the treatment will have to be withdrawn and the patient would be initiated on separate dosage forms [11]. Furthermore, narrow therapeutic index drugs or those that require frequent dose titrations are unsuitable for FDC regimens [12,13]. In the era of personalised medicine, it is clear that a novel platform that enables a flexible process for tailored dosing and drug combinations is required [14–17].

It is in this niche that three-dimensional printing (3DP) offers significant promise as a transformative technology [18–23]. Three-dimensional printing is an additive manufacturing technique that fabricates objects from a computer-aided design (CAD) file in a layer-by-layer manner [24–28]. Owing to its flexibility, 3DP allows the combination of multiple materials in a single dosage form with different geometries [29–33]. Since the drugs are physically separated, it is possible to adjust doses and release profiles individually as well as to co-formulate drugs that may potentially interact [12,34–38]. Indeed, previous studies have 3D printed polypills containing paracetamol and caffeine with varying designs (multi-layered and DuoCaplet), enabling specific release profiles to be attained depending on the position of the drug in the caplet, independent of drug solubility [39]. Khaled. et al. fabricated a 3D printed polypill containing five drugs that were released in two different profiles [40]. The same group incorporated three different drugs within a single 3D printed tablet using a semisolid extrusion-based printer, each of which have a distinct release profile depending on their spatial location [41].

The most widely used 3DP technique in pharmaceuticals is fused deposition modelling (FDM), which involves the use of drug-loaded polymer filaments as feedstock that are heated and deposited layer-by-layer [42–47]. However, most commercially available FDM printers can only print with a limited number of filaments, and hence, enabling a maximum deposition of a limited number of spatially separated drugs [35]. Stereolithographic (SLA) 3DP is an alternative technology hitherto relatively unexplored for pharmaceutical applications. It works by using a laser to photocure a liquid resin, comprising a photopolymerisable monomer and a photoinitiator that upon exposure to light initiates polymerisation of the monomer [48]. Stereolithographic 3DP offers some key advantages over other 3DP technologies including avoidance of thermal degradation [28,49], improved resolution and higher accuracy [50], and is also considered a faster method than FDM or selective laser sintering (SLS) 3DP processes [51]. Further information about the SLA process has been described elsewhere [52].

By blending a drug into the resin, SLA 3DP has previously been used to make tablets [52] and hydrogels [53] and its versatility has allowed the exploration of how geometric parameters influence drug release kinetics [54]. Thus far, however, no such work has demonstrated the ability for SLA to produce polypills, likely due to the difficulty in printing spatially-separated layers. A particular challenge relates to the software and hardware of commercially available SLA printers, which does not allow for multi-resin printing.

In this work, for the first time, we have overcome this limitation of SLA printing by developing an SLA printer that is capable of printing multi-layered tablets. We exemplify its use by printing a polypill 3D-printed tablet (printlet) containing six different model drugs (paracetamol, naproxen, caffeine, aspirin, prednisolone, and chloramphenicol), some of which are commonly administered together to improve their efficacy. The spatial separation of the drugs was determined with Raman microscopy and the modification of drug release rates upon changing polypill geometry (cylindrical and ring shapes) and excipient addition was evaluated using dissolution tests. Critically, this work has generated a new SLA pharmaceutical printing process, revolutionising the manufacture of polypills and treatment pathways for patients.

2. Materials and Methods

The model drugs paracetamol (MW = 151.2 g/mol), acetylsalicylic acid (MW = 180.2 g/mol), naproxen (MW = 252.2 g/mol), chloramphenicol (MW = 323.1 g/mol), and caffeine (MW = 194.2 g/mol) were purchased from Sigma–Aldrich Ltd. (Gillingham, UK) and prednisolone (MW = 360.4 g/mol) was purchased from Severn Biotech Ltd. (Kidderminster, UK).

Polyethylene glycol diacrylate (PEGda, average MW 575 g/mol) and diphenyl (2,4,6-trimethylbenzoyl) phosphine oxide (TPO) were purchased from Sigma-Aldrich Ltd. (Gillingham, UK). The salts for preparing the buffer dissolution media were purchased from VWR International Ltd., Poole, UK. All materials were used as received.

2.1. 3D Printing

PEGda was used as the photopolymerisable monomer and TPO as the photoinitiator (PI). The compositions of the formulations are shown in Table 1.

Table 1. Compositions (% w/w) of the initial resins for printing.

Material \ Formulation	Type I (% w/w)	Type II (% w/w)	Type III (% w/w)
PEGda	89	89	44.5
PEG300	-	-	44.5
TPO	1	1	1
Drug	10	10	10

Each formulation was prepared by dissolving the drug and the PI in liquid PEGda and PEG300 when applicable. The components were added into a beaker under constant stirring until complete dissolution of the powders in the polymer(s). Then each solution was poured into a resin tray for printing.

All printlets were fabricated using a Form 1+ SLA 3D printer (Formlabs Inc., Somerville, MA, USA). The printer was equipped with a 405 nm laser able to fabricate objects with a resolution of 300 μm and a layer thickness of 25 μm, 50 μm, 100 μm or 200 μm. Printlets (a cylinder—10 mm diameter and 3 mm height, or a ring—10 mm diameter and 6 mm height) were designed in AutoCAD®® 2017 (Autodesk Inc, San Rafael, CA, USA) and exported as a stereolithographic file (.stl) (Figure 1) to the Preform Software v.2.3.3 OpenFL, (Formlabs Inc., Somerville, MA, USA).

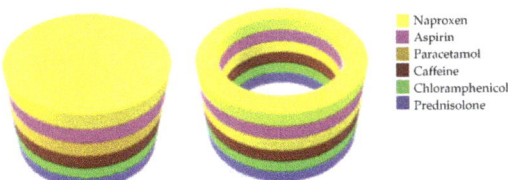

Figure 1. 3D designs of the printlets. Type I: Cylinder (**left**, 10 mm diameter and 3 mm height), Types II and III: Ring (**right**, 10 mm diameter and 6 mm height).

The printlets were fabricated keeping the order of the drugs in the polypill unchanged, having the drugs with the higher water solubility (paracetamol and caffeine) in the inner layers, whereas the drugs with the lowest water solubility (naproxen and prednisolone) were printed in the outer layers (Figure 1). Three forms of polypill were printed:

- Type I: Cylinder shape
- Type II: Ring shape
- Type III: Ring shape with a soluble filler (PEG 300)

The Form 1+ printer is designed to print homogeneous objects. To fabricate printlets with different drugs in discrete layers it is necessary to pause printing in order to change the resin formulation in the printing tray. Hence, the use of an application programming interface (OpenFL version of PreForm software) was required to enable the 3D printer to be manually communicated with.

The OpenFL version of the software PreForm was used to allow pausing of printing and raising of the build platform to enable switching of the resin tray. Once the resin tray was changed, the build plate was lowered to its previous position and printing was resumed. The required number of layers (6 blocks of layers of 0.5 mm for the cylinder tablets and 6 blocks of layers of 1 mm for the ring-shaped printlets) was then easily printed, with a deionised water rinse of the printed object between resins to avoid cross-contamination. After this, the platform was returned to its previous position to print the next block of layers until the polypill was completed.

The printlets were printed directly on the build platform at room temperature without supports.

2.2. Printlet Dimensions

The printlets were weighed and measured (width and height) using a digital calliper (0.150 mm PRO-MAX, Fowler, mod S 235 PAT). The measurements were performed in triplicate.

2.3. Raman Spectroscopy and Mapping

Samples were mounted and focused using a 50× objective on a Renishaw RA802 Pharmaceutical Analyser equipped with a 785 nm laser operating at 50% power (ca. 100 mW at sample). Spectral arrays were acquired with 26,000 spectra recorded over the surface of the sample using a step size of 50 µm in the x- (10.15 mm) and y- (6.5 mm) dimensions.

Processing was performed with Renishaw WiRE software using two approaches: (i) direct classical least-squares (DCLS) component matching to reference 3D prints of the pure drugs in the printing matrix and (ii) using direct classical least-squares (DCLS) component matching to reference spectra extracted from each of the 6 layers of the printed polypill layers.

Higher spatial resolution maps were acquired across the naproxen, aspirin, and paracetamol layers using the same basic acquisition parameters, with an increased spatial resolution achieved by acquiring spectral arrays with ca. 30,000 spectra recorded over a section of the sample (1 mm along x and 3 mm along y) using a step size of 10 µm.

2.4. X-ray Powder Diffraction (XRPD)

X-ray powder diffraction patterns of pure drugs and individual printed discs (23 × 1 mm) were recorded using a Rigaku MiniFlex 600 (Rigaku, The Woodlands, TX, USA) with a Cu Kα X-ray source (λ = 1.5418 Å) and accompanying software Miniflex Guidance Version 1.2.01. The intensity and voltage applied were 15 mA and 40 kV. The angular range of data acquisition was 3–40° 2θ, with a step size of 0.02° at a speed of 2° min^{-1}.

2.5. Determination of Drug Concentration in the Polypills

Printlets were crushed using a mortar and pestle with 50 mL of ethanol to enhance extraction of poorly water-soluble drugs, this solution was then taken to 1 L with deionised water and constantly stirred during 24 h. Samples of the solutions were filtered through a 0.45 µm filter (Millipore Ltd., Dublin, Ireland) and the amount of drug in solution was determined using HPLC (Hewlett Packard 1050 Series HPLC system, Agilent Technologies, Cheadle, UK).

The validated HPLC assay consisted of a stationary phase of an Eclipse 5 µm C18 column, 4.6 mm × 150 mm (Agilent, Santa Clara, CA, USA) and a mobile phase with a gradient elution system of ortho-phosphoric acid, pH = 2.7 (A) and acetonitrile (B) at 25 °C. The gradient system consisted of; 0–7.5 min linear change from A–B (87:13 v/v) to A–B (50:50 v/v) and kept until 8.5 min; then 8.5–9.5 min linear change to the initial conditions, A–B (87:13 v/v). The flow rate was kept at 1.5 mL/min and the injection volume was 20 µL. The eluent was screened at a wavelength of 263 nm. The retention times for the drugs were as follows: paracetamol, 2 min; caffeine, 2.6 min; aspirin, 5.2 min; chloramphenicol, 5.8 min; prednisolone, 6.15 min; and naproxen, 9.4 min (so a total elution time of 10 min). All measurements were made in duplicate.

2.6. Dynamic Drug Dissolution Testing Conditions

Drug dissolution profiles for the printlets were obtained with a USP II apparatus (Model PTWS, Pharmatest, Germany). The printlets were placed in 750 mL of 0.1 M HCl for 2 h to simulate the gastric compartment, and then transferred into 950 mL of modified Hanks (mHanks) bicarbonate physiological medium for 35 min (pH 5.6 to 7.4); and then in modified Krebs buffer (1000 mL) (pH 7 to 7.4 and then to 6.5). The modified Hanks buffer-based dissolution medium (136.9 mM NaCl, 5.37 mM KCl, 0.812 mM $MgSO_4 \cdot 7H_2O$, 1.26 mM $CaCl_2$, 0.337 mM $Na_2HPO_4 \cdot 2H_2O$, 0.441 mM KH_2PO_4, 4.17 mM $NaHCO_3$) forms an in situ modified Kreb's buffer by addition of 50 mL of pre-Krebs solution (400.7 mM $NaHCO_3$ and 6.9 mM KH_2PO_4) to each dissolution vessel [55,56].

The formulations were tested in the small intestinal environment for 3.5 h (pH 5.6 to 7.4), followed by pH 6.5 representing the colonic environment [55,57,58]. The medium is primarily a bicarbonate buffer in which bicarbonate (HCO^{3-}) and carbonic acid (H_2CO_3) co-exist in equilibrium, along with CO_2 (aq) resulting from dissociation of the carbonic acid. The pH of the buffer is controlled by an Auto pH System™ [59,60], which consists of a pH probe connected to a source of carbon dioxide gas (pH-reducing gas), as well as to a supply of helium (pH-increasing gas), controlled by a control unit. The control unit is able to provide a dynamically adjustable pH during testing (dynamic conditions) and to maintain a uniform pH value over the otherwise unstable bicarbonate buffer pH.

The paddle speed of the USP-II was fixed at 50 rpm and the tests were conducted at 37 ± 0.5 °C ($n = 3$). Sample of the dissolution media (1 mL) was withdrawn and the drug concentration was determined by HPLC using the method described above.

2.7. Determination of Swelling Ratio (SR) for Individual Layers

Three-dimensional printed blocks of layers for each formulation were quickly rinsed with deionised water then blotted with filter paper to remove any uncured liquid formulation and water on the surface immediately following fabrication, then they were weighed (W_i). The cylinders were then placed into 0.1 M HCl for 2 h, then transferred to modified Hanks (mHanks) bicarbonate physiological medium for 22 h at 37 °C to simulate the dissolution test conditions. At specific time points the excess water was carefully wiped off and the layers were weighed (W_s). The SR was calculated using the following equation:

$$SR = \frac{W_s}{W_i} \tag{1}$$

3. Results and Discussion

3.1. 3D Printing Process

For the first time, it was possible to modify a commercial SLA 3D printer in order to fabricate a series of polypill printlets containing six drugs and in unique geometries (Type I: cylindrical and Types II and III: ring-shaped; Figure 2). The commercially available Form 1+ printer has the functionality to only create homogeneous objects composed of single resins, making it impossible for the production of printed dosage forms containing spatially-separated active ingredients. In order to achieve multi-resin printing, it was identified that the printer would need to be paused, the build platform raised, and the resin tray removed and replaced with a new resin formulation. Although the 3D printer PreForm software does have the functionality to pause printing at any point during the fabrication process, the build platform currently remains in the same position (where either the object or the platform itself are within the resin tray), physically obstructing the change of the resin tray or the material within it.

In order to overcome this challenge, we re-designed the printer software to enable a controlled raising and lowering of the build platform once printing was paused, facilitating manual changing of the resin in the printer tray. To achieve this, the Form 1+ printer software was manually modified using the OpenFL version of PreForm software, which is an application programming interface for the Form 1 and Form 1+ FormLabs 3D printers. An application programming interface is a group of functions, commands, protocols, and objects that allows programmers to create software or interact with an external system (the 3D printer in this case) without having to write a code from scratch. Here, the software was modified to include command inputs that enabled the following six steps to be carried out: (1) the resin formulation was printed using SLA; (2) the printing process was paused upon layer completion; (3) the build platform was raised, enabling resin tray removal; (4) the resin tray was replaced which included a different resin formulation; (5) the build plate was lowered to its previous position and; (6) printing was resumed to create the next formulation layer.

In this way, multiple polypill printlets could be easily fabricated in 30 min, with the order of drugs in the layers controlled by the resin formulation in the tank at any particular point. The customised print settings (with six laser passes for the first layer to ensure adhesion and two for the rest) used allowed the successful production of printlets directly on the build platform, achieving good adhesion without significantly affecting the dimensions. Crucially, this approach avoids material wastage and potential dose variation compared with other methods that utilise supports for adhesion to the build platform that need to be removed and discarded post-printing.

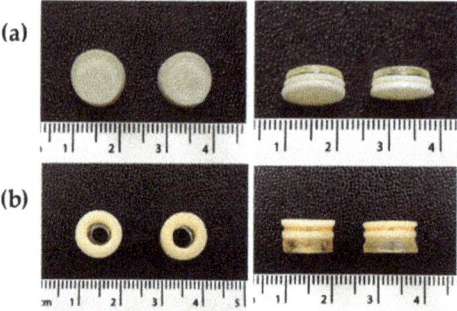

Figure 2. Polypill printlet (**a**) Type I (cylinder shape) and (**b**) Type II (ring shape). The Type III formulation was visually identical to Type II, and hence, has not been included here. The scale is in cm.

3.2. Physical Characteristics

3.2.1. Drug Distribution and Solid-State Characteristics

Raman spectroscopy has previously been used to evaluate the spatial distribution and phase of drugs within tablets, and as such, was used here to map a cross-sectional surface of a multi-layered 3D-printed flat polypill [61]. Processing of the arrays using DCLS component matching to produce false colour representations of distribution shows the presence of the six drugs within the six layers of the polypill (Figure 3), highlighting the success in utilising SLA to print separate resin formulations within separate compartments.

However, detailed interrogation of individual Raman spectra within the mapped areas leads us to note that there is evidence of "diffusion" of certain drugs (naproxen, aspirin, and paracetamol) between the layers which was not anticipated through visual examination of the white light microscopic image which shows a distinct boundary between each. Further mapping activities were performed, focusing on the three layers containing naproxen, aspirin, and paracetamol. These spectral arrays were acquired with a significantly higher resolution over a reduced area, i.e., 1 mm in x by 3 mm in the s-dimensions to better understand the distribution of drug in this area (Section 2.3). Figure 4a–c show DCLS processing of these arrays using pure printed drug references (i.e., containing one drug plus printing matrix) to demonstrate this diffusion effect between these three layers. It is reasonably clear to see that the principle drug content is within the layer containing that drug, but there is evidence of the drug diffusing into the next layers with an attenuating signal, i.e., a diminishing concentration.

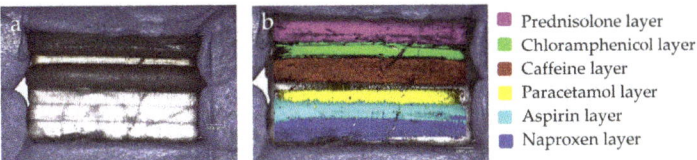

Figure 3. Visual imaging of a Type I polypill, using (**a**) optical light microscopy and (**b**) Raman mapping. The images show the spatial separation of layers.

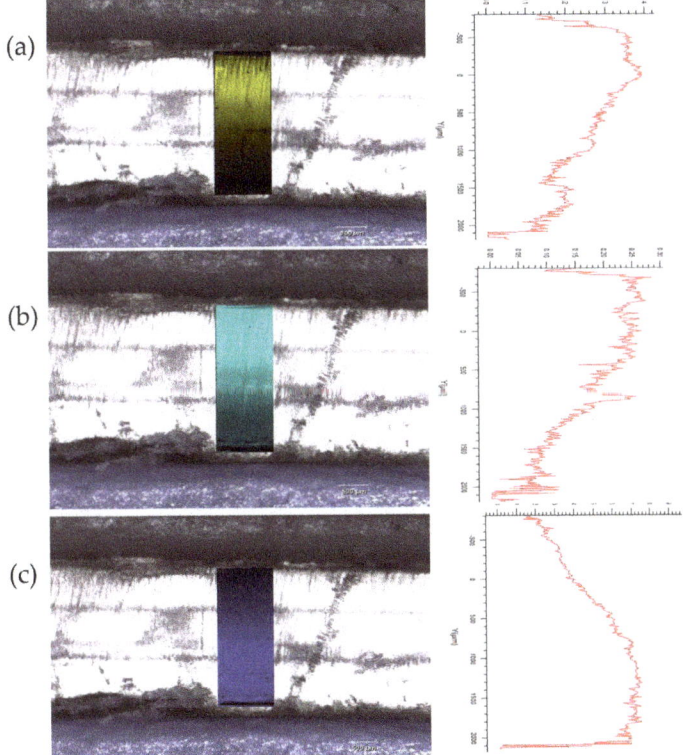

Figure 4. Raman mapping of a Type I polypill across the naproxen, aspirin, and paracetamol layers with an increased spatial resolution (30,000 spectra across 1 mm in x by 3 mm in y. (**a**) Shows the partial diffusion of paracetamol into the adjacent layers; (**b**) shows the partial diffusion of aspirin into the adjacent layers; and (**c**) shows the partial diffusion of naproxen into the adjacent layers.

Conversely, caffeine and prednisolone were localised solely within their respective layers, with no evidence of any diffusion. Furthermore, these drugs have appeared to act as a barrier to diffusion of the other layers, e.g., there is no evidence of the paracetamol diffusing into the caffeine layer, whereas it does diffuse into the aspirin layer. Evidence of this differential diffusion effect is presented in Figure 5, where distribution of each drug is evaluated by plotting DCLS match across the y-dimension of the mapped polypill.

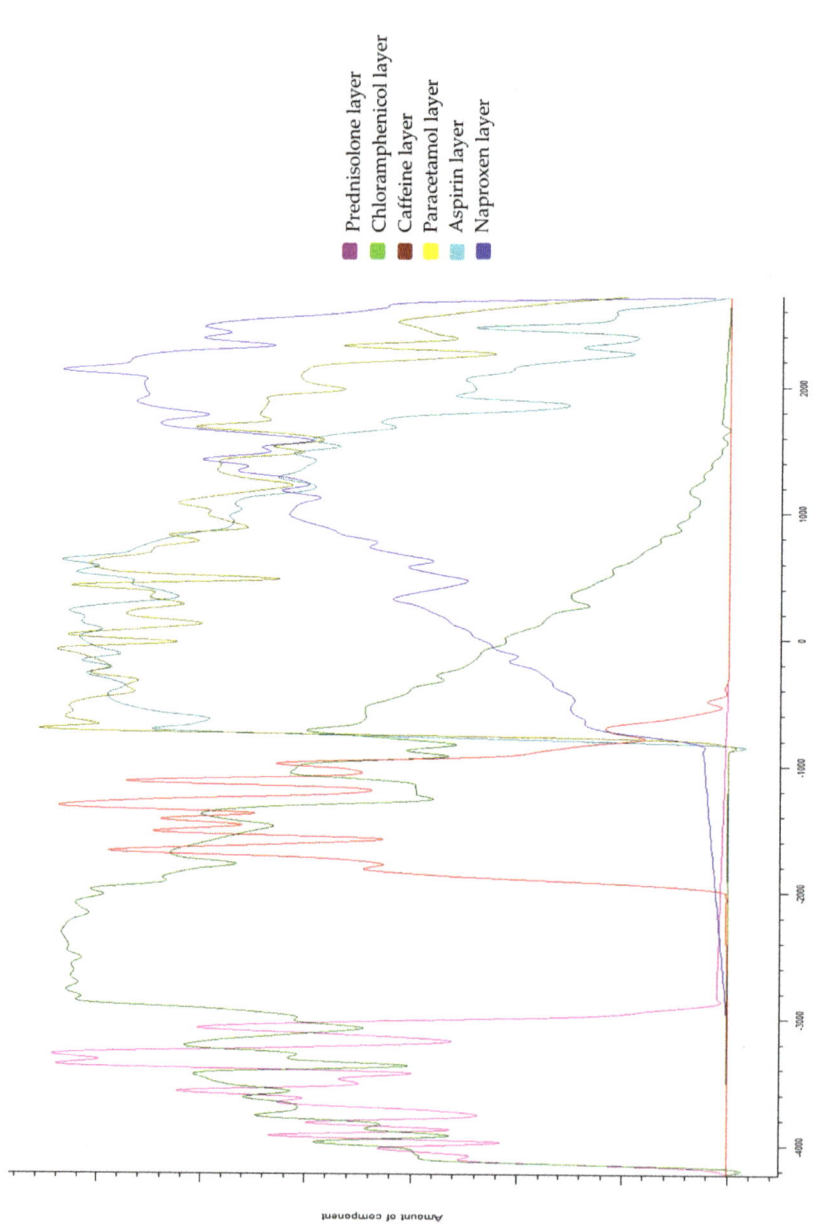

Figure 5. Drug distribution profiles in the Y-dimension of the polypill showing the diffusion between layers in the paracetamol, aspirin, and naproxen layers, with a tight distribution in the caffeine and prednisolone layers.

This phenomenon was hypothesised to be due to the phase of the drugs within the printed polypill; post-printing, the layers containing paracetamol, naproxen, aspirin, and chloramphenicol were visually clear with a glassy appearance and the prednisolone and caffeine formulations were white (opaque), which was an initial indicator for differences in solid-state characteristics (Figure 2). These findings were further interrogated using XRPD (Figure 6).

Indeed, four of the drugs (aspirin, paracetamol, naproxen, and chloramphenicol) were found to be in the amorphous phase due to the absence of sharp peaks in the XRPD spectra (Figure 6b,d–f respectively). Conversely, prednisolone and caffeine were found to be present in the crystalline phase (Figure 6a,c respectively). Specifically, several crystalline peaks were found post-printing for caffeine (at 12.6, 27.2, and 28.0 2θ) and for prednisolone, one crystalline peak was observed at 16.4 2θ. In both cases, consistent peak shifts of ~+1 2θ was apparent, which was attributed to the stress–strain influence, or the change in height presentation, of a printed disc versus the raw powder.

Previous studies have highlighted that amorphous drug materials have a higher propensity to diffuse across polymeric matrices [62]. As such, it is likely that in this study the amorphous drugs (aspirin, paracetamol, naproxen, and chloramphenicol) are diffusing across the layers more readily compared with the crystalline drugs (caffeine and prednisolone), which remain in their respective layers. Stabilising drugs in their amorphous phase as a solid dispersion is favourable for low solubility drugs due to the potential for an increase in drug solubility and bioavailability.

3.2.2. Printlet Dimensions and Weight Variation

In order to evaluate the effect of drug addition on the resin printability, the consistency in weight and dimensions of the polypill printlets was evaluated (target dimensions: 3 mm × 10 mm for the cylinders and 6 mm × 10 mm for the rings) (Table 2). In general, all the formulations yielded slightly wider diameters than their corresponding targets, ranging from 10.73 mm to 11.07 mm. In general, height and weight variation were higher for Type I cylindrical printlets compared with Type II and III ring-shaped printlets. This variability in mass could be due to the multiple factors both from the liquid formulation and the settings of the printer. The number of laser passes for each printed layer and the laser power directly affect the curing depth, and hence, the properties of the printed layer [63]. Hence, the parameters need to be optimised for each resin type. It should also be noted that the difference in the target and real dimensions could be adjusted by simply scaling the electronic object. HPLC was used to evaluate drug content of the polypills post-printing. Drug loading was found to range between 85–104%, which is within the acceptable range for content uniformity (85–115%) set by the British Pharmacopoeia.

Table 2. Dimension and weight data for the polypills.

Type I		
Width (mm) ± %CV	Height ± SD (mm)	Weight ± SD (mg)
10.99 ± 1.0	2.81 ± 9.8	329 ± 13.6
Type II		
Width (mm) ± %CV	Height ± SD (mm)	Weight ± SD (mg)
11.07 ± 0.1	6.12 ± 0.03	501.13 ± 6.3
Type III		
Width (mm) ± %CV	Height ± SD (mm)	Weight ± SD (mg)
10.73 ± 0.18	6.12 ± 0.02	553 ± 8.9

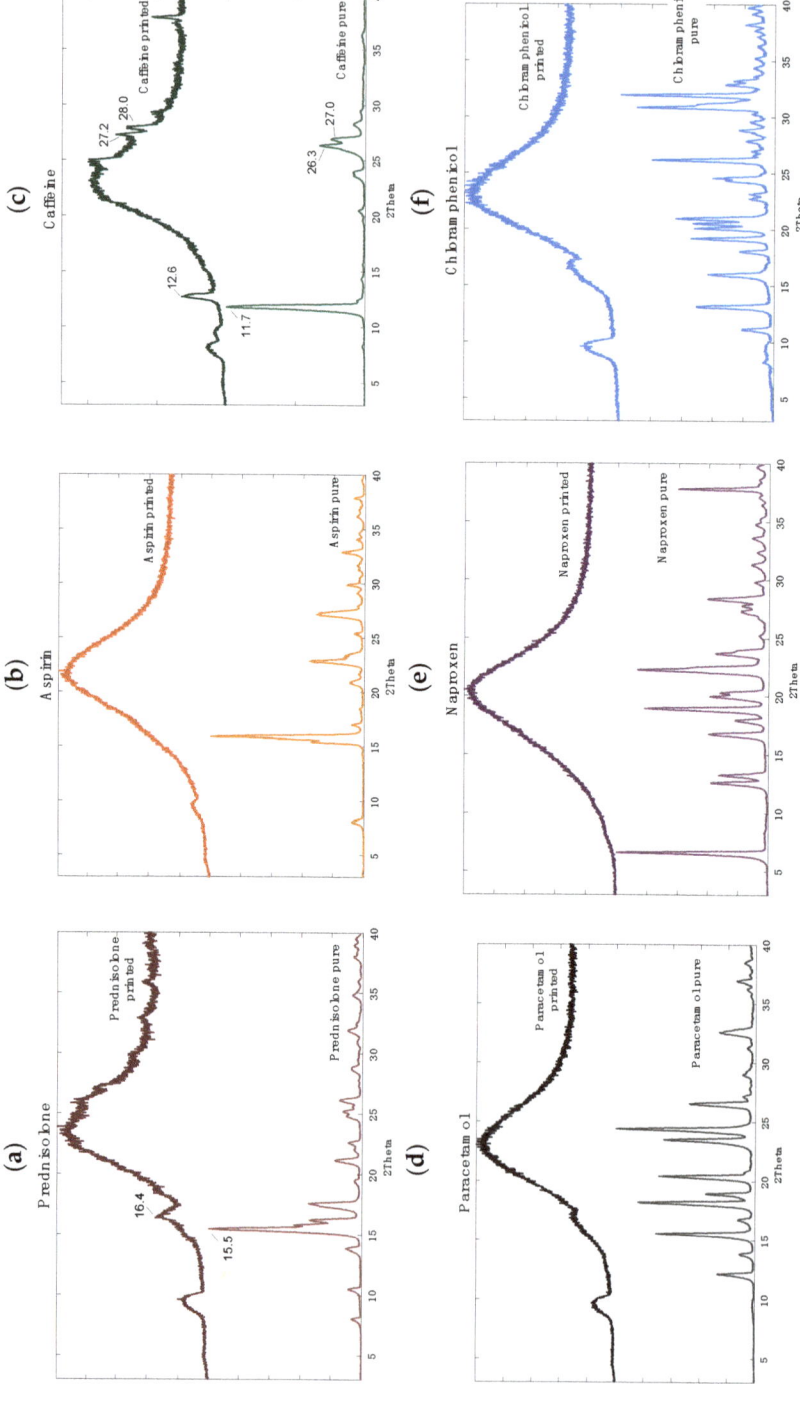

Figure 6. X-ray powder diffractograms of pure and printed drugs: (a) prednisolone, (b) aspirin, (c) caffeine, (d) paracetamol, (e) naproxen and (f) chloramphenicol.

3.3. Drug Release Studies

The effect of geometry and excipient addition on drug release was evaluated for each of the three polypill types (Figure 7). For polypill Type I (standard cylindrical shape), none of the drugs reached 100% release after 20 h (range 22–80% release) (Figure 7a). Interestingly, it was observed that the printlets swelled and remained intact at the bottom of the dissolution vessel. SEM images were used to evaluate the surface morphology of the cylindrical polypill before and after swelling (data not shown). Due to the cross-linking of the monomers within the polymeric matrix, the "dry" polypill exhibited a compact surface under SEM imaging, whereas several pores were visible on the surface of a swollen polypill exposed to dissolution medium. These results highlight that the mechanism for drug release from SLA tablets is via diffusion of the water into the printlet, followed by the solubilisation and diffusion of drug through micropore channels within the polymeric matrix.

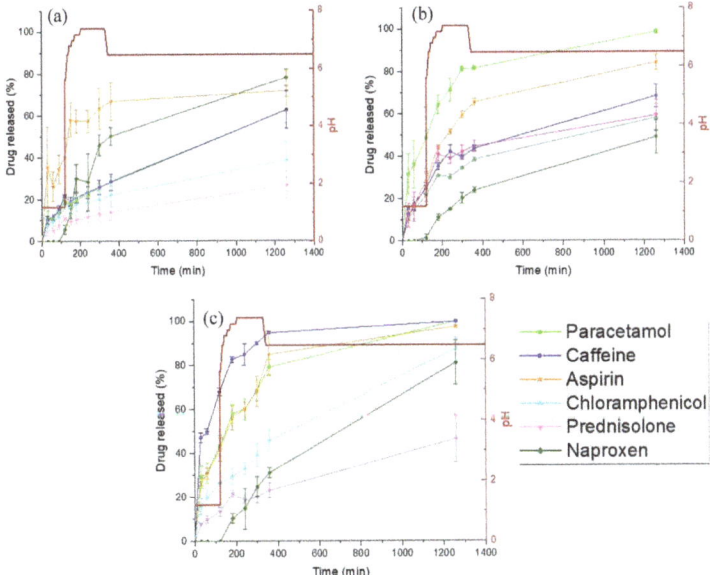

Figure 7. Drug dissolution profiles for the 3D printed polypills: (**a**) Type 1 cylindrical polypill; (**b**) Type II ring-shaped polypill; and (**c**) Type III ring-shaped polypill + PEG 300.

In order to increase dissolution rate, polypill Type II was designed to have a ring-shaped geometry in order to increase the formulation surface area (and hence dissolution rate). For the water-soluble drugs (placed in the inner layers) the rate of release was enhanced by the presence of a hole in the polypill due to the increased exposure to the dissolution medium (paracetamol 60% versus 95%, and caffeine 60% versus 65% for polypill Type I and II, respectively) (Figure 7b). However, for the lower solubility drugs placed in the outer layers (naproxen and prednisolone), the presence of the hole did not significantly change the drug release profile, likely due to the low water solubility of the drugs.

As such, polypill Type III was formulated and designed in order to evaluate the impact of a soluble filler (PEG 300) on dissolution. PEG 300 is commonly used a solubilising agent in oral formulations, as such, it was hypothesised that its inclusion would increase drug solubility, and hence, release. It was found that the addition of PEG 300 increased drug release substantially compared with polypill Type I (for paracetamol, caffeine, and aspirin ~100% release was achieved after 20 h, and for chloramphenicol and naproxen release was increased to >80%) (Figure 7c). For prednisolone, drug release was increased to 45%; however, it did not achieve complete release after 20 h. It was noted before that poorly soluble drugs like prednisolone are not completely released when incorporated within sustained release devices. This has been attributed mainly to its poor solubility in water and dissolution rate of the drug in a hydrophilic matrix, and, as seen in the XRPD data, could be due to the presence of prednisolone in the crystalline phase (Figure 6) [64].

For prednisolone in particular, Di Colo. et al. noted that the swelling ratio (SR) of the hydrogel had a great influence on the dissolution and diffusion of the drug [65]. To evaluate this concept here, the SR at 24 h and the time to maximum SR was calculated for each of the 3D-printed drug layers (Table 3). The results show that the overall SR values for the different printed layers were similar (~1.1), indicating that the formulations exhibited analogous cross-linking densities despite the difference in drug incorporation. However, the maximum value for swelling ratio for each formulation was reached at different time points (caffeine at 300 min; prednisolone at 240 min; chloramphenicol at 120 min; and the rest at 24 h). Although the maximum SR for the prednisolone layer was reached at 240 min, drug release was not increased beyond this time in the dissolution studies, and hence, in this case was not deemed to be the most significant factor to hindering prednisolone release.

Table 3. Swelling ratios of the individual 3D-printed layers after 24 h in water. * Indicates maximum swelling occurred before 24 h (caffeine 300 min, prednisolone 240 min, chloramphenicol 120 min).

Drug	Swelling Ratio
Paracetamol	1.21 ± 0.07
Aspirin	1.15 ± 0.03
Naproxen	1.18 ± 0.03
Prednisolone *	1.11 ± 0.05
Chloramphenicol *	1.05 ± 0.02
Caffeine *	1.17 ± 0.02

Another possible explanation for the unexpected release behaviour of prednisolone is that it could have a higher affinity for the polymer than for the aqueous media used in the dissolution test. To evaluate this concept, drug diffusion studies were carried out, whereby placebo 3D printed tables were placed into saturated solutions of either prednisolone or caffeine for drug-loading via passive diffusion over a period of 14 days. Results showed that the amount of drug released in fresh media from the loaded 3D-printed tablets was ~3 times higher for prednisolone than for caffeine (data not shown). This suggests that a higher amount of prednisolone was able to diffuse and reside within the cross-linked PEGda networks compared with caffeine, likely due to the higher affinity of prednisolone to the polymer. As well as its poor aqueous solubility, this explains why prednisolone is not readily released from the 3D-printed tablet matrix. Such results highlight the need for continued drug screening and resin formulation optimisation to ensure drug release is appropriately controlled for tailoring to individual patient needs.

4. Conclusions

For the first time, a commercial SLA 3D printer was successfully modified to enable multi-resin printing for the fabrication of bespoke and tailored polypills containing six different active ingredients. The printer platform was optimised such that printing could be paused, the resin tray removed, and replaced with different resin formulations. Using this technique, a number of different polypill geometries (cylindrical and ring-shaped) and formulation compositions (with and without a soluble filler) were produced that demonstrated acceptable physicochemical characteristics and differing drug release profiles. Although the drug formulations were suitable for 3D printing, further research is needed to determine the most optimal printer settings for each formulation to achieve accurate dimensions, and thus dosing, and for achieving specific drug release profiles when required. Crucially, this study shows the potential of SLA 3D printing for fabricating multi-layered polypills to improve personalisation for patients.

Author Contributions: Conceptualization, P.R.-M., A.G., A.W.B. and S.G.; Methodology, P.R.-M., A.G., A.W.B., R.T and S.G.; Software, P.R.-M. and X.X; Validation, P.R.-M. and X.X.; Formal analysis, P.R.-M., S.J.T. and R.T.; investigation, P.R.-M., X.X., S.J.T., A.A. and R.T.; Resources, P.R.-M., S.J.T., A.A., X.X. and R.T.; Data curation, P.R.M, X.X., S.J.T. and A.A.; writing—original draft preparation, S.J.T. and P.R.-M.; Writing—review and editing, S.J.T, A.G, A.W.B., S.G. and R.T.; visualization, P.R.-M., A.A., X.X. and S.J.T.; Supervision, S.J.T., A.G., A.W.B, R.T. and S.G.; Project administration, A.G., A.W.B. and S.G.

Funding: The authors thank the Engineering and Physical Sciences Research Council (EPSRC), UK for their financial support (EP/L01646X).

Acknowledgments: The authors would like to thank Tim Smith (Renishaw, UK) for his help in acquiring Raman data using their demonstration RA802 In Wotton-Under-Edge.

Conflicts of Interest: The authors declare no conflict of interest. The co-authors A.G., S.G. and A.W.B. are directors of FabRx Ltd. The company had no role in the design of the study; in the collection, analyses, or interpretation of data; in the writing of the manuscript, and in the decision to publish the results.

References

1. Fonseca, V.; Rosenstock, J.; Patwardhan, R.; Salzman, A. Effect of Metformin and Rosiglitazone Combination Therapy in Patients With Type 2 Diabetes Mellitus. *JAMA* **2000**, *283*, 1695–1702. [CrossRef] [PubMed]
2. Gradman, A.H.; Basile, J.N.; Carter, B.L.; Bakris, G.L. Combination therapy in hypertension. *J. Am. Soc. Hypertens.* **2010**, *4*, 42–50. [CrossRef] [PubMed]
3. Cruz, A.T.; Garcia-Prats, A.J.; Furin, J.; Seddon, J.A. Treatment of Multidrug-resistant Tuberculosis Infection in Children. *Pediatr. Infect. Dis. J.* **2018**, *37*, 831–834. [CrossRef] [PubMed]
4. Weverling, G.J.; Lange, J.M.; Jurriaans, S.; Prins, J.M.; Lukashov, V.V.; Notermans, D.W.; Roos, M.; Schuitemaker, H.; Hoetelmans, R.M.; Danner, S.A.; et al. Alternative multidrug regimen provides improved suppression of HIV-1 replication over triple therapy. *AIDS* **1998**, *12*, F117–F122. [CrossRef] [PubMed]
5. Payne, R.A.; Avery, A.J. Polypharmacy: One of the greatest prescribing challenges in general practice. *Br. J. Gen. Pract.* **2011**, *61*, 83. [CrossRef] [PubMed]
6. Bangalore, S.; Kamalakkannan, G.; Parkar, S.; Messerli, F.H. Fixed-dose combinations improve medication compliance: A meta-analysis. *Am. J. Med.* **2007**, *120*, 713–719. [CrossRef]
7. Castellano, J.M.; Sanz, G.; Penalvo, J.L.; Bansilal, S.; Fernandez-Ortiz, A.; Alvarez, L.; Guzman, L.; Linares, J.C.; Garcia, F.; D'Aniello, F.; et al. A polypill strategy to improve adherence: Results from the FOCUS project. *J. Am. Coll. Cardiol.* **2014**, *64*, 2071–2082. [CrossRef]
8. Connor, J.; Rafter, N.; Rodgers, A. Do fixed-dose combination pills or unit-of-use packaging improve adherence? A systematic review. *Bull. World Health Organ.* **2004**, *82*, 935–939.
9. Yusuf, S.; Pais, P.; Afzal, R.; Xavier, D.; Teo, K.; Eikelboom, J.; Sigamani, A.; Mohan, V.; Gupta, R.; Thomas, N. Effects of a polypill (Polycap) on risk factors in middle-aged individuals without cardiovascular disease (TIPS): A phase II, double-blind, randomised trial. *Lancet* **2009**, *373*, 1341–1351.
10. Patel, A.; Shah, T.; Shah, G.; Jha, V.; Ghosh, C.; Desai, J.; Khamar, B.; Chakraborty, B.S. Preservation of Bioavailability of Ingredients and Lack of Drug-Drug Interactions in a Novel Five-Ingredient Polypill (Polycap™). *Am. J. Cardiovasc. Drugs* **2010**, *10*, 95–103. [CrossRef]
11. Webster, R.; Castellano, J.M.; Onuma, O.K. Putting polypills into practice: Challenges and lessons learned. *Lancet* **2017**, *389*, 1066–1074. [CrossRef]
12. Alomari, M.; Vuddanda, P.R.; Trenfield, S.J.; Dodoo, C.C.; Velaga, S.; Basit, A.W.; Gaisford, S. Printing T3 and T4 oral drug combinations as a novel strategy for hypothyroidism. *Int. J. Pharm.* **2018**, *549*, 363–369. [CrossRef] [PubMed]
13. Tian, P.; Yang, F.; Xu, Y.; Lin, M.-M.; Yu, L.-P.; Lin, W.; Lin, Q.-F.; Lv, Z.-F.; Huang, S.-Y.; Chen, Y.-Z. Oral disintegrating patient-tailored tablets of warfarin sodium produced by 3D printing. *Drug Dev. Ind. Pharm.* **2018**, *44*, 1918–1923. [CrossRef] [PubMed]
14. Vuddanda, P.R.; Alomari, M.; Dodoo, C.C.; Trenfield, S.J.; Velaga, S.; Basit, A.W.; Gaisford, S. Personalisation of warfarin therapy using thermal ink-jet printing. *Eur. J. Pharm. Sci.* **2018**, *117*, 80–87. [CrossRef] [PubMed]
15. Goyanes, A.; Chang, H.; Sedough, D.; Hatton, G.B.; Wang, J.; Buanz, A.; Gaisford, S.; Basit, A.W. Fabrication of controlled-release budesonide tablets via desktop (FDM) 3D printing. *Int. J. Pharm.* **2015**, *496*, 414–420. [CrossRef] [PubMed]

16. Alomari, M.; Mohamed, F.H.; Basit, A.W.; Gaisford, S. Personalised dosing: Printing a dose of one's own medicine. *Int. J. Pharm.* **2015**, *494*, 568–577. [CrossRef] [PubMed]
17. El Aita, I.; Breitkreutz, J.; Quodbach, J. On-demand manufacturing of immediate release levetiracetam tablets using pressure-assisted microsyringe printing. *Eur. J. Pharm. Biopharm.* **2019**, *134*, 29–36. [CrossRef] [PubMed]
18. Basit, A.W.; Gaisford, S. *3D Printing of Pharmaceuticals*; Springer International Publishing: Cham, Switzerland, 2018.
19. Awad, A.; Fina, F.; Trenfield, S.J.; Patel, P.; Goyanes, A.; Gaisford, S.; Basit, A.W. 3D Printed Pellets (Miniprintlets): A Novel, Multi-Drug, Controlled Release Platform Technology. *Pharmaceutics* **2019**, *11*, 148. [CrossRef]
20. Vithani, K.; Goyanes, A.; Jannin, V.; Basit, A.W.; Gaisford, S.; Boyd, B.J. A Proof of Concept for 3D Printing of Solid Lipid-Based Formulations of Poorly Water-Soluble Drugs to Control Formulation Dispersion Kinetics. *Pharm. Res.* **2019**, *36*, 102. [CrossRef]
21. Vithani, K.; Goyanes, A.; Jannin, V.; Basit, A.W.; Gaisford, S.; Boyd, B.J. An Overview of 3D Printing Technologies for Soft Materials and Potential Opportunities for Lipid-based Drug Delivery Systems. *Pharm. Res.* **2018**, *36*, 4–24. [CrossRef]
22. Linares, V.; Casas, M.; Caraballo, I. Printfills: 3D printed systems combining fused deposition modeling and injection volume filling. Application to colon-specific drug delivery. *Eur. J. Pharm. Biopharm.* **2019**, *134*, 138–143. [CrossRef] [PubMed]
23. Hsiao, W.-K.; Lorber, B.; Reitsamer, H.; Khinast, J. 3D printing of oral drugs: A new reality or hype? *Expert Opin. Drug Deliv.* **2017**, 1–4. [CrossRef] [PubMed]
24. Awad, A.; Trenfield, S.J.; Goyanes, A.; Gaisford, S.; Basit, A.W. Reshaping drug development using 3D printing. *Drug Discov. Today* **2018**, *23*, 1547–1555. [CrossRef] [PubMed]
25. Fina, F.; Madla, C.M.; Goyanes, A.; Zhang, J.; Gaisford, S.; Basit, A.W. Fabricating 3D printed orally disintegrating printlets using selective laser sintering. *Int. J. Pharm.* **2018**, *541*, 101–107. [CrossRef] [PubMed]
26. Fina, F.; Goyanes, A.; Gaisford, S.; Basit, A.W. Selective laser sintering (SLS) 3D printing of medicines. *Int. J. Pharm.* **2017**, *529*, 285–293. [CrossRef] [PubMed]
27. Goyanes, A.; Det-Amornrat, U.; Wang, J.; Basit, A.W.; Gaisford, S. 3D scanning and 3D printing as innovative technologies for fabricating personalized topical drug delivery systems. *J. Control. Release* **2016**, *234*, 41–48. [CrossRef]
28. Kadry, H.; Wadnap, S.; Xu, C.; Ahsan, F. Digital light processing (DLP) 3D-printing technology and photoreactive polymers in fabrication of modified-release tablets. *Eur. J. Pharm. Sci.* **2019**, *135*, 60–67. [CrossRef]
29. Fina, F.; Goyanes, A.; Madla, C.M.; Awad, A.; Trenfield, S.J.; Kuek, J.M.; Patel, P.; Gaisford, S.; Basit, A.W. 3D printing of drug-loaded gyroid lattices using selective laser sintering. *Int. J. Pharm.* **2018**, *547*, 44–52. [CrossRef] [PubMed]
30. Sadia, M.; Arafat, B.; Ahmed, W.; Forbes, R.T.; Alhnan, M.A. Channelled tablets: An innovative approach to accelerating drug release from 3D printed tablets. *J. Control. Release* **2018**, *269*, 355–363. [CrossRef]
31. Isreb, A.; Baj, K.; Wojsz, M.; Isreb, M.; Peak, M.; Alhnan, M.A. 3D printed oral theophylline doses with innovative 'radiator-like' design: Impact of polyethylene oxide (PEO) molecular weight. *Int. J. Pharm.* **2019**, *564*, 98–105. [CrossRef]
32. Siyawamwaya, M.; du Toit, L.C.; Kumar, P.; Choonara, Y.E.; Kondiah, P.P.P.D.; Pillay, V. 3D printed, controlled release, tritherapeutic tablet matrix for advanced anti-HIV-1 drug delivery. *Eur. J. Pharm. Biopharm.* **2019**, *138*, 99–110. [CrossRef] [PubMed]
33. Kavanagh, O.N.; Albadarin, A.B.; Croker, D.M.; Healy, A.M.; Walker, G.M. Maximising success in multidrug formulation development: A review. *J. Control. Release* **2018**, *283*, 1–19. [CrossRef] [PubMed]
34. Genina, N.; Boetker, J.P.; Colombo, S.; Harmankaya, N.; Rantanen, J.; Bohr, A. Anti-tuberculosis drug combination for controlled oral delivery using 3D printed compartmental dosage forms: From drug product design to in vivo testing. *J. Control. Release* **2017**, *268*, 40–48. [CrossRef] [PubMed]
35. Pereira, B.C.; Isreb, A.; Forbes, R.T.; Dores, F.; Habashy, R.; Petit, J.-B.; Alhnan, M.A.; Oga, E.F. 'Temporary Plasticiser': A novel solution to fabricate 3D printed patient-centred cardiovascular 'Polypill' architectures. *Eur. J. Pharm. Biopharm.* **2019**, *135*, 94–103. [CrossRef] [PubMed]

36. Sadia, M.; Isreb, A.; Abbadi, I.; Isreb, M.; Aziz, D.; Selo, A.; Timmins, P.; Alhnan, M.A. From 'fixed dose combinations' to 'a dynamic dose combiner': 3D printed bi-layer antihypertensive tablets. *Eur. J. Pharm. Sci.* **2018**. [CrossRef] [PubMed]
37. Trenfield, S.J.; Awad, A.; Goyanes, A.; Gaisford, S.; Basit, A.W. 3D Printing Pharmaceuticals: Drug Development to Frontline Care. *Trends Pharmacol. Sci.* **2018**, *39*, 440–451. [CrossRef] [PubMed]
38. Gioumouxouzis, C.I.; Baklavaridis, A.; Katsamenis, O.L.; Markopoulou, C.K.; Bouropoulos, N.; Tzetzis, D.; Fatouros, D.G. A 3D printed bilayer oral solid dosage form combining metformin for prolonged and glimepiride for immediate drug delivery. *Eur. J. Pharm. Sci.* **2018**, *120*, 40–52. [CrossRef] [PubMed]
39. Goyanes, A.; Wang, J.; Buanz, A.; Martinez-Pacheco, R.; Telford, R.; Gaisford, S.; Basit, A.W. 3D Printing of Medicines: Engineering Novel Oral Devices with Unique Design and Drug Release Characteristics. *Mol. Pharm.* **2015**, *12*, 4077–4084. [CrossRef] [PubMed]
40. Khaled, S.A.; Burley, J.C.; Alexander, M.R.; Yang, J.; Roberts, C.J. 3D printing of five-in-one dose combination polypill with defined immediate and sustained release profiles. *J. Control. Release* **2015**, *217*, 308–314. [CrossRef] [PubMed]
41. Khaled, S.A.; Burley, J.C.; Alexander, M.R.; Yang, J.; Roberts, C.J. 3D printing of tablets containing multiple drugs with defined release profiles. *Int. J. Pharm.* **2015**, *494*, 643–650. [CrossRef] [PubMed]
42. Awad, A.; Trenfield, S.J.; Gaisford, S.; Basit, A.W. 3D printed medicines: A new branch of digital healthcare. *Int. J. Pharm.* **2018**, *548*, 586–596. [CrossRef] [PubMed]
43. Beck, R.C.R.; Chaves, P.S.; Goyanes, A.; Vukosavljevic, B.; Buanz, A.; Windbergs, M.; Basit, A.W.; Gaisford, S. 3D printed tablets loaded with polymeric nanocapsules: An innovative approach to produce customized drug delivery systems. *Int. J. Pharm.* **2017**, *528*, 268–279. [CrossRef] [PubMed]
44. Goyanes, A.; Fernández-Ferreiro, A.; Majeed, A.; Gomez-Lado, N.; Awad, A.; Luaces-Rodríguez, A.; Gaisford, S.; Aguiar, P.; Basit, A.W. PET/CT imaging of 3D printed devices in the gastrointestinal tract of rodents. *Int. J. Pharm.* **2018**, *536*, 158–164. [CrossRef] [PubMed]
45. Zhang, J.; Feng, X.; Patil, H.; Tiwari, R.V.; Repka, M.A. Coupling 3D printing with hot-melt extrusion to produce controlled-release tablets. *Int. J. Pharm.* **2017**, *519*, 186–197. [CrossRef] [PubMed]
46. Kollamaram, G.; Croker, D.M.; Walker, G.M.; Goyanes, A.; Basit, A.W.; Gaisford, S. Low temperature fused deposition modeling (FDM) 3D printing of thermolabile drugs. *Int J Pharm* **2018**, *545*, 144–152. [CrossRef] [PubMed]
47. Pietrzak, K.; Isreb, A.; Alhnan, M.A. A flexible-dose dispenser for immediate and extended release 3D printed tablets. *Eur. J. Pharm. Biopharm.* **2015**, *96*, 380–387. [CrossRef]
48. Alhnan, M.A.; Okwuosa, T.C.; Sadia, M.; Wan, K.W.; Ahmed, W.; Arafat, B. Emergence of 3D Printed Dosage Forms: Opportunities and Challenges. *Pharm. Res.* **2016**, *33*, 1817–1832. [CrossRef]
49. Goyanes, A.; Buanz, A.B.M.; Hatton, G.B.; Gaisford, S.; Basit, A.W. 3D printing of modified-release aminosalicylate (4-ASA and 5-ASA) tablets. *Eur. J. Pharm. Biopharm.* **2015**, *89*, 157–162. [CrossRef]
50. Gardan, J. Additive manufacturing technologies: State of the art and trends. *Int. J. Prod. Res.* **2016**, *54*, 3118–3132. [CrossRef]
51. Vitale, A.; Cabral, J. Frontal Conversion and Uniformity in 3D Printing by Photopolymerisation. *Materials* **2016**, *9*, 760. [CrossRef]
52. Wang, J.; Goyanes, A.; Gaisford, S.; Basit, A.W. Stereolithographic (SLA) 3D printing of oral modified-release dosage forms. *Int. J. Pharm.* **2016**, *503*, 207–212. [CrossRef] [PubMed]
53. Martinez, P.R.; Goyanes, A.; Basit, A.W.; Gaisford, S. Fabrication of drug-loaded hydrogels with stereolithographic 3D printing. *Int. J. Pharm.* **2017**, *532*, 313–317. [CrossRef] [PubMed]
54. Martinez, P.R.; Goyanes, A.; Basit, A.W.; Gaisford, S. Influence of Geometry on the Drug Release Profiles of Stereolithographic (SLA) 3D-Printed Tablets. *AAPS PharmSciTech* **2018**. [CrossRef] [PubMed]
55. Fadda, H.M.; Merchant, H.A.; Arafat, B.T.; Basit, A.W. Physiological bicarbonate buffers: Stabilisation and use as dissolution media for modified release systems. *Int. J. Pharm.* **2009**, *382*, 56–60. [CrossRef] [PubMed]
56. Liu, F.; Merchant, H.A.; Kulkarni, R.P.; Alkademi, M.; Basit, A.W. Evolution of a physiological pH6.8 bicarbonate buffer system: Application to the dissolution testing of enteric coated products. *Eur. J. Pharm. Biopharm.* **2011**, *78*, 151–157. [CrossRef]
57. Goyanes, A.; Hatton, G.B.; Basit, A.W. A dynamic in vitro model to evaluate the intestinal release behaviour of modified-release corticosteroid products. *J. Drug Deliv. Sci. Technol.* **2015**, *25*, 36–42. [CrossRef]

58. Goyanes, A.; Hatton, G.B.; Merchant, H.A.; Basit, A.W. Gastrointestinal release behaviour of modified-release drug products: Dynamic dissolution testing of mesalazine formulations. *Int. J. Pharm.* **2015**, *484*, 103–108. [CrossRef]
59. Merchant, H.A.; Frost, J.A.; Basit, A.W. Apparatus and Method for Testing Medicaments. U.S. Patent 15/392,113, 20 April 2014.
60. Merchant, H.A.; Goyanes, A.; Parashar, N.; Basit, A.W. Predicting the gastrointestinal behaviour of modified-release products: Utility of a novel dynamic dissolution test apparatus involving the use of bicarbonate buffers. *Int. J. Pharm.* **2014**, *475*, 585–591. [CrossRef]
61. Trenfield, S.J.; Goyanes, A.; Telford, R.; Wilsdon, D.; Rowland, M.; Gaisford, S.; Basit, A.W. 3D printed drug products: Non-destructive dose verification using a rapid point-and-shoot approach. *Int. J. Pharm.* **2018**, *549*, 283–292. [CrossRef]
62. Yonemochi, E.; Sano, S.; Yoshihashi, Y.; Terada, K. Diffusivity of amorphous drug in solid dispersion. *J. Therm. Anal. Calorim.* **2013**, *113*, 1505–1510. [CrossRef]
63. Corcione, C. Development and Characterization of Novel Photopolymerizable Formulations for Stereolithography. *J. Polym. Eng.* **2014**, *34*, 85–93. [CrossRef]
64. Rao, V.M.; Haslam, J.L.; Stella, V.J. Controlled and complete release of a model poorly water-soluble drug, prednisolone, from hydroxypropyl methylcellulose matrix tablets using (SBE)7m-β-cyclodextrin as a solubilizing agent. *J. Pharm. Sci.* **2001**, *90*, 807–816. [CrossRef] [PubMed]
65. Di Colo, G.; Baggiani, A.; Zambito, Y.; Mollica, G.; Geppi, M.; Serafini, M.F. A new hydrogel for the extended and complete prednisolone release in the GI tract. *Int. J. Pharm.* **2006**, *310*, 154–161. [CrossRef] [PubMed]

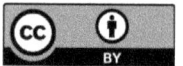

© 2019 by the authors. Licensee MDPI, Basel, Switzerland. This article is an open access article distributed under the terms and conditions of the Creative Commons Attribution (CC BY) license (http://creativecommons.org/licenses/by/4.0/).

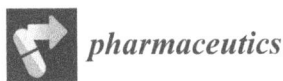

Article

3D Printed Pellets (Miniprintlets): A Novel, Multi-Drug, Controlled Release Platform Technology

Atheer Awad [1], Fabrizio Fina [1], Sarah J. Trenfield [1], Pavanesh Patel [1], Alvaro Goyanes [2,3,*], Simon Gaisford [1,2] and Abdul W. Basit [1,2,*]

1. Department of Pharmaceutics, UCL School of Pharmacy, University College London, 29-39 Brunswick Square, London WC1N 1AX, UK; atheer.awad.15@ucl.ac.uk (A.A.); fabrizio.fina.14@ucl.ac.uk (F.F.); sarah.trenfield.16@ucl.ac.uk (S.J.T.); pavanesh.patel.14@ucl.ac.uk (P.P.); s.gaisford@ucl.ac.uk (S.G.)
2. FabRx Ltd., 3 Romney Road, Ashford, Kent TN24 0RW, UK
3. Departamento de Farmacología, Farmacia y Tecnología Farmacéutica, R + D Pharma Group (GI-1645), Universidade de Santiago de Compostela, 15782 Santiago de Compostela, Spain
* Correspondence: a.goyanes@fabrx.co.uk (A.G.); a.basit@ucl.ac.uk (A.W.B.)

Received: 3 February 2019; Accepted: 25 March 2019; Published: 29 March 2019

Abstract: Selective laser sintering (SLS) is a single-step three-dimensional printing (3DP) process that can be leveraged to engineer a wide array of drug delivery systems. The aim of this work was to utilise SLS 3DP, for the first time, to produce small oral dosage forms with modified release properties. As such, paracetamol-loaded 3D printed multiparticulates, termed miniprintlets, were fabricated in 1 mm and 2 mm diameters. Despite their large surface area compared with a conventional monolithic tablet, the ethyl cellulose-based miniprintlets exhibited prolonged drug release patterns. The possibility of producing miniprintlets combining two drugs, namely paracetamol and ibuprofen, was also investigated. By varying the polymer, the dual miniprintlets were programmed to achieve customised drug release patterns, whereby one drug was released immediately from a Kollicoat Instant Release matrix, whilst the effect of the second drug was sustained over an extended time span using ethyl cellulose. Herein, this work has highlighted the versatility of SLS 3DP to fabricate small and intricate formulations containing multiple active pharmaceutical ingredients with distinct release properties.

Keywords: three dimensional printing; additive manufacturing; 3D printed drug products; printlets; personalised medicines; personalized pharmaceuticals; multiple units; spheroids; beads; acetaminophen

---

1. Introduction

Three-dimensional printing (3DP) is a revolutionary additive manufacturing technology that can transform 3D designs into real objects by sequential layering [1]. Its applications are broad, ranging from aviation and automobiles to human organs and implants [2,3]. Unlike conventional production methods, 3DP has the capability to accurately distribute materials, facilitating the production of medications with individualised doses [4,5] and polypills with multiple active pharmaceutical ingredients (APIs), wherein each drug can be placed in a different layer [6] or compartment [7]. In addition, this technology can create highly precise dosage forms with varying shapes [8] and sizes [9,10], enabling the local delivery of drugs to specified organs [11–13] and offering versatile drug release modes [14,15]. Within healthcare, 3DP is forecast to transition medication production from centralised facilities to decentralised spaces, such as clinics, hospitals and local pharmacies [16,17]. More specifically, this technique could be implemented as a digitised production tool for the remote design, development and dispensing of bespoke medications optimised to each patient's needs [18,19].

Selective laser sintering (SLS) is a rapid 3DP process that offers a one-step, solvent-free method for production [20,21]. This technology utilises a laser beam to selectively bind powdered materials together to produce 3D objects in a layered manner [22]. To date, SLS has shown great flexibility, enabling it to fabricate a wide array of dosage forms, with different shapes [23] and release characteristics ranging from orally-disintegrating tablets [24] to immediate and modified release dosage forms [25]. The high precision of the laser permits the printing of very detailed lattice structures with controllable internal architectures, which are otherwise impossible to produce using conventional production methods [26–28]. The high resolution of the SLS 3DP system may render this technology suitable for the preparation of multiparticulate drug delivery systems.

Compared with single-unit dosage forms, multiparticulate systems offer a more attractive means for dosing flexibility, with additional therapeutic benefits to the patients [29]. As an example, multiple-unit dosage forms can be divided into desired doses without necessitating alteration of the formulation or manufacturing process. They also have a more reproducible and predictable journey through the gastrointestinal tract. For example, the spreading of multi-unit medicines means that the formulation will be more exposed to fluids during its transit; thus, multiparticulates are free to disperse in the gastrointestinal tract, which can maximise drug release and drug absorption. Moreover, in the presence of food, the gastric emptying of these systems is considered to be more uniform when compared to single-oral dosage units [30]. Furthermore, given that recent studies have shown that some dosage forms, having a similar size to enteric coated size 9 capsules, do not actually empty from the stomach of small rodents [31], the use of multiparticulate systems provides a clear advantage over other pharmaceutical products. As such, these dosage forms are suited for administration to various animal species, where they can be printed in dimensions and doses personalised to the model, making them applicable throughout the whole drug development pathway.

An important challenge in formulating small dosage forms lies in the difficulty of controlling the drug release from the polymeric matrices and the low drug loading potential in comparison with conventional manufacturing processes [32]. A potential benefit of the SLS technology lies in its laser sintering process, which fuses the drug and polymer particles together, producing a strong coherence between the particles and sustaining the drug release from the molten matrix. Moreover, the high resolution of the laser beam enables the printing of very small and detailed units. In fact, the additive nature of the process offers the advantage of higher control over the composition and content distribution within the printed formulations, which in turn may render this technology highly accurate and reproducible, enabling it to produce multi-drug iterations with distinct and uniform dosing. The discrete separation of the APIs resolves problems associated with compatibility and physical interaction, which are a major setback in most multi-drug formulations. More notably, the ease of preparation of the SLS feedstock makes the overall process quick, user-friendly and economical.

Hence, the aim of this study was to investigate the suitability of SLS 3DP for manufacturing small dosage forms with modified release properties, herein termed miniprintlets. Paracetamol-loaded miniprintlets with sustained drug release kinetics were created in two different sizes (1 mm and 2 mm in diameter), to evaluate the effect of changing the size on in vitro dissolution. SLS was further used for the dual printing of miniprintlets with two rate-controlling systems incorporating two model drugs, paracetamol and ibuprofen. To our knowledge, this work is the first to report the engineering of such small and intricate 3D printed formulations containing multiple APIs with distinct release properties.

2. Materials and Methods

Paracetamol USP grade (MW 151.16 g/mol, solubility in water at 37 °C: 21.80 g/L) and ibuprofen (sodium salt; MW 228.26 g/mol, solubility in water: 100 g/L) (both from Sigma-Aldrich, Poole, UK) were used as model drugs. Ethyl cellulose N7 was obtained from Ashland, Schaffhausen, Switzerland and Kollicoat Instant Release (IR) was obtained from BASF, Ludwigshafen, Germany. Candurin Gold Sheen was purchased from Merck, Darmstadt, Germany. The salts for preparing the buffer dissolution media were purchased from VWR International Ltd., Leicestershire, UK.

2.1. Printing Process

All the powders were sieved using a 150 µm sieve prior to their use to permit a better flow of the powder particles in the chamber, resulting in a better printing procedure [33]. For all the formulations, 100 g of a mixture of drug and excipients were blended using a mortar and pestle (Table 1). 3% Candurin Gold Sheen was added to the formulations to enhance energy absorption from the laser and aid printability. The single miniprintlets were loaded with 5% paracetamol, whereas the dual miniprintlets contained 6.5% paracetamol and 3.5% ibuprofen, which is the ratio at which combinations containing these drugs tend to be at. Powder mixtures were transferred to a desktop SLS printer (Sintratec Kit, AG, Brugg, Switzerland) to fabricate the oral dosage formulations. 123D Design (Version 14.2.2, Autodesk Inc., San Rafael, CA, USA) was used to design the templates of the spherical miniprintlets (1 mm and 2 mm in diameter). The 3D models were exported as a stereolithography (.stl) file into the 3D printer Sintratec central software (Version 1.1.13, Sintratec, AG, Brugg, Switzerland). The dual miniprintlets consisted of two distinct regions, wherein the one region had immediate release properties and the other region exhibited sustained release (Figure 1). As such, to prevent the mixing of the two powders and permit precise control over the content of each region, the reservoir platform was kept empty and instead, the powders were manually added to the building platform before the start of each layer. From our observation, the manual addition of the powder slightly lengthened the printing process, as the freshly added layer required additional heating prior to the start of the printing. The dual miniprintlets were fabricated in two different configurations; in configuration A (Con A), paracetamol was mixed with Kollicoat IR (Par/KIR region) and ibuprofen was with ethyl cellulose (Ibu/EC region). Comparatively, in configuration B (Con B), the positions of the drugs were switched and paracetamol was mixed with ethyl cellulose (Par/EC region), whilst ibuprofen was with Kollicoat IR (Ibu/KIR region).

Table 1. Compositions of the single and dual miniprintlets.

Miniprintlets *	Paracetamol (Par)	Ibuprofen (Ibu)	Kollicoat Instant Release (KIR)	Ethyl Cellulose (EC)
Single	5%	-	-	92%
Dual–Con A				
Par/KIR	6.5%	-	56.5%	-
Ibu/EC	-	3.5%	-	30.5%
Dual–Con B				
Ibu/KIR	-	3.5%	30.5%	-
Par/EC	6.5%	-	-	56.5%

* All formulations contain 3% w/w Candurin® Gold Sheen.

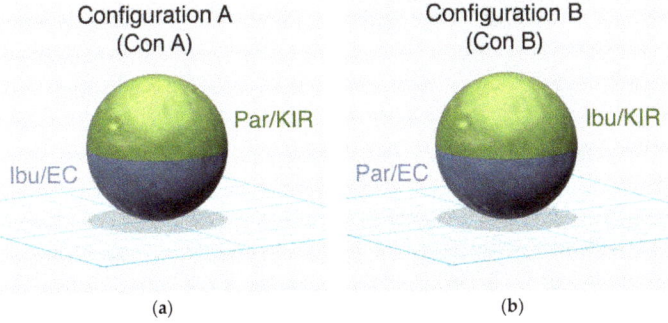

Figure 1. Schematic representation of the compositions of (**a**) configuration A and (**b**) configuration B of the dual miniprintlets.

Powder in the reservoir platform (150 mm × 30 mm × 150 mm) of the printer was moved to the building platform (150 mm × 30 mm × 150 mm) by a sled, producing a flat and homogeneously distributed layer of powder. The chamber and surface printing temperatures for all the miniprintlets were 100 °C and 120 °C, respectively. A 2.3 W blue diode laser (445 nm), with a scanning speed of 50 mm/s, was activated to sinter the powder on to the building platform based on the STL file. At this point, the reservoir platform moved up, the building platform moved down, and the sled distributed a thin layer of powder on top of the previous layer. This process was repeated layer-by-layer until the object was completed. The powder was then removed from the chamber and sieved using a 710 μm sieve to recover the miniprintlets. For each batch, 100 miniprintlets were printed at a time. Before the start of printing, the printer required ~10 min to warm up the platforms; the time was, however, reduced to 2–3 min in successive printing jobs, as the printer was able to maintain the heat within its chamber.

2.2. Thermal Analysis

Differential scanning calorimetry (DSC) was used to characterise the powders and the drug-loaded miniprintlets. DSC measurements were performed with a Q2000 DSC (TA instruments—Waters LLC, New Castle, DE, USA) at a temperature range of 0 °C to 200 °C and a heating rate of 10 °C/min. Calibration for cell constant and enthalpy was performed with indium (T_m = 156.6 °C, ΔH_f = 28.71 J/g), according to the manufacturer's instructions. Nitrogen was used as a purge gas with a flow rate of 50 mL/min for all the experiments. Data were collected with TA Advantage software for Q series (Version 2.8.394) and analysed using TA Instruments Universal Analysis 2000 (TA instruments—Waters LLC, New Castle, DE, USA). All melting temperatures are reported as extrapolated onset unless otherwise stated. TA aluminium pans and lids (Tzero) were used with an average sample mass of 3–5 mg.

For thermogravimetric analysis (TGA), average samples of 8–10 mg of raw drugs, polymers and powder mixtures were heated at a temperature range of 50 °C to 500 °C and a heating rate of 10 °C/min in open aluminium pans using a Discovery TGA (TA instruments—Waters LLC, New Castle, DE, USA). Nitrogen, at a flow rate of 25 mL/min, was used as a purge gas. Data were collected and analysed using TA Instruments Trios software (Version 4.5.0.5), where the percentage mass loss with respect to temperature was calculated.

2.3. X-ray Powder Diffraction (XRPD)

Discs of 23 mm diameter × 1 mm height made from the mixtures of drugs and excipients were 3D printed and analysed. Samples of pure drugs, polymers and powder mixtures were also analysed. The X-ray powder diffraction patterns were obtained in a Rigaku MiniFlex 600 (Rigaku, Wilmington, MA, USA) using a Cu Kα X-ray source (λ = 1.5418 Å). The intensity and voltage applied were 15 mA and 40 kV, respectively. The angular range of data acquisition was 3–40° 2θ, with a stepwise size of 0.02° at a speed of 2°/min.

2.4. Characterisation of the Miniprintlets

2.4.1. Determination of the Miniprintlets Morphology

The diameter of the miniprintlets was measured using a digital caliper. For the weight and diameter measurements, 5 and 10 miniprintlets were used, respectively, from each formulation. For the diameter measurements, the average of the longest and shortest distances was used for each miniprintlet.

2.4.2. Scanning Electron Microscopy (SEM)

Surface images of the 2 mm miniprintlets were taken with a scanning electron microscope (SEM, JSM-840A Scanning Microscope, JEOL GmbH, Freising, Germany). All samples for SEM testing were coated with carbon (~30–40 nm).

2.4.3. X-ray Micro Computed Tomography (Micro-CT)

A high-resolution X-ray micro computed tomography (Micro-CT) scanner (SkyScan1172, Bruker-microCT, Kontich, Belgium) was used to three-dimensionally visualise the internal structure and calculate the density of the miniprintlets. In this study, 2 mm dual miniprintlets were scanned with a resolution of 2000 × 1048 pixels. 3D imaging was performed by rotating the object through 180° with steps of 0.4° and four images were recorded for each of those. Image reconstruction was performed using NRecon software (Version 1.7.0.4, Bruker-microCT) and 3D model rendering and viewing were performed using the associate program CT-Volume software (Version 2.3.2.0). The collected data were analysed using Analyzer (Version 1.16.4.1), where maps of different colours were used to represent the density of the miniprintlets.

2.4.4. Determination of Drug Content

In total, 20–25 mg of miniprintlets from each size were placed in separate volumetric flasks containing 10 mL of methanol. For the dual miniprintlets, single miniprintlets consisting of the individualised composition of each region were printed using the same parameters and were used for the drug content testing. Miniprintlets consisting of Kollicoat IR were dissolved in 10 mL of water, whereas the miniprintlets consisting of ethyl cellulose were dissolved in 10 mL of methanol. Samples of solution were then filtered through 0.22 µm filters (Millipore Ltd., Cork, Ireland) and the drug concentrations were determined with high-performance liquid chromatography (HPLC) (Hewlett Packard 1050 Series HPLC system, Agilent Technologies, Cheshire, UK). The validated HPLC assay entailed injecting 20 µL samples for analysis, using a mobile phase with a gradient elution system of (A) acetonitrile and (B) 0.1% formic acid in distilled water, through an Eclipse plus C18 3.5 µm column, 4.6 × 100 mm (Zorbax, Agilent technologies, Cheshire, UK), maintained at 40 °C. The mobile phase was pumped at a flow rate of 1 mL/min under the following gradient program: 0–2 min, 15% A; 2–8 min, 15–55% A; 8–25 min, 55% A; 25–26 min, 55–15% A. The eluents were screened at a wavelength of 230 nm, where the retention times for paracetamol and ibuprofen were 2.57 min and 14.36 min, respectively. The tests were done in triplicate.

2.5. In-Vitro Dissolution Testing

Drug dissolution profiles for the miniprintlets were obtained with a USP-II apparatus (Pharmatest PTWS 100, Haiburg, Germany): (1) 250 mg of miniprintlets were placed within in-house sinkers and dissolved in 750 mL of 0.1 M HCl for 2 h to simulate gastric residence time, and (2) were then transferred into 950 mL of modified Hanks (mHanks) bicarbonate physiological medium for 35 min (pH 5.6 to 7); (3) and in modified Krebs buffer (1000 mL) (pH 7 to 7.4 and then to 6.5). The modified Hanks buffer-based dissolution medium [34] (136.9 mM NaCl, 5.37 mM KCl, 0.812 mM $MgSO_4.7H_2O$, 1.26 mM $CaCl_2$, 0.337 mM $Na_2HPO_4.2H_2O$, 0.441 mM KH_2PO_4, 4.17 mM $NaHCO_3$) forms an in-situ modified Kreb's buffer [35] through the addition of 50 mL of pre-Krebs solution (400.7 mM $NaHCO_3$ and 6.9 mM KH_2PO_4) to each dissolution vessel.

The miniprintlets were tested in the small intestinal environment for 3.5 h (pH 5.6 to 7.4) [36]. The medium is primarily a bicarbonate buffer in which bicarbonate (HCO_3^-) and carbonic acid (H_2CO_3) co-exist in equilibrium, along with CO_2 (aq) resulting from dissociation of the carbonic acid. The pH of the buffer is controlled by an Auto pH System^{TM} [37,38], which consists of a pH probe connected to a source of carbon dioxide gas (pH-reducing gas), as well as to a supply of helium (pH-increasing gas), controlled by a control unit. The control unit is able to provide a dynamically adjustable pH during testing (dynamic conditions) and to maintain a uniform pH value over the otherwise unstable bicarbonate buffer pH. The paddle speed of the USP-II was fixed at 50 rpm and the tests were conducted at 37 ± 0.5 °C (n = 3). The percentage of drug released from the miniprintlets was determined using HPLC, as described in Section 2.4.4.

3. Results and Discussion

SLS 3DP was successfully utilised to create miniprintlets in two different diameters, 1 mm and 2 mm. Paracetamol was employed as the model drug and ethyl cellulose was employed as the main polymer matrix. A laser scanning speed of 50 mm/s was selected because it was found to provide enough energy for the effective bonding of consecutive printing layers, while maintaining the desired shape and dimensions of the miniprintlets. The time needed to print one batch of 100 miniprintlets of 1 mm was ~2 min, whereas the time need to print one batch of 2 mm miniprintlets was ~2 min and 40 s.

Dual miniprintlets for multi-drug therapy were also fabricated, incorporating paracetamol and ibuprofen in different layers. Like the single miniprintlets, the dual miniprintlets were printed in two different sizes, 1 mm and 2 mm. The dual miniprintlets were prepared in two different configurations, wherein one drug was dispersed in Kollicoat IR, a polyvinyl alcohol/polyethylene glycol graft copolymer with immediate release characteristics, and the other drug was dispersed in ethyl cellulose. Paracetamol and ibuprofen were selected as model drugs since previous studies have shown that the combination of both drugs has a greater synergistic efficacy compared with their individual use [39,40]. The time needed to print one batch of 100 dual miniprintlets of 1 mm was ~2 min and 30 s, whereas for 2 mm miniprintlets, it was ~3 min and 40 s. The time is slightly higher than for the single miniprintlets due to the manual addition of the powders, which required additional surface heating.

Despite their small sizes, all the miniprintlets showed high uniformity in weight and diameter (Table 2). Generally, the 1 mm miniprintlets displayed a higher precision in weight when compared to the 2 mm miniprintlets. In terms of diameter, the dual miniprintlets appeared to have more precise values, wherein Con B has been shown to be more accurate when compared to theoretical diameter measurements. The 1 mm single miniprintlets, on the other hand, had the least precise and accurate readings.

Table 2. Characteristics of the miniprintlets (SD—standard deviation).

Miniprintlets	Weight (mg ± SD)	Diameter (mm ± SD)	Paracetamol Content (% ± SD)	Ibuprofen Content (% ± SD)
Single				
1 mm	0.84 ± 0.03	1.14 ± 0.06	101.1 ± 0.5	-
2 mm	3.90 ± 0.13	1.99 ± 0.06	96.9 ± 0.2	-
Dual–Con A				
1 mm	0.67 ± 0.03	1.04 ± 0.02	100.1 ± 1.5 *	99.4 ± 1.0 *
2 mm	4.27 ± 0.15	2.03 ± 0.02	98.5 ± 1.5 *	99.6 ± 1.4 *
Dual–Con B				
1 mm	0.50 ± 0.02	1.01 ± 0.04	99.2 ± 0.2 *	98.3 ± 1.1 *
2 mm	4.10 ± 0.08	2.00 ± 0.03	96.6 ± 0.5 *	100.2 ± 1.5 *

* The following values were calculated by printing single miniprintlets with compositions identical to the corresponding region being tested.

HPLC analysis showed that the drug content values were in agreement with the theoretical drug loadings in all the miniprintlets, confirming that no significant drug loss occurred during the printing process (Table 2), thus confirming the high accuracy and reproducibility of the SLS process. TGA data of the drugs, polymers and powder mixtures predicted that all the components would remain stable and no degradation of the drugs and excipients was likely to occur at the printing temperatures (≤ 120 °C) (Figure 2).

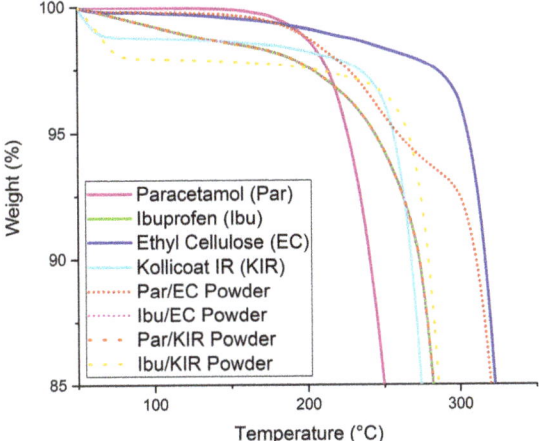

Figure 2. Thermogravimetric analysis (TGA) results of the raw drugs, polymers and powders prior to printing.

DSC and XRPD analysis of the drug, polymers and powder mixtures prior to printing, and of the miniprintlets, were performed to determine the physical state of the drugs and the degree of their incorporation within the polymers (Figures 3 and 4). Before printing, the DSC data showed that the raw paracetamol powder exhibited a melting endotherm at approximately 168 °C, indicative of form I [41]. The raw ibuprofen powder exhibited a broad endotherm at 100 °C, indicative of dehydration, and a sharp melting endotherm at approximately 200 °C, indicative of a racemic conglomerate, which melts at 199 °C [42]. The DSC data of the Par/EC miniprintlets showed a small melting endotherm at approximately 168 °C, demonstrating that paracetamol still exists in its crystalline form. The Par/KIR, Ibu/EC and Ibu/KIR miniprintlets, on the other hand, showed no evidence of melting endotherms, indicating that the drugs are either molecularly dispersed within the polymers or dissolved within the polymers as the temperature increases during the DSC process. Corroborating with the results obtained by DSC, the X-ray diffractograms of the Par/EC discs demonstrated that paracetamol was partially crystalline in the miniprintlets (Figure 4b). For Par/KIR, paracetamol showed less crystalline peaks in the printed discs, indicating that it had been converted to an amorphous state (Figure 4a). Interestingly, the Par/KIR and Ibu/KIR discs showed an increase in crystalline peaks, attributed to Kollicoat IR, which could be due to its exposure to heat during the sintering process [43].

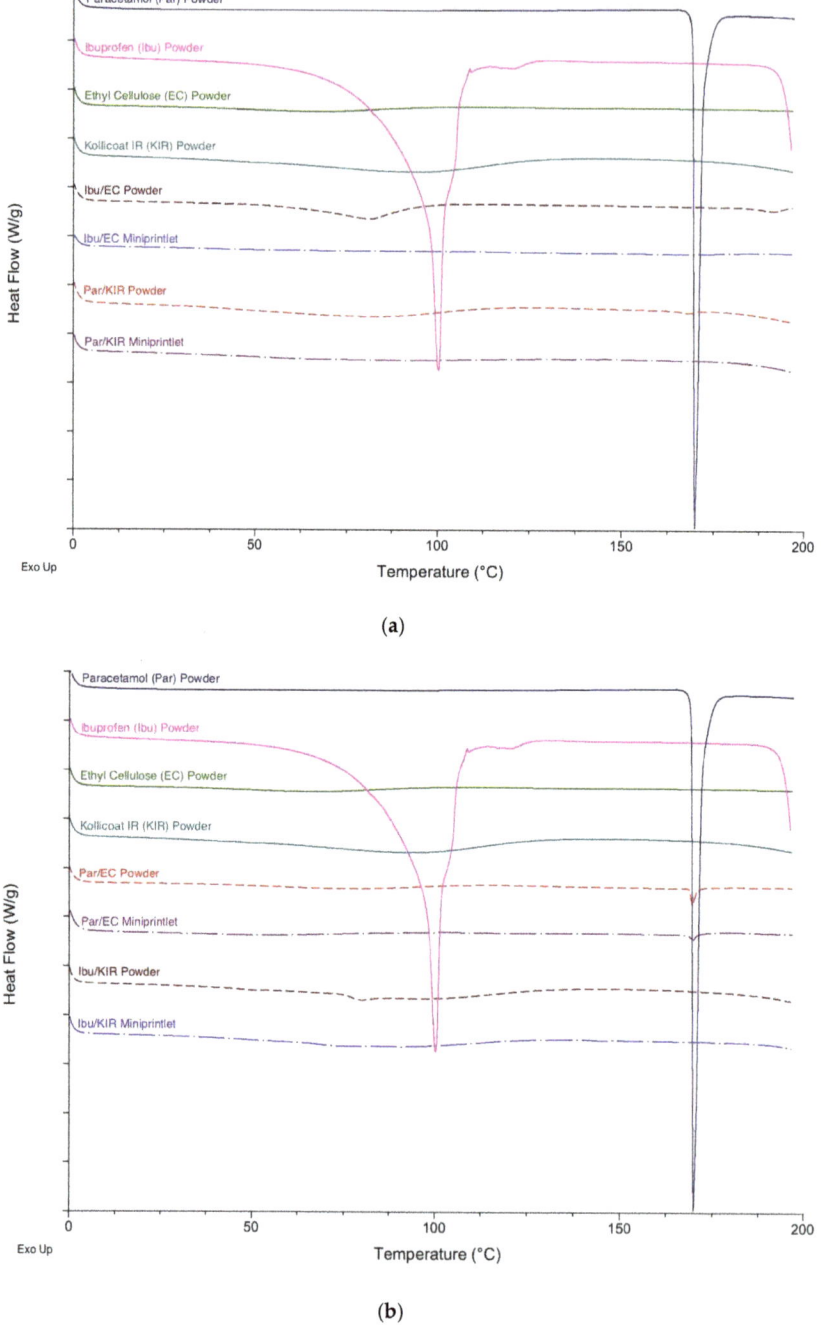

Figure 3. Differential scanning calorimetry (DSC) thermograms of the pure drugs, polymers and powder mixture prior to printing and the miniprintlets used in (**a**) Con A and (**b**) Con B of the dual miniprintlets.

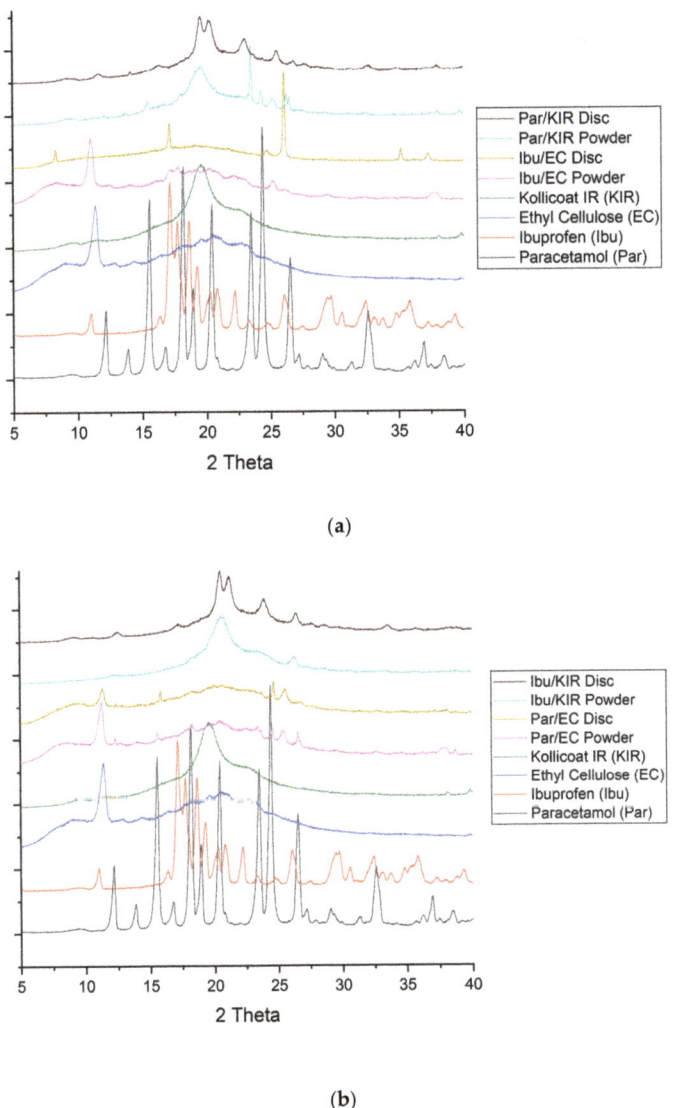

Figure 4. X-ray diffractograms of the drugs-excipients prior to printing and the 3D printed discs used in (**a**) Con A and (**b**) Con B of the dual miniprintlets.

X-ray micro-CT was used to visualise the 3D structures of the dual miniprintlets (Figure 5). A clear distinction between the two sections can be seen in both configurations, confirming that the two drug regions did not mix during the printing process. The Kollicoat IR regions were denser than the ethyl cellulose regions and are shown in a yellow colour in the images, whereas the ethyl cellulose regions had a dark purple colour. SEM images of the miniprintlets validate the micro-CT results and provide visual confirmation of the differences of the laser effect on the two polymers, even though the same sintering parameters were used (Figure 6). The image of the single miniprintlet shows that ethyl cellulose undergoes a more intense sintering process, where less particles are seen on the surface (Figure 6a). The Con A dual miniprintlets, on the other hand, show two distinct regions, including a molten Ibu/EC region and a Par/KIR sintered region (Figure 6b). As such, it can be concluded that Kollicoat IR undergoes a low intensity sintering process, and thus, a higher space volume between the particles was formed and spherical polymer particles can be distinctively observed on the surface. This can be explained by the difference in the particle shape of each polymer, wherein the Kollicoat IR particles were round, causing them to have less surface area available for contact with nearby particles. On the other hand, the ethyl cellulose particles had irregular, flaky shapes with higher surface area in contact with surrounding particles (Figure 6). The Con B dual miniprintlets also showed two distinct regions, wherein the Ibu/KIR region had bigger round particles indicative of Kollicoat IR and the Par/EC region had irregular particles indicative of paracetamol.

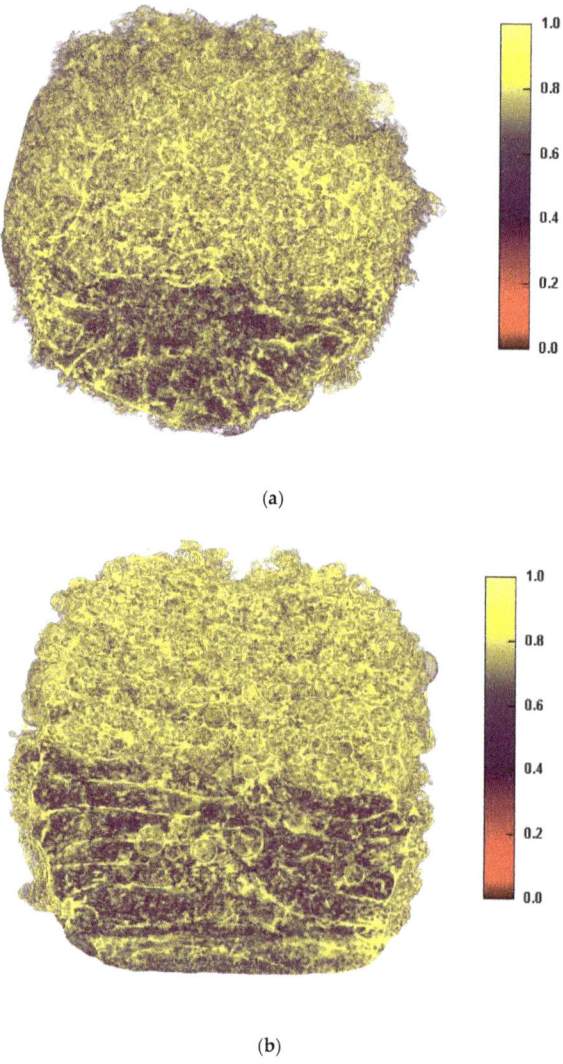

Figure 5. Cross-sectional x-ray micro computed tomography (CT) images of (**a**) Con A and (**b**) Con B of the 2 mm dual miniprintlets. The yellow regions represent the Kollicoat Instant Release (KIR) regions, whereas the dark purple regions are the ethyl cellulose (EC) regions. The scale bar is representative of density.

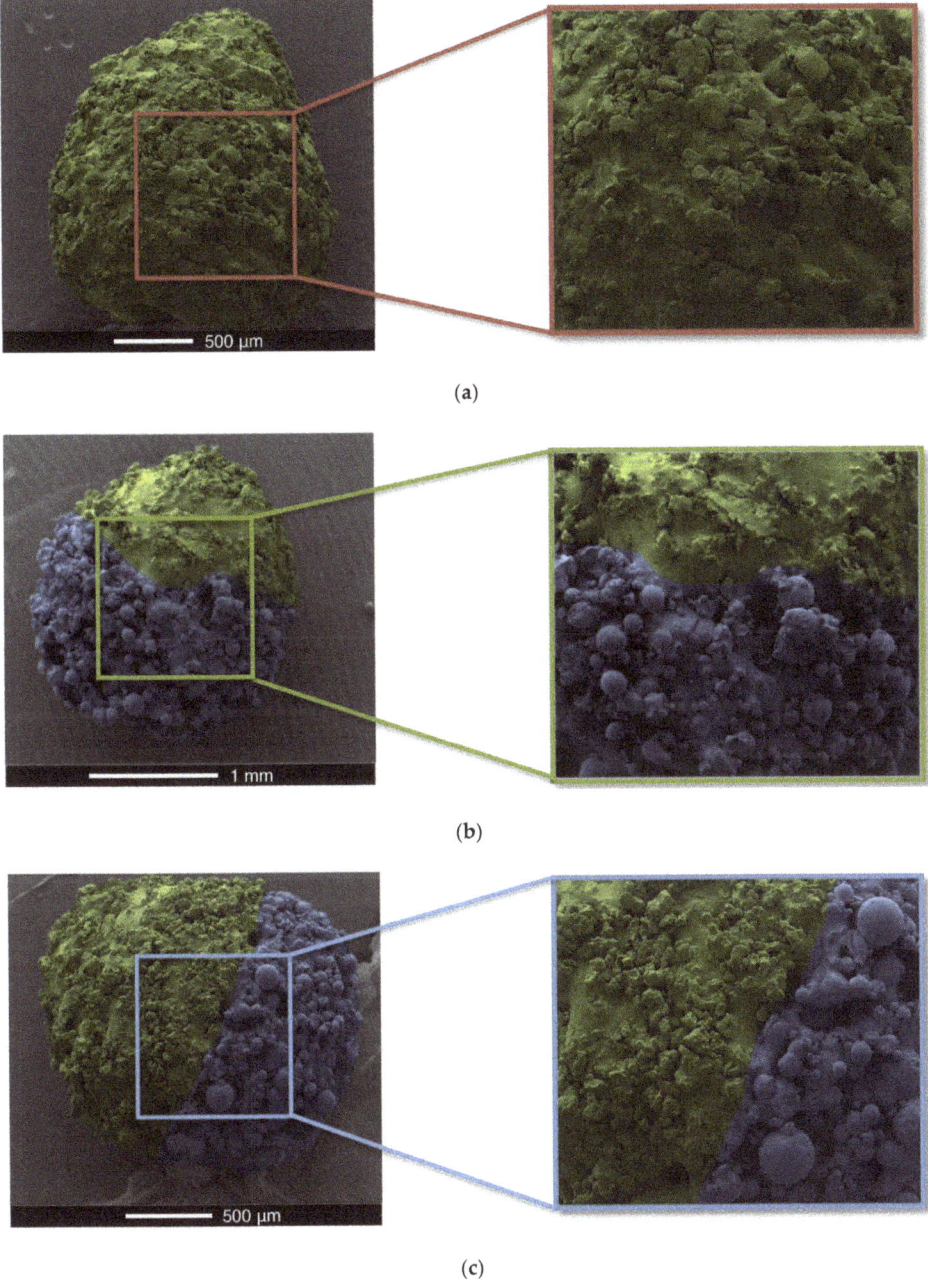

Figure 6. Scanning electron microscopy (SEM) images of the 2 mm (**a**) single miniprintlet, and (**b**) Con A and (**c**) Con B of the dual miniprintlets. The yellow regions represent the EC regions, whereas the blue regions represent the KIR regions.

Drug dissolution profiles from the miniprintlets were obtained using a dynamic in vitro model, which simulates gastric and intestinal conditions of the gastrointestinal tract (Figure 7) [44]. Despite their larger surface area compared with large monolithic systems, all of the single miniprintlets exhibited sustained and slow paracetamol release, with a drug release of 88% and 61% from the 1 mm and 2 mm miniprintlets, respectively, after 24 h (Figure 7a). As expected, the drug release rate from the miniprintlets was reduced when increasing the diameter. In a previous study, ethyl cellulose has shown very slow release, where only 20% paracetamol was released after 24 h from cylindrical printlets [26]. As such, this shows that the miniprintlets are more suited as a drug delivery platform for SLS printing using ethyl cellulose as the main polymer matrix. Indeed, this can be correlated to the increased surface area resulting from the reduction in diameter of the respective miniprintlets.

In the dual miniprintlets incorporating two drugs, interestingly, the release profile of paracetamol from the Par/EC region of the 2 mm dual miniprintlets was similar to the 1 mm single miniprintlets, further highlighting that the addition of another region does not affect the original release of the drug and that the two regions maintain their distinct release properties. Regarding Kollicoat IR, owing to the immediate release properties of the polymer, paracetamol was completely released from the Par/KIR region of the Con A dual miniprintlets within 30 min. Additionally, 20% and 15% ibuprofen was released from the Ibu/EC region of the 1 mm and 2 mm Con A dual miniprintlets within the first 2 h, respectively, from the EC layer (Figure 7b). These percentages are probably lower than that of the Par/EC region due to the low solubility of ibuprofen in acidic medium. After being exposed to intestinal conditions (pH 5.6–7.4), acceleration in the dissolution rate was observed, wherein 91% and 79% ibuprofen was released from the 1 mm and 2 mm Con A dual miniprintlets within 24 h, respectively. A similar effect caused by the low drug solubility in acidic medium was seen in the behaviour of Ibu/KIR formulations (Con B), where only 15% and 10% of the drug was released from the 1 mm and 2 mm dual miniprintlets in the first 2 h, respectively (Figure 7c). Once exposed to intestinal conditions, the drug was completely released within 5 min. Par/EC, on the other hand, behaved differently, whereby 50% and 46% was released in the acidic medium from the 1 mm and 2 mm Con B dual miniprintlets, respectively. Under intestinal conditions, a sustained effect was observed, where 99% and 84% of paracetamol was released from the 1 mm and 2 mm Con B dual miniprintlets after 24 h, respectively.

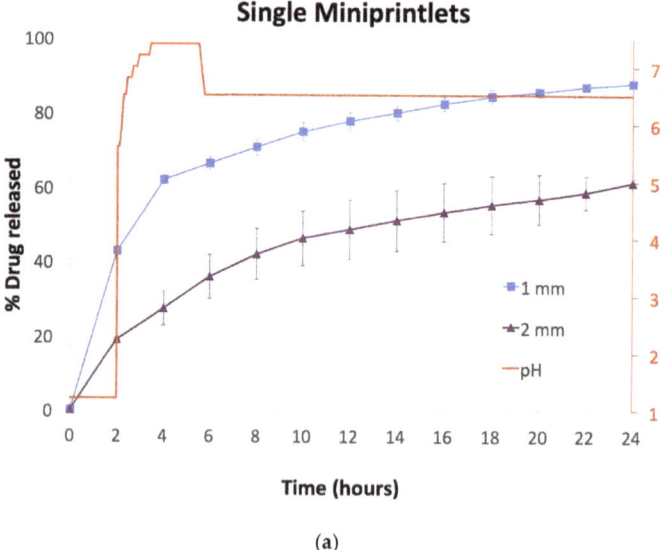

(a)

Figure 7. Cont.

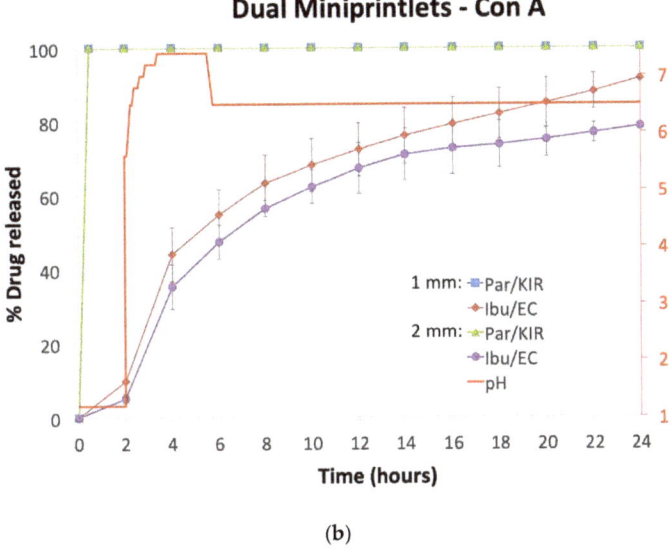

(b)

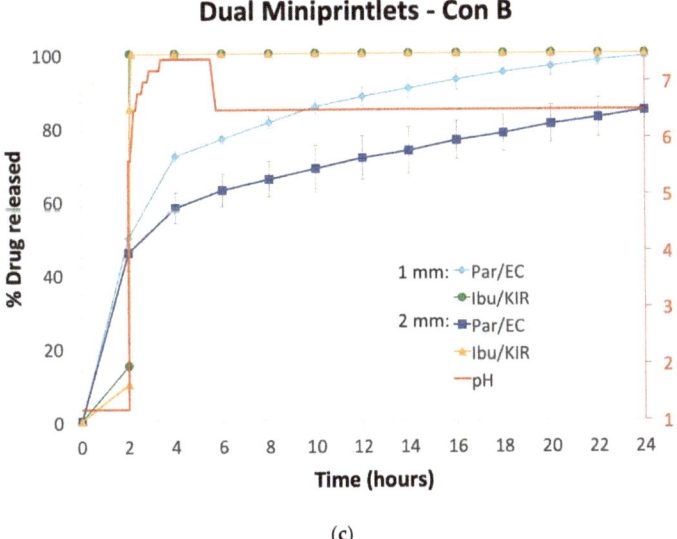

(c)

Figure 7. Drug dissolution profiles of the (**a**) single miniprintlets, and (**b**) Con A and (**c**) Con B of the dual miniprintlets. The red line shows the pH values of the media under acidic conditions for 2 h, followed by intestinal conditions using dynamic dissolution apparatus.

Conventionally, the production of controlled release multiparticulate systems has been achieved through the use of extrusion-spheronisation and coating [45]. However, this is a multi-step process that is time-consuming and costly, requiring dedicated equipment. Conversely, the SLS technology is a single process that sinters powder particles together using a laser sintering process. As such, the strong coherence between the drug particles and the polymer matrix results in a more sustained release and reduces the amount of drug initially released. Moreover, the use of a slow laser scanning speed increases the duration of the effect of the laser on the powder, allowing more energy to be transmitted, resulting in a higher degree of sintering and consequently sustaining the drug release [46,47]. Unlike coating, damage to the surface of the miniprintlets does not affect their release properties, as the drugs are uniformly dispersed in a matrix structure and are not covered by a protective layer. Moreover, in the case of coating, the drug release becomes generally fast once the coating ruptures or dissolves, whereas in this matrix system, the drug release remains constant [48]. This can be explained by the insoluble nature of ethyl cellulose, whereby the drug molecules diffuse through the matrix. Compared with a single-unit dosage form, risks of dose-dumping and peak plasma fluctuations are minimised with this multiparticulate system, as each miniprintlet acts as a separate drug depot, having an individualised drug dose and release mechanism [49]. In particular, this could benefit narrow therapeutic index drugs, which are characterised by having a small difference between the therapeutic and toxic doses, wherein improper dosing could lead to undesirable adverse effects or inefficient therapy [50].

The use of dual miniprintlets offers the choice of combining multiple APIs, where each drug could have a different release profile within the same miniprintlet. The formulation of the miniprintlets in a combination of instant and extended release forms could offer benefits, such as convenient dosing with a lower frequency of intake [51], while providing longer lasting analgesic and antipyretic effects. As such, drug combinations with different doses, having the same ratio of APIs, could be prepared to suit the need of patients from different age groups [52,53]. The development of a patient-centric platform could be particularly beneficial for paediatric and geriatric patients, where dose adjustments are needed due to variations in pharmacodynamic and pharmacokinetic characteristics [54]. In contrast to previously proposed pathways for personalised medications, the use of the miniprintlet platform is much simpler and more efficient, as it does not require altering of the shape or dimensions of the dosage form, both of which could affect the drug release [55,56]. The use of this novel approach could enhance the treatment regime, moving it away from a 'one size fits all' approach toward personalised medicines, which are safer and more effective [57].

4. Conclusions

In this work, we demonstrated that miniprintlets prepared using SLS 3DP offer a novel drug delivery approach with high flexibility and control over the drug content and release properties. Fine-tuning of the therapeutic effect can be achieved by modulating parameters such as the dimensions and matrix composition, which in turn can be leveraged to produce multi-drug systems. To our knowledge, this study is the first to demonstrate the possibility of combining two rate-controlling systems in such small and intricate pharmaceutical dosage forms, enabling the individual programming of each drug. As such, this emphasises the value of this technology, making it favourable over other commercial fabrication systems for the production of pharmaceuticals.

Author Contributions: Conceptualization, A.A., F.F., S.J.T., A.G., S.G. and A.W.B.; Data curation, A.A., F.F. and S.J.T.; Formal analysis, A.A. and F.F.; Investigation, A.A., F.F., S.J.T. and P.P.; Methodology, A.A., F.F., A.G., S.G. and A.W.B.; Project administration, A.G., S.G. and A.W.B.; Resources, A.A., F.F., S.J.T., A.G. and P.P.; Software, A.A. and F.F.; Supervision, A.G., S.G. and A.W.B.; Validation, A.A., F.F. and P.P.; Visualization, A.A.; Writing—original draft, A.A.; Writing—review & editing, A.A., F.F., S.J.T., A.G., S.G. and A.W.B.

Funding: This research received no external funding.

Acknowledgments: The authors would like to acknowledge the assistance provided by John Frost to modify the printer's platform and Andrew Weston's help with the SEM imaging.

Conflicts of Interest: The authors declare no conflict of interest. The co-authors A.G., S.G. and A.B. are directors of FabRx Ltd. The company had no role in the design of the study; in the collection, analyses, or interpretation of data; in the writing of the manuscript, and in the decision to publish the results.

References

1. Basit, A.W.; Gaisford, S. *3D Printing of Pharmaceuticals*, 1st ed.; Springer International Publishing: Berlin, Germany, 2018. [CrossRef]
2. Barnatt, C. *3D Printing*, 3rd ed.; CreateSpace Independent Publishing Platform: Scotts Valley, SC, USA, 2016.

3. Murphy, S.V.; Atala, A. 3D bioprinting of tissues and organs. *Nat. Biotechnol.* **2014**, *32*, 773–785. [CrossRef] [PubMed]
4. Arafat, B.; Qinna, N.; Cieszynska, M.; Forbes, R.T.; Alhnan, M.A. Tailored on demand anti-coagulant dosing: An in vitro and in vivo evaluation of 3D printed purpose-designed oral dosage forms. *Eur. J. Pharm. Biopharm.* **2018**, *128*, 282–289. [CrossRef]
5. Verstraete, G.; Samaro, A.; Grymonpré, W.; Vanhoorne, V.; Van Snick, B.; Boone, M.N.; Hellemans, T.; Van Hoorebeke, L.; Remon, J.P.; Vervaet, C. 3D printing of high drug loaded dosage forms using thermoplastic polyurethanes. *Int. J. Pharm.* **2018**, *536*, 318–325. [CrossRef]
6. Okwuosa, T.C.; Pereira, B.C.; Arafat, B.; Cieszynska, M.; Isreb, A.; Alhnan, M.A. Fabricating a shell-core delayed release tablet using dual fdm 3D printing for patient-centred therapy. *Pharm. Res.* **2017**, *34*, 427–437. [CrossRef] [PubMed]
7. Maroni, A.; Melocchi, A.; Parietti, F.; Foppoli, A.; Zema, L.; Gazzaniga, A. 3D printed multi-compartment capsular devices for two-pulse oral drug delivery. *J. Control. Release* **2017**, *268*, 10–18. [CrossRef]
8. Fu, J.; Yu, X.; Jin, Y. 3D printing of vaginal rings with personalized shapes for controlled release of progesterone. *Int. J. Pharm.* **2018**, *539*, 75–82. [CrossRef]
9. Goyanes, A.; Scarpa, M.; Kamlow, M.; Gaisford, S.; Basit, A.W.; Orlu, M. Patient acceptability of 3D printed medicines. *Int. J. Pharm.* **2017**, *530*, 71–78. [CrossRef]
10. Arafat, B.; Wojsz, M.; Isreb, A.; Forbes, R.T.; Isreb, M.; Ahmed, W.; Arafat, T.; Alhnan, M.A. Tablet fragmentation without a disintegrant: A novel design approach for accelerating disintegration and drug release from 3D printed cellulosic tablets. *Eur. J. Pharm. Sci.* **2018**, *118*, 191–199. [CrossRef]
11. Liang, K.; Carmone, S.; Brambilla, D.; Leroux, J.C. 3D printing of a wearable personalized oral delivery device: A first-in-human study. *Sci. Adv.* **2018**, *4*, eaat2544. [CrossRef]
12. Melocchi, A.; Inverardi, N.; Uboldi, M.; Baldi, F.; Maroni, A.; Pandini, S.; Briatico-Vangosa, F.; Zema, L.; Gazzaniga, A. Retentive device for intravesical drug delivery based on water-induced shape memory response of poly(vinyl alcohol): Design concept and 4D printing feasibility. *Int. J. Pharm.* **2019**. [CrossRef] [PubMed]
13. Kollamaram, G.; Croker, D.M.; Walker, G.M.; Goyanes, A.; Basit, A.W.; Gaisford, S. Low temperature fused deposition modeling (FDM) 3D printing of thermolabile drugs. *Int. J. Pharm.* **2018**, *545*, 144–152. [CrossRef] [PubMed]
14. Kadry, H.; Al-Hilal, T.A.; Keshavarz, A.; Alam, F.; Xu, C.; Joy, A.; Ahsan, F. Multi-purposable filaments of hpmc for 3D printing of medications with tailored drug release and timed-absorption. *Int. J. Pharm.* **2018**, *544*, 285–296. [CrossRef] [PubMed]
15. Beck, R.C.R.; Chaves, P.S.; Goyanes, A.; Vukosavljevic, B.; Buanz, A.; Windbergs, M.; Basit, A.W.; Gaisford, S. 3D printed tablets loaded with polymeric nanocapsules: An innovative approach to produce customized drug delivery systems. *Int. J. Pharm.* **2017**, *528*, 268–279. [CrossRef]
16. Janssen, R.B.I.; Moolenburgh, E.; Posthumus, B. TNO: The Impact of 3-D Printing on Supply Chain Management. Available online: http://3din.nl/wp-content/uploads/2014/02/TNO-Whitepaper-3-D-Printing-and-Supply-Chain-Management-April-2014-web.pdf (accessed on 2 March 2019).
17. Awad, A.; Trenfield, S.J.; Goyanes, A.; Gaisford, S.; Basit, A.W. Reshaping drug development using 3D printing. *Drug Discov. Today* **2018**, *23*, 1547–1555. [CrossRef] [PubMed]
18. Kaae, S.; Lind, J.L.M.; Genina, N.; Sporrong, S.K. Unintended consequences for patients of future personalized pharmacoprinting. *Int. J. Clin. Pharm.* **2018**. [CrossRef]
19. Zema, L.; Melocchi, A.; Maroni, A.; Gazzaniga, A. Three-dimensional printing of medicinal products and the challenge of personalized therapy. *J. Pharm. Sci.* **2017**, *106*, 1697–1705. [CrossRef]
20. Rowe, C.W.; Katstra, W.E.; Palazzolo, R.D.; Giritlioglu, B.; Teung, P.; Cima, M.J. Multimechanism oral dosage forms fabricated by three dimensional printing. *J. Control. Release* **2000**, *66*, 11–17. [CrossRef]
21. Fina, F.; Gaisford, S.; Basit, A.W. Powder bed fusion: The working process, current applications and opportunities. In *3D Printing of Pharmaceuticals*, 1st ed.; Basit, A.W., Gaisford, S., Eds.; Springer International Publishing: Berlin, Germany, 2018; pp. 81–105. [CrossRef]
22. Eosoly, S.; Brabazon, D.; Lohfeld, S.; Looney, L. Selective laser sintering of hydroxyapatite/poly-ε-caprolactone scaffolds. *Acta Biomaterialia* **2010**, *6*, 2511–2517. [CrossRef] [PubMed]

23. Trenfield, S.J.; Goyanes, A.; Telford, R.; Wilsdon, D.; Rowland, M.; Gaisford, S.; Basit, A.W. 3D printed drug products: Non-destructive dose verification using a rapid point-and-shoot approach. *Int. J. Pharm.* **2018**, *549*, 283–292. [CrossRef]
24. Fina, F.; Madla, C.M.; Goyanes, A.; Zhang, J.; Gaisford, S.; Basit, A.W. Fabricating 3D printed orally disintegrating printlets using selective laser sintering. *Int. J. Pharm.* **2018**, *541*, 101–107. [CrossRef] [PubMed]
25. Fina, F.; Goyanes, A.; Gaisford, S.; Basit, A.W. Selective laser sintering (SLS) 3D printing of medicines. *Int. J. Pharm.* **2017**, *529*, 285–293. [CrossRef]
26. Fina, F.; Goyanes, A.; Madla, C.M.; Awad, A.; Trenfield, S.J.; Kuek, J.M.; Patel, P.; Gaisford, S.; Basit, A.W. 3D printing of drug-loaded gyroid lattices using selective laser sintering. *Int. J. Pharm.* **2018**, *547*, 44–52. [CrossRef] [PubMed]
27. Williams, J.M.; Adewunmi, A.; Schek, R.M.; Flanagan, C.L.; Krebsbach, P.H.; Feinberg, S.E.; Hollister, S.J.; Das, S. Bone tissue engineering using polycaprolactone scaffolds fabricated via selective laser sintering. *Biomaterials* **2005**, *26*, 4817–4827. [CrossRef] [PubMed]
28. Duan, B.; Wang, M.; Zhou, W.Y.; Cheung, W.L.; Li, Z.Y.; Lu, W.W. Three-dimensional nanocomposite scaffolds fabricated via selective laser sintering for bone tissue engineering. *Acta Biomaterialia* **2010**, *6*, 4495–4505. [CrossRef]
29. Ghebre-Selassie, I. *Multiparticulate Oral Drug Delivery*; Taylor & Francis: Oxford, UK, 1994.
30. Davis, S.S.; Hardy, J.G.; Taylor, M.J.; Whalley, D.R.; Wilson, C.G. A comparative study of the gastrointestinal transit of a pellet and tablet formulation. *Int. J. Pharm.* **1984**, *21*, 167–177. [CrossRef]
31. Goyanes, A.; Fernández-Ferreiro, A.; Majeed, A.; Gomez-Lado, N.; Awad, A.; Luaces-Rodríguez, A.; Gaisford, S.; Aguiar, P.; Basit, A.W. Pet/ct imaging of 3D printed devices in the gastrointestinal tract of rodents. *Int. J. Pharm.* **2018**, *536*, 158–164. [CrossRef] [PubMed]
32. Kim, J.-Y.; An, S.-H.; Rhee, Y.-S.; Park, C.-W.; Park, E.-S. A comparative study between spray-drying and fluidized bed coating processes for the preparation of pramipexole controlled-release microparticles for orally disintegrating tablets. *Dry. Technol.* **2014**, *32*, 935–945. [CrossRef]
33. Yap, C.Y.; Chua, C.K.; Dong, Z.L.; Liu, Z.H.; Zhang, D.Q.; Loh, L.E.; Sing, S.L. Review of selective laser melting: Materials and applications. *Appl. Phys. Rev.* **2015**, *2*, 041101. [CrossRef]
34. Liu, F.; Merchant, H.A.; Kulkarni, R.P.; Alkademi, M.; Basit, A.W. Evolution of a physiological pH 6.8 bicarbonate buffer system: Application to the dissolution testing of enteric coated products. *Eur. J. Pharm. Biopharm.* **2011**, *78*, 151–157. [CrossRef]
35. Fadda, H.M.; Basit, A.W. Dissolution of ph responsive formulations in media resembling intestinal fluids: Bicarbonate versus phosphate buffers. *J. Drug Deliv. Sci. Technol.* **2005**, *15*, 273–279. [CrossRef]
36. Goyanes, A.; Hatton, G.B.; Basit, A.W. A dynamic in vitro model to evaluate the intestinal release behaviour of modified-release corticosteroid products. *J. Drug Deliv. Sci. Technol.* **2015**, *25*, 36–42. [CrossRef]
37. Merchant, H.A.; Frost, J.; Basit, A.W. Apparatus and Method for Testing Medicaments. Patent PCT/GB2013/051145, 7 November 2013.
38. Merchant, H.A.; Goyanes, A.; Parashar, N.; Basit, A.W. Predicting the gastrointestinal behaviour of modified-release products: Utility of a novel dynamic dissolution test apparatus involving the use of bicarbonate buffers. *Int. J. Pharm.* **2014**, *475*, 585–591. [CrossRef] [PubMed]
39. Moore, P.A.; Hersh, E.V. Combining ibuprofen and acetaminophen for acute pain management after third-molar extractions. *J. Am. Dent. Assoc.* **2013**, *144*, 898–908. [CrossRef] [PubMed]
40. Mehlisch, D.R.; Aspley, S.; Daniels, S.E.; Bandy, D.P. Comparison of the analgesic efficacy of concurrent ibuprofen and paracetamol with ibuprofen or paracetamol alone in the management of moderate to severe acute postoperative dental pain in adolescents and adults: A randomized, double-blind, placebo-controlled, parallel-group, single-dose, two-center, modified factorial study. *Clin. Ther.* **2010**, *32*, 882–895. [CrossRef]
41. Sibik, J.; Sargent, M.J.; Franklin, M.; Zeitler, J.A. Crystallization and phase changes in paracetamol from the amorphous solid to the liquid phase. *Mol. Pharm.* **2014**, *11*, 1326–1334. [CrossRef]
42. Zhang, G.G.Z.; Paspal, S.Y.L.; Suryanarayanan, R.; Grant, D.J.W. Racemic species of sodium ibuprofen: Characterization and polymorphic relationships. *J. Pharm. Sci.* **2003**, *92*, 1356–1366. [CrossRef] [PubMed]
43. Janssens, S.; Anné, M.; Rombaut, P.; Van den Mooter, G. Spray drying from complex solvent systems broadens the applicability of kollicoat IR as a carrier in the formulation of solid dispersions. *Eur. J. Pharm. Sci.* **2009**, *37*, 241–248. [CrossRef] [PubMed]

44. Goyanes, A.; Hatton, G.B.; Merchant, H.A.; Basit, A.W. Gastrointestinal release behaviour of modified-release drug products: Dynamic dissolution testing of mesalazine formulations. *Int. J. Pharm.* **2015**, *484*, 103–108. [CrossRef] [PubMed]
45. Ghebre-Sellassie, I.; Knoch, A. Pelletization techniques. In *Encyclopedia of Pharmaceutical Technology*; Swarbrick, J., Ed.; Informa Healthcare USA, Inc.: New York, NY, USA, 2007; Volume 3, pp. 2651–2663.
46. Lee, H.; Lim, C.H.J.; Low, M.J.; Tham, N.; Murukeshan, V.M.; Kim, Y.-J. Lasers in additive manufacturing: A review. *Int. J. Precis. Eng. Manuf.-Green Technol.* **2017**, *4*, 307–322. [CrossRef]
47. Neubert, V.; Czelusniak, T.; Lohrengel, A.F.; Higa, C.L.; Amorim, F. Selective laser sintering of mo-cuni composite to be used as edm electrode. *Rapid Prototyp. J.* **2014**, *20*, 59–68. [CrossRef]
48. Goyanes, A.; Fina, F.; Martorana, A.; Sedough, D.; Gaisford, S.; Basit, A.W. Development of modified release 3D printed tablets (printlets) with pharmaceutical excipients using additive manufacturing. *Int. J. Pharm.* **2017**, *527*, 21–30. [CrossRef]
49. Dukić-Ott, A.; Thommes, M.; Remon, J.P.; Kleinebudde, P.; Vervaet, C. Production of pellets via extrusion–spheronisation without the incorporation of microcrystalline cellulose: A critical review. *Eur. J. Pharm. Biopharm.* **2009**, *71*, 38–46. [CrossRef] [PubMed]
50. Trenfield, S.J.; Awad, A.; Goyanes, A.; Gaisford, S.; Basit, A.W. 3D printing pharmaceuticals: Drug development to frontline care. *Trends Pharmacol. Sci.* **2018**, *39*, 440–451. [CrossRef]
51. Gioumouxouzis, C.I.; Baklavaridis, A.; Katsamenis, O.L.; Markopoulou, C.K.; Bouropoulos, N.; Tzetzis, D.; Fatouros, D.G. A 3D printed bilayer oral solid dosage form combining metformin for prolonged and glimepiride for immediate drug delivery. *Eur. J. Pharm. Sci.* **2018**, *120*, 40–52. [CrossRef] [PubMed]
52. Awad, A.; Trenfield, S.J.; Gaisford, S.; Basit, A.W. 3D printed medicines: A new branch of digital healthcare. *Int. J. Pharm.* **2018**, *548*, 586–596. [CrossRef] [PubMed]
53. Palo, M.; Holländer, J.; Suominen, J.; Yliruusi, J.; Sandler, N. 3D printed drug delivery devices: Perspectives and technical challenges. *Expert Rev. Med. Devices* **2017**, *14*, 685–696. [CrossRef]
54. Breitkreutz, J.; Boos, J. Paediatric and geriatric drug delivery. *Expert Opin. Drug Deliv.* **2007**, *4*, 37–45. [CrossRef]
55. Martinez, P.R.; Goyanes, A.; Basit, A.W.; Gaisford, S. Influence of geometry on the drug release profiles of stereolithographic (SLA) 3D-printed tablets. *AAPS PharmSciTech* **2018**, *19*, 3355–3361. [CrossRef] [PubMed]
56. Sadia, M.; Arafat, B.; Ahmed, W.; Forbes, R.T.; Alhnan, M.A. Channelled tablets: An innovative approach to accelerating drug release from 3D printed tablets. *J. Control. Release* **2018**, *269*, 355–363. [CrossRef]
57. Vithani, K.; Goyanes, A.; Jannin, V.; Basit, A.W.; Gaisford, S.; Boyd, B.J. An overview of 3D printing technologies for soft materials and potential opportunities for lipid-based drug delivery systems. *Pharm. Res.* **2018**, *36*, 4. [CrossRef]

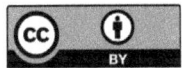

© 2019 by the authors. Licensee MDPI, Basel, Switzerland. This article is an open access article distributed under the terms and conditions of the Creative Commons Attribution (CC BY) license (http://creativecommons.org/licenses/by/4.0/).

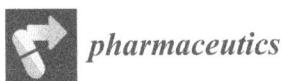

Article

Optimization and Prediction of Ibuprofen Release from 3D DLP Printlets Using Artificial Neural Networks

Marijana Madzarevic [1,*], Djordje Medarevic [1], Aleksandra Vulovic [2,3], Tijana Sustersic [2,3], Jelena Djuris [1], Nenad Filipovic [2,3] and Svetlana Ibric [1,*]

1. Department of Pharmaceutical Technology and Cosmetology, Faculty of Pharmacy, University of Belgrade, 450 Vojvode Stepe Str., 11221 Belgrade, Serbia; djordje.medarevic@pharmacy.bg.ac.rs (D.M.); jelena.djuris@pharmacy.bg.ac.rs (J.D.)
2. Department for Applied Mechanics and Automatic Control, Faculty of Engineering, University of Kragujevac, 6, Sestre Janjic Str., 34000 Kragujevac, Serbia; aleksandra.vulovic@kg.ac.rs (A.V.); tijanas@kg.ac.rs (T.S.); fica@kg.ac.rs (N.F.)
3. Bioengineering Research and Development Center (BioIRC), 6 Prvoslava Stojanovica Str., 34000 Kragujevac, Serbia
* Correspondence: marijana.madzarevic@pharmacy.bg.ac.rs (M.M.); svetlana.ibric@pharmacy.bg.ac.rs (S.I.)

Received: 20 September 2019; Accepted: 12 October 2019; Published: 18 October 2019

Abstract: The aim of this work was to investigate effects of the formulation factors on tablet printability as well as to optimize and predict extended drug release from cross-linked polymeric ibuprofen printlets using an artificial neural network (ANN). Printlets were printed using digital light processing (DLP) technology from formulations containing polyethylene glycol diacrylate, polyethylene glycol, and water in concentrations according to D-optimal mixture design and 0.1% w/w riboflavin and 5% w/w ibuprofen. It was observed that with higher water content longer exposure time was required for successful printing. For understanding the effects of excipients and printing parameters on drug dissolution rate in DLP printlets two different neural networks were developed with using two commercially available softwares. After comparison of experimental and predicted values of in vitro dissolution at the corresponding time points for optimized formulation, the R^2 experimental vs. predicted value was 0.9811 (neural network 1) and 0.9960 (neural network 2). According to difference f_1 and similarity factor f_2 (f_1 = 14.30 and f_2 = 52.15) neural network 1 with supervised multilayer perceptron, backpropagation algorithm, and linear activation function gave a similar dissolution profile to obtained experimental results, indicating that adequate ANN is able to set out an input–output relationship in DLP printing of pharmaceutics.

Keywords: three-dimensional printing; additive manufacturing; digital light processing technology; printlets; neural networks; optimization; prediction

1. Introduction

Three-dimensional printing (3DP) is an additive manufacturing process that allows the fabrication of three-dimensional solid objects of virtually any shape from a 3D model file [1–3]. The basic mechanism for most types of 3D printing is the same (layer-by-layer production of 3D objects from digital designs) [4], but the difference lies in input materials and operating principles. There are several types of 3D printing technologies: fused deposition modeling (FDM)—based on extrusion [5], selective laser sintering (SLS)—based on powder bed fusion [6], stereolithography (SLA), and digital light processing technology (DLP)—based on photopolymerization of the resin and others [2]. SLA 3D printing was the first rapid prototyping method developed and perhaps the most popular due to its superior resolution and accuracy [7]. DLP is a "sister technology" to SLA as the only significant difference between these technologies is the light source used to cure the resin. SLA printers use lasers combined with galvanometers to cure the resin while in DLP 3D printers, the light source is a specially developed digital light projector screen. Due to the presence of this screen, DLP is generally considered to be faster and more efficient than SLA [8]. The main drawbacks of SLA and DLP technology are the limited number of photocrosslinkable polymers that are available for medical applications, and these materials are currently not on the generally recognized as safe (GRAS) list of excipients [9].

Research in the field of oral drug delivery using SLA and DLP is still very limited. Wang et al. who fabricated 4-aminosalicylic acid and paracetamol loaded printlets, showed no drug degradation during the 3D printing process. [7]. In the study by Martinez et al. percentage of water in the initial formulation was varied, showing that the crosslinking density is slightly modified as the water content increases (up to 30%) and this dilution with water did not seem to significantly affect the speed at which the drug was released [9]. Influence of geometry on the drug release profiles was investigated by Martinez et al. [10]. In the study by Kadry et al. theophylline, as a model drug, and two photoreactive polymers, polyethylene glycol diacrylate (PEGDA) and polyethylene glycol dimethacrylate (PEGDMA), were used. Polymer concentration was varied to produce sturdy printlets with minimum polymer concentration applying, for the first time, DLP technology [11]. Optimization techniques have not yet been applied in 3D DLP fabrication and optimization of solid oral dosage forms.

The most frequently used optimization technique is design of experiments (DoE), but with the development of computer science, artificial neural network (ANN) have attracted a lot of attention. Despite the advantages of DoE-based polynomial model fitting, often the developed models show bad fit resulting to a poor optimum estimation. An alternative approach that has been successfully applied in cases where conventional DoE methods prove inadequate is the use of feed-forward ANNs [12]. Neural networks create their knowledge by detecting the patterns and relationships in data. It is a biologically inspired computer-based system formed from hundreds of single units, artificial neurons, connected with coefficients (units) which constitute the neural structure. The artificial neuron takes one or more inputs and creates an output, which is passed on to another neuron. One of the most useful advantages of artificial neural networks is their ability to generalize. The multilayered perceptron (MLP) neural network is one of the simplest ANNs and consists of an input layer, output layer, and one or more hidden layers of neurons. During the 'training process' the system is able to establish the relationship between inputs and outputs using algorithms designed to alter the weights of the connections in the network to produce a desired signal flow. Although MLP has proved efficient in solving an important number of pharmaceutical development problems, no single software or modeling algorithm can solve 'all' problems [13–16]. There are a few examples in literature describing combination of DoE and ANN with recognized possibility as a powerful tool in predicting optimal conditions from a low number of experiments [17]. DoE enable determination of the quantitative relationship between selected input variables and responses while ANNs often exhibit superior performance in prediction of the responses for given values of inputs [18]. ANN can be used in completing one portion of data in the experimental design data pool, resulting in satisfying results for some outputs, considering the number of experimental data used for modeling [19].

The aim of this work was to investigate the effects of formulation factors on printability as well as to optimize and predict extended drug release from cross-linked polymeric ibuprofen printlets using ANN created in two different softwares. For a meticulous investigation of the effects of excipients on drug release, ANN was used because it is highly recommended to present the complicated relations and strong nonlinearity between different parameters [20]. The prediction and optimization method was applied to the development of ibuprofen extended-release 3D printlets using MLP and the backpropagation algorithm with linear and log-sigmoid activation functions.

2. Materials and Methods

PEGDA, average MW 700, was obtained from Sigma–Aldrich, Tokyo, Japan. Polyethylene glycol (PEG 400, average MW 400) was purchased from Fagron B.V., Rotterdam, The Netherlands. Ethanol, absolute was purchased from Honeywell Riedel-de-Haën™, Seelze, Germany and 2-propanol was obtained from Merck KGaA, Darmstadt, Germany. Ibuprofen (Ph. Eur. 9.0) was used as a model substance, PEGDA as the photopolymerizable monomer, while PEG 400 and water were used to alter the cross-linking density. PEG 400 is chemically similar to PEGDA and the difference is that does not have photopolymerizable terminal groups. Riboflavin (Ph. Eur. 9.0) was used as the photo-initiator. The photo-initiator converts to reactive radicals upon exposure to light to catalyze the polymerization of the formulation. In photopolymerization reactions different photo-initiators can be used, and riboflavin is reported as pharmacologically non-toxic photo-initiator [9,21,22].

2.1. Preparation of Photopolymer Solution

Based on preliminary experiments, lower and upper limits (% w/w) of each component were selected as follows: PEGDA (30.0–74.6%), PEG 400 (10.0–54.6%), water (10.0–30%), and amounts of ibuprofen and riboflavin were kept constant, 5.0% and 0.1% respectively. Eleven formulations were prepared according to D-optimal mixture design from Design Expert software 7.0.0 (Stat-Ease Inc., Minneapolis, MN, USA). Compositions of the formulations obtained by the software are given in Table 1. Firstly PEGDA, PEG 400, and ibuprofen were mixed with propeller mixer Heidolph RZR2020 (Heidolph, Schwabach, Germany) until complete dissolution (approximately 60 min). Riboflavin and water were added next, keeping the solution protected from light and with constant mixing until complete dissolution (approximately 45 min). Compositions of three test formulations were selected so that they differ from the previous 11 and were prepared in the same way. Approximately the same concentration of PEGDA and PEG 400 was selected in the placebo formulation. Percentage of water was varied from 10 to 30 in formulations F1–F11, based on which 15% of water was chosen in the placebo formulation.

Table 1. Composition (% w/w) of the initial resins used to print the printlets.

Formulation	PEGDA	PEG 400	Water	riboflavin	ibuprofen
F1	32.10	32.60	30.00	0.10	5.00
F2	30.00	44.10	20.50	0.10	5.00
F3	74.60	10.00	10.10	0.10	5.00
F4	62.40	21.80	10.50	0.10	5.00
F5	50.60	34.00	10.00	0.10	5.00
F6	65.80	11.20	17.70	0.10	5.00
F7	30.00	54.60	10.00	0.10	5.00
F8	58.10	10.00	26.60	0.10	5.00
F9	39.30	45.30	10.00	0.10	5.00
F10	46.20	23.10	25.40	0.10	5.00
F11	40.40	35.60	18.70	0.10	5.00
Test 1	35.00	47.90	12.00	0.10	5.00
Test 2	55.00	24.90	15.00	0.10	5.00
Test 3	65.00	7.90	22.00	0.10	5.00
F placebo	42.50	42.40	15.00	0.10	0.00

2.2. Printing Dosage Forms

In this study a DLP printer, based on photopolymerization process, was used for fabrication of solid oral dosage forms, called printlets. The DLP printer offers fast and efficient printing by projecting the light onto a whole layer at once, while the SLA printer prints each layer in a line by line pattern. The advantage of the Wanhao DLP printer is an open software and the possibility for adjustment of parameters for printing a particular mixture [11]. A schematic view of the printing process is shown in Figure 1. The template used to print the printlets (a cylinder, 10.00 mm diameter, 3.02 mm height) was designed with Autodesk Fusion 360 (Autodesk Inc, San Rafael, CA, USA) (Figure 2a) and exported as a stereolithography file (stl) into the 3D printer software (Creation Workshop X). All 3D printlets were printed with a Wanhao Duplicator 7 printer (Wanhao, Zhejiang, China) with layer thickness of 100 µm, bottom exposure 800 s, and 10 bottom layers. Trial-and error approach was used to establish exposure time for successful printing. In screening formulations, ibuprofen content was 5.0% and the water content was varied from 5.0% to 30.0%. The minimum exposure time which lead to solidification was selected. This criterion for exposure time allowed printing to be as short as possible.

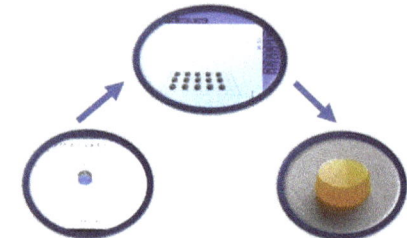

Figure 1. Digital light processing technology (DLP) printing process.

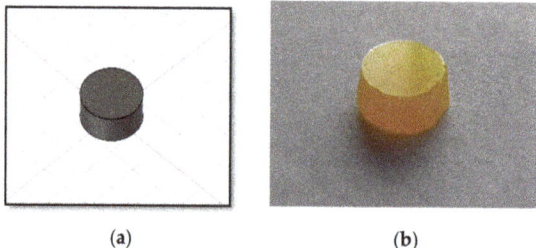

(a)   (b)

Figure 2. (a) 3D model of DLP printlet; (b) DLP printlet

2.3. Characterization of Printlets

2.3.1. Determination of Physical and Mechanical Properties

Three-D printed printlets were washed with 2-propanol to remove any uncured liquid formulation on the surface immediately after fabrication, then they were weighed and measured (diameter and thickness, $n = 10$) using a caliper. The breaking force of printlets ($n = 10$) was measured using a hardness tester Erweka TBH 125D (Erweka, Langen, Germany). Microscopic observations of placebo and optimal printlets were done under a polarized light microscope Olympus BX 51P (Olympus, Tokyo, Japan). Photos were acquired using cellSens Entry Version 1.14 software (Olympus, Tokyo, Japan).

2.3.2. Determination of Drug Concentration in 3DP Printlets

Printed printlets were crushed using mortar and pestle ($n = 3$), and 200 mg of the crushed printlet was diluted with 10 mL of ethanol. Samples were placed in an ultrasonic bath Bandelin–Sonorex RK102H (Sonorex–Bandelin, Berlin, Germany) at room temperature and sonicated for 15 min to enhance extraction of ibuprofen. At the end of sonification, dispersions were cooled to room temperature and then filtered through a 0.45 μm Millipore filter (Merck Millipore Ltd. Carrigtwohill, County Cork, Ireland) A sample of 250 μL of the solution was diluted to 50 mL with phosphate buffer pH 6.8. Amount of drug in solution was determined using UV–Vis spectroscopy Evolution 300 (Thermo–Fisher Scientific, Waltham, MA, USA) at the wavelength of 221 nm. Corresponding placebo samples were analyzed in order to nullify the possible effect of other printlet constituents on drug absorbance.

2.3.3. Dissolution Test Conditions

Drug release profiles were obtained using the paddle apparatus Erweka DT 600 (Erweka, Langen, Germany). The printlets were placed in 900 mL of phosphate buffer pH 6.8 for 8 h. The paddle speed of the USPII was fixed at 75 rpm, and the tests were conducted at 37 ± 0.5 °C. Buffer samples of 4 mL were withdrawn at predetermined time intervals, filtrated through a 0.45 µm Millipore filter (Merck Millipore Ltd. Carrigtwohill, County Cork, Ireland), and the absorbance of released ibuprofen was measured UV-spectrophotometrically at the wavelength of the relative maximum absorbance (221 nm). Studies were performed in triplicate.

2.3.4. Kinetic Model

A number of mathematical models have been proposed to describe drug release from pharmaceutical delivery systems [23,24]. Drug release profiles were fitted into four mathematical models including zero-order, first-order, Higuchi, and Korsmeyer–Peppas.

2.3.5. Differential Scanning Calorimetry (DSC)

DSC was used to study the thermal properties of placebo and optimal printlets. DSC analyses were performed on a DSC 1 differential scanning calorimeter Mettler Toledo AG (Analytical, Zurich, Switzerland). Accurately weighed 5–10 mg of samples (optimal and placebo formulation) were placed in pierced aluminum pans, and subjected to heating at 10 °C/min in the range of −50–200 °C under nitrogen purge gas flow of 50 mL/min. An empty pan was used as a reference.

2.4. Artificial Neural Network Modeling

To get better insight in an input–output relationship in DLP printing of ibuprofen printlets in ANN modeling, two artificial neural networks, using different commercially available software, were used. Each software has unique potential in solving problems.

(1) Neural Network 1. Commercially available STATISTICA 7.0 Neural Networks software (StatSoft Inc., Tulsa, OK, USA.) was used throughout the study. For prediction and optimization of ibuprofen release from 3D DLP printlets, supervised MLP and backpropagation algorithm with linear activation function were used. The data set was split into training (8 formulations), validation (2 formulations) and test (1 formulation) subsets. Amount of PEGDA, PEG 400, and water (% w/w) in formulations were selected as input factors affecting the release of ibuprofen. The cumulative percentage of ibuprofen release from 3D DLP printlets at time points of 1, 2, 4, 6, and 8 h was used as output data (Table S1). A trial and error approach, conducted by varying the number of layers and number of nodes in the hidden layer(s), was used to train the neural network. Learning rate and momentum were 0.6, the number of layers was varied from 3 to 10, and the number of nodes in the hidden layer(s) from 4 to 10. The criteria to choose the "best MLP model" were minimal test error and maximum coefficient of determination R^2 for observed vs. predicted values. After the training process, the prediction ability of the developed network was examined by external validation with the unseen samples of three test formulations.

(2) Neural Network 2. Another approach was the usage of commercial software MATLAB R2014b (The MathWorks, Inc., Natick, MA, USA) to investigate the combination of process and formulation factors on optimization of ibuprofen release. A supervised MLP network and backpropagation algorithm with linear and log-sigmoid activation functions were used for the prediction. Percentage of PEGDA, PEG 400, and water in formulations were selected as input factors affecting the release of ibuprofen, as well as exposure times (s). The cumulative percentage of ibuprofen released after 2, 4, 6, and 8 h was the output data (Table S2). The most optimal MLP model was chosen based on the maximum R and minimal normalized mean square error between the calculated and target output for the test data. After the training process was finished, the prediction was examined by external validation with the unseen test (optimal formulation).

2.5. Optimization of 3D Printed Printlets

D-optimal mixture design was established by data predicted using evaluated MLP, because this approach of using DoE-based modeling to decipher the black-box nature of the ANNs resulted in satisfying results. Data obtained using DoE enable the development of more accurate models and improve process understanding [19]. The desirability function approach has been proven to be a useful statistical tool, the most widely used in industry, for solving multi-variable problems and optimization of one or several responses [19,23]. The objective function, D(X), called the desirability function is used in this method. It reflects the desirable ranges for each response (di) from zero to one (least to most desirable respectively). The simultaneous objective function is a geometric mean of all transformed responses. The numerical optimization technique was used to generate the composition of formulation with desirable drug release. The criteria for the selection of the optimal formulation were the percentage of in vitro release at time points of 2, 4, 6, and 8 h—not more than 30%, 60%, and 70%, and not <80%, respectively. The importance of the first two goals was set with two pluses, and the importance of the next two goals was set with three pluses, as they were more significant. After determination of the optimal composition of the formulation, the formulation was prepared, characterized by dissolution test, and the obtained results from the dissolution test were compared with the predictions by neural network 1 and neural network 2. Predictability was expressed through calculation of the coefficient of determination (R^2), f_1 (difference factor) and f_2 (similarity factor). Difference and similarity factor are represented in Equations (1) and (2).

$$f_1 = \left(\frac{\sum_{t=1}^{n} |Rt - Tt|}{\sum_{t=1}^{n} Rt} \right) \times 100 \tag{1}$$

$$f_2 = 50 \times \log_{10} \left[\frac{100}{\sqrt{1 + \frac{\sum_{t=1}^{n}(Rt-Tt)^2}{n}}} \right] \tag{2}$$

where n is the number of dissolution sampling times, and Rt and Tt are the mean percent dissolved at each time point, t, for the experimental and predicted values of drug released, respectively.

3. Results and Discussion

3.1. Printing Process

With 5.0% of the water in screening formulations, printlets were successfully fabricated with an exposure time of 100 s. There was no solidification of the resins with lower exposure time. The increase in water content up to 10.1% required exposure time to be at least 400 s, and with 30.0% water in the formulation, printing was possible at exposure time of 800 s due to which the process lasted for a long time. The water content affected the exposure time to the light projector so that with the increase in the content of water in the formulation, longer exposure time was required, and that was criteria for setting printing parameters in the way presented in Table 2. The minimal exposure time which lead to solidification was selected to keep printing time as short as possible.

It was observed that for every formulation it is necessary to find adequate printing parameters with a trial and error approach because there is no guideline for process parameters selection for mixtures containing photopolymers for pharmaceutical application. A similar observation was reported in the study by Robles-Martinez et al. [24]. Exposure time for every formulation was longer than reported in the published paper by Kadry et al., but in this published paper 2-hydroxy-4'-(2-hydroxyethoxy)-2-methylpropiophenone was used as the photo-initiator, theophylline as the active substance, and the content of the formulation was different as well as their characteristics [11].

Table 2. Printing process parameters.

Formulation	Exposure Time (s)	Bottom Exposure (s)	Layer Thickness (mm)	Bottom Layers
F1	800.00	800.00	0.10	10.00
F2	800.00	800.00	0.10	10.00
F3	400.00	800.00	0.10	10.00
F4	400.00	800.00	0.10	10.00
F5	500.00	800.00	0.10	10.00
F6	600.00	800.00	0.10	10.00
F7	400.00	800.00	0.10	10.00
F8	800.00	800.00	0.10	10.00
F9	400.00	800.00	0.10	10.00
F10	800.00	800.00	0.10	10.00
F11	600.00	800.00	0.10	10.00
Test 1	400.00	800.00	0.10	10.00
Test 2	500.00	800.00	0.10	10.00
Test 3	600.00	800.00	0.10	10.00
F placebo	600.00	800.00	0.10	10.00

3.2. Characterization of Printlets

3.2.1. Physical and Mechanical Properties and Drug Content

A DLP printer was able to fabricate 3D printlets with ibuprofen similar to results obtained by Martinez et al [9]. A DLP printlet as well as a 3D model are presented in Figure 2. All fabricated printlets had a smooth surface and consistency in shape. Measured tablet weight, dimensions, hardness, and drug load (mean ± SD) are shown in Table 3.

For better determination of the effects of the formulation factors on obtained mechanical characteristics of printlets, the content of PEGDA, PEG 400, and water were evaluated as the input variables for D-optimal mixture design. Three responses, weight, hardness, and drug load, separately, were fitted to linear, quadratic, special cubic, and full cubic models. The best-fitting mathematical model was selected based on several statistical parameters including adjusted R-squared, predicted R-squared, and predicted residual sum of square (PRESS) (Table 4). The focus was on the model maximizing the adjusted R-squared and the predicted R-squared. The linear model was considered the best fitted model for each of the three responses.

Table 3. Measured tablet weight, dimensions, hardness, and drug load (mean ± SD).

Formulation	Weight (mg)	Diameter (mm)	Thickness (mm)	Hardness (N)	Drug Load (mg)
F1	387.00 ± 45.20	11.13 ± 0.62	3.00 ± 0.00	47.33 ± 3.21	24.11 ± 2.51
F2	378.00 ± 29.00	10.86 ± 0.31	3.09 ± 0.20	32.00 ± 17.00	23.00 ± 1.58
F3	323.40 ± 21.60	10.81 ± 0.31	3.00 ± 0.00	108.33 ± 23.71	15.00 ± 1.00
F4	296.70 ± 4.50	10.17 ± 0.26	3.02 ± 0.04	92.33 ± 29.02	14.40 ± 0.22
F5	354.40 ± 21.10	10.55 ± 0.38	3.00 ± 0.00	33.00 ± 4.58	22.30 ± 0.13
F6	278.90 ± 11.50	10.04 ± 0.09	3.00 ± 0.00	132.33 ± 18.88	18.30 ± 0.75
F7	345.10 ± 32.70	10.52 ± 0.32	2.99 ± 0.02	n.d.[1]	21.70 ± 2.05
F8	400.10 ± 42.90	12.40 ± 0.55	2.97 ± 0.23	29.67 ± 3.51	27.10 ± 2.91
F9	340.50 ± 19.50	10.60 ± 0.17	2.94 ± 0.13	19.00 ± 8.66	23.00 ± 1.13
F10	375.00 ± 28.70	11.53 ± 0.43	2.92 ± 0.11	37.00 ± 16.52	25.80 ± 1.98
F11	377.50 ± 37.30	11.40 ± 0.47	2.99 ± 0.12	35.00 ± 24.25	25.50 ± 2.53

[1] n.d. not determined

Mathematically, the relationship for the studied variables was expressed in the following Equations (3)–(5) in actual values. Dimensions of printlets were similar to 3D model but variation in mass and dimension became greater for printlets containing more water. From Equation (3), water had the greatest impact on weight. Water dilutes the formulation, reduces viscosity, and consequently the reproducibility of printing with SLA printer [9]. Instead of the advantages of the DLP printer, previously mentioned, the reproducibility problem with customized resins has not been overcome with this technology.

$$\text{weight} = 2.68392 \times PEGDA + 3.78589 \times PEG400 + 6.42698 \times \text{water} \tag{3}$$

$$\text{hardness} = 1.52104 \times PEGDA - 0.53285 \times PEG400 - 0.28236 \times \text{water} \tag{4}$$

$$\text{drug load} = 0.11399 \times PEGDA + 0.24544 \times PEG400 + 0.53252 \times \text{water} \tag{5}$$

From results and Equation (4) it was observed that the content of PEGDA affected the hardness of the printlets. For printlets with a higher content of PEGDA, greater force was required to break printlets. PEG 400 and water had negative effects. With a higher content of PEG 400 or water, a lower force was measured to break the printlet. Printlet F7 was too elastic, and the hardness tester could not break them. Content of ibuprofen in printlets was greatly affected by the amount of water, with higher water content higher drug content was observed. From Equation (5) there was also a positive effect of PEGDA and PEG 400 on drug load. In a research paper by Martinez et al. it had been demonstrated that the solubility of ibuprofen was increased with the presence of solvents like polyethylene glycol 300, which decreased the polarity of the aqueous solution [9]. Even if the represented mathematical models do not achieve high values of R^2 (R^2 values reached 0.58, 0.57, 0.62, respectively), information extracted through the analysis of the mathematical expressions can help to improve understanding of the effects of formulation factors on characteristics of printlets.

Table 4. Model summary statistics.

Weight	Linear	Quadratic	Special Cubic	Cubic
Adjusted R^2	0.4828	11,760.57	0.0573	0.5331
Predicted R^2	0.2042	−2.6704	−4.744	−15888.43
PRESS	11,760.57	54,239.56	84,882.21	2.35×10^8
Hardness	**Linear**	**Quadratic**	**Special Cubic**	**Cubic**
Adjusted R^2	0.4575	0.5454	0.4311	n.d.
Predicted R^2	0.0542	−1.4961	−4.3319	n.d.
PRESS	13,171.03	34,759.87	74,249.53	n.d.
Drug load	**Linear**	**Quadratic**	**Special Cubic**	**Cubic**
Adjusted R^2	0.5184	0.6846	0.6145	0.7212
Predicted R^2	0.2228	−0.1716	−0.8126	−9,486.5367
PRESS	139.12	209.72	324.46	1.70×10^6

[1] n.d. not determined

3.2.2. Dissolution Test

Dissolution profiles for all formulations are shown in Figure 3. Printlets fabricated with cross-linkable photoreactive polymers, such as PEGDA, remained intact throughout the dissolution test similar to published studies [11,25]. The fastest dissolution after 8 h was from formulation F7 (90.72 ± 5.06%) that had the highest concentration of PEG 400 (54.6% w/w), and the slowest dissolution after 8 h was from F8 (38.04 ± 1.41%) that had the lowest concentration of PEG 400 (10% w/w) and high concentration of PEGDA (58.1% w/w). In this study, it was observed that PEG 400 had a great influence on the drug release profile, as it was concluded in the study by Wang et al. [7] that changes in the ratio of PEGDA/PEG 300 played an important role in drug release rate. The reduction in the concentration of PEGDA probably increases the drug release rate because of the lower degree of cross-linking in the tablet matrix and increases in the proportion of PEG 400 affected the greater molecular mobility in the tablet core. Formulation F2 had a high concentration of PEG 400 (44.1% w/w) and the lowest concentration of PEGDA (30% w/w) but dissolution after 8 h was slower than expected (45.69 ± 0.61%) probably because of the interactions of excipients. The effect of excipients on ibuprofen released after 8 h of dissolution on a 3D surface plot is shown in Figure 4. Martinez at al. [9] showed that dissolution is the slowest from the formulation containing no water and gets faster as the water content is increased, but this clear proportion between water and dissolution rate could not be observed in this study. Martinez et al. used printing with the same process parameters for all formulations, but for the formulations and printer used in this study, it was necessary to adjust the exposure time. By comparing these observations, it can be concluded that not only excipients and their interactions but also printing process parameters could effect drug dissolution rate. Effects of excipients could not be evaluated just by observing modulation in their concentration; it was necessary to apply advanced software. Content of PEGDA, PEG 400, and water were evaluated as the input variables for D-optimal mixture design to determinate their effects on drug release, but the proposed mathematical model was not significant. Because the relationships between the drug release profile of 3D DLP printlets and formulation factors were not well understood, artificial neural networks were used for further research.

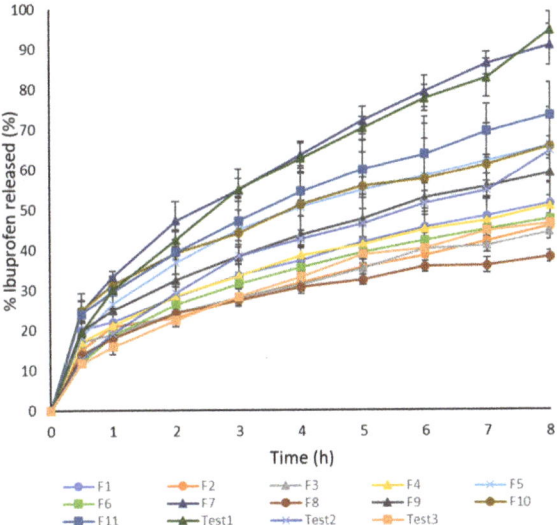

Figure 3. Dissolution profiles of ibuprofen printlets F1–F11 and Test 1–Test 3, Δ exposure time 400 s, × exposure time 500 s, ■ exposure time 600 s, • exposure time 800 s.

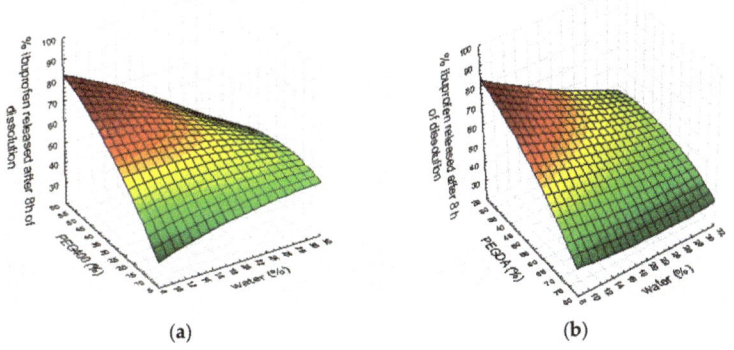

Figure 4. *Cont.*

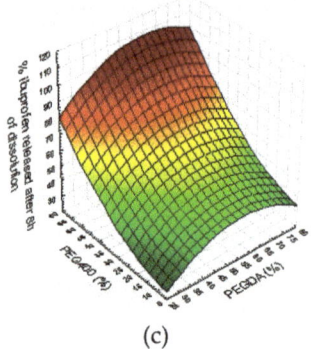

(c)

Figure 4. Interaction effect of excipients on ibuprofen released after 8 h of dissolution. (**a**) x- polyethylene glycol (PEG) 400 (%), y—water (%), (**b**) x—polyethylene glycol diacrylate (PEGDA) (%), y—water (%), (**c**) x—PEG 400 (%), y—PEGDA (%), z axis on all graphics—cumulative % of ibuprofen released after 8 h of dissolution test.

3.2.3. Drug Release Kinetic

To interpret the mechanism of drug release from the printlets, data were fitted into various kinetic models such as zero-order, first-order, the Higuchi equation, and the Korsemeyer–Peppas equation. The highest R^2 coefficient determines the suitable mathematical model that best describes drug release kinetics and n gave insights into the mechanism of drug release [26,27]. The most proper model fitted to data based on having the closest R^2 to 1 was the Higuchi model (R^2 was between 0.9746 to 0.9993 for all formulations, Table 5) meaning drug release was afforded through a diffusion process, square root time dependent. In formulations F2 and F the optimum was predominately zero order kinetics but R^2 for the Higuchi model was also high. The values of n less than 0.45 reveal that the diffusion pattern is a kind of Fickian diffusion and values of n between 0.45 and 0.89 reveal that the diffusion pattern is anomalous transport [28]. In the evaluated formulations there was predominately Fickian diffusion as a mechanism of drug release, and during the dissolution test no erosion or swelling of printlets was observed.

Table 5. Parameters obtained by fitting dissolution data to various mathematical models.

Formulation	Zero Order		First Order		Higuchi		Korsmeyer–Peppas		
	k_0	R^2	k_1	R^2	k_h	R^2	k_{kp}	R^2	n
F1	0.0707	0.9859	0.0021	0.9428	1.9807	0.9945	5.3769	0.9780	0.3588
F2	0.0643	0.9881	0.0022	0.9348	1.7921	0.9861	3.9965	0.9777	0.3843
F3	0.0614	0.9866	0.0021	0.9498	1.7126	0.9886	4.5005	0.9739	0.3619
F4	0.0727	0.9642	0.0023	0.8935	2.0614	0.9982	4.1796	0.9977	0.4024
F5	0.0997	0.9379	0.0025	0.8345	2.8606	0.9922	3.9337	0.9950	0.4609
F6	0.0744	0.9427	0.0026	0.8285	2.1292	0.9940	2.3934	0.9932	0.4895
F7	0.1445	0.9775	0.0027	0.8961	4.0722	0.9985	4.7498	0.9985	0.4767
F8	0.0510	0.9285	0.0020	0.8493	1.4654	0.9871	4.0217	0.9962	0.3671
F9	0.0856	0.9746	0.0023	0.9089	2.4164	0.9993	4.8273	0.9972	0.4027
F10	0.0857	0.9591	0.0020	0.8963	2.4347	0.9957	7.4583	0.9968	0.3489
F11	0.1082	0.9744	0.0023	0.9089	3.0557	0.9989	5.5710	0.9958	0.4147
Test 1	0.1552	0.9758	0.0031	0.8732	4.3715	0.9959	3.0129	0.9980	0.5535
Test 2	0.1045	0.9641	0.0031	0.8563	2.9500	0.9891	1.8925	0.9944	0.5656
Test 3	0.0776	0.9685	0.0029	0.8875	2.1940	0.9959	1.9670	0.9969	0.5144
F optimal	0.1286	0.9892	0.0029	0.9516	3.5609	0.9749	3.5776	0.9544	0.4872

k_0—zero order rate constant, k_1—first order rate constant, k_h—Higuchi dissolution constant, k_{kp}—Korsmeyer release rate constant, R^2—coefficient of determination, n—drug release exponent,

3.3. Development of Artificial Neural Network Models

(1) Neural network 1. In the process of creating the most appropriate neural network 1 it was found that increasing the number of layers decreased the coefficient of determination (Figure 5). One hidden layer is normally adequate to provide an accurate prediction and more than one hidden layer can be used for modeling complex problems [29]. Selected MLP had a minimum root mean square (RMS = 0.0296) and the highest coefficient of determination (R^2 = 0.9994) for obtained vs. predicted values of cumulative drug release for two formulations. Hence, a network consisting of three input and five output units, with eight hidden units arranged in a single hidden layer was selected. MLP was tested with a set of test data. Three test formulations (Test 1, 2, 3) were prepared and examined in the same test conditions as formulations F1–F11. A correlation plot was constructed of the experimentally obtained responses and those predicted by MLP. The square coefficient R^2 was 0.9478 (Figure 6a).

(2) Neural network 2. For the second version of the ANN, where exposure times were used as inputs as well as percentage of PEGDA, PEG 400, and water, correlation plots of predicted and obtained values of drug release for all formulations (training, validation, and test) showed that the MLP model had a regression plot with coefficient R^2 = 0.99877, which indicated that the optimum MLP model was reached (Figure 6b). An optimal neural network with neural network 2 was achieved using five hidden layers with the number of units being 5, 5, 6, 5, and 6 per layer. The data set consisted of training (90% of samples) and validation (10% of samples) subsets.

Architecture of developed neural networks is presented in Figure 7.

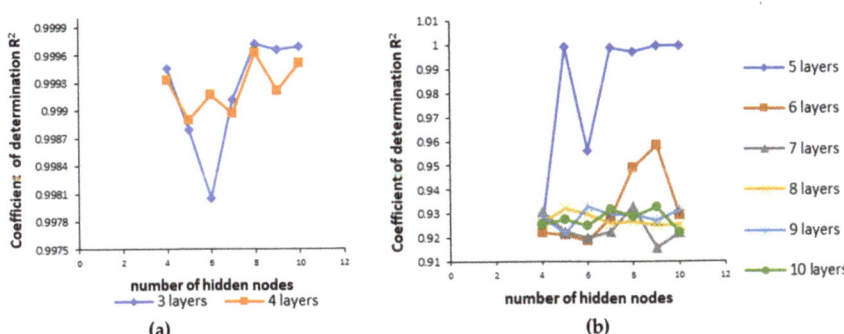

Figure 5. Coefficient of determination (R^2) for neural network 1 with different numbers of hidden nodes and layers (**a**) for 3 and 4 layers (**b**) for 5 to 10 layers.

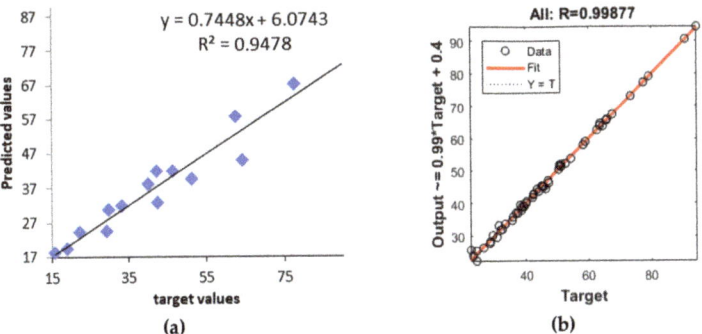

Figure 6. Predicted and experimental cumulative % of ibuprofen release (**a**) for the test dataset in neural network 1 and (**b**) for the whole dataset (training, validation, and test) in neural network 2.

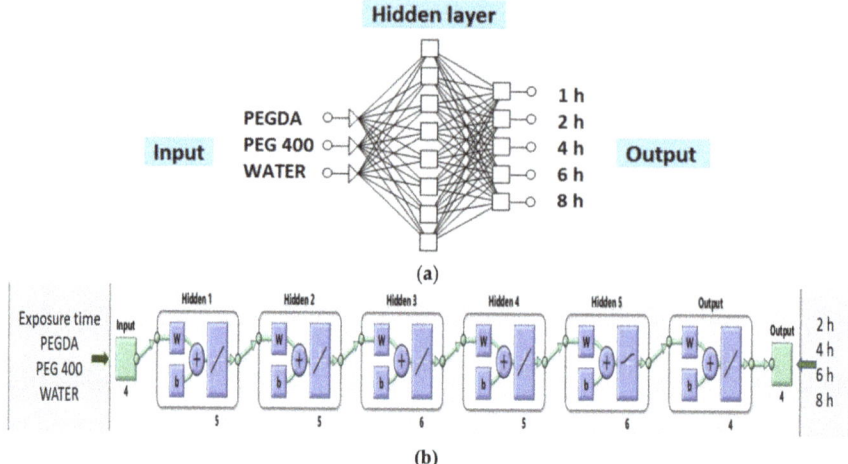

Figure 7. (a) Architecture of neural network 1 and (b) architecture of neural network 2.

3.4. Optimization and Characterization of Optimal Formulation

The optimal formulation according to the desirability function approach consisted of: PEGDA 30%, PEG 400 52.89%, water 12.02%, riboflavin 0.10%, and ibuprofen 5.00%, and printing was done in the same way as test formulations with exposure time of 400 s, bottom exposure 800 s, layer thickness 0.1, and 10 bottom layers. Predicted drug release at time points of 2, 4, 6, and 8 h was 41.96%, 63.34%, 70.00%, and 79.99% respectively. Fabricated optimal and appropriate placebo formulation was observed under a polarized light microscope and cross-sections are shown in Figure 8. On cross-section of printlets, layers were clearly visible which demonstrated the printing process, but inside of layers in both placebo and optimal printlet undefined structures could be observed. The reasons for their appearance have not been clarified.

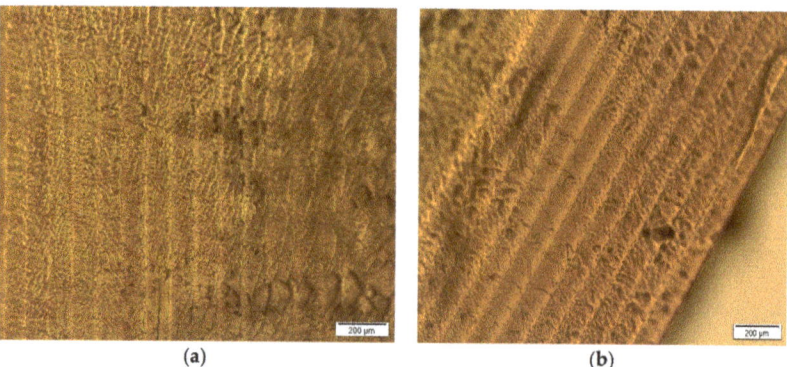

Figure 8. (a) Cross-section of placebo tablet; (b) cross-section of optimal tablet

DSC curves of placebo and optimal printlets are represented in Figure 9. The combination of a sharp peak near 0 °C and a broad peak below 0 °C was observed for the optimal printlet, suggesting co-existence of free and loosely bound water in this formulation. Loosely bound water is associated with non-freezing water and interacts weakly with the ether oxygen, a hydrogen bonded complex between water molecules similar to that in bulk water [30]. The broad endotherm near 100 °C in both placebo and optimal formulations reflects water loss upon heating [9]. No melt endotherm characteristics for ibuprofen are seen, indicating that the drug dissolves in the polymer and/or the water. The solubility of the drug is increased with the presence of solvents like PEG 400, which decreases the polarity of the aqueous solution [9,31]. The exothermic peak near −40°C present in optimal printlets and non-present in placeboes indicates a glass transition temperature of ibuprofen and the presence of ibuprofen in the amorphous phase [32,33].

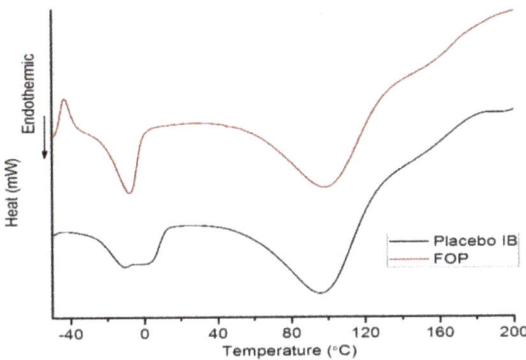

Figure 9. Differential scanning calorimetry (DSC) curves of placebo and optimal printlet.

A dissolution test was performed under the same conditions as the test formulations and results are represented in Table 6 and graphically in Figure 10. For the optimal ibuprofen DLP printlet, comparison of release profiles predicted by neural network 1 and neural network 2 and experimental results was done by calculation of f_1 and f_2. Obtained values for neural network 1 are $f_1 = 14.30$ and $f_2 = 52.15$, and for neural network 2 are $f_1 = 22.34$ and $f_2 = 44.91$.

Table 6. Predicted and experimental in vitro release values at time points of 2, 4, 6, and 8 h for optimal formulation of 3D DLP printlets.

Time (h)	Predicted Values (%) Neural Network 1	Predicted Values (%) Neural Network 2	Experimental Values (%)
2	41.96	45.37	29.85
4	63.34	62.77	51.18
6	70.00	76.66	65.73
8	79.99	88.46	76.60

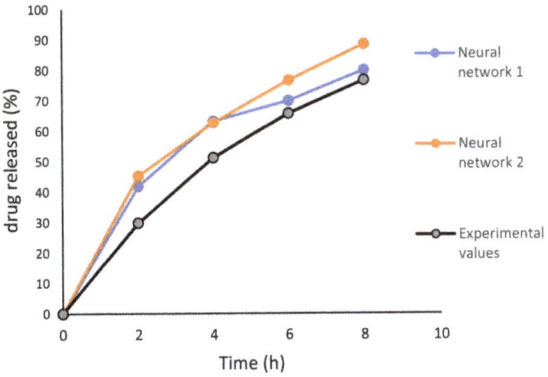

Figure 10. Experimental and predicted dissolution test profiles.

Two different neural networks were developed to test possibilities of understanding the effect of excipients on ibuprofen release. After comparison of predicted and experimental values of in vitro dissolution at the corresponding time points for optimized formulation, the R^2 experimental vs. predicted value was 0.9811 (neural network 1) and 0.9960 (neural network 2). These values are very close to 1.0, with neural network 2 having a slightly higher R^2 value compared to neural network 1. In machine learning, the correlation coefficient and coefficient of determination are usually adopted as evaluation metrics for regression problems. However, the correlation coefficient and the coefficient of determination cannot properly evaluate the performance of the pharmaceutical formulation prediction models. Thus, specific criteria suitable for pharmaceutics should be introduced to evaluate the model performance [34]. In vitro dissolution profiles can be compared by a model-independent method which includes the difference factor (f_1) and the similarity factor (f_2) [35]. Obtained values of f_1 and f_2 for neural network 1 and 2 showed that neural network 1 gave a similar dissolution profile to obtained experimental results. In developing an optimal formulation, the importance of the first two goals was set with two pluses, and the importance of the next two goals (drug release at 6 and 8 hours) was set with three pluses. From the profiles, it is visible that predicted values at 6 and 8 hours were closer to the real values. Neural network 2 was created with combination of formulation and process parameters. Generally, the main limitation regarding the neural networks is the small number of experiments available, as a higher number of experiments would increase the accuracy of the neural network and this will be done in future studies. ANN with possibilities to provide an understanding of the relationship of input–output variables and give better insights into the effects of excipients and process parameters on dissolution rate could help in optimization of formulating processes and printing printlets according to patient's needs.

There are a lot of printing process and formulation parameters and their effects on printlet characteristics are still unknown. Further research will be conducted with the aim to investigate the applicability of combination of ANN and DLP technologies for other drugs and to investigate the effect of formulation and process parameters on characteristics of printlets matrix created with 3D printing technology.

4. Conclusions

DLP technology, as a type of 3D printing technology, can be used for the production of extended-release ibuprofen printlets with PEGDA, PEG 400, and water as the main ingredients, and riboflavin as a photo-initiator. It is necessary to adjust printing parameters for every formulation because of the effect of excipients on the success of printing. The relationship between excipients and drug release in tested formulations is complex and non-linear. Artificial neural networks with their ability to generalize can be a useful tool for understanding the effects of excipients on printlets characteristics with the aim to print printlets with the desired drug release. No single software or modeling algorithm can solve "all" problems, but for better prediction and optimization, application of different softwares can be a helpful method. In this study it was demonstrated that adequate ANN is able to understand the input–output relationship in DLP printing of pharmaceutics.

Supplementary Materials: The following are available online at http://www.mdpi.com/1999-4923/11/10/544/s1: Table S1: Dataset for neural network 1 and Table S2: Dataset for neural network 2.

Author Contributions: Conceptualization M.M., D.M., J.D., A.V., T.S., N.F., and S.I.; methodology, M.M., D.M., J.D., A.V.,T.S., N.F., and S.I.; software, M.M., T.S., A.V., and S.I.; validation, M.M. and D.M.; formal analysis, M.M., T.S., and A.V.; investigation, M.M.; resources, N.F. and S.I.; data curation, M.M., T.S., and A.V.; writing—original draft preparation, M.M.; writing—review and editing, M.M., D.M., J.D., A.V., T.S., N.F., and S.I.; visualization, M.M. and D.M.; supervision, J.D., N.F., and S.I.; project administration, N.F. and S.I.

Funding: This work was done under the projects TR34007, III41007, and OI174028 from the Ministry of Education, Science, and Technological Development, Republic of Serbia. In addition, this study is supported by COST Action MP1404 SimInhalle 'simulation and pharmaceutical technologies for advanced patient-tailored inhaled medicines', supported by COST (European Cooperation in Science and Technology), www.cost.eu.

Conflicts of Interest: The authors declare no conflict of interest.

References

1. Goyanes, A.; Det-Amornrat, U.; Wang, J.; Basit AW. Gaisford, S. 3D scanning and 3D printing as innovative technologies for fabricating personalized topical drug delivery systems. *J. Control. Release* **2016**, *234*, 41–48. [CrossRef] [PubMed]
2. Norman, J.; Madurawe, R.D.; Moore, C.M.V.; Khan, M.A.; Khairuzzaman, A. A new chapter in pharmaceutical manufacturing: 3D-printed drug products. *Adv. Drug Deliv. Rev.* **2017**, *108*, 39–50. [CrossRef] [PubMed]
3. Awad, A.; Trenfield, S.J.; Goyanes, A.; Gaisford, S.; Basit, A.W. Reshaping drug development using 3D printing. *Drug Discov. Today* **2018**, *23*, 1547–1555. [CrossRef] [PubMed]
4. Zhang, J.; Vo, A.Q.; Feng, X.; Bandari, S.; Repka, M.A. Pharmaceutical Additive Manufacturing: a Novel Tool for Complex and Personalized Drug Delivery Systems. *AAPS PharmSciTech* **2018**, *19*, 3388–3402. [CrossRef] [PubMed]
5. Zhang, J.; Feng, X.; Patil, H.; Tiwari, R.V.; Repka, M.A. Coupling 3D printing with hot-melt extrusion to produce controlled-release tablets. *Int. J. Pharm.* **2017**, *519*, 186–197. [CrossRef] [PubMed]
6. Fina, F.; Madla, C.M.; Goyanes, A.; Zhang, J.; Gaisford, S.; Basit, A.W. Fabricating 3D printed orally disintegrating printlets using selective laser sintering. *Int. J. Pharm.* **2018**, *541*, 101–107. [CrossRef] [PubMed]
7. Wang, J.; Goyanes, A.; Gaisford, S.; Basit, A.W. Stereolithographic (SLA) 3D printing of oral modified-release dosage forms. *Int. J. Pharm.* **2016**, *503*, 207–212. [CrossRef]
8. Sadia, M.; Alhnan, M.A.; Ahmed, W.; Jackson, M.J. 3D printing of pharmaceuticals. In *Micro and Nanomanufacturing*; Springer Nature: Basel, Switzerland, 2017; Volume 2, pp. 467–498.
9. Martinez, P.R.; Goyanes, A.; Basit, A.W.; Gaisford, S. Fabrication of drug-loaded hydrogels with stereolithographic 3D printing. *Int. J. Pharm.* **2017**, *532*, 313–317. [CrossRef]
10. Martinez, P.R.; Goyanes, A.; Basit, A.W.; Gaisford, S. Influence of Geometry on the Drug Release Profiles of Stereolithographic (SLA) 3D-Printed Tablets. *AAPS PharmSciTech* **2018**, *19*, 3355–3361. [CrossRef]
11. Kadry, H.; Wadnap, S.; Xu, C.; Ahsan, F. Digital light processing (DLP)3D-printing technology and photoreactive polymers in fabrication of modified-release tablets. *Eur. J. Pharm. Sci.* **2019**, *135*, 60–67. [CrossRef]
12. Barmpalexis, P.; Kanaze, F.I.; Kachrimanis, K.; Georgarakis, E. Artificial neural networks in the optimization of a nimodipine controlled release tablet formulation. *Eur. J. Pharm. Biopharm.* **2010**, *74*, 316–323. [CrossRef] [PubMed]
13. Ibrić, S.; Djuriš, J.; Parojčić, J.; Djurić, Z. Artificial Neural Networks in Evaluation and Optimization of Modified Release Solid Dosage Forms. *Pharmaceutics* **2012**, *4*, 531–550. [CrossRef] [PubMed]
14. Agatonovic-Kustrin, S.; Beresford, R. Basic concepts of artificial neural network (ANN) modeling and its application in pharmaceutical research. *J. Pharm. Biomed. Anal.* **2000**, *22*, 717–727. [CrossRef]
15. Das, P.J.; Preuss, C.; Mazumder, B. Artificial Neural Network as Helping Tool for Drug Formulation and Drug Administration Strategies. In *Artificial Neural Network for Drug Design, Delivery and Disposition*; Elsevier Inc.: Amsterdam, The Netherlands, 2015; pp. 263–276. [CrossRef]
16. Landin, M.; Rowe, R.C. Artificial neural networks technology to model, understand, and optimize drug formulations. In *Formulation Tools for Pharmaceutical Development*; Woodhead Publishing: Oxford, UK, 2013; pp. 7–37. [CrossRef]
17. Havel, J.; Peña, E.M.; Rojas-Hernández, A.; Doucet, J.P.; Panaye, A. Neural networks for optimization of high-performance capillary zone electrophoresis methods. *J. Chromatogr. A.* **1998**, *793*, 317–329. [CrossRef]
18. Medarević, D.P.; Kleinebudde, P.; Djuriš, J.; Djurić, Z.; Ibrić, S. Combined application of mixture experimental design and artificial neural networks in the solid dispersion development. *Drug Dev. Ind. Pharm.* **2016**, *42*, 389–402. [CrossRef]
19. Miletić, T.; Ibrić, S.; Đurić, Z. Combined Application of Experimental Design and Artificial Neural Networks in Modeling and Characterization of Spray Drying Drug: Cyclodextrin Complexes. *Dry Technol.* **2014**, *32*, 167–179. [CrossRef]
20. Takahara, J.; Takayama, K.; Nagai, T. Multi-objective simultaneous optimization technique based on an artificial neural network in sustained release formulations. *J. Control. Release* **1997**, *49*, 11–20. [CrossRef]
21. Fouassier, J.P.; Lalev, J. Supramolecular Photochemistry Principles and Applications of Photochemistry. In *Handbook of Photochemistry and Photophysics of Polymeric Materials*; Wiley-VCH: Weinheim, Germany, 2012. [CrossRef]

22. Nguyen, A.K.; Gittard, S.D.; Koroleva, A.; Schlie, S.; Gaidukeviciute, A.; Chichkov, B.N.; Narayan, R.J. Two-photon polymerization of polyethylene glycol diacrylate scaffolds with riboflavin and triethanolamine used as a water-soluble photoinitiator. *Regen. Med.* **2013**, *8*, 725–738. [CrossRef]
23. Savic, I.; Nikolic, V.; Savic, I.; Nikolic, L.; Stankovic, M.; Moder, K. Optimization of total flavonoid compound extraction from camellia sinesis using the artificial neural network and response surface methodology. *Hem. Ind.* **2012**, *67*, 249–259. [CrossRef]
24. Robles-Martinez, P.; Xu, X.; Trenfield, S.; Awad, A.; Goyanes, A. 3D-Printing of a Multi-Layered Polypill containing Six Drugs using a Novel Stereolitographic Method. *Pharmaceutics* **2019**, *11*, 1–15. [CrossRef]
25. Clark, E.A.; Alexander, M.R.; Irvine, D.J.; Roberts, C.J.; Wallace, M.J.; Sharpe, S.; Wildman, R.D. 3D printing of tablets using inkjet with UV photoinitiation. *Int. J. Pharm.* **2017**, *529*, 523–530. [CrossRef] [PubMed]
26. Mhlanga, N.; Ray, S.S. Kinetic models for the release of the anticancer drug doxorubicin from biodegradable polylactide/metal oxide-based hybrids. *Int. J. Biol. Macromol.* **2015**, *72*, 1301–1307. [CrossRef] [PubMed]
27. Caccavo, D. An overview on the mathematical modeling of hydrogels' behavior for drug delivery systems. *Int. J. Pharm.* **2019**, *560*, 175–190. [CrossRef] [PubMed]
28. Ritger, L.P.A.; Peppas, N.A. Simple equation for description of solute release II. Fickian and anomalous release from swellable devices. *J. Control. Release.* **1987**, *5*, 37–42. [CrossRef]
29. Sun, Y.; Peng, Y.; Chen, Y.; Shukla, A.J. Application of artificial neural networks in the design of controlled release drug delivery systems. *Adv. Drug Deliv. Rev.* **2003**, *55*, 1201–1215. [CrossRef]
30. Jang, E.S.; Kamcev, J.; Kobayashi, K.; Yan, N.; Sujanani, R.; Dilenschneider, T.J.; Park., H.B.; Paul, D.R.; Freeman, B. Influence of water content on alkali metal chloride transport in cross-linked Poly(ethylene glycol) Diacrylate.1. Ion sorption. *Polymer* **2019**, *178*, 121554. [CrossRef]
31. Haddadin, R.; Qian, F.; Desikan, S.; Hussain, M.; Smith, R.L. Estimation of drug solubility in polymers via differential scanning calorimetry and utilization of the fox equation. *Pharm. Dev. Technol.* **2009**, *14*, 18–26. [CrossRef]
32. Hussain, A.; Smith, G.; Khan, K.A.; Bukhari, N.I.; Pedge, N.I.; Ermolina, I. Solubility and dissolution rate enhancement of ibuprofen by co-milling with polymeric excipients. *Eur. J. Pharm. Sci.* **2018**, *123*, 395–403. [CrossRef]
33. Dudognon, E.; Danède, F.; Descamps, M.; Correia, N.T. Evidence for a new crystalline phase of racemic Ibuprofen. *Pharm. Res.* **2008**, *25*, 2853–2858. [CrossRef]
34. Yang, Y.; Ye, Z.; Su, Y.; Zhao, Q.; Li, X.; Ouyang, D. Deep learning for in vitro prediction of pharmaceutical formulations. *Acta Pharm. Sin. B.* **2019**, *9*, 177–185. [CrossRef]
35. Diaz, D.A.; Colgan, S.T.; Langer, C.S.; Bandi, N.; Likar, M.D.; Van Alstine, L. Erratum to: Dissolution Similarity Requirements: How Similar or Dissimilar Are the Global Regulatory Expectations? *AAPS J.* **2016**, *18*, 792. [CrossRef] [PubMed]

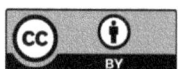

© 2019 by the authors. Licensee MDPI, Basel, Switzerland. This article is an open access article distributed under the terms and conditions of the Creative Commons Attribution (CC BY) license (http://creativecommons.org/licenses/by/4.0/).

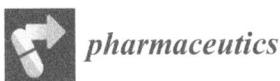

Article

Stencil Printing—A Novel Manufacturing Platform for Orodispersible Discs

Henrika Wickström [1,*], Rajesh Koppolu [2], Ermei Mäkilä [3], Martti Toivakka [2] and Niklas Sandler [1]

1. Pharmaceutical Sciences Laboratory, Åbo Akademi University, Tykistökatu 6A, 20520 Turku, Finland; niklas.o.sandler@gmail.com
2. Laboratory of Natural Materials Technology, Åbo Akademi University, Porthaninkatu 3, 20500 Turku, Finland; rajesh.koppolu@abo.fi (R.K.); martti.toivakka@abo.fi (M.T.)
3. Laboratory of Industrial Physics, University of Turku, Vesilinnantie 5, 20500 Turku, Finland; emmaki@utu.fi
* Correspondence: henrika.wickstrom@abo.fi

Received: 16 November 2019; Accepted: 16 December 2019; Published: 1 January 2020

Abstract: Stencil printing is a commonly used printing method, but it has not previously been used for production of pharmaceuticals. The aim of this study was to explore whether stencil printing of drug containing polymer inks could be used to manufacture flexible dosage forms with acceptable mass and content uniformity. Formulation development was supported by physicochemical characterization of the inks and final dosage forms. The printing of haloperidol (HAL) discs was performed using a prototype stencil printer. Ink development comprised of investigations of ink rheology in combination with printability assessment. The results show that stencil printing can be used to manufacture HAL doses in the therapeutic treatment range for 6–17 year-old children. The therapeutic HAL dose was achieved for the discs consisting of 16% of hydroxypropyl methylcellulose (HPMC) and 1% of lactic acid (LA). The formulation pH remained above pH 4 and the results imply that the drug was amorphous. Linear dose escalation was achieved by an increase in aperture area of the print pattern, while keeping the stencil thickness fixed. Disintegration times of the orodispersible discs printed with 250 and 500 µm thick stencils were below 30 s. In conclusion, stencil printing shows potential as a manufacturing method of pharmaceuticals.

Keywords: stencil printing; pharmacoprinting; orodispersible discs; orodisperible films

1. Introduction

Pharmaceuticals are predominantly produced according to a centralized and time-consuming batch processing approach [1]. This supply chain model allows production of only a few dose strengths in large volumes, which for the blockbuster drugs are chosen based on population level information [2]. Challenges may arise if a patient is treated with an active pharmaceutical ingredient (API) with a narrow therapeutic window or a varying pharmacokinetic or pharmacodynamic profile. In these cases, patients would benefit from a more personalized dosing tailored according to the patient's age, weight, body surface, gender, genetic profile, or treatment response [3,4]. A more pull-driven and personalized production of medicines could be possible if printing technologies would be utilized. Decentralized manufacturing of doses could result in added value when treating patients with medicines where tailoring and monitoring of the dose is critical. Printing technologies have for instance shown to allow simultaneous personalized dose preparation and identification [5].

Orodispersible films (ODFs) that disintegrate in the mouth have been developed to ease the administration of medicines to children and elderly that have difficulty swallowing pills [6]. Orodispersible films are conventionally manufactured using solvent casting and the formulation development is usually done on a smaller scale [7]. However, the film composition and the processing conditions need to be tuned when the production is moved from a laboratory scale to a continuous manufacturing process [8]. When manufacturing ODFs by solvent casting, the dosing can be adjusted by varying the wet film thickness during the manufacturing process or by varying the API content of the solution [9]. Dosing is achieved by cutting different areas of the film. The cutting is a critical step and it might also lead to product waste. A dosing device, which would improve the dosing flexibility, was developed to address this issue [10]. Electrospinning is another method, which has been utilized to produce ODFs [11]. Dosing flexibility is similarly achieved by cutting different areas of the electrospun film.

Impact, non-impact, and 3D printing technologies have been investigated as potential manufacturing methods of ODFs. If doses are manufactured utilizing printing technologies the critical dose cutting step is eliminated. Single dose units have either been made by depositing a drug containing ink formulation onto a placebo ODF or drug formulations directly onto a release liner or packaging material foil. High viscous solutions have been deposited onto ODFs by flexography (impact method) [12]. Low viscous drug solutions and suspensions have been deposited onto placebo ODFs by thermal, piezoelectric, and solenoid valve-based inkjet technology (non-impact methods) [13–17]. Especially inkjet printing has shown to allow accurate deposition of one or more APIs according to a digital design. Single unit ODF doses have been prepared by extruding a semi-solid ink formulation through a syringe using pressure assisted 3D printing according to a digital design [18]. Hot-melt extrusion has also been used to formulate solid filaments used in fused deposition modeling (FDM) 3D printers to produce ODFs [19]. Hot-melt ram extrusion 3D printing, which combines extrusion and printing, has also been explored to produce ODFs [20].

In solvent casting, flexographic, inkjet, and extrusion printing different solvents are used in the ink formulation, and consequently the formulations need to be dried. The use of organic solvents and the drying step has shown to have an impact on the mechanical properties of the ODFs [8]. Furthermore, the manufacturing method has also shown to have an impact on the mechanical properties; the ODFs made by solvent casting were more durable compared to ODFs prepared by FDM [19]. When considering using hot-melt extrusion as a manufacturing method of ODFs one needs to ensure that the API does not degrade by the heat of the manufacturing step. The manufacturing method needs to be chosen considering the physicochemical properties of the drug and the dosing range/flexibility needed.

Stencil printing is a potential manufacturing method of ODFs or orodispersible discs that has not been explored before. Previously in other industries the method has shown to be suited as both a point-of-need and low-cost high-throughput manufacturing process [21,22]. Stencil printing is an impact printing method that enables pattern transfer mediated by a stencil (Figure 1). Stencil printing is a variant of screen printing in which the ink is distributed through the open pores of a patterned mesh/screen. In stencil printing the ink is passed through the stencil apertures with the help of a blade or a squeegee and can either be built as a flatbed or rotary printing process. Stencil printing has lately been utilized to manufacture wearable electronics with resolutions reaching from mm to a few μm [23–25]. The inks that have been used for stencil printing of electronics are solder pastes, which contain metal particles of specific particle size ranges, and the rheological properties of the pastes have been investigated with regards to stencil printability [26,27]. In general, screen and stencil printing technologies have been utilized in various fields, since it allows printing onto various materials (i.e., textiles, metal, plastics, ceramics, and paper) [28].

The suitability of producing pharmaceuticals using stencil printing has not been studied before. Thus, this article will give insight about the potential of stencil printing of drug containing polymer inks in the manufacture of personalized dosage forms. Furthermore, ink formulation properties and factors affecting the printing process are investigated and discussed.

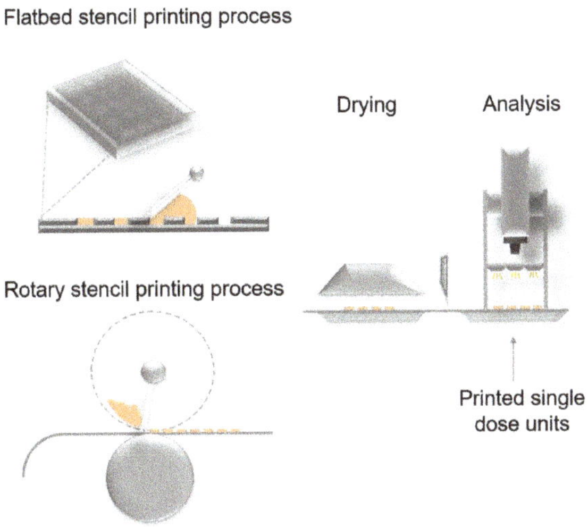

Flatbed stencil printing process

Figure 1. Planar and rotary stencil printing processes.

2. Materials and Methods

2.1. Stencil Printing Set-Up

The stencil printing can be built as a batchwise (flatbed) or a continuous (rotary) printing process (Figure 1) [28]. Critical variables affecting the stencil printing process have previously been identified and divided into the following categories: stencil, substrate, ink, printer, and environment [26]. In this proof of concept study prototype flatbed printer was used. The batchwise stencil printing set-up consisted of a drawdown coater (K202, RK Print-coat instruments Ltd., Royston, UK), a blade holder connected to a rod, a blade, and a frame. A Silhouette Curio crafting cutter (Silhouette America Inc., Lehi, UT, USA) was used to make stencils out of polyester films (125 µm; Melinex, Dupont Teijin Films, Cheste, VA, USA) and Teflon (PTFE Etraflon film) films (Figure 2A). Disc, square, and teardrop geometries were designed using the Silhouette studio v3. Software (Silhouette America Inc.) and the shapes were cut out from the films. The cut polyester stencil films were glued together to make 250, 500, 750, and 1000 µm thick stencils. The Teflon films were acquired with thicknesses of 250, 500, 1000, and 1500 µm. Stencils with varying stencil area (Ø 10.8, 14.4, 18.0, 21.6, and 25.2 mm) were only prepared for the disc geometry (Figure 2B).

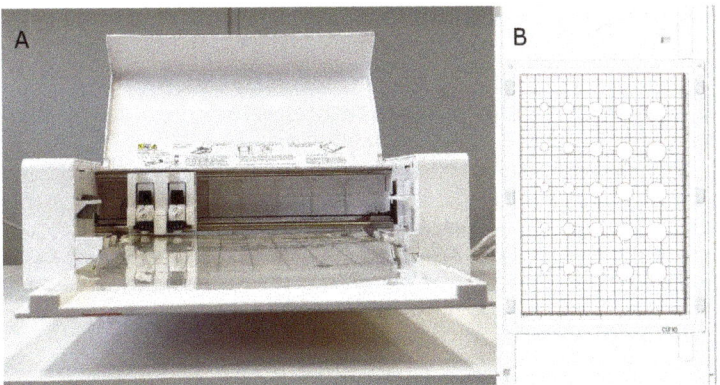

Figure 2. (**A**) A Silhouette Curio crafting cutter machine and (**B**) stencil aperture design.

2.2. Ink Formulation

Hydroxypropyl methylcellulose (HPMC) inks with polymer contents of 12–18% were prepared as placebo formulations. HPMC (Methocel E5 Premium LV, Dow, Bomlitz, Germany) was dissolved in a deionized water and ethanol (Etax Aa 99.5%, Altia Oyj, Rajamäki, Finland) solvent mixture (1:1, v/v) using high speed mixing. Glycerol (CAS 200-289-5, Fagron GmbH & Co. KG, Glinde, Germany) (1%) was used as a plasticizer. Erythrosin B (spirit soluble 95%, CAS 16423-68-0, Aldrich Chem. Co., Milwaukee, WI, USA) was added (1%, v/w) as colorant to the formulations. Formulation development was continued with the formulation that contained 16% of HPMC. Lactic acid (LA, 1%, v/w) (CAS 50-21-5, Sigma-Aldrich, Japan), was added to the 1:1 ethanol water solvent mixture to lower the pH and consequently allow haloperidol (HAL, CAS 52-86-8, Sigma, China) to dissolve. Table 1 lists the various combinations of ink formulations that were studied.

Table 1. The compositions of the formulations used.

Formulations	Lactic Acid (LA)	Haloperidol (HAL)
HPMC 16%	−	−
HPMC 16% LA	+	−
HPMC 16% LA HAL	+	+
HPMC 16% HAL	−	+

2.3. Stencil Printing

Printing of the orodispersible discs was performed at a speed of 259 mm/min using transparency films (Folex Imaging, Clear transparent X-10.0 film, 0.100 mm) as substrate/release liner. The ink was poured onto the 250, 500, 750, and 1000 µm thick stencils and was distributed with the help of a blade. Each printing pass generated 15 doses. The printed discs were dried overnight in an oven (T = 25 °C, RH % = 60).

2.4. Rheology

The dynamic viscosity and the thixotropic flow (time dependent recovery) of the inks were measured using a rheometer (Physica MCR 300, Paar Physica, Graz, Austria) connected with a thermostated bath and a temperature control unit (Techne RB-12A & TU-16D). The cone and plate measurement geometry (50 mm diameter and 2° angle) was used for the measurements. Prior to the measurements the samples were preconditioned for 1 min at a shear rate of 100 s^{-1} and then let to rest for 2 min. A shear rate ramp ranging from 0.1 to 1000 s^{-1} was applied to the samples (n = 3) at 25 °C. Thixotropy was evaluated with a step test in which the time dependent viscosity recovery is observed after applying a high-shear rate (500 s^{-1}) step change to a low constant shear rate 0.1 s^{-1}. Formulations containing 16% of HPMC were further studied.

2.5. Visual Print Evaluation

The spreading of inks HPMC 12–18% was studied by capturing images of discs dried overnight at 25 °C and relative humidity of 60%. The discs (Ø 18 mm) were printed with 250, 500, and 1000 µm thick stencils onto transparency film substrates. Images were captured using a mobile phone camera (OnePlus5T OnePlus Technology Ltd., Shenzhen, China) at a fixed height. Spreading of the inks with different polymer content on the substrates was analyzed based on the captured images using the ImageJ software. Before the image analysis was performed, the hue and saturation values of the image were adjusted, the scale was set, and the printed area with 12 discs was selected.

2.6. pH

The pH of the ink formulations and the printed discs was measured using a pH meter (FE20, Mettler Toledo AG, Schwerzenbach, Switzerland). For the surface pH of the discs (500 µm stencil, Ø

18 mm) 1 mL of distilled water was used to wet the surface and provide adequate contact with the electrode. The reading was taken after allowing the pH electrode to equilibrate for 1 min on the surface of the discs.

2.7. Disintegration

The test system consisted of a sample holder clamp to which the printed disc was attached. A smaller clip of 3 g was fixed to the bottom of the disc as a weight. The disintegration tests were performed using a static test set-up by immersing half of the disc ($n = 10$) and the weight into a beaker of 500 mL distilled water (37.0 ± 0.5 °C). The endpoint was recorded when the 3-gram clip reached the bottom of the disintegration beaker. The tests were performed under ambient conditions of samples conditioned overnight in 25 °C and 60% relative humidity. Discs (Ø 18 mm) printed using HPMC 12–18% placebo inks and 250, 500, 750, and 1000 µm thick stencils were analyzed.

2.8. Drug Assay

A HPLC (LaChrome, Merck Hitachi, Tokyo, Japan) system (Interface D7100, Pump L-7100, Autosampler L-7200, Detector L-7450, Shimadzu column oven CTO-10) was used for the quantification of the printed HAL doses. The separation was performed using an Intersil ODS-3.5 µm, 4.6 × 150 mm column (GL Sciences, Tokyo, Japan) with a pre-column (Guard Column E 10 mm) attached. The mobile phase consisted of 0.05% TFA in deionized water (CAS 76-05-1, Trifluoroacetic acid, Sigma-Aldrich, Germany) and 0.05% TFA in ACN (CAS 75-05-8, Acetonitrile, HPLC grade, Fisher Chemicals, Loughborough, UK) (65:35, v/v). The flow rate was 1 mL/min, injection volume was 10 µL, and detection wavelength was set at 243 nm.

2.9. Uniformity of Mass of Single-Dose Preparations

The stencil printed discs of different sizes (Ø 10.8, 14.4, 18.0, 21.6, and 25.2 mm) were conditioned for 12 h at 25 °C and 60% relative humidity before being weighed. A total of 20 units were chosen at random and weighed individually.

2.10. Uniformity of Content of Single Dose Preparations

The content uniformity of the stencil printed discs of different sizes (Ø 10.8, 14.4, 18.0, 21.6, and 25.2 mm) was determined ($n = 10$) in 100 mL of 1% lactic acid deionized water/EtOH solution (1:1, v/v) for 2 h at 150 rpm. Samples were withdrawn and analyzed as such according to the drug assay described above.

2.11. Polarized Light Microscopy

The stencil printed discs were imaged using a microscope with transmitted polarized light (Leica DM IRB microskopie and Systeme GmbH, Wezlar, Germany) with ×10/0.3 magnification (PL fluotar 506000). Images of starting materials and printed discs were captured using a OnePlus 5T mobile phone camera.

2.12. X-ray Powder Diffraction

The crystallinity of the printed disc components was studied with X-ray diffraction (XRD). The samples were placed on zero-background holders and scanned with PANalytical Empyrean diffractometer (Malvern Panalytical B.V., Almelo, the Netherlands) in θ/θ Bragg-Brentano geometry, using Cu Kα radiation with a PIXcel3D detector in scanning line mode. The scan was done for 2θ in a range of 5–50° with a step size of 0.013° using a step time of 60 s. The incident beam optics consisted of a 0.04 rad Soller slit and a fixed 1/4° divergence slit, while the diffracted beam optics included a 0.04 rad Soller slit.

2.13. Differential Scanning Calorimetry (DSC)

DSC measurements were carried out using a conventional DSC (Q 2000, TA instruments, USA). The printed samples were measured in Tzero aluminum pans with perforated (discs) and intact (raw materials) lids. Thermograms of the discs were recorded in a heat/isothermal/cool/heat cycle. The samples (5.1 ± 0.2 mg) were heated up to 100 °C with a rate of 10 °C/min, held at 100 °C at 5 min, cooled down to −40 °C at a rate of 10 °C/min and heated up to 200 °C using a rate of 10 °C/min. Thermograms of raw materials (5.03 ± 0.2 mg) were recorded as a ramp from 0 to 200 °C using a rate of 10°/min. The DSC was calibrated using sapphire crystals and indium.

2.14. Fourier Transform Infrared Spectroscopy (FTIR)

The FTIR spectra of the samples were obtained using Bruker Invenio R spectrometer (Bruker Optics GmbH, Ettlingen, Germany), equipped with a PA301 photoacoustic detector (Gasera Oy, Turku, Finland) using dried air as the carrier gas.

3. Results

3.1. Stencil Preparation

The polyester film (250 μm) was the material with the most favorable characteristics to be used as stencil material. The apertures and geometries were easily designed and cut from the polyester films. Since the stencil thickness and the aperture area of the stencils were the dose defining units, the possibility to vary these factors was of importance. Thicker stencils were produced by attaching 250 μm films on top of each other to make 250, 500, 750, and 1000 μm thick stencils. The stencils made of Teflon were not suitable because the thinnest films (250 and 500 μm) were not rigid enough, which caused challenges during the aperture emptying when the stencil was removed and the thickest (1000 and 1500 μm) were not flat enough. Thus, polyester was the best option as stencil material.

3.2. Ink Formulation Development

The suitability of producing variable dose strengths using a flatbed stencil printing process was studied. HAL was chosen as a model drug. The drug is used for treatment of schizophrenia and the therapeutic dose for 6–17 year-old children is 0.5–3 mg, while it is up to 10 mg once a day for adults [29]. HAL is known to be a CYP2D6 substrate and polymorphism of the liver enzyme between individuals has a large impact on the pharmacokinetics of the drug [30]. Genotype identification of the CYP2D6 substrate is estimated to be beneficial for 30–40% of patients, when selecting the active pharmaceutical ingredient or customizing the dose for an individual. Consequently, patients could benefit from having personalized doses printed of this specific drug.

HPMC was chosen as a matrix former since it is soluble in water and ethanol mixtures and remains stable in pH between 3–11. HAL is practically insoluble in water, slightly soluble in ethanol, and freely soluble in dilute acids [31]. Lactic acid (1%) was added to the formulation to enable the drug to dissolve. HAL is known to be stable in aqueous lactic acid solutions at room temperature [32] and known to be a saliva stimulant, which is of relevance when formulating an orodispersible drug formulation [33]. Erythrosine was chosen as colorant due to its good solubility in ethanol and glycerol was added as a plasticizer. The ink formulation is shown in Table 2.

Table 2. Ink formulation.

Ingredient	Function	Quantity (%)
HAL	API	1
HPMC E5	Matrix former	12–18
Erythrosine	Colorant	1
Glycerol	Plasticizer	3.5
Ethanol	Solvent	50
Lactic acid 1% (aq.)	Solvent, pH modifier, saliva stimulant	Ad 100

3.3. Ink Rheology and Printability

The rheological characteristics of the inks were determined by applying a shear ramp on the samples and by monitoring the time dependent recovery of the samples after application of a step change in shear rate. The HPMC 12–18% inks showed all Newtonian behavior between shear rates 0.1 and 100 s^{-1}. However, at higher shear rates the inks showed shear-thinning behavior. All inks had higher low shear viscosities than 1000 mPas; at a shear rate of 10 s^{-1} the viscosity of the inks HPMC 12, 14, 16, and 18% were 1240, 2177, 3660, and 6190 mPas, respectively (Figure 3A). The thixotropic flow of the inks was also investigated. All inks recovered quickly to their original viscosity levels after an applied high shear rate step of 500 s^{-1} for 30 s (Figure 3B). In general, the viscosity of the ink should be low enough to allow the blade to press and fill the ink through the apertures of the stencil, but high enough to retain its geometry when the stencil is removed. Ink formulations with HAL dissolved (HPMC 16% LA HAL) and dispersed (HPMC 16% HAL) were prepared, which enabled comparison of the rheological properties of inks with and without particles. The dispersed particles had an impact on the viscosity at low shear rates, while the HPMC 16% LA HAL formulation showed similar behavior as the HPMC 16% and HPMC 16% LA formulations with the same polymer content (Figure 4).

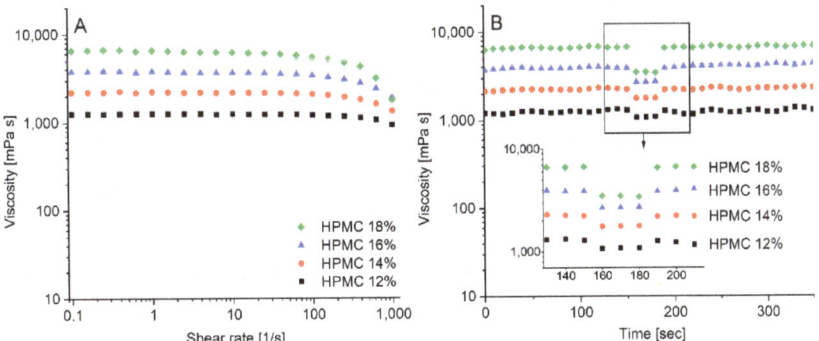

Figure 3. (**A**) Shear ramp of formulations containing 12–18% polymer ($n = 3 \pm$ std), (**B**) thixotropic flow measurements (shear rate: 0.1, shear rate: 500, shear rate: 0.1 s^{-1}, $n = 3 \pm$ std) for hydroxypropyl methylcellulose (HPMC) 12–18%.

The printability was evaluated in terms of aperture filling of different geometries and spreading of the ink onto the release liner. The aperture geometry was evaluated at a fixed printing speed (259 mm/min) and using a 500 µm stencil with disc, square, and teardrop apertures. No clear difference in aperture filling was observed between geometries when ink formulation HPMC 16% was printed under the above-mentioned conditions (Figure 5). However, at higher speeds differences could possibly be distinguished. It has been reported that the aperture geometry should be rotated 45° to the printing direction to ensure uniform filling of the apertures [34]. Taking this into account, the square and teardrop (printed from the sharper direction) should be preferred. However, the circular geometry is less prone to slumping, meaning that it has a greater ability to retain the printed shape.

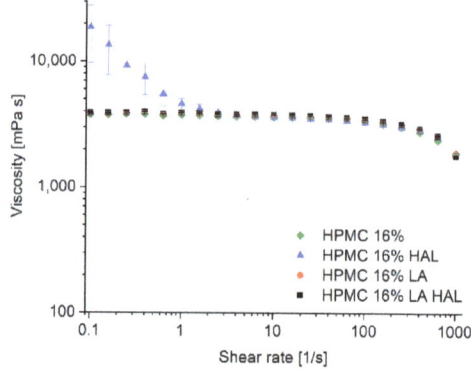

Figure 4. Shear ramp of HPMC 16% formulations (HAL = haloperidol, LA = lactic acid).

Figure 5. Stencil printed discs of 3 geometries using ink formulation HPMC 16% (500 μm stencil height).

Next, the spreading of the inks onto the release liner was studied. Inks were printed using stencils with circular apertures (Ø 18 mm) and stencil thicknesses of 250, 500, and 1000 μm. The spreading of the ink onto the release liner was evaluated based on image analysis done after allowing the samples to dry for 24 h at 25 °C and 60% relative humidity. The lower the ink viscosity and the higher the stencil thickness, the more the ink spread on the transparency film/release liner (Figure 6). Formulations containing less than 16% of HPMC were seen to spread more than 15% from the original stencil aperture area of 254.57 mm^2. Due to the low viscosity of the inks some spreading was expected. Higher print quality could also be achieved by making fine pitch stencils by laser cutting.

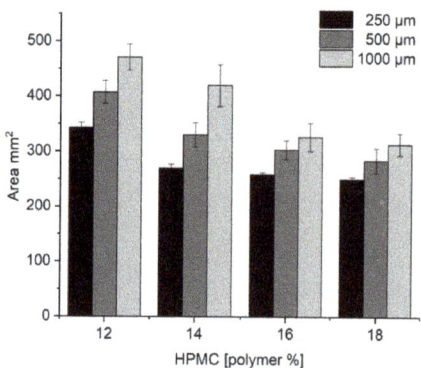

Figure 6. Area from printed Ø 18 mm discs analyzed using ImageJ ($n = 12$) for formulations with increasing polymer content and stencil height.

3.4. Disintegration of Discs

The disintegration times of the discs (Ø 18 mm) containing 12–18% of HPMC and printed using 250 μm stencil were below 4 s and for 500 μm stencils below 28 s (Figure 7). The disintegration results of the discs prepared using the 500 μm stencil fulfilled the specification threshold of 30 s for orodispersible tablets. The European Pharmacopeia 9th edition (Ph. Eur. 9th) does not contain any specifications regarding disintegration times of ODFs. The disintegration times for the 12, 14, 16, and 18% of HPMC discs printed with the thickest stencil 1000 μm were 29 ± 5, 49 ± 18, 140 ± 37, and 200 ± 30 s, respectively. Based on these disintegration results and on the results from the spreading tests in Section 3.2, the formulation containing 16% of HPMC was further studied.

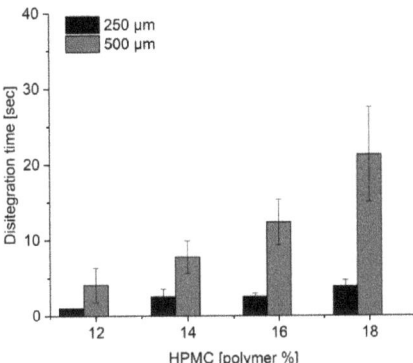

Figure 7. Disintegration time (s) for 18 mm disc formulations ($n = 10$) with increasing polymer content (12–18%) and 250 and 500 μm thick stencils.

3.5. pH of Ink Formulations and Disc Surfaces

The impact of HAL and LA on the formulation pH was investigated. LA lowered the pH of the ink formulation to 3–4, whereas the addition of HAL increased the pH. The surface pH of the stencil printed discs was determined to be above 4 (Table 3). ODFs with a surface pH of 4.5–6.5 have been investigated not to cause local irritation of the mucosa in the mouth [35]. Drug delivery of slightly acidic ODFs is less likely to cause harm the mucosa compared to mucoadhesive buccal films that are attached for a longer time to the mucosal membrane [36].

Table 3. Ink formulation and disc surface pH (average ± standard deviation) (21.5 ± 1 °C).

Formulation	Ink Formulation ($n = 3$)	Surface pH ($n = 3$)
HPMC 16%	7.10 ± 0.02	6.02 ± 0.28
HPMC 16% LA	3.23 ± 0.06	4.18 ± 0.45
HPMC 16% LA HAL	4.24 ± 0.09	4.08 ± 0.15
HPMC 16% HAL	8.00 ± 0.06	5.59 ± 0.14

3.6. Quantification of Haloperidol by HPLC

HAL was detected using HPLC. The method used showed to be linear ($R^2 = 0.999$) within a concentration range of 1–50 μg/mL. The detection limit (LOD) was 0.38 μg/mL and quantification limit (LOQ) was 1.15 μg/mL. The retention time of HAL was 4.5 min (capacity factor 2). The method was seen to be reproducible and the samples were seen to remain stable (Supplementary Materials Table S1).

3.7. Uniformity of Mass and Content

The printed discs fulfilled the requirements of mass uniformity stated in Ph. Eur. 9th. No mass unit deviated more than 10% from the average mass. The printed discs also fulfilled the content uniformity requirements. Each individual content was between 85–115% of the average content. Linear dose escalation was seen for the discs with various aperture areas printed with a 500 µm stencil (R^2 = 0.9961) (Table 4). The mass and dose escalation were not precisely doubled as the stencil thickness increased in the following range: 250–500–1000 µm. The amount of paste transferred is dependent on the aperture size and pressure [37]. Repetition of the dose escalation study could be done in the future with a stencil printer where the pressure could be set and monitored. Furthermore, the removal of the stencil should also be automated to minimize human error.

Table 4. Uniformity of mass (n = 20, average ± standard deviation) and uniformity of content (n = 10, average ± standard deviation) of discs (Ø 10.8–25.2 mm) printed with HPMC 16% LA HAL and 500 µm stencil.

Discs (Ø mm)	Uniformity of Mass (mg ± sd)	Uniformity of Content (mg ± sd)
10.8	10.78 ± 0.20	0.49 ± 0.01
14.4	18.70 ± 0.53	0.87 ± 0.02
18.0	29.43 ± 0.83	1.43 ± 0.03
21.6	42.59 ± 1.11	1.97 ± 0.04
25.2	55.30 ± 1.34	2.56 ± 0.07

3.8. Polarized Light Microscopy

The starting material as well as printed discs were studied under the polarized light microscope (Figure 8). The crystal morphology of HPMC was acicular, while the HAL was platy. The particle size of HAL was larger compared to the HPMC polymer. HPMC was almost entirely dissolved in the solvent mixtures with and without LA (HPMC 16% and HPMC 16% LA). The pH drop caused by LA enabled HAL to dissolve, while it remained dispersed in the neutral polymer matrix (HPMC 16% HAL). Lower pH was shown to lighten the red color of erythrosine, which is due to its predominantly unionized form at a pH below 4.5 [38]. Consequently, the colorant was less soluble and provided lower color intensity in the solvent mixtures containing LA.

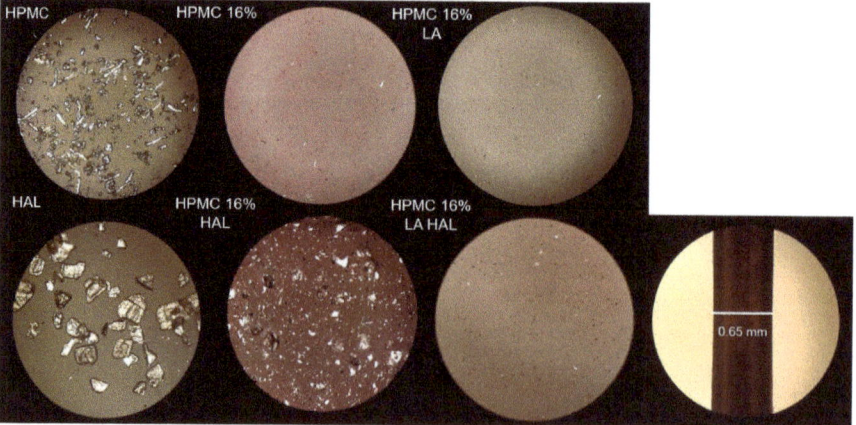

Figure 8. Polarized light microscopy of raw materials HPMC and haloperidol (HAL) and printed discs HPMC 16%, HPMC 16% lactic acid (LA), HPMC 16% LA HAL, and HPMC 16% HAL (magnification ×10), stencil height 500 µm.

3.9. X-ray Diffraction

The printed formulation with HAL dispersed in the polymer matrix (HPMC 16% HAL) showed small diffraction peaks at 12.8, 14.9, 19.9, and 25.9 (Figure 9). These peaks correspond to those observed in the initial crystalline HAL. The HPMC powder was amorphous as suggested by the broad halos near 10° and 20° with a small diffraction peak at 31.9°, which is typical for the polymer. The physical mixture of HAL/HPMC (1/16) correspondingly showed the attenuated reflections related to the pure API on the amorphous HPMC background, suggesting limited interaction between the API and the polymer when only mixed. The printed formulation HPMC 16% LA HAL was amorphous. Consequently, the small addition of LA made the solvent mixture more acidic, which in turn enabled the drug to dissolve.

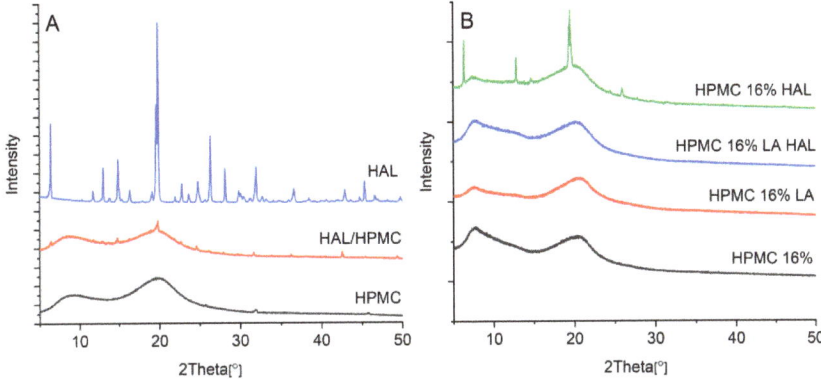

Figure 9. (**A**) X-ray diffractogram of powders HAL, HPMC, and physical mixture HAL/HPMC (1/16) and (**B**) printed discs of HPMC 16%, HPMC 16% LA, HPMC 16% LA HAL, and HPMC 16% HAL.

3.10. Differential Scanning Calorimetry (DSC)

For reference purposes, the thermal behavior of the pure HAL and HPMC were analyzed with DSC. The crystalline HAL expectedly underwent melting at 150.8 °C with an enthalpy of fusion, ΔH_{fus} = 140.5 J/g (Figure 10). The pure HPMC, as the XRD diffractogram suggested, did not indicate any phase transitions in the utilized temperature range, showing only a glass transition occurring at ca. 174–175 °C. Only a slight shift in the melting onset of HAL was observed for the physical mixture, as the phase transition began at 149.5 °C. The DSC results from the ink formulations supported the observations made with the XRD. The only disc where crystalline HAL could be detected was the HPMC 16% HAL with a melting point of 144.6 °C and heat of fusion of 2.78 J/g.

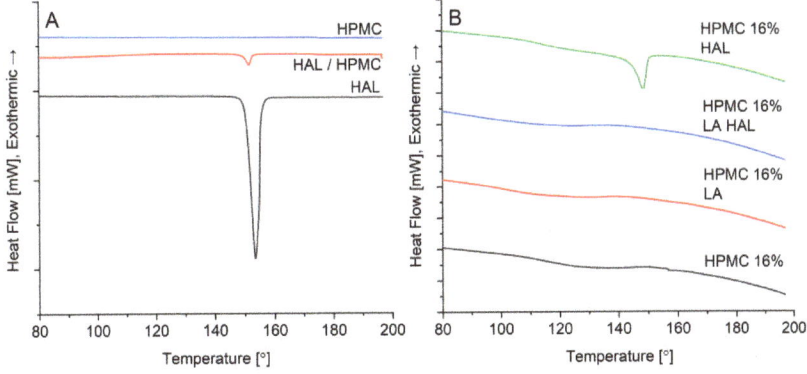

Figure 10. Thermograms of the (**A**) pure components and their physical mixture in 1:16 w/w ratio (HAL/HPMC) and (**B**) printed discs of HPMC 16%, HPMC 16% LA, HPMC 16% LA HAL, and HPMC 16% HAL, (stencil thickness 500 μm).

3.11. Fourier Transform Infrared Spectroscopy

The carbonyl stretch in HAL at 1681 cm^{-1} could be distinguished in the printed HPMC 16% LA HAL discs where the drug was dissolved in the ink (Figure 11) [39]. However, the peak was not detected for the HPMC 16% HAL discs with crystals. Because the XRD and DSC results showed amorphization of the HPMC 16% LA HAL, one would expect to see a shift in the carbonyl group of the HAL due to hydrogen bond formation. However, this could not be confirmed with the FTIR measurements. The peak at 1728 cm^{-1} (carbonyl stretch of the acid) belonging to lactic acid was distinguished for printed discs of the HPMC 16% LA and HPMC 16% LA HAL formulations [40].

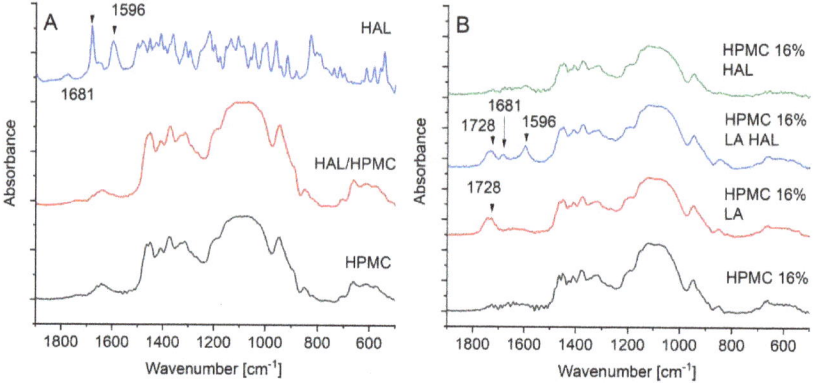

Figure 11. Infrared spectra of (**A**) pure HAL, HPMC, and physical mixture of HAL/HPMC (1/16) and (**B**) printed discs of HPMC 16%, HPMC 16% LA, HPMC 16% LA HAL, and HPMC 16% HAL.

4. Discussion

The suitability of producing pharmaceuticals using stencil printing was explored. Polymer-based ink formulations were developed and printed according to the predefined geometries cut from the stencil to prepare personalized doses of HAL. The stencils were the dose defining units; different doses were varied by aperture areas and stencil heights. The higher the viscosity of the ink formulation, the less spreading of the solution occurred after printing. Thus, ink solutions with dynamic viscosities >3000 mPas (shear rate 10 s^{-1}) were the most favorable formulations for stencil printing. Formulations with dynamic viscosities of at least 1000 mPas (shear rate 6 s^{-1}) have been successfully used to produce ODFs by solvent casting [8]. The viscosity of the ink formulation is of major importance in solvent casting, since it affects the API content per cm^2. It is less critical in stencil printing, since the dose and the volume printed is defined by the aperture of the stencil.

This study shows that a pull-driven and batchwise production of personalized doses utilizing stencil printing technology and a polymer-based ink formulation was possible. A printing speed of 259 mm/min was used to manufacture 15 doses at a time, while solvent casting speeds of 17–339 mm/min have been used to manufacture ODFs [8]. The solvent cast film needs to be cut to make personalized doses. Cutting, which has been defined as a critical process parameter, might also cause drug waste. Thus, printing is more suited for the production for personalized doses.

The placebo discs printed using the 250 and 500 µm thick stencils disintegrated completely within 5 and 30 s, respectively. These results are in line with disintegration results of HPMC ODFs found in literature [41].

The robustness of the stencil printing process could be improved by automating the stencil movement and ink distribution steps. Addition of a drying unit to the plate on which the printing is performed and optimization of the drying time would speed up the process. Since the ink formulations used in this study were comparable with solvent casting formulations, drying was also considered as the time limiting step for the stencil printing process. Automated batchwise printing, drying, and analysis unit could be used for manufacturing personalized doses.

Alternatively, the production capacity of stencil printing could be improved if the solvent amount of the ink formulation would be reduced. Particles are often included in the inks or pastes used for manufacturing of electronics using stencil printing technology and the pastes show usually non-Newtonian behavior and have higher viscosities [26]. Adjustment of the solder paste rheology have been reported to enable high print resolution [23–25]. The rheology can be adjusted by varying the particle size, distribution, and shape, as well as the solvents and the viscosity controlling agents [42]. Development of a paste with higher solid content of an API with small particle size and narrow size distribution could be done in the future. The advantages of the orodispersible dosage form could remain by printing a pastier ink onto a placebo ODF or onto a porous substrate to ease administration. However, ink optimization would need to be conducted to ensure accurate print quality and ink compatibility with the substrate. This alternative could suit continuous and high-throughput manufacturing of stencil printed dosage forms with a more restricted dosing flexibility. However, to develop a robust stencil printing process that enables the production of dosage forms that fulfill the quality requirements set by regulatory authorities entails interplay among engineering, formulation development, and quality assurance.

5. Conclusions

This study demonstrated that a polymer-based HAL ink formulation could be printed using a batchwise stencil printing process to prepare orodispersible HAL dosage forms for children within a therapeutic dose range and fulfilling both mass and content uniformity requirements. The polymer-based inks were Newtonian at shear rates below $100~s^{-1}$ and recovered quickly to the original viscosity level after application of a high shear rate step. X-ray and DSC results suggest that HAL was amorphous for the printed formulation HPMC 16% LA HAL and crystalline for the printed formulation HPMC 16% HAL, without LA.

Supplementary Materials: The following are available online at http://www.mdpi.com/1999-4923/12/1/33/s1. Table S1. Repeatability, reproducibility and sample stability of the HPLC method.

Author Contributions: H.W. managed the project, as well as planned and executed the research, acquired the funding, and wrote the article. E.M. assisted with the FTIR and X-ray measurements at the University of Turku. R.K. and M.T. brought expertise to the stencil printing and rheology parts of the article. N.S. and M.T. supervised the research. All authors reviewed the article. All authors have read and agreed to the published version of the manuscript.

Funding: This research was funded by the Finnish Cultural Foundation/Suomen Kulttuurirahasto Grant number: 00181173.

Acknowledgments: The authors thank DOW Germany for the Methocel E5 Premium LV.

Conflicts of Interest: The authors declare no conflict of interest.

References

1. Srai, J.S.; Badman, C.; Krumme, M.; Futran, M.; Johnston, C. Future supply chains enabled by continuous processing—Opportunities and challenges. May 20–21, 2014 Continuous Manufacturing Symposium. *J. Pharm. Sci.* **2015**, *104*, 840–849. [CrossRef] [PubMed]
2. Al-Metwali, B.; Mulla, H. Personalised dosing of medicines for children. *J. Pharm. Pharmacol.* **2017**, *69*, 514–524. [CrossRef] [PubMed]
3. Florence, A.T.; Lee, V.H. Personalised medicines: More tailored drugs, more tailored delivery. *Int. J. Pharm.* **2011**, *415*, 29–33. [CrossRef] [PubMed]
4. Jorgensen, A.L.; Prince, C.; Fitzgerald, G.; Hanson, A.; Downing, J.; Reynolds, J.; Zhang, J.E.; Alfirevic, A.; Pirmohamed, M. Implementation of genotype-guided dosing of warfarin with point-of-care genetic testing in three UK clinics: A matched cohort study. *BMC Med.* **2019**, *17*, 76. [CrossRef] [PubMed]

5. Edinger, M.; Bar-Shalom, D.; Sandler, N.; Rantanen, J.; Genina, N. QR encoded smart oral dosage forms by inkjet printing. *Int. J. Pharm.* **2018**, *536*, 138–145. [CrossRef] [PubMed]
6. Arya, A.; Chandra, A.; Sharma, V.; Pathak, K. Fast dissolving oral films: An innovative drug delivery system and dosage form. *Int. J. ChemTech Res.* **2010**, *2*, 576–583.
7. Hoffmann, E.M.; Breitenbach, A.; Breitkreutz, J. Advances in orodispersible films for drug delivery. *Expert Opin. Drug Deliv.* **2011**, *8*, 299–316. [CrossRef]
8. Thabet, Y.; Breitkreutz, J. Orodispersible films: Product transfer from lab-scale to continuous manufacturing. *Int. J. Pharm.* **2018**, *535*, 285–292. [CrossRef]
9. Woertz, C.; Kleinebudde, P. Development of orodispersible polymer films containing poorly water soluble active pharmaceutical ingredients with focus on different drug loadings and storage stability. *Int. J. Pharm.* **2015**, *493*, 134–145. [CrossRef]
10. Niese, S.; Breitkreutz, J.; Quodbach, J. Development of a dosing device for individualized dosing of orodispersible warfarin films. *Int. J. Pharm.* **2019**, *561*, 314–323. [CrossRef]
11. Song, Q.; Guo, X.; Sun, Y.; Yang, M. Anti-solvent Precipitation Method Coupled Electrospinning Process to Produce Poorly Water-Soluble Drug-Loaded Orodispersible Films. *Aaps Pharmscitech* **2019**, *20*, 273. [CrossRef] [PubMed]
12. Janßen, E.M.; Schliephacke, R.; Breitenbach, A.; Breitkreutz, J. Drug-printing by flexographic printing technology—A new manufacturing process for orodispersible films. *Int. J. Pharm.* **2013**, *441*, 818–825. [CrossRef] [PubMed]
13. Genina, N.; Fors, D.; Palo, M.; Peltonen, J.; Sandler, N. Behavior of printable formulations of loperamide and caffeine on different substrates—Effect of print density in inkjet printing. *Int. J. Pharm.* **2013**, *453*, 488–497. [CrossRef] [PubMed]
14. Buanz, A.B.; Saunders, M.H.; Basit, A.W.; Gaisford, S. Preparation of personalized-dose salbutamol sulphate oral films with thermal ink-jet printing. *Pharm. Res.* **2011**, *28*, 2386. [CrossRef]
15. Wickström, H.; Hilgert, E.; Nyman, J.; Desai, D.; Şen Karaman, D.; de Beer, T.; Sandler, N.; Rosenholm, J. Inkjet printing of drug-loaded mesoporous silica nanoparticles—A platform for drug development. *Molecules* **2017**, *22*, 2020. [CrossRef]
16. Planchette, C.; Pichler, H.; Wimmer-Teubenbacher, M.; Gruber, M.; Gruber-Wölfler, H.; Mohr, S.; Mohr, S.; Tetyczka, C.; Hsiao, W.-K.; Paudel, A.; et al. Printing medicines as orodispersible dosage forms: Effect of substrate on the printed micro-structure. *Int. J. Pharm.* **2016**, *509*, 518–527. [CrossRef]
17. Alomari, M.; Vuddanda, P.R.; Trenfield, S.J.; Dodoo, C.C.; Velaga, S.; Basit, A.W.; Gaisford, S. Printing T3 and T4 oral drug combinations as a novel strategy for hypothyroidism. *Int. J. Pharm.* **2018**, *549*, 363–369. [CrossRef]
18. Sjöholm, E.; Sandler, N. Additive manufacturing of personalized orodispersible warfarin films. *Int. J. Pharm.* **2019**, *564*, 117–123. [CrossRef]
19. Musazzi, U.M.; Selmin, F.; Ortenzi, M.A.; Mohammed, G.K.; Franzé, S.; Minghetti, P.; Cilurzo, F. Personalized orodispersible films by hot melt ram extrusion 3D printing. *Int. J. Pharm.* **2018**, *551*, 52–59. [CrossRef]
20. Jamróz, W.; Kurek, M.; Łyszczarz, E.; Szafraniec, J.; Knapik-Kowalczuk, J.; Syrek, K.; Paluch, M.; Jachowicz, R. 3D printed orodispersible films with Aripiprazole. *Int. J. Pharm.* **2017**, *533*, 413–420. [CrossRef]
21. Kay, R.; Desmulliez, M. A review of stencil printing for microelectronic packaging. *Solder. Surf. Mt. Technol.* **2012**, *24*, 38–50. [CrossRef]
22. Martín-Yerga, D.; Álvarez-Martos, I.; Blanco-López, M.C.; Henry, C.S.; Fernández-Abedul, M.T. Point-of-need simultaneous electrochemical detection of lead and cadmium using low-cost stencil-printed transparency electrodes. *Anal. Chim. Acta* **2017**, *981*, 24–33. [CrossRef] [PubMed]
23. Kay, R.W.; De Gourcuff, E.; Desmulliez, M.P.Y.; Jackson, G.J.; Steen, H.A.H.; Liu, C.; Conway, P.P. Stencil printing technology for wafer level bumping at sub-100 micron pitch using Pb-free alloys. In Proceedings of the Electronic Components and Technology, Lake Buena Vista, FL, USA, 31 May 2005; pp. 848–854.
24. Lazarus, N.; Bedair, S.S.; Kierzewski, I.M. Ultrafine pitch stencil printing of liquid metal alloys. *ACS Appl. Mater. Interfaces* **2017**, *9*, 1178–1182. [CrossRef] [PubMed]
25. Yin, D.; Jiang, N.R.; Liu, Y.F.; Zhang, X.L.; Li, A.W.; Feng, J.; Sun, H.B. Mechanically robust stretchable organic optoelectronic devices built using a simple and universal stencil-pattern transferring technology. *Light Sci. Appl.* **2018**, *7*, 35. [CrossRef]

26. Amalu, E.H.; Ekere, N.N.; Mallik, S. Evaluation of rheological properties of lead-free solder pastes and their relationship with transfer efficiency during stencil printing process. *Mater. Des.* **2011**, *32*, 3189–3197. [CrossRef]
27. Krammer, O.; Gyarmati, B.; Szilágyi, A.; Illés, B.; Bušek, D.; Dušek, K. The effect of solder paste particle size on the thixotropic behaviour during stencil printing. *J. Mater. Process. Technol.* **2018**, *262*, 571–576. [CrossRef]
28. Kipphan, H. *Handbook of Print Media: Technologies and production Methods*; Springer Science & Business Media: Berlin/Heidelberg, Germany, 2001; pp. 55–58.
29. Lääketietokeskus. Available online: https://laakeinfo.fi/Medicine.aspx?m=1360&d=3098906 (accessed on 16 November 2019).
30. Ingelman-Sundberg, M. Genetic polymorphisms of cytochrome P450 2D6 (CYP2D6): Clinical consequences, evolutionary aspects and functional diversity. *Pharm. J.* **2005**, *5*, 6. [CrossRef]
31. *European Pharmacopoeia*, 9th ed.; Council of Europe: Strasbourg, France, 2016.
32. Öler, M.; Hakyemez, G. Investigations of some physicochemical properties of haloperidol which may affect its activity. *J. Clin. Pharm. Ther.* **1988**, *13*, 341–349. [CrossRef]
33. Ream, R.L.; Moore, D.M. Saliva stimulating chewing gum composition, Patent and Trademark Office. U.S. Patent 4,088,788, 8 May 1978.
34. Huang, B.; Lee, N.C. Solder bumping via paste reflow for area array packages. In Proceedings of the 27th Annual IEEE/SEMI International Electronics Manufacturing Technology Symposium, San Jose, CA, USA, 17–18 July 2002; pp. 1–17.
35. Yehia, S.A.; El-Gazayerly, O.N.; Basalious, E.B. Fluconazole mucoadhesive buccal films: In vitro/in vivo performance. *Curr. Drug Deliv.* **2009**, *6*, 17–27. [CrossRef]
36. Perumal, V.A.; Lutchman, D.; Mackraj, I.; Govender, T. Formulation of monolayered films with drug and polymers of opposing solubilities. *Int. J. Pharm.* **2008**, *358*, 184–191. [CrossRef]
37. Pan, J.; Tonkay, G.L.; Storer, R.H.; Sallade, R.M.; Leandri, D.J. Critical variables of solder paste stencil printing for micro-BGA and fine-pitch QFP. *IEEE Trans. Electron. Packag. Manuf.* **2004**, *27*, 125–132. [CrossRef]
38. Maing, I.Y.; Parliment, T.H.; Soukup, R.J. Stabilization of erythrosine in aqueous acidic food systems, Patent and Trademark Office. U.S. Patent 4,133,900, 9 January 1979.
39. Cassanas, G.; Morssli, M.; Fabregue, E.; Bardet, L. Vibrational spectra of lactic acid and lactates. *J. Raman Spectrosc.* **1991**, *22*, 409–413. [CrossRef]
40. Saluja, H.; Mehanna, A.; Panicucci, R.; Atef, E. Hydrogen bonding: Between strengthening the crystal packing and improving solubility of three haloperidol derivatives. *Molecules* **2016**, *21*, 719. [CrossRef] [PubMed]
41. Preis, M.; Gronkowsky, D.; Grytzan, D.; Breitkreutz, J. Comparative study on novel test systems to determine disintegration time of orodispersible films. *J. Pharm. Pharmacol.* **2014**, *66*, 1102–1111. [CrossRef]
42. Nguty, T.A.; Ekere, N.N.; Adebayo, A. Correlating solder paste composition with stencil printing performance. In Proceedings of the Twenty Fourth IEEE/CPMT International Electronics Manufacturing Technology Symposium (Cat. No. 99CH36330), Austin, TX, USA, 19 October 1999; pp. 304–312.

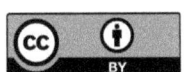

© 2020 by the authors. Licensee MDPI, Basel, Switzerland. This article is an open access article distributed under the terms and conditions of the Creative Commons Attribution (CC BY) license (http://creativecommons.org/licenses/by/4.0/).

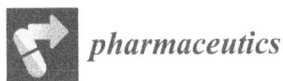

Article

Embedded 3D Printing of Novel Bespoke Soft Dosage Form Concept for Pediatrics

Katarzyna Rycerz [1,2], Krzysztof Adam Stepien [1,2], Marta Czapiewska [1,3], Basel T. Arafat [4], Rober Habashy [1], Abdullah Isreb [1], Matthew Peak [5] and Mohamed A. Alhnan [6,*]

1. School of Pharmacy and Biomedical Sciences, University of Central Lancashire, Preston, Lancashire PR1 2HE, UK; katarzyna.rycerz7@gmail.com (K.R.); krzysztof.stepien@wum.edu.pl (K.A.S.); marta.czapiewska@cm.umk.pl (M.C.); robo_85@hotmail.com (R.H.); AIsreb@uclan.ac.uk (A.I.)
2. Faculty of Pharmacy with the Laboratory Medicine Division, Medical University of Warsaw, 02-091 Warsaw, Poland
3. Faculty of Pharmacy, Department of Pharmaceutical Technology, Collegium Medicum in Bydgoszcz, Nicolaus Copernicus University in Toruń, Toruń, Jurasza 2 St., 85-089 Bydgoszcz, Poland
4. Faculty of Medical Sciences and Public Health, Anglia Ruskin University, Chelmsford CM1 1SQ, UK; Basel.arafat@anglia.ac.uk
5. Paediatric Medicines Research Unit, Alder Hey Children's NHS Foundation Trust, Liverpool L12 2AP, UK; Matthew.Peak@alderhey.nhs.uk
6. Institute of Pharmaceutical Sciences, School of Cancer and Pharmaceutical Sciences, King's College London, London SE1 9NH, UK
* Correspondence: Alhnan@kcl.ac.uk; Tel.: +44-(0)20-7848-7265

Received: 20 October 2019; Accepted: 18 November 2019; Published: 26 November 2019

Abstract: Embedded three-dimensional printing (e-3DP) is an emerging method for additive manufacturing where semi-solid materials are extruded within a solidifying liquid matrix. Here, we present the first example of employing e-3DP in the pharmaceutical field and demonstrate the fabrication of bespoke chewable dosage forms with dual drug loading for potential use in pediatrics. Lego^{TM}-like chewable bricks made of edible soft material (gelatin-based matrix) were produced by directly extruding novel printing patterns of model drug ink (embedded phase) into a liquid gelatin-based matrix (embedding phase) at an elevated temperature (70 °C) to then solidify at room temperature. Dose titration of the two model drugs (paracetamol and ibuprofen) was possible by using specially designed printing patterns of the embedded phase to produce varying doses. A linearity [R^2 = 0.9804 (paracetamol) and 0.9976 (ibuprofen)] was achieved between percentage of completion of printing patterns and achieved doses using a multi-step method. The impact of embedded phase rheological behavior, the printing speed and the needle size of the embedded phase were examined. Owning to their appearance, modular nature, ease of personalizing dose and geometry, and tailoring and potential inclusion of various materials, this new dosage form concept holds a substantial promise for novel dosage forms in pediatrics.

Keywords: personalized medicine; additive manufacturing; complex structures; tablets; patient-specific; structural design; gums

1. Introduction

With increasing regulatory incentives for pediatric formulation development and focus in delivering patient-centred health care, developing age-appropriate formulations is gaining increased interest [1] from the pharmaceutical sector. Within Europe, the pediatric regulation on improving medicines for children was amended to include a requirement to evaluate the acceptability of formulations of medicines for children seeking a marketing authorization. There have been increasing efforts to provide high-quality, effective, and safe formulations for children [2]. The use of unlicensed and off-label medicines in pediatrics is extensive [3]. A lack of age-appropriate formulations for children means that available medicines are frequently modified to achieve an intended dose and/or administration to the child [3]. For example, tablets may need to be split by healthcare professionals or families to achieve an intended dose, with the potential for significant under- or over-dosing [4,5].

Chewable jelly or jelly-like oral doses have been proposed as easy-to-handle and to swallow for the elderly population and are often prepared using gelatin, glycogelatin, and caseinate [6]. The inclusion of drug in the structure provides an opportunity for taste masking and avoids the need for drinking water [7]. Several products of chewable gels and dosage forms are commercially available, particularly for the delivery of vitamins [8], mineral supplements [9], nutrition [10], as well as for the treatment of osteoporosis [11,12]. However, formulating chewable oral doses is often associated with challenges regarding drug stability and the capacity for higher doses.

Several reports have showed the potential of 3D printing in controlling dosage [13,14], drug combination [15–17], and proposed modification of pediatric-friendly shapes [18–21]. However, there are limited examples of using 3D printing for fabrication of patient-specific chewable oral dosage forms. Stereolithographic 3D printing can also produce gel tablets [22]; however, developing oral dosage forms with this approach is hindered by the difficulty of acceptance by regulatory bodies of necessary polymer initiators required for 3D printing. Fused deposition modeling (FDM) 3D printing has also been used to produce child-friendly shapes and has achieved improved taste-masking [18]. In a recent report, Goyanes et al. (2019) provided personalized chewable formulations prepared by direct ink writing of pectin-based gel for the treatment of maple syrup urine disease. Such an approach requires a formulation change to accommodate each model drug.

Embedded 3D printing (e-3DP) is an emerging technology that allows the free form fabrication of multiminerals with complex structures. The method involves extruding a viscoelastic ink (embedded phase) using a deposition nozzle at a predefined path into a solidifying reservoir (embedding phase). Following printing, the reservoir is solidified usually through a curing method to form a monolithic structure. e-3DP has been used for production of highly programmable and seamless structures such as wearable electronics [23]. Applying this approach in the pharmaceutical field holds the opportunity of providing a modular system of a generic matrix that embeds one or more drugs at individualized doses to meet the need of one or a small number of patients. The aim of this work is to apply e-3DP to pharmaceutical grade material to craft bespoke oral concept chewable dosage forms for pediatrics. Lego™-like bricks made of chewable soft material were produced by applying novel printing patterns of model drug suspension (embedded phase) into a liquid gelatin-based matrix (embedding phase). We studied the impact of printing materials composition, process parameters and demonstrated the system ability of providing bespoke dosage control and dual drug release by manipulating printing patterns. The two model drugs (paracetamol and ibuprofen) are often used in combination or alternately for the treatment of febrile children [24–26].

2. Materials and Methods

2.1. Materials

Ibuprofen (grade 25) was donated by BASF (Burgbernheim, Germany). Paracetamol (≥99.0%) and gelatin were purchased from Sigma-Aldrich (Darmstadt, Germany). Glycerol EP was supplied by J.M. Loveridge Ltd. (Andover, UK). Locust bean gum (from *Ceratonia siliqia* seeds) were purchased from Sigma-Aldrich (Poole, UK). Food dyes (Brilliant Blue and Lake Allura Red) were supplied by FastColours LLP (Huddersfield, UK).

2.2. Preparation of Embedding and Embedded Materials

Each oral dosage form was composed of ibuprofen or paracetamol powder suspension in locust gum solution (paste) and embedding medium (gelatin-based gel).

2.2.1. Embedding Medium

An optimized weight ratio of water: glycerol: gelatin (45:25:30) was used as a thermo-responsive embedding medium. Initially, water was heated to 75 °C followed by the addition of gelatin, with stirring, until complete dissolution.

2.2.2. Embedded Drug Paste

A solution of 2.98% w/w locust bean (at temperature 80 °C) was used to suspend model drug particles in the medium. For paracetamol, suspensions (100 g) were prepared at different drug concentrations: 20%, 30%, 40%, 50%, or 60% in locust bean solution. For ibuprofen, suspensions (100 g) were prepared at different drug concentrations: 16%, 22%, 28%, 34%, or 40% w/w in locust bean solution. The suspensions were colored by adding 5 mg of Brilliant Blue (paracetamol) and Lake Allura Red (ibuprofen) and manually stirred for 2 min for homogenization. Following rheological and experimental printing (Section 2.6), the concentrations of 40% (paracetamol) and 28% (ibuprofen) were chosen as default for printing oral doses.

2.3. Modification of Dual FDM 3D Printer

In order to develop a process of manufacturing novel soft dosage forms via e-3DP, a MakerBot Replicator Experimental 2X dual FDM 3D printer (MakerBot Industries, Brooklyn, NY, USA) was modified as highlighted in Supplementary Data, Figure S1. The 3D printer has two FDM nozzle heads. The right extruder/head of the dual 3D printer was replaced by a syringe-based liquid dispenser. The design for the dispenser was obtained from an open-source design (Thingiverse, 2017) and the different parts were produced by 3D printing using a M2 MakerGear FDM 3D printer and acrylonitrile butadiene styrene (ABS) filaments (MakerGear LLC, Beachwood, OH, USA). The dispenser head was installed and equipped with either a 2.5 mL or a 10 mL syringe. A Nema 17 1.5 A 4-lead stepper motor (MakerBot Industries, Brooklyn, NY, USA) was connected to the motherboard using the default housing connectors [26].

2.4. Design of Template and Pattern

The template design was produced by 3D printing using a M2 MakerGear FDM 3D printer and ABS filaments (MakerGear LLC) and Simplify 3D software (Simplify 3D LLC, Cincinnati, OH, USA). A Lego™-like design was chosen to test proof-of-concept that a complex shape and a design familiar to children could be produced using e-3DP. A Lego™-like template was printed using polylactic acid (PLA) filament (MakerBot). The design of the pattern for printing the paste with active substance was prepared using Autodesk® 3ds Max® Design version 2018 (Autodesk Inc., San Rafael, CA, USA). The design was saved in STL format and imported to Simplify 3D software (version 4.1) (Simplify 3D LLC, Cincinnati, OH, USA). During experimentation, printing the paste with the active substance in the desired pattern was carried out using a modified MakerBot Replicator Experimental 2X and using Simplify 3D software. The dimensions for the embedded printing pattern were: X × Y × Z = 20 × 29.52 × 0.45 mm and were optimized to fit within a gelatin-based Lego™-like brick (40 × 25 × 15 mm). For 25%, 50%, and 75% printing patterns, the designs had identical X and Z dimensions whilst the Y axis was 8.1, 15, or 22.5 mm, respectively. Printing the full design (100%) corresponded to doses of approximately 107 and 115 mg for ibuprofen and paracetamol, respectively. In order to demonstrate the capacity of the system for printing lower and higher doses, the printing pattern was printed at 25%, 50%, or 75% of the full design for smaller doses and the design was repeated twice (200%) or three times (300%) to achieve larger doses. All printing patterns were printed within identical Lego™-like templates as detailed above.

2.5. Embedded 3D Printing Process

Two methods of embedding the printing patterns in the gelatin matrix were performed:

2.5.1. One-Step Embedded 3D Printing

To embed a drug suspension pattern into warm gelatin, the embedding medium was first heated to approximately 70 °C and cast into a Lego™ shape template and placed on the printing plate of the 3D printer heated to 75 °C. Parameters (positions, dimensions, printing speed, extrusion multiplier) were programmed in the Simplify3D software. Prior to printing the embedded layer(s), the building platform was heated to 75 °C and gelatin was poured into the template. The G-code was modified to allow the needle tip to start extrusion at a height of 4 mm from the bottom of the design. The extrusion multiplier was set at 10.0 and the size of the needle was G16. The printing patterns were assessed at the following needle speeds: 50, 55, 60, or 65 mm/min.

2.5.2. Multi-Step Embedded 3D Printing

Embedding the drug into the structure was performed using three steps: (i) casting liquid gelatin solution (6 mL) inside the template and left to cool to solidify; (ii) printing the drug-paste (embedded phase) on the surface of the semi-solid gelatin; and (iii) covering the drug-paste with a second portion (5 mL) of liquid gelatin. In order to allow the printing of two model drugs at two separate specific levels, the printing was carried out by casting 4 mL of embedding phase followed by paracetamol printing and then an additional 3 mL of embedding phase. Following the printing of the ibuprofen layer, a final layer of gelatin (4 mL) was cast.

The following settings were used: retraction distance 1 mm, retraction speed 1200 mm, extrusion width manual 0.4 mm, outline direction: inside to outside, and movement speed $x - y$ 500 mm/min and z:150 mm/min. Infill printing speeds of 45, 50, 55, or 60 mm/s and extrusion multiplier of 3×, 5×, or 10×, and luer lock needle head with different nozzle sizes of G15, G16, and G17 (McMaster Ltd., Chicago, IL, USA) were screened. Following the analysis of a range of different printing parameters, the following parameters, 55 mm/min, nozzle size G16, and extrusion multiplier 5× were chosen as default to print different paracetamol and ibuprofen doses.

2.6. Rheological Studies of Embedded Material

A shear Physica MCR 102 rheometer (Anton Paar, Ostfildern, Germany) was used in oscillation mode with a parallel plate configuration (plate diameter = 25 mm). The gap between the plate and the base was set at 0.5 mm. An amplitude sweep test was performed to determine the linear viscoelastic region (LVR). Afterwards, frequency sweep tests were performed at a strain amplitude of 1% (well within the LVR region) and an angular frequency range from 100 to 0.1 rad/sec. Measurements were taken at room temperature. Power law fit was used in the linear shear thinning area of the obtained rheological data to measure the shear-thinning index (n) and the consistency coefficient (k):

$$\eta = k\gamma^{(n-1)} \qquad (1)$$

where η is the viscosity, γ is the shear rate, and k is the consistency coefficient which measures the material's resistance to flow at low rate.

2.7. Scanning Electron Microscopy (SEM)

The surface and cross-sections of drug loaded oral dosages were assessed using a Quanta-200 SEM microscope at 20 kV. Samples were coated under vacuum with a gold coater JFC-1200 Fine Coater (Jeol, Tokyo, Japan). In addition, photographs of tablets were acquired using a Canon EOS-1D Mark IV (Canon Ltd., Tokyo, Japan).

2.8. Drug Contents Using HPLC

A HPLC method was used for simultaneous detection of paracetamol and ibuprofen. Agilent 1260 HPLC system (Agilent Technologies, Waldbronn, Germany) was employed using 35:65 v/v mixture of

0.1% orthophosphoric acid solution (pH 2.2) and acetonitrile as a mobile phase and a Kinetex 3.5 µm XB-C18 (100 × 4.6 mm) column (Phenomenex, Aschaffenburg, Germany). An injection volume of 2.0 µL at wavelength 210 nm, column temperature of 45 °C and a flow rate of 0.5 mL/min was used. The retention times were 1.9 and 4.2 min for paracetamol and ibuprofen, respectively, and the stop time was 5 min. A calibration curve for each of paracetamol (up to 500 mg/L) and ibuprofen (up to 320 mg/L) was plotted and yielded linearity regression co-efficients of $R^2 = 0.9987$ and 0.9990 with limits of detection of 22.2 and 11.2 mg/L and limits of quantification of 37.4 and 73.8 mg/L for paracetamol and ibuprofen, respectively.

2.9. Dissolution Test for Oral Doses

To study in vitro theophylline release for 3D printed oral dosages, an AT 7 Smart USP II dissolution test apparatus (Sotax AG, Aesch, Switzerland) was used. Each oral dose contained a dual dose of 80 mg ibuprofen and 200 mg paracetamol. A dissolution medium of 900 mL phosphate buffer BP (pH 7.2) at 37 ± 0.5 °C with a paddle speed of 50 rpm was used for 2 h. The dissolution medium was chosen according to USP 31 monograph for ibuprofen tablets [27]. Each experiment was carried out in triplicate. Samples were collected at 0, 5, 10, 15, 20, 25, 30, 35, 40, 45, 50, 60, 70, 80, 90, 100, 110, and 120 min intervals and drug concentration was determined using HPLC as specified in Section 2.8.

2.10. Statistical Analysis

To assess the relative influences of needle size, speed of needle movement, and extrusion multiplier, standard multiple linear regression was applied using IBM SPSS Statistics software version 25 (Chicago, IL, USA). Initial data analysis indicated no violation of the assumptions of normality, linearity, multicollinearity, and homoscedasticity.

3. Results and Discussion

3.1. Development of Embedded Phase for Pharmaceutical e-3DP

To achieve a successful e-3DP, both the embedding and embedded phases need to meet specific criteria. The embedded phase is usually required to be: (i) a shear-thinning yield stress fluid [28]; (ii) a controllable flow from the nozzle; (iii) immersible/low miscibility with embedding phase, (iv) of equal or similar density to the embedding phase; and (v) chemically compatible with the embedding material. Moreover, the embedding phase (often referred to as a matrix) should have thixotropic properties or be curable and solidify or increase in viscosity following the embedding process. Satisfying these stringent criteria is a major challenge to apply this emerging method in the pharmaceutical field.

In this work, e-3DP enabled the encapsulation of model drugs in pre-specified shapes into an embedding material. Figure 1 illustrates the production of the proposed embedded dosage form. We adapted pharmaceutical materials to match the technical needs of e-3DP, which often requires the use of heat- or UV light-curable materials [29,30] to increase the rigidity of the embedding phase to solid or semi-solid states. Although these processes might yield a functional material, they are likely to face significant regulatory and commercial hurdles when approval is sought for oral use. Therefore, an alternative approach was tested using widely available, biodegradable, and commonly used approved excipients: gelatin and glycerol [31,32]. The combination of these excipients yields a matrix that is semi-solid at room temperature, but liquified at 75 °C when in contact with the printing plate. The inclusion of glycerol provides a sweet taste and facilitates the matrix dissolution in the gastric medium.

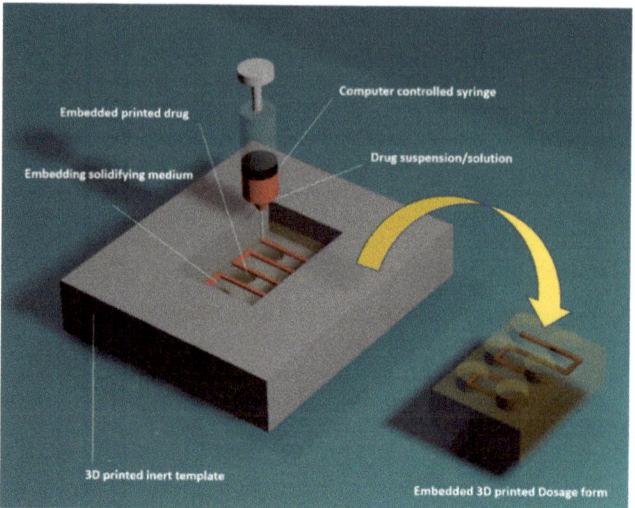

Figure 1. Schematic of production of embedded 3D printing of an oral dosage form using a Lego™-like design as a template. Drug paste (embedded phase) is extruded in a pre-determined path into a gelatin-based matrix (embedding phase) to yield a chewable dosage form.

Locust bean gum, a non-anionic polysaccharide biopolymer that is extracted from Carob tree seeds [33], has been used as a suspending agent for the embedded phase. The fabrication process was carefully developed to achieve a balance between the ease of flow of the embedded ink from the nozzle and the rapid solidification on/within the embedding phase upon application. To optimize this, a series of paracetamol and ibuprofen pastes (drug particle suspension in Locust bean gum solution) of increasing concentrations was prepared and the rheological behavior of these suspensions was assessed (Figure 2). In general, the viscosity of gum and suspensions decreased with increasing shear rate (Figure 2) and reflected the shear-thinning behavior of the inks used. The gum (drug-free) showed a viscosity with a consistency coefficient (k) value of 1.7235 Pa.S corresponding to blank suspensions. However, following the addition of paracetamol and ibuprofen, the k values increased reflecting the increase in viscosity of these suspensions (28% ibuprofen and 40% paracetamol, corresponding to k values of 17.022 and 10.304 Pa.S, respectively). At these drug concentrations, a consistent flow was maintained when the suspension-filled syringe was loaded onto the 3D printer. However, a further increase in the concentration of ibuprofen or paracetamol in the suspension resulted in an excessive rise in the viscosity of the suspension; therefore, rendering the suspension non-extrudable under the printing conditions. Hence, optimized concentrations of 40% paracetamol and 28% ibuprofen were used as default conditions for printing. The shear-thinning behavior of gum has been reported in previous studies and is linked to the entanglement of the polymeric chains in the solution [34]. This observation was supported by the results of the rheological study carried on the solutions containing either ibuprofen or paracetamol. This rheological behavior can be attributed to the β-D-mannose backbone with (1,6) linked α-D-galactose substitution, where mannose units within the structures have been proposed to allow self-assembly.

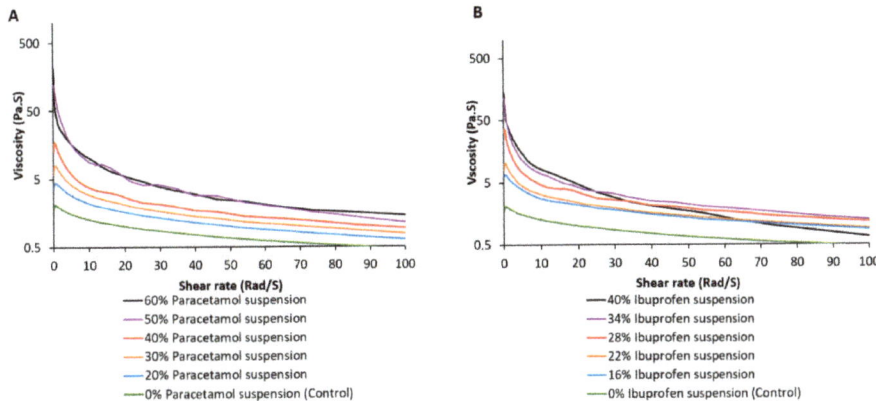

Figure 2. Impact of (**A**) paracetamol and (**B**) ibuprofen concentration on the rheological behavior of the applied ink (embedded phase).

3.2. Single- and Multi-Stage e-3DP

Printing patterns were specifically designed to be included within gelatin-based Lego™-like bricks (Figure 1). The printing pattern is composed of a series of repeated parallel lines and right angles to create sufficient space between the paralleled lines to be filled with gelatin. The design was proposed to fit within 3 mm margins in the gelatin bricks. Initially, a single stage e-3DP was assessed (Figure 3A). However, this resulted in the formation of irregular lines and deviation from the pre-defined path (Supplementary data, Figure S2) as well as unreproducible printing patterns in each product (Supplementary data, Figure S3).

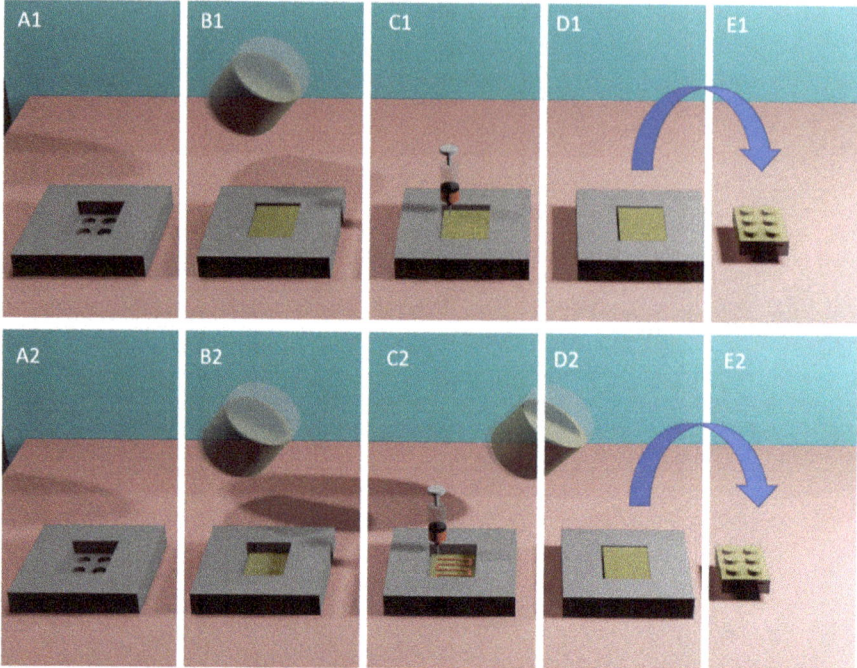

Figure 3. e-3DP process was carried out using (i) Single-stage printing: a 3D printed template (**A1**) is initially filled with gelatin-based matrix liquid at 70 °C (**B1**) and the drug paste is extruded instantly into the the liquified matrix (**C1**). The template is then cooled to room temperature (**D1**), and (**E1**) oral dosage form is extracted from the template; or (ii) Two stage printing: (**A2**) template is initially filled with gelatin-based matrix liquid at 70 °C and (**B2**) the template is cooled to room temperature, (**C2**) the drug paste is extruded onto the surface of the solidified gelatin-based matrix and (**D2**) the secondary layer of gelatin matrix is cast on the template surface, (**E2**) following cooling to room temperature, the dosage form is extracted.

In order to generate a more reproducible extrusion that mimics the printing patterns as per CAD design, an alternative multi-stage printing method was devised (Section 2.4), where the embedded phase (ink) is extruded on the surface of an initial layer of gelatin that is cast prior to printing. The dosage form is completed by applying a secondary layer of gelatin (Figure 3B) to fully seal the embedded phase within the gelatin matrix. This method yielded an improved printing path (Figure 4). An explanation for such improvement might a reduced resistance of the ink flow from the nozzle into atmosphere air (compared to gelatin solution) which prevented irregularity in the final printed drug patterns. Several printing parameters were assessed to define the optimized printing parameters with least variability in dosing.

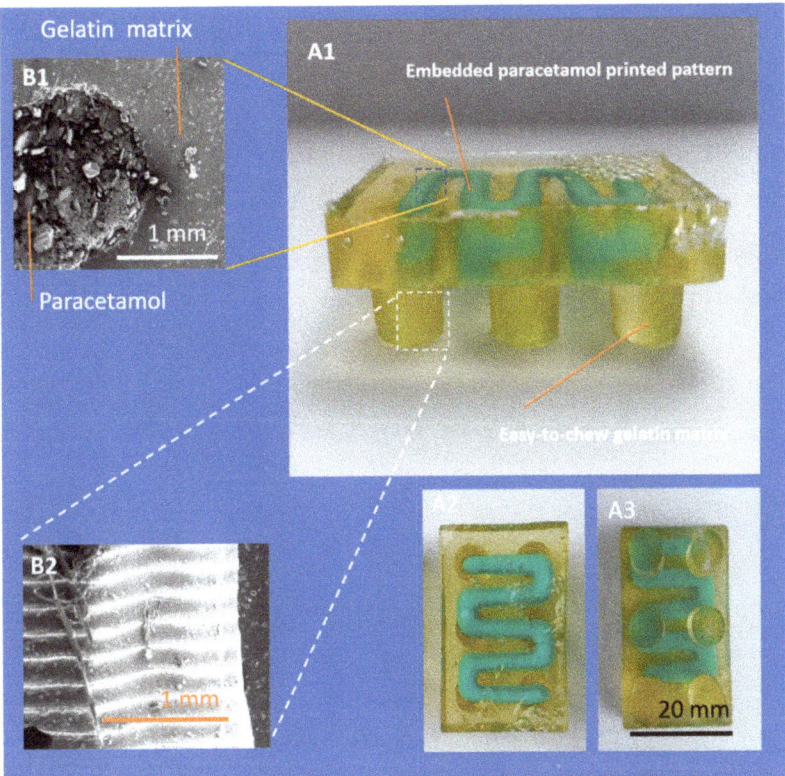

Figure 4. Photographs of (**A1**) side, (**A2**) front, and (**A3**) back view of Lego™-like soft gelatin with embedded paracetamol dose. SEM images of (**B1**) cross-section embedding and embedded matrix and (**B2**) surface of gelatin-based matrix.

3.3. Impact of Printing Parameters on Drug Dosing Amount and Accuracy

The impact of the speed of movement of the printer nozzle is highlighted in Figure 5 and Table 1, where reducing the speed of printing generally resulted in an increase in the amount of dispensed paracetamol using the same printing patterns. This might be a result of extrusion of a larger amount of material (at the same flow rate) with a longer time available to complete the shape. When a larger needle size was used, it resulted in extrusion of higher doses with reduced resistance from the increased internal diameter of the needle.

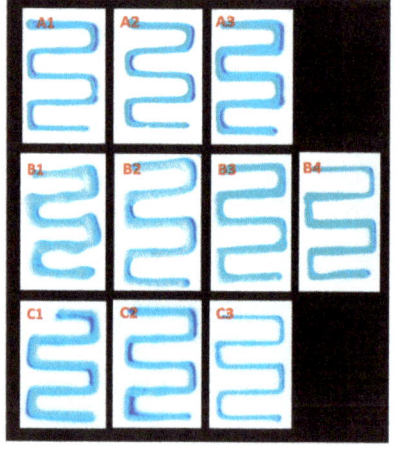
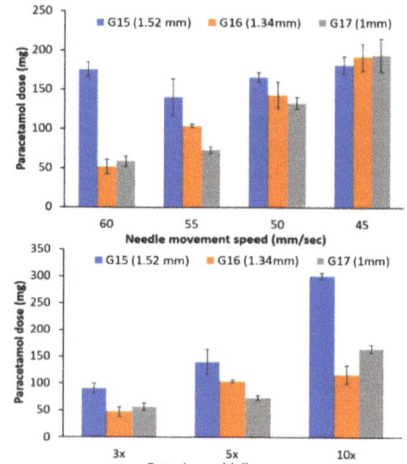

Figure 5. Impact of process setting on printing pattern of paracetamol paste (embedded phase): extrusion multiplier (**A1**) 3, (**A2**) 5, and (**A3**) 10. Speed of needle head: (**B1**) 45, (**B2**) 50, (**B3**) 55, and (**B4**) 60 mm/min. Needle size (**C1**) G15, (**C2**) G16, and (**C3**) G17.

Table 1. Impact of needle size, extrusion multiplier, and speed of the needle movement on the dose paracetamol in mg (100% of printing pattern).

Extrusion Multiplier *	Needle Size G15 (1.52 mm) ±SD	SD%	Needle Size G16 (1.34 mm) ±SD	SD%	Needle Size G17 (1 mm) ±SD	SD%
3×	90.8 ± 4.3	4.7%	47.4 ± 4.2	5.1%	56.5 ± 6.9	12.2%
5×	140.3 ± 23.3	16.6%	103.6 ± 2.1	2%	73.3 ± 4.4	6%
10×	300.8 ± 9.4	3.12%	116.6 ± 7.2	6.2%	165.2 ± 22.4	13.6%
Speed (mm/sec) **						
60	175.5 ± 9.0	5.1%	51.8 ± 9.1	17.6%	59.2 ± 6.7	11.3%
55	140.3 ± 23.3	16.6%	103.6 ± 2.1	2%	73.3 ± 4.4	6%
50	165.8 ± 6.2	3.7%	143.2 ± 16.9	11.8%	133.0 ± 7.3	5.5%
45	181.4 ± 11.0	6.1%	191.5 ± 17.2	9%	194.0 ± 21.3	10.9%

* The speed of the nozzle movement was fixed at 55 mm/sec. ** Extrusion multiplier was fixed at 5×.

One important factor in dose dispensing is the extruder multiplier (an empirical value that is proportional to the extrusion rate), which appeared to determine the doses dispensed for each needle size (Table 1). It is essential to co-ordinate these process parameters to achieve successful printing. For instance, a fast-moving needle with a limited extrusion rate will result in incomplete and voided structure, while a slow moving needle with an exaggerated extrusion rate will result in an overfilled lump. An optimized extrusion multiplier of 5×, a needle size of G16 (internal diameter of 1.3 mm) and a needle speed of 55 mm/sec yielded the most reproducible printing patterns with the narrowest standard deviation (SD% = 2%). Hence, these parameters were selected as a default setting for further testing. Under these settings, reproducible doses of 116.6 mg and 107.4 mg of paracetamol and ibuprofen, respectively, were achieved.

To quantify the relative impact of these different printing parameters, standard multi-linear regression was used and yielded the following equation:

$$\text{Dispensed dose (mg)} = 267.36 + 17.4\ \text{ExM} - 6.88\ V + 105.4\ \emptyset \tag{2}$$

where ExM is extrusion multiplier, V is the speed of needle movement (mm/sec), and Ø is the inner diameter of needle (mm). The equation highlights that dispensed dose is increased by a larger extrusion multiplier and needle size and is reduced by a faster needle speed. The multiple regression model indicated that extrusion multiplier (standardized coefficient β = 0.572, $p < 0.002$) and needle speed (β = −0.499, $p < 0.005$) are the most influential factors, followed by needle size (β = −0.374, $p < 0.05$). The model was able to describe 67.6% of the variance (F (3, 17) = 11.824, $p < 0.0005$). Other process factors such as retraction amount and speed may also influence the dispensed dose.

In order to establish the ability of the system to produce a different range of doses, the printing pattern was clipped or duplicated at different proportions (Figure 6). For instance, to achieve smaller doses, printing patterns were trimmed reduced to 25%, 50%, or 75% to cover dose ranges of 16–77 mg and 12–76 mg of paracetamol and ibuprofen, respectively. To achieve higher doses, the printing design was repeated following the same printing path twice or three times followed by an elevation of height at 0.5 mm after each layer (Table 2). Figure 6 shows rendered images and photographs of the printed patterns using this approach for both paracetamol and ibuprofen. For both model drugs, good linearity [R^2 = 0.9804 (paracetamol) and 0.9976 (ibuprofen)] was achieved between the percentage of printed patterns and the achieved doses. The negative intercept values in the trendline equations suggest that there is a reduced extruded ink in small size designs, e.g., at 25% of design pattern. This could be a direct result of the shear-thinning behavior of the ink, where dynamic viscosity is high at the beginning of the printing process before it is reduced as ink flow continues. Another source of variation in the dispensed dose could result from resistance to ink flow by the layer already extruded from the needle nozzle while printing the next layer. This could be mitigated by careful adjustment of the height that the needle travels on z-axis following deposition of each layer. For this technology to be adopted in a clinical setting, the precision of dosing needs to be improved. This could be achieved by enhancing the retraction mechanism in both nozzle design and software.

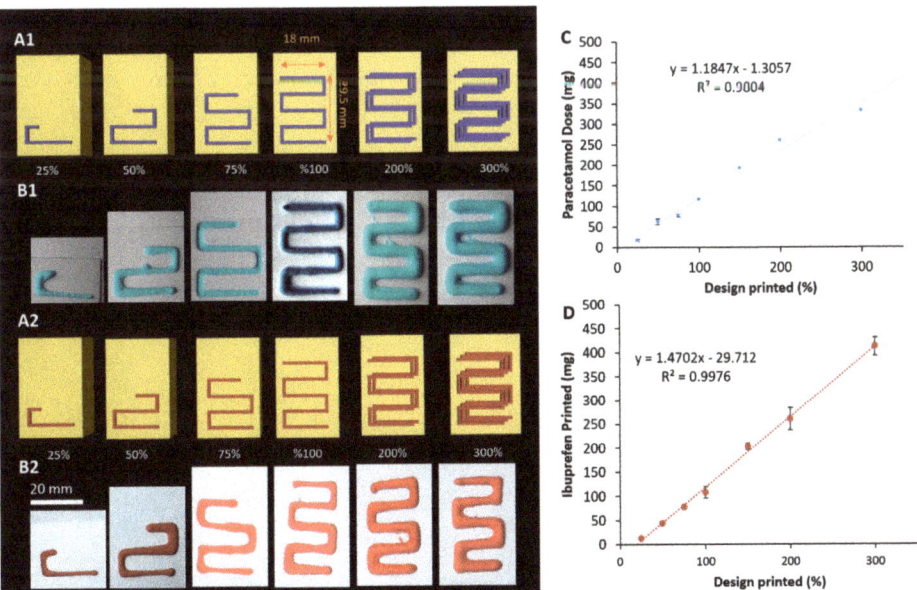

Figure 6. Rendered [(**A1**) and (**A2**)] and photograph [(**B1**) and (**B2**)] images of printing patterns for paracetamol and ibuprofen. Linearity between the printing pattern percentages and achieved doses for (**C**) paracetamol and (**D**) ibuprofen, respectively.

Table 2. Dosing of paracetamol and ibuprofen using different percentages of the printing pattern.

Printing Pattern	Paracetamol Dose (mg) ±SD	SD%	Ibuprofen Dose (mg) ± SD	SD%
25%	16.1 ± 2.7	16.9%	12.1 ± 1.0	8.1
50%	61.7 ± 5.1	8.2%	44 ± 1.9	4.4
75%	77 ± 12.2	15.8%	77 ± 4.0	5.2
100%	116.7 ± 7.0	6.0%	107.4 ± 12.1	11.3
200%	259.4 ± 16.8	6.5%	260.3 ± 23.6	9.1
300%	329.8 ± 6.4	2%	411.9 ± 19.2	4.7

The system enables different printing patterns for dose titration without the need for altering the concentration of the embedded phase or changing the formulation or the volume of the external embedding phase. Such a challenge is often faced when relatively large drug loading needs to be incorporated in gel structure.

3.4. Drug Release from 3D Printed Oral Doses

Another important aspect for an age-appropriate dosage form is the ability to accommodate different drugs in a minimal number of doses. Paracetamol and ibuprofen have frequently been used in combination for management of numerous pediatric conditions such as fever, post-operative pain, and pain relief [35–38]. The concept described herein has potential clinical utility under circumstances when combined rather than alternate therapy is required. The ability of the technology to easily produce drug combinations at variable ratios in a single oral dosage form is of great interest. In addition, reducing the number of individual medicines into a single dosage form is appealing to families, minimizing the need to adhere to several drug administrations which can lead to missed, omitted, or dual doses. Figure 7 demonstrates ibuprofen and paracetamol release from gelatin Lego™-like bricks. The pH of the dissolution medium was selected as recommended by USP pharmacopial monograph for ibuprofen and was within the reported range of salivary pH in healthy individuals [39]. Upon introduction in dissolution medium, the gelatin-based matrix will dissolve quickly, leaving a paste of printed drug patterns to dissolve at a slower rate.

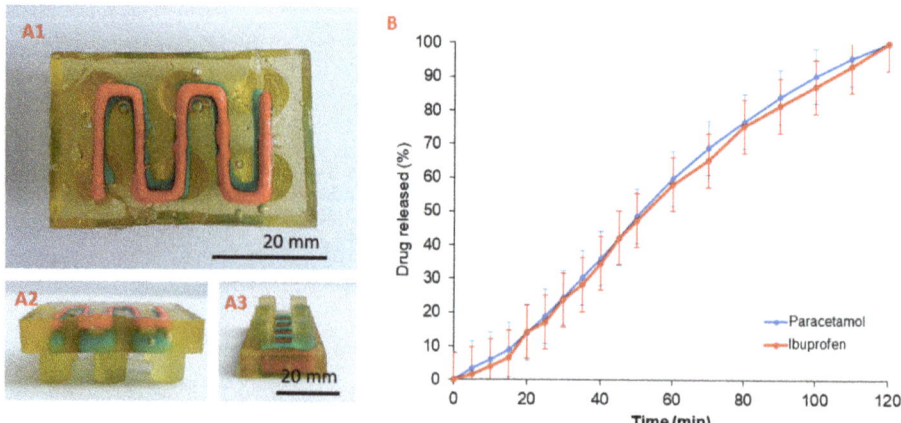

Figure 7. (**A1**) Bottom and [(**A2**) and (**A3**)] side views of oral concept gelatin-based dosage form for paracetamol (blue) and ibuprofen (red). (**B**) Drug release from the dosage form in simulated intestinal fluids (pH 7.2) using USP II dissolution test (n = 3, 50 rpm, error bar represents standard deviation).

It is interesting to highlight that both drugs were released at similar rate despite the relatively higher solubility of paracetamol compared to ibuprofen at intestinal pH (approximately 20.9 versus 3.9 g/L, respectively) [40,41]. This may be due to the slow dissolution of locust bean gum, a galactomanon that acts as a gel former in the embedded phase. It is likely that the release patterns of both drugs were governed by drug diffusion through diffusing spaces within the network of macromolecular chains [42,43]. In the future, it will be possible to manipulate drug release by applying different 'ink' matrixes to accommodate for different release patterns.

One potential advantage of applying e-3DP for production of chewable products is the possibility of encapsulation of drug paste in an acceptable gelatin matrix. Although some of the embedded materials are likely to be in contact with taste buds in the tongue, the system can potentially reduce the extent and the duration of such interaction, hence providing some advantage for bitter drugs. Another important novelty aspect in this concept dosage form is its modular nature that can include individualized drugs (single or combination) and doses in a single chewable form, hence offering the possibility for more complex dosing regimens and high levels of individualization. For example, the possibility of titrating the relative doses of paracetamol and ibuprofen in a single dosage form is an advancement on the current options available for circumstances in which combination therapy is indicated.

4. Conclusions

We have demonstrated the potential of using e-3DP for the delivery of bespoke concept chewable soft dosage forms for use in different age groups including children. The soft nature and sweet taste of the matrix may help patients with swallowing difficulties or palatability challenges. Compared to traditional oral disintegrating tablets and soft gels, the method allows independent design of both shell and core materials without modifying the external embedded matrix composition. In addition, by manipulating the geometry of printing patterns, simultaneous dosing and drug release of two different active pharmaceutical ingredients was achieved. Moving forward, the use of other liquid inks as an embedding phase (for example, hydrogels, suspension of nanoparticles, therapeutic biologics) offers the possibility of extending e-3DP printing to plethora of patient specific oral drug delivery systems.

Supplementary Materials: The following are available online at http://www.mdpi.com/1999-4923/11/12/630/s1. Figure S1. Modification of dual FDM 3D printer to accommodate a liquid/semisolids dispenser (right) in combination with FDM 3D printer head (left). Figure S2. Soft dosage forms with paracetamol paste inside (blue line) fabricated via one-step e-3DP with different printing speeds: (A) 50, (B) 60, (C) 65, and (D) 70 mm/min. Figure S3. Soft dosage forms with paracetamol inside (blue line) fabricated via one-step e-3DP with printing speed of 55.0 mm/min.

Author Contributions: Investigation, K.R., K.A.S., and M.C.; Formal analysis, B.T.A. and A.I.; Investigation, R.H.; Supervision and writing—review and editing, M.P.; Software, writing—original draft preparation, visualization, and supervision, M.A.A.

Funding: This research received no external funding.

Conflicts of Interest: The authors declare no conflict of interest.

References

1. Liu, F.; Ranmal, S.; Batchelor, H.K.; Orlu-Gul, M.; Ernest, T.B.; Thomas, I.W.; Flanagan, T.; Tuleu, C. Patient-centred pharmaceutical design to improve acceptability of medicines: Similarities and differences in paediatric and geriatric populations. *Drugs* **2014**, *74*, 1871–1889. [CrossRef]
2. Ranmal, S.R.; Cram, A.; Tuleu, C. Age-appropriate and acceptable paediatric dosage forms: Insights into end-user perceptions, preferences and practices from the Children's Acceptability of Oral Formulations (CALF) Study. *Int. J. Pharm.* **2016**, *514*, 296–307. [CrossRef] [PubMed]
3. Turner, M.A.; Catapano, M.; Hirschfeld, S.; Giaquinto, C.; Global Research in Paediatric. Paediatric drug development: The impact of evolving regulations. *Adv. Drug Deliv. Rev.* **2014**, *73*, 2–13. [CrossRef] [PubMed]

4. Madathilethu, J.; Roberts, M.; Peak, M.; Blair, J.; Prescott, R.; Ford, J.L. Content uniformity of quartered hydrocortisone tablets in comparison with mini-tablets for paediatric dosing. *BMJ Paediatr. Open* **2018**, *2*, e000198. [CrossRef] [PubMed]
5. Saimbi, S.; Madden, V.; Stirling, H.; Yahyouche, A.; Batchelor, H. Comparison of Hydrocortisone 10 Mg Tablets: Tablet Hardness Optimised for Adult Use Has Negative Consequences for Paediatric Use. *Arch. Dis. Child.* **2016**, *101*, e2. [CrossRef] [PubMed]
6. Hanawa, T.; Watanabe, A.; Tsuchiya, T.; Ikoma, R.; Hidaka, M.; Sugihara, M. New oral dosage form for elderly patients: Preparation and characterization of silk fibroin gel. *Chem. Pharm. Bull. (Tokyo)* **1995**, *43*, 284–288. [CrossRef] [PubMed]
7. Dairaku, M.; Togashi, M. Development of Air Push Jelly Formulation. *Yakuzaigaku (J. Pharm. Sci. Technol. Jpn.)* **2005**, *65*, 209–214.
8. Wagner, C.L.; Shary, J.R.; Nietert, P.J.; Wahlquist, A.E.; Ebeling, M.D.; Hollis, B.W. Bioequivalence Studies of Vitamin D Gummies and Tablets in Healthy Adults: Results of a Cross-Over Study. *Nutrients* **2019**, *11*. [CrossRef]
9. Adult Multivitamin Gummies Tablet, Chewable. Available online: https://www.webmd.com/drugs/2/drug-163130/adult-multivitamin-gummies-oral/details (accessed on 2 May 2019).
10. Koga, C.C.; Lee, S.Y.; Lee, Y. Consumer Acceptance of Bars and Gummies with Unencapsulated and Encapsulated Resveratrol. *J. Food Sci.* **2016**, *81*, S1222–S1229. [CrossRef]
11. Imai, K. Alendronate sodium hydrate (oral jelly) for the treatment of osteoporosis: Review of a novel, easy to swallow formulation. *Clin. Interv. Aging* **2013**, *8*, 681–688. [CrossRef]
12. Kunisaki, C.; Tanaka, Y.; Kosaka, T.; Miyamoto, H.; Sato, S.; Suematsu, H.; Yukawa, N.; Sato, K.; Izumisawa, Y.; Akiyama, H.; et al. A Comparative Study of Intravenous Injection Form and Oral Jelly Form of Alendronate Sodium Hydrate for Bone Mineral Disorder after Gastrectomy. *Digestion* **2017**, *95*, 162–171. [CrossRef] [PubMed]
13. Isreb, A.; Baj, K.; Wojsz, M.; Isreb, M.; Peak, M.; Alhnan, M.A. 3D printed oral theophylline doses with innovative 'radiator-like' design: Impact of polyethylene oxide (PEO) molecular weight. *Int. J. Pharm.* **2019**, *564*, 98–105. [CrossRef] [PubMed]
14. Okwuosa, T.C.; Soares, C.; Gollwitzer, V.; Habashy, R.; Timmins, P.; Alhnan, M.A. On demand manufacturing of patient-specific liquid capsules via co-ordinated 3D printing and liquid dispensing. *Eur. J. Pharm. Sci.* **2018**, *118*, 134–143. [CrossRef] [PubMed]
15. Oblom, H.; Zhang, J.; Pimparade, M.; Speer, I.; Preis, M.; Repka, M.; Sandler, N. 3D-Printed Isoniazid Tablets for the Treatment and Prevention of Tuberculosis-Personalized Dosing and Drug Release. *AAPS Pharm. Sci. Tech.* **2019**, *20*, 52. [CrossRef] [PubMed]
16. Pereira, B.C.; Isreb, A.; Forbes, R.T.; Dores, F.; Habashy, R.; Petit, J.B.; Alhnan, M.A.; Oga, E.F. 'Temporary Plasticiser': A novel solution to fabricate 3D printed patient-centred cardiovascular 'Polypill' architectures. *Eur. J. Pharm. Biopharm.* **2019**, *135*, 94–103. [CrossRef] [PubMed]
17. Sadia, M.; Isreb, A.; Abbadi, I.; Isreb, M.; Aziz, D.; Selo, A.; Timmins, P.; Alhnan, M.A. From 'fixed dose combinations' to 'a dynamic dose combiner': 3D printed bi-layer antihypertensive tablets. *Eur. J. Pharm. Sci.* **2018**, *123*, 484–494. [CrossRef] [PubMed]
18. Scoutaris, N.; Ross, S.A.; Douroumis, D. 3D Printed "Starmix" Drug Loaded Dosage Forms for Paediatric Applications. *Pharm. Res.* **2018**, *35*, 34. [CrossRef]
19. Preis, M.; Oblom, H. 3D-Printed Drugs for Children-Are We Ready Yet? *AAPS Pharm. Sci. Tech.* **2017**, *18*, 303–308. [CrossRef]
20. Awad, A.; Trenfield, S.J.; Gaisford, S.; Basit, A.W. 3D printed medicines: A new branch of digital healthcare. *Int. J. Pharm.* **2018**, *548*, 586–596. [CrossRef]
21. Alhnan, M.A.; Okwuosa, T.C.; Sadia, M.; Wan, K.W.; Ahmed, W.; Arafat, B. Emergence of 3D Printed Dosage Forms: Opportunities and Challenges. *Pharm. Res.* **2016**, *33*, 1817–1832. [CrossRef]
22. Martinez, P.R.; Goyanes, A.; Basit, A.W.; Gaisford, S. Fabrication of drug-loaded hydrogels with stereolithographic 3D printing. *Int. J. Pharm.* **2017**, *532*, 313–317. [CrossRef] [PubMed]
23. Khan, S.; Ali, S.; Bermak, A. Recent Developments in Printing Flexible and Wearable Sensing Electronics for Healthcare Applications. *Sensors (Basel)* **2019**, *19*. [CrossRef] [PubMed]

24. Luo, S.; Ran, M.; Luo, Q.; Shu, M.; Guo, Q.; Zhu, Y.; Xie, X.; Zhang, C.; Wan, C. Alternating Acetaminophen and Ibuprofen versus Monotherapies in Improvements of Distress and Reducing Refractory Fever in Febrile Children: A Randomized Controlled Trial. *Paediatr. Drugs* **2017**, *19*, 479–486. [CrossRef] [PubMed]
25. Paul, I.M.; Sturgis, S.A.; Yang, C.; Engle, L.; Watts, H.; Berlin, C.M., Jr. Efficacy of standard doses of Ibuprofen alone, alternating, and combined with acetaminophen for the treatment of febrile children. *Clin. Ther.* **2010**, *32*, 2433–2440. [CrossRef] [PubMed]
26. Wong, T.; Stang, A.S.; Ganshorn, H.; Hartling, L.; Maconochie, I.K.; Thomsen, A.M.; Johnson, D.W. Combined and alternating paracetamol and ibuprofen therapy for febrile children. *Evid. Based Child Health* **2014**, *9*, 675–729. [CrossRef]
27. Convention, U. *United States Pharmacopia 31-NF*; Unider States Pharmacopial Convention: Rockville, MD, USA, 2007.
28. Grosskopf, A.K.; Truby, R.L.; Kim, H.; Perazzo, A.; Lewis, J.A.; Stone, H.A. Viscoplastic Matrix Materials for Embedded 3D Printing. *ACS Appl. Mater. Interfaces* **2018**, *10*, 23353–23361. [CrossRef]
29. Muth, J.T.; Vogt, D.M.; Truby, R.L.; Menguc, Y.; Kolesky, D.B.; Wood, R.J.; Lewis, J.A. Embedded 3D printing of strain sensors within highly stretchable elastomers. *Adv. Mater.* **2014**, *26*, 6307–6312. [CrossRef]
30. Truby, R.L.; Wehner, M.; Grosskopf, A.K.; Vogt, D.M.; Uzel, S.G.M.; Wood, R.J.; Lewis, J.A. Soft Somatosensitive Actuators via Embedded 3D Printing. *Adv. Mater.* **2018**, *30*, e1706383. [CrossRef]
31. Foox, M.; Zilberman, M. Drug delivery from gelatin-based systems. *Expert. Opin. Drug Deliv.* **2015**, *12*, 1547–1563. [CrossRef]
32. Young, S.; Wong, M.; Tabata, Y.; Mikos, A.G. Gelatin as a delivery vehicle for the controlled release of bioactive molecules. *J. Control. Release* **2005**, *109*, 256–274. [CrossRef]
33. Kennedy, J.R.; Kent, K.E.; Brown, J.R. Rheology of dispersions of xanthan gum, locust bean gum and mixed biopolymer gel with silicon dioxide nanoparticles. *Mater. Sci. Eng. C. Mater. Biol. Appl.* **2015**, *48*, 347–353. [CrossRef] [PubMed]
34. Alves, M.M.; Antonov, Y.A.; Goncalves, M.P. Phase equilibria and mechanical properties of gel-like water-gelatin-locust bean gum systems. *Int. J. Biol. Macromol.* **2000**, *27*, 41–47. [CrossRef]
35. Kokki, H. Nonsteroidal anti-inflammatory drugs for postoperative pain: A focus on children. *Paediatr. Drugs* **2003**, *5*, 103–123. [CrossRef] [PubMed]
36. Malya, R.R. Does combination treatment with ibuprofen and acetaminophen improve fever control? *Ann. Emerg. Med.* **2013**, *61*, 569–570. [CrossRef]
37. Sjoukes, A.; Venekamp, R.P.; van de Pol, A.C.; Hay, A.D.; Little, P.; Schilder, A.G.; Damoiseaux, R.A. Paracetamol (acetaminophen) or non-steroidal anti-inflammatory drugs, alone or combined, for pain relief in acute otitis media in children. *Cochrane Database Syst. Rev.* **2016**, *12*, CD011534. [CrossRef]
38. Wong, T.; Stang, A.S.; Ganshorn, H.; Hartling, L.; Maconochie, I.K.; Thomsen, A.M.; Johnson, D.W. Cochrane in context: Combined and alternating paracetamol and ibuprofen therapy for febrile children. *Evid. Based Child Health* **2014**, *9*, 730–732. [CrossRef]
39. Baliga, S.; Muglikar, S.; Kale, R. Salivary pH: A diagnostic biomarker. *J. Indian Soc. Periodontol.* **2013**, *17*, 461–465. [CrossRef]
40. Rivera-Leyva, J.C.; Garcia-Flores, M.; Valladares-Mendez, A.; Orozco-Castellanos, L.M.; Martinez-Alfaro, M. Comparative Studies on the Dissolution Profiles of Oral Ibuprofen Suspension and Commercial Tablets using Biopharmaceutical Classification System Criteria. *Indian J. Pharm. Sci.* **2012**, *74*, 312–318. [CrossRef]
41. Shaw, L.R.; Irwin, W.J.; Grattan, T.J.; Conway, B.R. The effect of selected water-soluble excipients on the dissolution of paracetamol and Ibuprofen. *Drug Dev. Ind. Pharm.* **2005**, *31*, 515–525. [CrossRef]
42. Parvathy, K.S.; Susheelamma, N.S.; Tharanathan, R.N.; Gaonkar, A.K. A simple non-aqueous method for carboxymethylation of galactomannans. *Carbohydr. Polym.* **2005**, *62*, 137–141. [CrossRef]
43. Sierakowski, M.R.; Milas, M.; Desbrieres, J.; Rinaudo, M. Specific modifications of galactomannans. *Carbohydr. Polym.* **2000**, *42*, 51–57. [CrossRef]

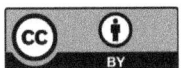 © 2019 by the authors. Licensee MDPI, Basel, Switzerland. This article is an open access article distributed under the terms and conditions of the Creative Commons Attribution (CC BY) license (http://creativecommons.org/licenses/by/4.0/).

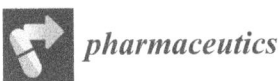

Article

Towards Printed Pediatric Medicines in Hospital Pharmacies: Comparison of 2D and 3D-Printed Orodispersible Warfarin Films with Conventional Oral Powders in Unit Dose Sachets

Heidi Öblom [1,*], Erica Sjöholm [1], Maria Rautamo [1,2] and Niklas Sandler [1]

1. Pharmaceutical Sciences Laboratory, Åbo Akademi University, Artillerigatan 6A, 20520 Åbo, Finland
2. HUS Pharmacy, HUS Helsinki University Hospital, Stenbäcksgatan 9B, 00290 Helsingfors, Finland
* Correspondence: heidi.oblom@abo.fi; Tel.: +358-2-215-4001

Received: 19 June 2019; Accepted: 11 July 2019; Published: 14 July 2019

Abstract: To date, the lack of age-appropriate medicines for many indications results in dose manipulation of commercially available dosage forms, commonly resulting in inaccurate doses. Various printing technologies have recently been explored in the pharmaceutical field due to the flexible and precise nature of the techniques. The aim of this study was, therefore, to compare the currently used method to produce patient-tailored warfarin doses at HUS Pharmacy in Finland with two innovative printing techniques. Dosage forms of various strengths (0.1, 0.5, 1, and 2 mg) were prepared utilizing semisolid extrusion 3D printing, inkjet printing and the established compounding procedure for oral powders in unit dose sachets (OPSs). Orodispersible films (ODFs) drug-loaded with warfarin were prepared by means of printing using hydroxypropylcellulose as a film-forming agent. The OPSs consisted of commercially available warfarin tablets and lactose monohydrate as a filler. The ODFs resulted in thin and flexible films showing acceptable ODF properties. Moreover, the printed ODFs displayed improved drug content compared to the established OPSs. All dosage forms were found to be stable over the one-month stability study and suitable for administration through a naso-gastric tube, thus, enabling administration to all possible patient groups in a hospital ward. This work demonstrates the potential of utilizing printing technologies for the production of on-demand patient-specific doses and further discusses the advantages and limitations of each method.

Keywords: warfarin; 3D printing; semisolid extrusion 3D printing; inkjet printing; orodispersible film; oral powder; pediatric; hospital pharmacy; personalized medicine; on-demand manufacturing

1. Introduction

The lack of suitable dosage forms or doses for children is a common situation in hospital wards [1]. To date, there are no commercially manufactured age-appropriate oral formulations containing warfarin sodium (WS) available for children, especially for neonates and infants. Warfarin is an anticoagulant with a narrow therapeutic index [2,3], which for pediatrics is used to prevent and treat thrombotic events in identified risk groups such as patients suffering from cancer, short bowel syndrome, and patients with a central venous catheter for administration of total parenteral nutrition [3]. The therapy involves dose titration and monitoring of the International Normalized Ratio (INR) [2]. Achieving the right dose often requires manipulation of tablets as WS is commercially available in Finland only as conventional tablets in strengths of 3 and 5 mg. A common way of tailoring the dose in hospital wards is by splitting the tablet into halves or quarters, which then further may be crushed and dissolved or dispersed before administration if the patient is unable to swallow tablets or in cases where the drug is administered through a naso-gastric tube. Splitting of tablets into halves or even smaller parts does not always result in uniform pieces regarding weight and drug content, which might lead to variability in doses and absorbed drug amounts resulting in a risk for under- or overdosing [4–7]. An alternative to tablet splitting is compounding of oral liquids, capsules, or oral powders in unit dose sachets (OPS) at the hospital pharmacy [8]. The dosing flexibility is better for oral liquids than for OPS or capsules. A disadvantage of oral liquids is, on the other hand, the stability, which usually is shorter for liquid dosage forms than for compounded solid dosage forms. The compounding of oral liquids might also require the use of excipients that can be harmful to children. Oral powders, capsules, and segments of tablets are dissolved or dispersed in a liquid before administration or alternatively given with food. For many hospitalized children the medication is given through an enteral feeding tube, which require the drug to be in liquid form or formulated in such a way that it easily can be dissolved or dispersed prior to administration. The fact that some patients have fluid restrictions further affect the requirements for the administration of dosage forms.

A need for tailored doses as well as dosage forms that are easy to administer to children has led to the development of new formulations such as mini-tablets and orodispersible films (ODFs) [9–11]. Both dosage forms are shown to be suitable for infants aged 6–23 months and preschool children aged 2–6 years [12–14]. ODFs are thin, rapidly dissolving or disintegrating polymer films that are administered directly into the mouth where they stick to the tongue or palatal [9,15]. The administration does not require water intake, making it a good alternative for patients with fluid restrictions or patients that are unable to swallow conventional tablets [9]. Disintegration time, as well as, film thickness and stickiness, has been identified as key acceptability characteristics for ODFs in healthy young adults [15]. Different methods mentioned in the literature for the production of ODFs are solvent casting, hot-melt extrusion, semisolid casting, solid dispersion extrusion, rolling, and printing technology methods, such as flexographic printing, semisolid extrusion 3D printing (EXT), and inkjet printing (IJP) onto edible substrates [16–20].

Novel three dimensional (3D) printed dosage forms have been presented in the literature as a potential way of manufacturing accurate, personalized doses for pediatric patients in hospital pharmacy settings [21]. Individual preferences, for instance, size, color, and shape of the printed dosage form are features that affect the acceptability of a dosage form [22]. By printing personalized medicines and considering an individual child's preferences as well as the need for individual doses, it would be possible to improve the patient centricity of hospital pharmacy compounding. 3D printing is a manufacturing technique that uses a computer-aided design (CAD) to deposit layers of material on top of each other producing 3D objects [19]. Examples of potential printing technologies for pharmaceutical manufacturing are flexographic printing, fused deposition modeling (FDM), EXT and 2D or 3D IJP [21,23,24]. Flexographic printing technology has successfully been used to produce drug-loaded ODFs [16]. FDM, also known as fused filament fabrication (FFF), is one of the most extensively investigated printing methods in the pharmaceutical field. The FDM process uses high temperatures to melt the thermoplastic drug-loaded polymer filament used as feedstock material, which is why the method may be unsuitable for thermolabile active pharmaceutical ingredients (API) and polymers [23,25]. Depending on the choice of polymer as well as the design of the dosage form, both immediate and sustained release formulations can be manufactured by means of FDM [26]. EXT, also called pressure-assisted microsyringe printing method (PAM), utilizes a semisolid formulation, e.g., gel or paste, as starting material [27,28]. The formulation is loaded in a syringe and extruded through the nozzle, by, e.g., pressurized air to form a solid dosage form. Immediate release tablets containing levetiracetam [28] and paracetamol [29] have been produced by means of EXT. The deposition of API containing ink onto edible substrates as well as jetting a binder solution onto a powder bed to form solid objects are two methods where IJP is explored for production of dosage forms [21,23]. Readers interested in more detailed information regarding printing methods explored in the pharmaceutical field are referred to the following reviews [21,30].

Recently studies have been conducted to produce personalized doses of warfarin by means of printing. Tian et al. have printed oral disintegrating tablets of WS using the binder jetting technique [31].

A binder liquid was sprayed from a nozzle on a powder bed, and the process was repeated in several layers until the desired dose of the tablet was achieved. Vuddanda et al. were able to produce ODFs with IJP technology [32]. A modified commercial printer was used to deposit a 300 mg/mL warfarin solution onto different sizes of edible substrates made of hydroxypropyl methylcellulose (HPMC), glycerol, and water, resulting in ODFs containing two different doses of warfarin. Additionally, EXT has been utilized to print ODFs containing various doses of WS using hydroxypropyl cellulose (HPC) as a film-forming agent [33]. Another approach to produce tailored doses of warfarin containing ODFs, by traditional solvent casting rather than utilizing printing techniques, has recently been presented by Niele et al. [34]. A long ODF placed in a tape dispenser enabled administration of personalized warfarin doses by tearing off a piece of ODF corresponding to a specific dose.

This study aims to compare the use of EXT and IJP with the conventional manufacturing method for compounding OPSs to produce various doses of warfarin. It further seeks to evaluate the quality and stability of the IJP and EXT printed ODFs as well as the OPSs prepared at a hospital pharmacy. To the best of our knowledge, there are no previous studies where the content uniformity of printed dosage forms would have been compared to traditional pharmacy compounded dosage forms like OPSs. The content uniformity and dose accuracy were expected to be better for the printed dosage forms than the oral powders as IJP is considered a very accurate method to prepare low-dose drugs, whereas OPSs or capsules have shown some inaccuracy in previous studies [20,21,35]. The ease of use was assessed by the suitability to administer the prepared dosage forms through a naso-gastric tube, describing how well the administration needs of the wards can be met. The risk for medication errors in drug administration was addressed by inkjet printing a QR code onto the ODFs. The final aim of this study was to evaluate the suitability of the utilized printing methods for extemporaneous compounding in a hospital pharmacy environment.

2. Materials and Methods

2.1. Materials

The anticoagulant warfarin was the drug investigated in the present study. Warfarin sodium (WS) loaded into the orodispersible films (ODFs) was acquired from Sigma-Aldrich (St. Louis, MO, USA), and the WS present in the compounded oral powders in unit dose sachets (OPSs) was obtained from commercial Marevan forte 5 mg tablets (Orion Pharma, Espoo, Finland). Lactose monohydrate (parve granules, Oriola, Espoo, Finland) was used as a filler in the OPS together with the ground tablets. Hydroxypropylcellulose (HPC, Klucel™ EXF, MW 80,000), which was used as a film-forming agent for both the EXT and IJP ODFs, was kindly donated by Ashland (Schaffhausen, Switzerland). Quinoline yellow (Sigma-Aldrich, Bangalore, India) and propylene glycol (PG) $\geq$ 99.5% (Sigma-Aldrich, St. Louis, MO, USA) were added to the IJP ink due to their respective properties as a colorant and viscosity/surface tension modifier. Ethanol $\geq$ 94% (Etax A, Altia, Helsinki, Finland) and purified water (Milli-Q water, Millipore SA-67120, Millipore, Molsheim, France) were used for analytics and as solvents in the polymer and ink solutions.

2.2. Methods

2.2.1. Manufacturing of Personalized Doses

Target doses of 0.1, 0.5, 1, and 2 mg, were prepared by three different manufacturing methods. Two new innovative manufacturing methods in the pharmaceutical field, namely semi-solid extrusion 3D printing (EXT) and 2D inkjet printing (IJP), were compared to the established manufacturing method for oral powder unit dose sachets (OPSs) compounded at HUS Pharmacy, the hospital pharmacy of HUS Helsinki University Hospital (HUS) and subsequently used at New Children's Hospital in Finland. The drug and the dose levels were selected based on an analysis of compounded OPSs at HUS Pharmacy in the year of 2018, which revealed that 1075 out of the 13,000 OPS manufactured at

HUS Pharmacy contained the drug WS. The analysis additionally showed that the compounded WS doses were between 0.1 and 2.3 mg, where the most frequently compounded doses were 0.5 and 1 mg.

2.2.2. Film Designs

Squared films with four different aimed doses were designed (Table 1) using a computer-aided design software (Inventor Professional software, version 2019, Autodesk, San Rafael, CA, USA) for the EXT ODFs and PowerPoint (version 2016, Microsoft Office, Microsoft Corporation, Redmond, WA, USA) for the IJP ODFs. EXT and IJP films were designed to have the same size, however, the printed area was designed to be slightly smaller for the IJP film to allow for manual cutting of the film after the printing step. A cutting template with the final size of the IJP film was also designed in PowerPoint. The EXT ODF designs were saved as .stl files and imported into the slicer software (RepertierHost v1.6.1, Hot-World GmbH and Co. KG, Willich, Germany) where the print settings were set, and the g-code was generated. The IJP designs were saved as .bmp files and imported into the printing software where the printing parameters were determined.

Table 1. Designed geometries for the ODFs.

Target Dose (mg)	Total Film Length (mm)	EXT ODF		IJP ODF
		Height (mm)	Volume (mm^3)	Printed Length (mm)
0.1	5 × 5	0.1	2.5	4.4 × 4.4
0.5	11.2 × 11.2	0.1	12.5	9.8 × 9.8
1	15.8 × 15.8	0.1	25	13.9 × 13.9
2	22.4 × 22.4	0.1	50	19.7 × 19.7

The film sizes were determined based on the assumption of what could be handled by a nurse at the hospital as well as physical considerations of pediatrics. The smallest film size was restricted by the size still manageable to handle, and the biggest film was limited by the size of a child's mouth. The different sizes for the EXT ODFs were designed to increase in volume in the same ratio as the dose escalation in order to enable the use of the same printing solution for manufacturing of all sizes. The final sizes of the IJP ODFs were designed to be equal to the sizes designed for the EXT, as displayed in Table 1.

2.2.3. Semisolid Extrusion 3D Printing

Printing Solution

The drug concentration in the HPC solution was determined by printing films ($n = 6$) of all designed sizes using a placebo HPC solution. The wet weight of the printed films was used to calculate the percent WS needed in the polymer solution to obtain the targeted doses. The average WS drug load for all of the different sizes based on the calculations was the selected drug load.

The placebo printing solution for the EXT was prepared by dissolving 15% (w/w) HPC in an ethanol and purified water mixture (ratio 1:1). The drug-loaded printing solution was prepared in a similar manner where 1.5% (w/w) WS and 15% (w/w) HPC were dissolved in a mixture of ethanol and purified water (ratio 1:1). The solutions were left on a magnetic stirrer overnight at room temperature to allow the polymer to fully dissolve.

Semisolid Extrusion 3D Printing

The prepared printing solutions were transferred into 10 mL disposable syringes attached to a single-use 25 G electro-polished tip (1/4" Techcon TE Needle, Ellsworth adhesives, Norsborg, Sweden). The Biobots 1 (Biobot, Philadelphia, PA, USA) EXT equipped with an air compressor was used to print both placebo and drug-loaded ODFs. Films were printed on pieces of transparency sheets with a set pressure of 25 PSI and a printing layer height of 0.1 mm. One vertical shell was printed, and the outlines were subsequently filled in using a rectilinear fill pattern with a 45° fill angle, an infill density of 100% and an infill overlap of 15%. All printing steps were conducted with a speed of 8 mm/s. Within each batch, one film was printed at a time, and the films were let to dry overnight in room temperature.

EXT films were printed on three different days, referred to as batch 1, 2, and 3, to evaluate the day-to-day and batch variability of the manufacturing method. The same printing solution was used for printing of all batches in order to obtain information regarding the robustness of the technique rather than differences possibly originating from the preparation of the print solution. As the same solution was used for printing on three different days (day 1, 2, and 4), the stability of the drug-loaded printing solution stored in room temperature was determined by UV-spectrophotometry (Lambda 35, PerkinElmer, Singapore, Singapore) at 207 nm.

2.2.4. Inkjet Printing

Preparation of Solvent Cast Printing Substrates

The polymeric substrates used in the IJP process were prepared by solvent casting. A drug-free HPC solution was prepared in the same manner as described for the placebo EXT ODFs and subsequently cast into films with a wet thickness of 600 μm utilizing a film applicator (Multicator 411, Erichsen, Hemer, Germany). The films were cast on top of transparency sheets (clear transparent X-10.0, Folex, Germany) and allowed to dry in room temperature minimum overnight (some longer, due to the printing of batches on different days).

Ink Formulation

The 100 mg/g WS ink solution for the IJP was obtained by dissolving WS (10% (w/w)) in the ink base consisting of a mixture of purified water (5% (w/w)), PG (27% (w/w)) and ethanol (57.99% (w/w)) (Table 2). The colorant quinoline yellow (0.01% (w/w)) was added to the ink solution in order to better visualize the printed area. A placebo ink was prepared in the same ratio as the drug-loaded ink, which was used for the production of placebo-imprinted ODFs needed for the analytics. Both inks were stored in the fridge at 4 °C. As for the EXT, the stability of the ink over multiple days was determined in a preliminary study by UV-spectrophotometry (Lambda 35, PerkinElmer, Singapore) at 207 nm.

Table 2. Ink compositions for IJP.

Substance	Drug-Loaded Ink (w/w %)	Placebo Ink (w/w %)
Warfarin sodium	10	-
Quinoline yellow	0.01	0.01
PG	27	27
Water	5	5
Ethanol	Ad 100	Ad 100

Inkjet Printing

Inkjet printing was performed with a PixDro LP50 piezoelectric printer (Roth and Rau, Eindhoven, Netherlands) equipped with a print head with 128 nozzles (SL-128 AA, Fujifilm, Tokyo, Japan) and a camera for visualization of the jetted droplets. The printing resolution was set to 720 dpi based on calculations of the target dose, estimated droplet volume, ink concentration, as well as the size of the printed area. Printing was conducted with a jetting frequency of 1400 Hz, a voltage of 80 V, an ink pressure of −18 mbar and a pulse shape of 3-16-5 μs. The prepared ink (drug or drug-free) was filtered (0.45 μm polypropylene membrane syringe filter, VWR International, Radnor, PA, USA) and used to imprint the prefabricated solvent cast HPC films according to the premade designs using 40–60 nozzles, a quality factor of 3 and bi-directional printing. One printing run resulted in 32 printed films of a certain size that were allowed to dry in ambient conditions overnight and subsequently cut with a scalpel according to a template in order to obtain the final size.

2.2.5. Compounding of Oral Powders in Unit Dose Sachets

The OPSs, each individual sachet weighing 200 mg, were compounded at the manufacturing unit at HUS Pharmacy in the same routinely manner as when OPSs are prepared and delivered for patients at the hospital. Three batches per dose were manufactured on three different days. The batch size was 30 OPSs except for the last batch of the 2 mg doses, where the batch size was 120 OPSs.

The OPSs were manufactured following the standard operating procedures of HUS Pharmacy for extemporaneously prepared OPSs. A pharmacist prepared the masses, and a technician or pharmacist weighed the individual sachets. Marevan forte 5 mg tablets were crushed in a mortar and ground with a pestle to a fine powder. Lactose monohydrate was added in geometric amounts to receive the final concentration and amount needed for each dose and batch size. The content of the individual sachets was weighed into waxed powder papers (Herra Järvisen Verstas Oy, Helsinki, Finland) using an analytical balance (MettlerToledo XP204, Greifensee, Switzerland). All sachets were labeled and packed in plastic ziplock bags.

2.2.6. Identification Labeling using Printed Quick Response (QR) Codes

ODFs prepared by IJP and EXT were imprinted with a quick response (QR) code containing vital information about the dosage form, such as type of dosage form, API, strength, manufacturing date, expiration date, as well as the batch number. The QR code was generated utilizing the free online QR generator (goQR.me, Foundata GmbH, Karlsruhe, Germany), saved as a .bmp file and imported into the printing software. A placebo ink containing 1% (w/w) brilliant blue G dissolved in the ink base consisting of 27% (w/w) PG, 5% (w/w) purified water, and 67% (w/w) ethanol was used for printing the QR code.

The same IJP and print head as utilized for the printing of the IJP ODFs was used to print the QR code. The ink was filtered through a 0.45 μm polypropylene membrane syringe filter (VWR International, Radnor, PA, USA) to remove any undissolved particles and bi-directional printing was conducted with a pulse shape of 3-16-5, a jetting frequency of 1700 Hz, a voltage of 80V, and an ink pressure of −18 mbar. The QR code was printed with one nozzle, a quality factor 1 and a resolution of 400 dpi. The readability of the imprinted QR code on the ODFs was evaluated using QR reader for iPhone (version 6.8, Tapmedia Ltd., UK) and QR Code Reader (version 1.0.7, Google Commerce Ltd., Dublin, Ireland) for android.

2.2.7. Weight, Thickness, and Appearance of Dosage Forms

The overall appearance of the prepared dosage forms was evaluated visually. The thickness of the ODFs was measured at 5 locations (all corners and the middle of the film) utilizing a caliper (CD-6"CX, Mitutoyo, Kawasaki, Japan) and the weight of the ODFs was determined using an analytical balance (AND GH-252, A and D Instruments Ltd., Tokyo, Japan). The weight and thickness of the ODFs used in the content analysis were chosen to represent the respective batches (average ± SD, $n = 10$).

2.2.8. Mechanical Testing

The mechanical properties of the produced ODFs were investigated using a TA-XTplus (Stable Micro Systems, Godalming, UK) texture analyzer equipped with a 10 kg load cell. The largest ODFs ($n = 5$) were one at a time clamped between the Perspex film support platform and the aluminum circular top plate (Film support rig HDP/FSR, Stable Micro Systems). The spherical probe (ø 5 mm, SMS P/5S, Stable Micro Systems) was used to puncture the film with a constant speed of 1 mm/s until reaching the target distance of 5 mm (EXT films) or 15 mm (IJP films). The acquisition of data started when the trigger force of 0.049 N was reached, and the maximum applied force and penetration depth (mm) into the film before rupturing was recorded. Experiments were conducted at ambient conditions.

2.2.9. Surface pH

The surface pH of the prepared EXT and IJP ODFs (drug-loaded and placebo) as well as of the prepared OPSs was determined in room temperature by placing one 2 mg dosage form in a small glass vial and adding 1 mL of purified water. The electrode of the pH meter (Mettler Toledo FE20, Mettler Toledo AG, Greifensee, Switzerland) was lowered into the solution, and the surface pH was determined after being immersed for 1 min and 15 min, respectively. Measurements for each formulation were performed in triplicate.

2.2.10. Moisture Content

The moisture content of the prepared dosage forms ($n = 3$) was investigated utilizing a moisture analyzer (Radwag Mac 50/NH, Radom, Poland). The sample with a target dose of 2 mg was placed on an aluminum pan, and the mass % weight loss corresponding to moisture evaporation was recorded as the sample was heated up to 120 °C. The end point of the measurement was set to when the change of mass had reached equilibrium and was less than 1 mg/min.

2.2.11. Disintegration

The disintegration time of the ODFs was investigated using the Petri dish method. The films were analyzed with regards to thickness and weight prior to the disintegration test. 10 mL of purified water was pipetted into a Petri dish, and the ODF was subsequently dropped on top of the liquid surface using tweezers. The time for the film to completely rupture in the middle into smaller film pieces utilizing this static method was recorded and reported as the time for the film to disintegrate. In other words, swelling (in any direction) of the film or small pieces wearing off at the edges was not defined as the endpoint.

2.2.12. Drug Content

Drug content of the prepared doses was determined to evaluate the amount of drug obtained in the final dosage form utilizing the different manufacturing techniques. Briefly, one ODF or OPS was placed in 100 mL of purified water and shaken (Multi-shaker PSU 20, Biosan, Latvia) at 50 rpm for a minimum of 3 h. Samples were diluted when necessary, and the absorbance was subsequently spectrophotometrically (Lambda 35, PerkinElmer, Singapore, Singapore) analyzed at 207 nm. The absorption of the drug-free ODFs at 207 nm, consisting of either a HPC film or a HPC placebo-ink imprinted film, was used as a baseline for the measurements. For the filtered (0.2 µm cellulose acetate syringe filter) OPSs, the absorbance of purified water at 207 nm was considered as the baseline. Ten replicates of all prepared doses were analyzed for each batch and manufacturing method. For stability, ten replicates of the largest target dose were analyzed at each stability time point.

Uniformity of content of single-dose preparations (UC) was calculated according to the European Pharmacopeia (Ph. Eur. 9.0) 2.9.6, test B [36]. The test complies with requirements if not more than one individual content is outside 85 and 115% of average content, and none is outside 75 and 125% of average content. If two or three individual dosage units are outside 85–115% of average content, a further 20 units should be tested. The test fails to comply with requirements if more than three individual contents are outside 85–115% of average content. Moreover, the prepared dosage forms were analyzed with regards to uniformity of dosage units as described in Ph. Eur. 2.9.40. The acceptability constant $k = 2.4$ ($n = 10$) and $T = 100\%$ were used to calculate the acceptance values (AV). The AV (L1) should be ≤ 15.0 to meet the requirements. In this study, the acceptance UC and AV were based on ten replicates, an additional 20 dosage forms were not analyzed.

2.2.13. In Vitro Dissolution

In vitro drug release studies were conducted for the pure drug as received, as well as for the prepared doses from the three different manufacturing techniques (EXT, IJP, and OPS) to study the drug release behavior of the dosage forms. The thickness and weight of the ODFs was documented prior to the dissolution study as well as the weight of the OPSs. The ODFs were placed in dissolution baskets and inserted in 250 mL glass bottles containing 100 mL of purified water, while the oral powder in the sachets were emptied from the sachets directly into the bottles. The bottles were kept on a shaking water bath at 37 °C and 50 rpm throughout the dissolution study. At each predetermined time point, 3 mL of media was manually withdrawn, and 3 mL of fresh media was added. The absorbance of the withdrawn solutions was measured at 207 nm using a UV–VIS spectrophotometer (Lambda 35, PerkinElmer, Singapore). The withdrawn solutions from the OPS samples were filtered through a 0.2 μm cellulose acetate syringe filter (rinsed with 30 mL of purified water prior to use) in order to remove undissolved particles. Samples were measured in triplicate, and the percent drug released was calculated based on the results obtained from the content measurements.

As a comparison to the manual dissolution, dosage forms with the highest drug load (target dose of 2 mg) were additionally studied utilizing an automated setup (Sotax AT 7smart, Basel, Switzerland). The ODFs were accurately weighed an inserted into baskets, while the oral powders from the OPSs were directly poured into the vessels filled with 500 mL of purified water at 37 ± 0.5 °C. The basket rotated with a speed of 50 rpm, and samples of the release media were automatically withdrawn at predefined time-points with the use of a pump (Sotax CY 6, Basel, Switzerland), filtered (glass microfiber filter GF/B, GE Healthcare Life Sciences, Little Chalfont, UK) and the absorbance measured at 207 nm utilizing an on-line UV–VIS spectrophotometer (Lambda 35, PerkinElmer, Singapore). The average percent drug release ($n = 3$) was once again calculated based on the results from the content measurements.

2.2.14. Evaluation of Drug Administration through a Naso-Gastric Tube

The administration of the produced dosage forms through a naso-gastric tube was mimicked to ensure that it would be possible to administer the prepared dosage forms to all patients at hospital wards. The amount of water used for administrating one OPS dose is not clearly standardized at HUS, but typically, the volume is as small as possible. To simulate the process used at the hospital ward, each dosage form was placed in a disposable plastic medicine cup and 2 mL purified water was added. The medicine cup was shaken for approximately 2 min whereafter the solution was administered into the naso-gastric tube (Nutricia Flocare pur tube, CH 6/60, inner diameter 1.1 mm, Nutricia Medical Devices BV, Zoetermeer, Netherlands) with the help of a disposable syringe and subsequently collected into a 100 mL volumetric flask. After administration of the dosage form, the naso-gastric tube was flushed with 2 mL of purified water, which likewise was collected in the volumetric flask. Purified water ad 100 mL was added, and the WS content was measured utilizing the same UV–VIS spectroscopy method as described in drug content measurement (Section 2.2.12). Three replicates of the largest target dose for all three manufacturing methods were tested.

2.2.15. Attenuated Total Reflectance Fourier Transform Infrared (ATR-FTIR)

The infrared spectra of the raw materials, physical mixtures, and the prepared dosage forms were obtained using an Attenuated Total Reflectance Fourier Transform Infrared (ATR-FTIR) spectroscopy (Spectrum Two, PerkinElmer Inc., Beaconsfield, UK). The samples were placed on top of the diamond (IJP ODFs with the printed side facing the diamond), and a force of 75 N was applied during the measurement to attain a good signal. Samples were measured from 4000 to 400 cm^{-1} with four accumulations at a resolution of 4 cm^{-1}. Spectra were obtained in duplicate, and a third measurement was performed in cases where differences were observed during the first two measurements. The software Spectrum (version 10.03.02, PerkinElmer) was used for acquisition of the spectra and for further data treatment utilizing baseline correction, normalization, and data tune-up.

2.2.16. Differential scanning calorimetry (DSC)

Differential scanning calorimetry (DSC) was utilized to evaluate the thermal properties of the samples using the Q2000 (TA Instruments, New Castle, DE, USA). Samples weighing 3.0 ± 0.1 mg were analyzed in sealed Tzero aluminum pans from −20 to 230 °C with a heating rate of 10 °C/min. The OPSs were only heated up to 220 °C to avoid further degradation of the sample. Measurements were performed in duplicate and in triplicate if differences were observed during the first two runs. Nitrogen was used as purge gas with a flow rate of 50 mL/min during all measurements. The data was analyzed utilizing the TA Universal Analysis software (version 4.5A, TA Instruments).

2.2.17. Stability

The stability of the EXT ODFs, IJP ODFs, and OPSs was investigated by visual inspection, mechanical analysis (of ODFs), UV–VIS spectroscopy (drug content), DSC, and ATR-FTIR. The EXT ODFs were stored in a Petri dish throughout the stability period and the IJP ODFs sheets were stacked on top of each other with a transparency sheet in between the printed samples and further covered with aluminum foil. The OPSs were stored in open ziplock bags as an external package. All samples were stored in ambient conditions in a cupboard protected from light. The temperature and relative humidity was tracked during the period using a humidity and temperature USB data logger (wk057, Wisemann Klein SL, Barcelona, Spain). Samples were analyzed at predefined time points, namely at day 1, 7, 14, 21, and 28.

3. Results and Discussion

3.1. Manufacturing of Personalized Doses

In the initial phase of the study, 60 formulations (data not shown) were screened with regards to their film-forming capacity as well as suitability to be processed into personalized ODFs by means of printing. A film-forming solution that was suitable for both the utilized printing techniques was desired in order to identify differences in the final dosage form originating from the printing methods rather than the formulation itself. A simple formulation consisting of the drug and HPC dissolved in a mixture of purified water and ethanol was chosen due to the excellent film-forming capacity of HPC, which resulted in clear, flexible films without the need of plasticizers. The printed formulations consisted of as few excipients as possible as a preference expressed by the medical doctors at HUS, however, disintegrants, saliva stimulating agents, sweeteners, taste masking agents, flavors, colorants, etc., may be introduced in the formulation to further tailor the properties of the ODF or to fulfill individual preferences of a patient. The amounts used of these types of ingredients are typically quite low in ODFs [37–39], and it is, therefore, unlikely that addition of these materials dramatically would change the printability nor the quality of the printed ODFs. As EXT and IJP nonetheless are techniques that require different properties of the formulation to be printable, the idea was to use the same HPC solution (15% w/w) as a substrate for IJP which subsequently was imprinted with a drug ink and which in the case of EXT was drug-loaded and printed into ODFs in a single step.

The OPSs were produced according to the standard operating procedure at HUS Pharmacy in order to be able to compare the OPSs in use at the hospital with the recently explored innovative 2D and 3D printing techniques.

3.1.1. Semisolid Extrusion Printing

The different sized ODFs were successfully manufactured according to the pre-made design utilizing EXT (a video of the printing process can be found in Video S1). The drug-concentration required in the printing solution was calculated based on the wet weight of the printed placebo ODFs and the target dose of the ODFs. Six films of each size (target dose of 0.1, 0.5, 1, and 2 mg) were printed and immediately weighed (Table 3). The average calculated drug concentration of the four different sizes was selected as the drug concentration in the solution used for EXT printing. The correlation between the wet weight and size (mm^3) of the printed placebo films as well as the subsequently dried films was 1 and 0.9998, respectively, suggesting that the weight of the prepared ODFs could be a reliable and easily accessible quality assurance method that could be utilized in a hospital setting as further confirmed in the drug content section.

Table 3. Wet and dry weights of the placebo EXT ODFs used to determine the drug load in the printing solution.

Target Dose	Wet Weight (mg)	Dry Weight (mg)	Theoretical Drug Concentration (%)
0.1	7.7 ± 0.1	1.2 ± 0.1	1.3
0.5	32.0 ± 0.2	5.3 ± 0.1	1.6
1	63.6 ± 0.5	10.5 ± 0.1	1.6
2	124.9 ± 1.2	21.4 ± 0.1	1.6
R^2	1	0.9998	Average 1.5

The used EXT utilizes pressurized air to force the solution out of the syringe. In this study, the aimed pressure was 25 PSI and the actual pressure was noted to be 24.8 ± 0.1 at the beginning of the printing process (when pressing start). One discovered drawback with the used printer was that it was difficult to attain the set pressure and even during printing of a single ODF the pressure would typically fluctuate. As pressure is one of the most important parameters to determine how much material is deposited per unit time, it may result in ODFs with fluctuating drug amount. Other factors to take into account when using an EXT 3D printer is that the distance between the syringe tip and the build platform will have an impact on the amount of solution that is being deposited. Furthermore, the length of the tip and the amount of solution in the syringe was seen to have an effect on the pressure required and the amount of solution being deposited. Consequently, at least all of these factors should be standardized or monitored to achieve ODFs with similar properties.

3.1.2. Inkjet Printing

The IJP ODFs were successfully produced in three subsequent steps involving, solvent casting of the substrate, deposition of the drug-loaded ink on the dry cast polymer sheet by means of IJP and finally drying overnight and cutting into the final size using a cutting template and a scalpel. A slightly modified ink from Genina et al. [40] was developed according to the requirements of the added components as well as the printer. A high concentration WS ink (100 mg/g) was used to enable printing of the desired dose in a single layer rather than using a multiple printing cycle approach as printing of a single layer was expected to decrease the manufacturing time and simultaneously act as visual quality control to spot non-printed areas. To achieve the target dose by printing a single layer, the dpi was calculated as described in the methods section. No clogging of the nozzles was observed during printing with the described ink formulation, even though recrystallization during printing of high concentration inks containing solvents that are easily evaporated may be of concern for IJP [40].

3.1.3. Manufacturing Times

One of the cornerstones of personalized medicine is that a single or a few doses could be tailored according to a patient's need at a specific time. Batches in personalized medicine are, therefore, typically small, as dose adjustments frequently may occur in order to achieve better treatment outcomes [26]. The manufacturing times for the different manufacturing methods were, hence, recorded to get an understanding of how time-consuming the production of a single dose would be.

The comparison of manufacturing times is somewhat challenging as the different techniques require different steps. In the case that these novel manufacturing techniques would become established manufacturing methods in, e.g., a hospital pharmacy setting, it would be desirable that the substrates, printing solutions, etc., would be contract manufactured and delivered to the hospital, where minor preparation steps such as addition of the desired API could be done. Based on that assumption, the noted manufacturing times in this study were the actual time it took for the printer to print the drug-loaded ODFs (not the preparation of, e.g., printing substrate or solution) whereas for the OPSs the manufacturing time included all the steps included in the SOP. The time to print a single ODF utilizing the two different printing techniques are shown in Table 4. The EXT ODFs were printed one at a time and the time was recorded from pressing start until the print head was returned to its starting position. The manufacturing time for a single IJP ODF was calculated based on all the printed batches consisting of 32 doses per batch.

Table 4. Manufacturing times for EXT ODFs and IJP ODFs. The manufacturing time includes the actual printing time, not premanufacturing steps nor drying times of films. For inkjet printing 51 ± 9 nozzles were used for target doses 0.1, 0.5, and 1 mg and 45 ± 7 nozzles for a target dose of 2 mg.

Target Dose	Manufacturing Time	
	EXT ODF	IJP ODF
0.1	42 s	3 ± 1 s
0.5	1 min 9 s	7 ± 1 s
1	1 min 44 s	13 ± 2 s
2	2 min 53 s	18 ± 3 s

The time required to print the IJP ODFs depended on the amount of used nozzles, in most cases so that an increased amount of used nozzles would lead to a decreased printing time. However, especially when printing the smaller sizes also the specific nozzles selected were observed to have an impact on the printing time as the print head in certain cases needs to move further to be able to use the chosen nozzles, thus understandably increasing the print time. Recording of manufacturing times showed that IJP was a faster technique than EXT, however, factors such as maintenance and cleaning require more time for the IJP compared to the EXT at least in a laboratory setting when the printer is not continuously running. The EXT printer utilizes disposable syringes and does not require a cleaning procedure in the same extent as the IJP printer, which needs to be flushed with a suitable solvent after use in order to ensure that contamination between different drugs and/or formulations do not occur. Printing of multiple films at once with the used EXT printer will reduce the manufacturing time as the transparency sheet does not need to be changed in between. It was furthermore noticed that the printing time for the smallest EXT ODFs with a target dose of 0.1 mg was, in total, 42 s from pressing start until the print head was returned to its starting position, where the actual print time stood for only 10 s. Printing of multiple EXT ODFs simultaneously may, however, be more challenging than printing only one ODF at a time due to, e.g., an unleveled build platform. This may affect the print quality and could result in increased fluctuations between the manufactured ODFs. Additionally, the print area in the used printer is relatively small, restricting the amount of ODFs printed at once.

One batch of OPSs consisted of 30 unit dose sachets except for the last batch of 2 mg OPSs, where the batch size was 120 units. Measured manufacturing times included the time to prepare the powder mass as well as the time to weigh all individual doses into powder papers and subsequently closing and labeling them. Preparation of the total mass for one batch of OPSs took 11.4 ± 2.6 min. The batch size did not affect the time needed to prepare the mass. Weighing of the OPSs took 31.7 ± 7.2 min for a batch of 30 units, whereas the time increased to 100 min for the batch of 120 units. Preparing dose powders in unit dose sachets does not require any premanufacturing steps or laborsome cleaning procedures as the manufacturing equipment, such as the pestle and mortar, are machine-washed after use.

3.1.4. Identification Labeling Using Printed QR Codes

Dried EXT and IJP ODFs were successfully imprinted with readable QR codes (video of the printing process can be found in Video S2) revealing the suitability to utilize IJP for enclosing information regarding the dosage form as also previously shown by Edinger et al. [41]. The QR code was printed directly on the ODFs with edible ink (Figure 1). QR codes are already in use for dosage forms prepared at HUS Pharmacy, but until now containing a limited amount of information (product number and batch number) and only present on the batch-specific label on the secondary package, not on a single dosage form.

The information incorporated in the QR code could easily be tailored according to the requirements or desires of the hospital. When manufacturing on-demand dosage forms tailored according to the need of the patient, patient information could beneficially be included in the QR code. An example of information that could be included is demonstrated in Figure 2. Incorporation of patient information in the QR code of the dosage form would allow the nurse to scan the code as an additional patient safety measure prior to administration to the patient. By doing that, it could, e.g., be ensured that the dose is intended for the specific patient, that the medication still should be given to the patient and the nurse would easily access information regarding how the doctor intended the dosage form to be administered. As patient information is classified as sensitive information, it should be handled securely according to the latest national legislation and general data protection regulations (GDPR). QR codes containing any sensitive information, such as patient information, should, therefore, have restricted access. In theory, this could be solved by the use of passwords and linkage to the patient database, which would require the same login information as otherwise used to access patient information. By linking the QR code, for example, to a database, it opens up the opportunity to include an increased amount of information without the QR code itself getting too detailed and, thus, minimizing the risk for the code to not be easily readable. Readers interested in the benefits and opportunities of QR-encoded dosage forms outside the hospital setting are referred to the interesting discussion by Edinger et al. [41].

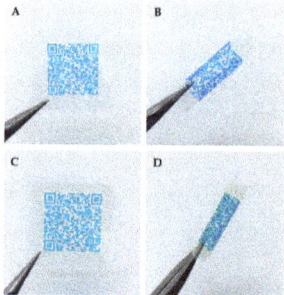

Figure 1. (**A**) EXT drug-loaded ODF imprinted with a QR code containing information about the dosage form and (**B**) the same EXT ODF rolled up to visualize the flexibility of the film. (**C**) IJP drug-loaded ODF with a printed QR code and (**D**) the flexible ODF is subsequently coiled up for illustrative purposes.

API: warfarin sodium
Strength: 0.1 mg
Patient: Baby Doe
Social security number: 010119A0101
Age: 4 months
Weight: 5.2 kg (21.3.2019)
Indication: anticoagulant
Dose: 0.1 mg ODF in the morning
Treatment duration/re-evaluation: until 30.3.2019
Administration: One 0.1 mg ODF placed on the tongue
Prescribing doctor: Dr. John Doe
Manufacturing unit: HUS Pharmacy
Manufacturing date: 21.3.2019
Expiration date: 21.4.2019
Excipients: purified water, ethanol 94%, HPC EXF, brilliant blue
Storage conditions: store protected from light

Figure 2. Example of the information that could be included in the QR code.

3.2. Physical Appearance and Mechanical Properties of the Dosage Forms

The ODFs prepared by means of EXT resulted in clear, thin films with a slight wavy structure if inspected closely. The small waves originated from the printing process where the ODFs were built up one line at a time subsequently adhering to the previous and resulting in the final ODF. The weight and thickness of the respective batches and sizes can be found in Table A1. The IJP ODFs were slightly thicker than the EXT ODFs due to the nature of IJP. The printing substrates were cast with a wet thickness of 600 µm, resulting in films that were slightly thicker than the dried EXT ODFs in order to be able to absorb the jetted ink without dissolving the substrate. As a result, the IJP ODFs were also found to weigh more. The manual cutting of the IJP films into their final size resulted in surprisingly small weight differences of the films within a batch. However, a difference in weight should not have an impact on the drug content in the IJP ODFs as they were designed to have a drug-free area around the film, as demonstrated in Table 1. The OPSs consisted of a powder mixture of pink larger particles (ground tablets) and white smaller lactose monohydrate particles. Pictures of all the prepared dosage forms can be seen in Figure 3.

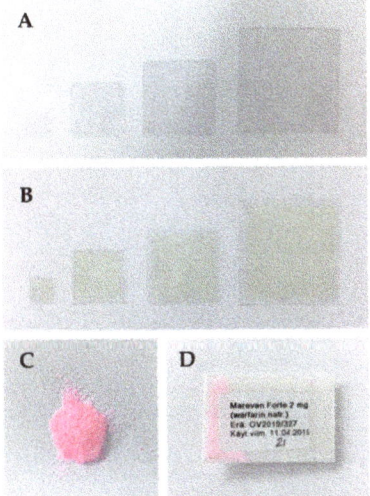

Figure 3. Pictures of the prepared dosage forms: (**A**) EXT ODFs; (**B**) IJP ODFs; (**C**) oral powder; and (**D**) OPS.

The mechanical properties of the prepared ODFs were investigated as ODFs should possess sufficient handling properties to ensure that they are not damaged during any of the steps involved preceding the administration of the dosage form [42]. Figure 4 displays the measured burst strength representing the maximum tolerated force (N) on the ODF before rupturing as well as the burst distance (mm) representing the flexibility of the ODF. The strongest ODFs were found to be the placebo IJP ODFs, which were prepared by solvent casting. The placebo IJP ODFs were observed to withstand over two times more force before rupturing compared to the placebo EXT ODFs, which may be explained by the fact that the placebo IJP ODFs also revealed a greater thickness. Moreover, the manufacturing method of the two placebo films differs, allowing the IJP ODF to be perfectly flat while the EXT ODF is built up one line at a time making the film slightly wavy. This may result in a more brittle film but, on the other hand, enable other advantages, such as fast disintegration compared to the solvent cast film (placebo IJP ODF) as will be discussed later.

Incorporation of the drug in the EXT ODFs appeared to only slightly decrease the strength of the ODFs, however, the burst distance decreased, and they were found to be the most brittle ODFs in this study. The ODFs to elongate the greatest before rupturing were the drug-loaded IJP ODFs. One-day-old WS IJP ODFs revealed an elongation distance of 5.61 ± 0.35 mm before rupturing, which is more than double (2.6 ± 0.2 mm) what was measured for the placebo IJP ODFs that served as the printing substrate. Introduction of the printing ink, hence, clearly showed an impact on the mechanical properties of the IJP ODFs. Additional moisture as well as PG, which both are known to have a plasticizing effect, seems to explain this behavior. Plasticizers typically interact with the polymer chains present in the formulation resulting in increased chain mobility and, consequently, a decreased glass transition temperature, which in terms of mechanical properties is seen as ODFs with improved plastic and elastic properties [43]. The drug-loaded EXT ODFs were much more brittle, bending 1.2 ± 0.1 mm (at day 1) before breaking, further indicating that both the manufacturing technique as well as the additional liquid applied during IJP influences the mechanical properties of the ODFs. The thickness of the films will to some extent have an impact on these results, but as can be seen in Table A2, the film thickness alone is not the reason to the differences between the formulations.

No major differences in the mechanical properties of the ODFs were witnessed during the one-month follow-up period for the EXT ODFs. Nevertheless, a tendency where the drug-loaded EXT ODFs show a decreased burst strength and burst distance one week after manufacturing may indicate that the ODFs were not completely dry after allowing to dry one day in room temperature. Another suggestion is that the films mechanical properties change according to the relative humidity. This can, however, not be supported by the placebo EXT ODFs and further studies are required to fully understand this phenomenon. The drug-loaded IJP ODFs show a trend where they over time become somewhat more brittle and simultaneously can resist a greater force before breaking, possibly due to slow evaporation of the deposited ink at room temperature. The conclusion of the mechanical study is that all prepared ODFs were possible to handle without breaking the dosage forms, however, further modifications such as changing the ODF thickness, addition/removal of plasticizer, etc., can be made to alter the properties of the ODFs if desired.

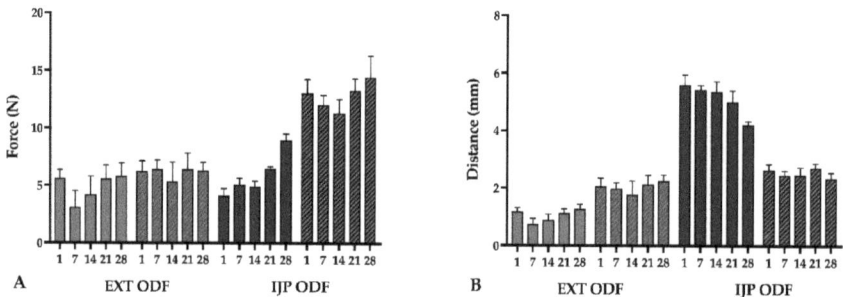

Figure 4. (**A**) Burst strength representing the maximum force (N) and (**B**) burst distance representing the elongation (mm) of the ODF before rupturing. Drug-loaded ODFs are shown as colored columns and placebo ODFs are presented as colored columns with a pattern. Data is shown as average ± SD, $n = 5$ for each time point.

3.3. Surface pH

The surface pH of ODFs is commonly investigated to ensure that the pH of the dosage form is in the range of physiological saliva (5.8–7.4). An ODF with a pH largely differing from this may cause local mucosal irritation and discomfort for the patient [39]. The ODFs prepared in this study all revealed a neutral pH (Table 5) indicating that no local side effects should be encountered at the administration site. The OPSs showed a pH of 9.36 ± 1.62 after being in contact with water for 1 min, perchance making it too alkaline for pleasant administration of the dose. However, the pH decreased and was in the neutral range (7.34 ± 0.19) after allowing the OPS to further dissolve for 14 min suggesting that the OPSs should be fully dissolved/dispersed before administration to avoid possible irritation when administered with a small amount of water.

Table 5. Surface pH of the drug-loaded 2 mg and corresponding placebo dosage forms after 1 min and 15 min, respectively, average ± SD, n = 3. WS = warfarin sodium, P = placebo.

Sample	Surface pH	
	1 min	15 min
EXT WS ODF	7.13 ± 0.13	7.07 ± 0.05
EXT P ODF	6.94 ± 0.10	6.43 ± 0.28
IJP WS ODF	7.37 ± 0.28	7.05 ± 0.03
IJP P ODF	7.03 ± 0.23	6.35 ± 0.21
OPS WS	9.36 ± 1.62	7.34 ± 0.19

3.4. Moisture Content

The moisture content of pharmaceutical products is important to investigate as moisture present in dosage forms may have a negative effect on the physico-chemical, chemical, as well as microbiological stability of the final product [44]. However, some moisture present in ODFs is typically desired due to the plasticizing effect of water, as completely dry films tend to be brittle and have reduced handleability. Depending on the film-forming polymer used, excipients such as glycerol, PG, polyethylene glycol, sorbitol, macrogols of low molecular mass, citrates, and phtalates may be added due to their plasticizing effect of the ODFs [45,46]. However, it is important to keep in mind that plasticizers may alter the properties of the ODFs in multiple ways, e.g., the taste and mechanical properties of the ODF may be affected. Additionally, plasticizers have a tendency to absorb water, which is why a very high amount of plasticizer added to the formulation may result in similar stability issues as discussed above due to the absorbed water. ODFs with a too high a moisture content have also been described as sticky [39].

In this study, the moisture content of the dosage forms was studied using a moisture analyzer. The moisture content in the studied samples may originate from residual solvent from the manufacturing process or due to the hygroscopic nature of one or multiple components present in the formulation. The prepared dosage forms showed a mass loss of 9.36 ± 2.53% (EXT drug-loaded ODFs), 10.5 ± 2.45% (EXT placebo ODFs), 12.39 ± 1.68% (IJP drug-loaded ODFs), 9.13 ± 4.05% (IJP placebo ODFs) and 2.38 ± 0.26% (OPSs), as shown in Figure 5. As expected, the ODFs possessed a higher moisture content than the OPSs due to the introduction of moisture during the manufacturing process. Moreover, the ODFs were dried and stored in ambient condition allowing the hygroscopic HPC to absorb moisture from the surrounding air [47]. The drug-loaded IJP ODFs revealed the highest moisture content, which can be described by the fact that these ODFs consisted of a substrate corresponding to the placebo EXT ODF, which subsequently was imprinted with the drug-loaded ink. In addition to introducing further liquid to the dosage form, the ink contained 27% (w/w) PG, which is known for its plasticizing effect and therefore also its ability to hold water and it has been reported that ODFs with plasticizers, such as PG, showed increased moisture uptake [48]. Consequently, the drug-loaded IJP ODFs would likely require a longer drying time to allow further evaporation of solvents. The difference in moisture content between the placebo and drug-loaded IJP ODFs may, furthermore, be explained by the fact that the IJP placebo ODFs were prepared in advance and had an increased drying time compared to the drug-loaded IJP ODF that only dried overnight. Further studies would be needed to get in-depth information regarding the most suitable drying time and conditions for the prepared ODFs regardless of the manufacturing method.

Nair et al. [49] have stated that an ideal ODF should have a moisture content of less than 5%. In this study, all of the prepared ODFs failed to comply with that limit. However, the EXT ODFs and IJP ODFs were easy to handle and did not stick to gloves during handling. The IJP ODFs were observed to slightly stick to the packing material (transparency sheet between the printed sheets) indicating that the drying time preferably should be increased conceivably due to the high amount of PG present in the ink as discussed above. However, the brief stability study conducted did not indicate degradation of the drug, suggesting that the amount of moisture present in the formulations did not affect the stability of the drug during the studied period.

Lactose monohydrate is a substance with low hygroscopicity meaning it has a low tendency to absorb moisture from the surroundings. It typically has a moisture content of about 5%, which is in agreement with the low moisture content of the OPSs (2.38 ± 0.26%), as they largely consist of this filler. The water present in lactose monohydrate being tightly bound in the crystal lattice makes it chemically inert and not likely to interact with the drug present [50], indicating that moisture should not be a problem for the compounded OPSs.

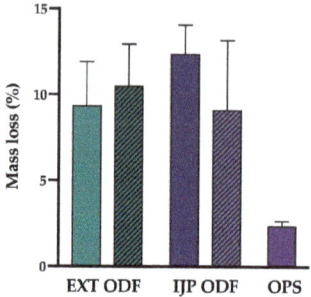

Figure 5. The moisture content reported as mass % weight loss of the sample, for the prepared dosage forms. Results presented as average ± SD, $n = 3$. Drug-loaded ODFs are shown as colored columns and placebo ODFs are presented as colored columns with a pattern.

3.5. Disintegration of Orodispersible Films

Rapid disintegration of ODFs is crucial due to the nature of the dosage form. Thus far, there are no specified methods or acceptance values available in the Ph. Eur. for testing the disintegration behavior of ODFs [36]. The limits available for orodispersible tablets (ODTs), stating that ODTs should disintegrate within 180 s, have therefore generally also been used for the novel ODFs [51]. In this study, all prepared ODFs complied with the disintegration limit described (Table A3). The different sizes of the EXT ODFs all disintegrated in less than 40 s. The IJP ODFs revealed an increased disintegration time (> 84 s), which can be explained by these ODFs being thicker compared to the EXT ODFs. Another difference originates from the manufacturing method, where the EXT ODFs have small waves originating from how the rectilinear infill was printed. These small lines likely result in an increased surface area and faster wetting of the ODF as compared the completely flat solvent cast film. The same phenomena, where a fast disintegration of fused deposition 3D-printed ODFs compared to solvent cast ODFs has recently been reported [52]. The drug-loaded ODFs required slightly longer time to disintegrate than the drug-free ODFs for both manufacturing methods, which may be explained by the presence of the drug in the formulation as also previously reported [37]. No major difference in the disintegration behavior of the ODFs was observed during the stability study (Table A4).

The OPSs could not be analyzed with this disintegration method as the dosage form already is in powder form. An attempt was nonetheless made to use the same method to identify the disintegration time of the ground Marevan particles as their pink color easily could be identified in the powder blend. The particles did not fully dissolve within 10 min and, therefore, the experiment was stopped. However, the Marevan particles dissolved instantly when the Petri dish was shaken after the experiment was stopped.

It is worth noticing that the disintegration method used in this study is a static method and the ODFs would likely disintegrate faster upon shaking. Additionally, the utilized Petri dish method allows the ODF to be wetted from only one side, which possibly results in slower disintegration. However, the method was selected, as no special equipment was needed. Furthermore, the film did not stick to the surface of the Petri dish with the chosen method, which might otherwise give false results. Since there is no standardized method in the Ph. Eur. it makes it difficult to compare disintegration results from different studies. Most importantly, even though a static method was selected in this study, all ODFs disintegrated within 180 s.

3.6. Drug Content

The drug content was determined for 10 dosage forms of each dose, batch, and manufacturing method and the measured content was compared to the target dose (Figure 6). Uniformity of content of single-dose preparations (UC) was determined in order to evaluate the precision of the used methods. Moreover, the acceptance value (AV) according to the Ph. Eur. was calculated, where dosage forms showing AV values of ≤ 15 comply with the set limit. Independent of the manufacturing method, all dosage forms prepared in the various batches were shown to comply with the limits stated for UC in the Ph. Eur. for the two largest doses containing 1 and 2 mg of WS (Table A1). Additionally, all ODFs passed the test for UC for the 0.5 mg dose, whereas one batch of the OPSs failed the test, having one unit outside ±25%, and another batch would have required testing of additional 20 OPSs since two individual contents were outside ±15% limits. For the 0.1 mg dose, two out of three batches for both EXT and IJP ODFs, as well as OPSs, fulfilled the requirements for the UC. For both the EXT and IJP ODFs the largest deviation from average content was more than 25% in one batch resulting in failure to comply with the set limit. For one batch of OPSs, an additional 20 units should have been analyzed to determine if the particular batch would pass or not. These results reveal that dose fluctuation occurs for low-dose dosage forms, but as the dose increases, all the studied manufacturing methods were able to produce repeatable dosage forms within the batch. However, between batches, differences in the average drug content and drug amount compared to the target dose were seen for all the manufacturing methods, as shown in Table A1. For the smallest dose (0.1 mg) the average drug content was 0.10–0.14 mg for EXT ODFs, 0.07–0.09 mg for IJP ODFs, and 0.05–0.09 mg for OPSs. Expressed as percentage of drug amount compared to target dose, the amount of WS varied between 72% and 140% for the EXT ODFs, between 52% and 112% for the IJP ODFs and between 36% and 104% for OPSs for the 0.1 mg dose when taking into account all the individual dosage forms manufactured in all three batches. This shows that in case of low-dose WS dosage forms, there can be a large fluctuation in the received dose for the child between the same dosage form prepared in different batches, which greatly may impact the treatment outcome. As the dose increases, the accuracy compared to the target dose also improves, and the fluctuation diminishes. For the 2 mg WS dose, the amount of drug compared to target dose was between 100.5–109.3% for EXT ODFs, 93.1–109.4% for IJP ODFs and 100.2–116.3% for OPSs when data from all batches are included.

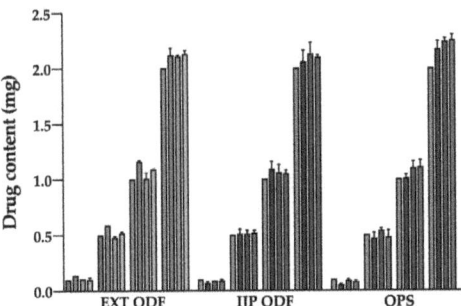

Figure 6. Drug content of the aimed doses of 0.1, 0.5, 1, and 2 mg for the prepared batches and various manufacturing techniques. Gray columns represent the target dose and the following columns represents batch 1, 2, and 3, respectively, for each manufacturing method. Data are presented as the average ± SD, $n = 10$.

EXT was found to be the method that fulfilled the criteria for AV for most of the doses and batches, indicating that the method showed best accuracy and precision regarding uniformity of the active substance among dosage units. The smaller the target dose, the more often the prepared dosage forms prepared by different techniques failed to comply with the AV as displayed in Table A1. Both utilized printing methods were, however, shown to be promising manufacturing methods for production of personalized doses when compared to the method currently used at the hospital pharmacy for preparation of tailored doses.

EXT ODFs revealed a linear correlation between the dry weight of the film and the drug content (mg) in the film. Batch 1, 2, and 3 were found to have R^2 values of 0.9996, 1, and 0.9999, respectively, suggesting that the weight of the dry EXT ODF could be used as an easily accessible tool for quality control in a hospital setting. EXT showed AV values ≥ 40 for two out of the three printed batches of the smallest ODF (target dose of 0.1 mg). This could, however, be anticipated already when calculating the drug concentration in the printing solution as the calculations revealed that the concentration should have been lower for the smallest size than for the rest of the sizes (Table 3). This suggests that to achieve acceptable AV values for the smallest sized EXT ODFs, an optimization of the g-code, design, or the drug concentration of the printing solution should preferably be made, while the other sizes may be printed with the used settings and drug concentration. It was additionally observed that the wet weight of the printed ODFs would deviate from the normal at the beginning of the printing session. This could also be an explanation to why the smallest size EXT ODFs showed high AV, as this strength was the first to be printed in each batch. However, additional studies would be needed to investigate this in a more structured manner.

During IJP of batch 1, some problems were observed as the ink was not stable in the printer before the printing process was started, which could be seen as disappearing droplets during the printing step. This may be explained by (partial) drying of the print head between printing session as it has been seen that the used print head works best if it constantly is kept wet. The printing process proceeded smoothly for batch 3, where the same nozzles could be used for printing of all different sizes and sheets, which directly shows in the drug content results as generally small AV. IJP has previously been described as a method suitable for manufacturing of low-dose dosage forms. However, in many conducted studies, only a single or a few nozzles have been used [53–55] compared to 40–60 nozzles used in this study, which will have an impact on the manufacturing time and further may impact the drug content. Independent of the amount of nozzles used, dosage forms with a drug amount deviating from the theoretical calculated amount have been reported [56]. As the dpi, used to obtain the target dose, is calculated based on the droplet size of the jetted droplets, a change in the average droplet size will directly have an impact on the amount of drug deposited in a certain area. In this study, the approach to utilize a high number of nozzles was preferred to decrease the printing time. However, as modest optimization regarding the ink and printing parameters was conducted in this study, the printing results were seen to differ depending on the nozzles used (placement in the print-head), especially during printing of batch 1. Furthermore, with an increased number of nozzles utilized a greater possibility of variation in droplet volume is introduced. Therefore, close attention should be paid to the droplet size of the used nozzles. Further development and optimization of the printing parameters to obtain droplets with a standard deviation as small as possible would likely improve the results for the IJP dosage forms. Moreover, the droplet volume of all nozzles intended to be used should preferably be investigated in a more systematic and automated approach than what was done in this study, where nozzles deviating too much from the average droplet volume would be excluded.

Regarding the optimization of the OPS, pure drug together with the filler lactose monohydrate could be used instead of the Marevan tablet. This would enable a more homogeneous blend as the particle size of the two materials would be more similar. Alternatively, improved grinding of the tablets and blending of the final mixture in a standardized manner would likely help to improve the content uniformity as well as decrease batch to batch variability.

The study revealed that even though the accuracy in some cases was a bit off, the precision was still excellent, seen as a small standard deviation of the drug content within the same batch. This indicates that the printing techniques are suitable techniques for manufacturing of personalized dosage forms even though some optimizations regarding dosage form design, printing parameters or formulation may need to be carried out to further excel the results. As a conclusion, the innovative ODFs prepared by means of printing were shown to be equally good and even improved with regard to uniformity of dosage units, than the OPSs currently used in a hospital setting.

The stability study revealed that the drug amount was kept unchanged during the studied period, even though small fluctuations were seen between the weeks that most likely originates from normal standard deviations within one batch (Figure 7). All the dosage forms with a target dose of 2 mg fulfilled the UC throughout the one-month period (Table A5). Furthermore, both the EXT ODFs and IJP ODFs showed satisfactory acceptance values, whereas the OPSs displayed slightly too high AV values for each week. This suggests that all of the prepared dosage forms may be used after storage at least for one month in a non-controlled environment, as typically is the case in a hospital ward.

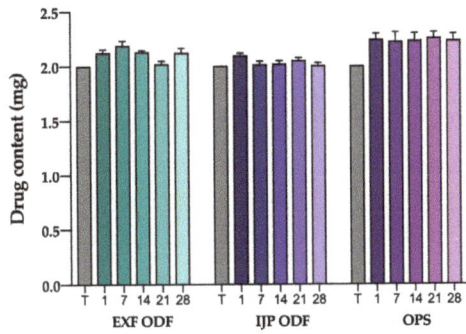

Figure 7. Stability of the manufactured dosage forms with a target dose of 2 mg at time points 1, 7, 14, 21, and 28 days. The gray columns represent the target dose of 2 mg. Data shown as average ± SD, $n = 10$.

3.7. In Vitro Dissolution

To date, neither the Ph. Eur. or United States Pharmacopeia (USP) specify the dissolution setup nor the requirements for fulfillment of the developed ODF, making it difficult to compare results from different studies. This is a known dilemma in the field of novel ODFs, and to further emphasize this, Speer et al. have recently demonstrated how different conditions and dissolution setups affect the in vitro drug release properties of ODFs [57].

In this study, the manually conducted in vitro dissolution studies revealed that all dosage forms with a target dose of 2 mg released 80% of the drug within the first 30 min (Figure 8). Both EXT and IJP ODFs displayed a similar drug release behavior. As expected, the OPS was the formulation with the fastest drug release, as the drug in this formulation was present in ground tablets, thus enabling a rapid release of the water-soluble drug due to a large surface area. On the contrary, for the ODFs, the drug present on the surface of the dosage form could immediately be released, while the rest was released once the polymer network was ruptured. When HPC particles undergo hydration, a viscous gel layer is formed, which inhibits further wetting from the inside and resulting in a slower drug release [47]. The thin manufactured ODFs were seen to disintegrate quickly. However, a complete drug release was not observed until around 30 min, leading to the suggestion that the drug particles after the ODF ruptured into smaller pieces, still were embedded in the polymer matrix. The size of the ODFs or OPSs were not observed to have a pronounced impact on the drug release, which is in line with the results obtained in the disintegration study.

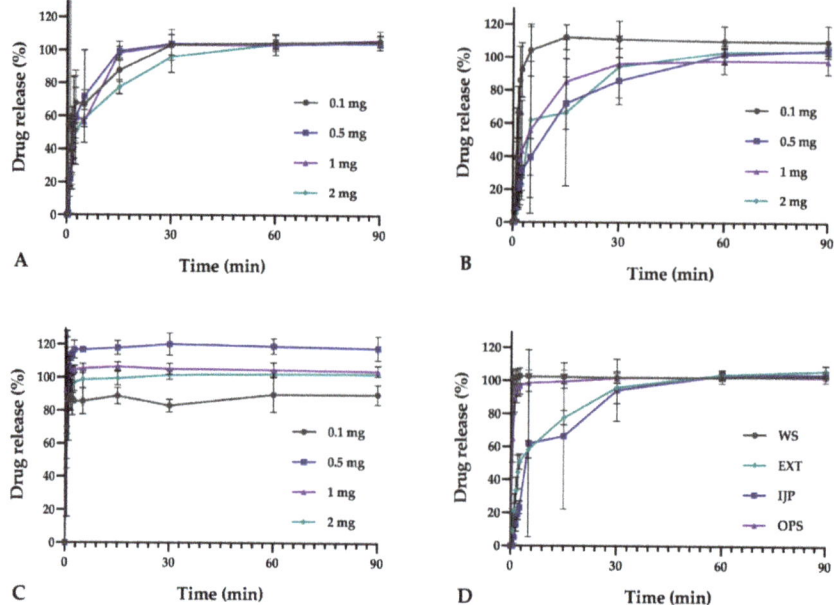

Figure 8. In vitro drug release of the prepared dosage forms in 100 mL of purified water, average ± SD (n = 3); (**A**) EXT ODFs, (**B**) IJP ODFs, (**C**) OPSs, and (**D**) an overview of all manufacturing methods and pure drug for the 2 mg dose.

When the on-line dissolution was conducted in 500 mL of purified water, the dissolution of the drug was faster for all formulations due to the increased amount of liquid and improved stirring compared to the manual setup. The EXT ODF and OPS with a target dose of 2 mg displayed an 80% drug release within the two first min of the experiment. Corresponding drug release for the IJP ODF was 4 min (Figure 9). This underpins the difference in results gained from the different setups as previously discussed. An automated setup is a more robust method due to decreased human errors and would, therefore, be favorable. However, the on-line dissolution setup could not be used for the smallest dosage forms in this study due to a low dose in the dosage form and a large volume of media required. A harmonized dissolution method tailored for ODFs would, therefore, be desired to excel the research of ODFs.

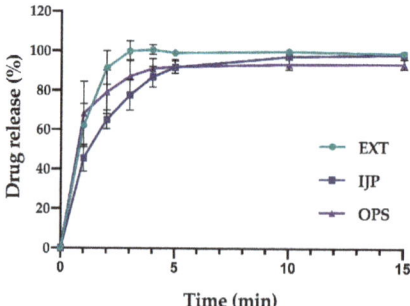

Figure 9. On-line in vitro drug release (%) of the different dosage forms conducted in 500 mL of purified water at 50 rpm, average ± SD, n = 3.

3.8. Evaluation of Drug Administration through a Naso-Gastric Tube

ODFs are normally administered directly into the mouth where they rapidly disintegrate. However, in hospital wards, there might occasionally be a need for the dosage form to be administered through an enteral feeding tube. Therefore, it must be possible to dissolve the dosage form in a small amount of water and subsequently administer it through the naso-gastric tube without the dissolved formulation blocking the tube. The simulation of drug content passing through the naso-gastric tube was performed to investigate the drug amount obtained after administration through the tube. The average amount of WS passing through the tube was compared to the average content measured for the same batch of each dosage form. The average drug amount passing through the naso-gastric tube was 92% for the OPSs, 84% for EXT ODFs and 75% for IJP ODFs (Table 6). Previous studies have shown, that from OPSs containing the drug dipyridamole and lactose as a filler, the amount of drug passing through a naso-gastric tube was 77.5–86.1% depending on the particle size of the filler (< 355 μm vs. < 250 μm) [35]. In size 0 gelatin capsules containing WS and lactose (particle size < 355 μm), the corresponding amount was 96.4%. The use of celluloses (MCC and SMCC) as filler increased the drug loss and occasional blockage of the tube was identified. In this study, no visual blockage of the tube was observed. However, the slightly lower amounts of WS passing through the naso-gastric tube for printed dosage forms suggest that the viscosity of the dissolved HPC films made the solution stick to the surface of the cup and tubing to a higher extent than for the lactose-containing OPSs. The prepared IJP ODFs contained an increased amount of polymer due to increased thickness compared to the EXT ODFs. This in combination with the fact that the IJP ODFs additionally contained PG, seem to have an impact on the drug amount passing through the naso-gastric tube in the studied setup. Some of the drug loss can also be explained by the fact that the syringe tip did not reach every corner of the cup, suggesting that interpersonal differences will occur when administering the dose in this manner.

Table 6. Content of warfarin sodium passing through the naso-gastric tube after dissolving/dispersing the different dosage forms in 2 mL of water. Results presented as the average ± SD, $n = 3$.

Dosage Form	Average Content (mg)	Content Compared to Average Batch Content (%)
EXT ODF	1.78 ± 0.05	84
IJP ODF	1.57 ± 0.12	75
OPS	2.07 ± 0.06	92

3.9. ATR-FTIR

The ATR-IR spectra of pure substances, physical mixtures as well as OPS, drug-loaded and placebo EXT and IJP ODFs are presented in Figure 10. The physical mixture of HPC and the drug showed bands attributed to HPC (3431 cm^{-1}, 2969 cm^{-1}) [58] as well as WS (1663 cm^{-1}, 1453 cm^{-1}, 1323 cm^{-1}, 1720 cm^{-1}, 759 cm^{-1} and 704 cm^{-1}) [32,59,60]. For the drug-loaded EXT ODF, similar bands as to pure WS were seen at 1326 cm^{-1}, 701 cm^{-1}, 760 cm^{-1}, and the broad peak characteristic for pure HPC was present at 3600–3100 cm^{-1} [61]. The placebo EXT ODF revealed the broad peak ranging from 3600–3100 cm^{-1} and further bands at 1452 cm^{-1} and 1326 cm^{-1}, suggesting that these may not be attributed to WS in the drug-loaded EXT ODF. As expected, the spectra of the placebo IJP ODF and placebo EXT ODF were identical as the formulation was the same in both placebo dosage forms, only the manufacturing process into ODFs differed. Moreover, drug-free IJP ODFs imprinted with placebo ink showed identical spectra as the placebo IJP ODF prior to printing, even though new components, such as PG and colorant were present in the imprinted placebo sample, leading to the suggestion that the difference in spectra between the drug-loaded IJP ODF compared to the drug-loaded EXT ODF may be a result of some interaction between the drug and the components in the ink. Bands attributed to WS were seen at 759 cm^{-1} and 700 cm^{-1}. The only characteristic band for WS identified for the OPS was located at 760 cm^{-1}. This band was, however, also found for pure lactose monohydrate.

The spectra for the OPSs as well as the Marevan tablet were almost identical to the spectra of lactose monohydrate, which may be explained by the fact that lactose monohydrate was in all formulations present in a much larger ratio than the drug.

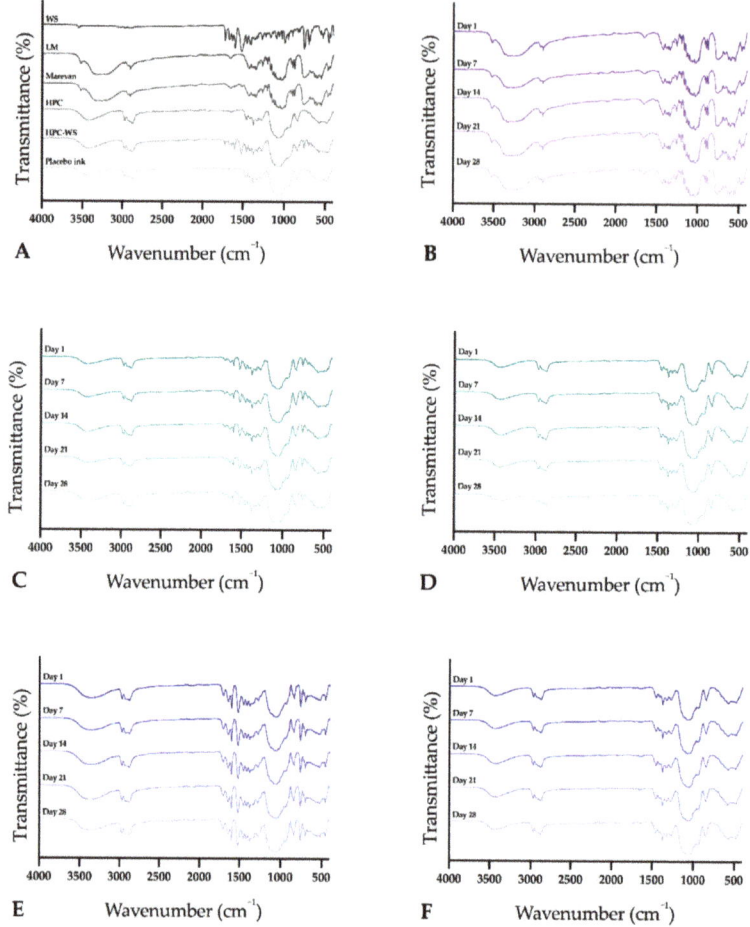

Figure 10. FT-IR spectra for (**A**) raw materials and/or starting materials; (**B**) OPS; (**C**) drug-loaded EXT; (**D**) placebo EXT ODF; (**E**) drug-loaded IJP ODF; and (**F**) placebo IJP ODF. The graphs present the spectra for the prepared drug-loaded and placebo dosage forms for day 1, 7, 14, 21, and 28.

No significant spectral shifts, differences in band intensity, or completely dilution of bands were observed for any of the dosage forms during the stability study, indicating that no major change in intermolecular interaction occurs during storage up to one month.

3.10. DSC

The thermal properties of the raw materials, physical mixtures, and final dosage forms were investigated once for the raw materials and over a one month period for the prepared dosage forms in order to gain information about how the thermal properties of the dosage forms change upon storage. WS showed a small and broad endothermic event with an onset at 36.5 °C and peak max at 74.1 °C followed by another larger endothermic event identified as the melting of the drug with onset and peak max at 177.7 and 192.7 °C, respectively (Figure 11).

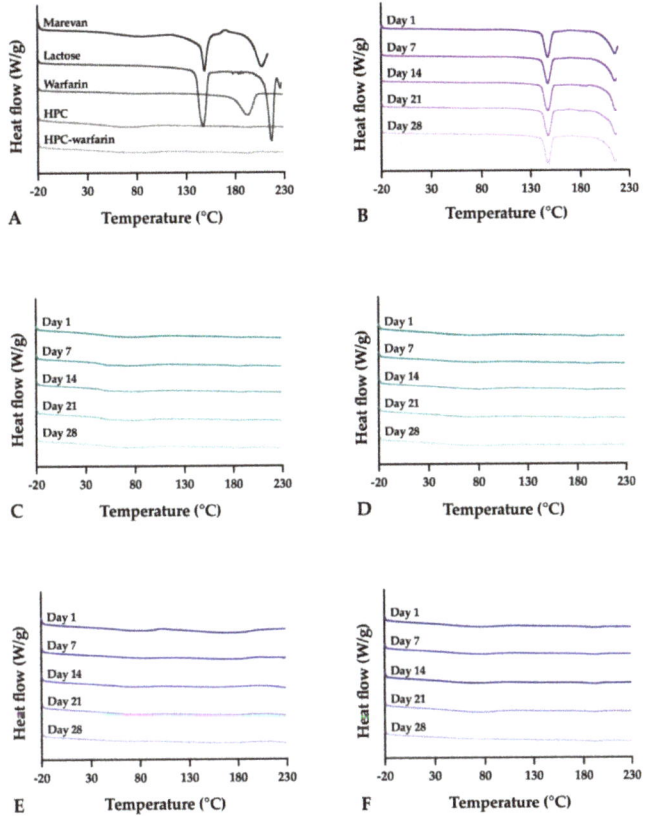

Figure 11. Thermograms (exo up) for (**A**) raw materials and the physical mixture of HPC and warfarin sodium; (**B**) OPS; (**C**) drug-loaded EXT ODF; (**D**) placebo EXT ODF; (**E**) drug-loaded IJP ODF; and (**F**) placebo IJP ODF over a one-month period.

The placebo EXT ODFs revealed a broad peak in the range of around 20–100 °C attributed to dehydration of water from the hygroscopic polymer followed by a small melting peak with an onset at 170.6 °C and a peak max located at 190.6 °C, which correlates to pure HPC prior to processing. Drug-loaded EXT ODFs revealed similar endothermic event, revealing a melting onset at 168.1 °C and a peak max at 185.0 °C. The addition of WS in the formulation resulted in a slight melt point depression compared to pure polymer, which may be explained by the interaction of the drug and the polymer leading to a reduction of the chemical potential of the system. However, no evident melting peak for the drug was seen, suggesting that the drug was not present in a crystalline form. The thermographs for IJP placebo ODFs were as expected, similar to the placebo EXT ODF and pure HPC, indicating that the solvent casting process does not affect the thermal properties of the polymer. Imprinting placebo IJP ODFs with drug-loaded ink resulted in broadening of the second endothermic event, which typically started immediately after the first one. The melt point depression and broadening of the melting event may be explained by the additional materials present in the IJP ODFs compared to the EXT ODFs such as PG acting as a plasticizer in the formulation. The OPSs revealed a sharp melting peak onset at 141.6 °C and peak max at 147.3 °C followed by decomposition of the material. The endothermic events correspond to lactose monohydrate used as a filler in the OPSs. Lactose monohydrate has been reported to lose the crystallization water at temperatures above 100 °C, complemented by a change in the crystalline structure of the material as it becomes anhydrous [50]. At 140 °C, the loss of water is completed, whereafter the material decomposes, thus explaining what was seen on the thermograms for the OPS. Due to the presence of lactose monohydrate in the formulation for the OPSs, no further conclusions could be drawn regarding the drug as the formulation decomposed prior to the melting of WS.

The thermograms of the different dosage forms prepared were not seen to change during storage for four weeks leading to the conclusion that the dosage forms may be given an expiration date of at least one month after manufacturing, which also is supported by the results in the drug content section.

3.11. Stability

A stability study was conducted over four weeks in order to assess the stability of the prepared dosage forms. OPSs were stored in sachets, which is how they are stored at the hospital, whereas single ODFs were not packed in a final packaging, exposing them to fluctuating humidities and temperatures. These conditions were thought to mimic the worst case scenario of how extemporaneously compounded on-demand medicines could be stored at the hospital wards. As the idea of personalized medicines is that small batches are prepared due to possible changes in the treatment, one month was considered to be a long enough follow-up period. All of the prepared dosage forms were found to be stable or possess acceptable properties during the one-month long stability study. The dosage forms were subjected to temperatures and relative humidities ranging from 19.6 to 21.5 °C and 13.0 to 32.9%, respectively. More detailed information regarding the results from the stability study is discussed in the different results sections of the manuscript.

3.12. Suitability of Manufacturing Methods in a Hospital Pharmacy Setting

The evaluation of the suitability of two different printing technologies as manufacturing methods for extemporaneously prepared medicines in hospital pharmacy setting was made based on aspects of patient safety, manufacturability, ease of administration, and GMP compliance adapting perspectives found in the literature [22,23]. Both advantages and limitations were identified with all manufacturing methods and dosage forms prepared in this study.

Recognized advantages for all investigated dosage forms in this study were the results of content uniformity and the one-month stability. EXT further showed promising results for uniformity of dosage units, and both EXT and IJP ODFs displayed good mechanical properties and fast disintegration. All dosage forms were suitable for administration through a naso-gastric tube, whereas the ODFs additionally have the option to be administered directly into a child's mouth. The inkjet printing method was successfully used to imprint QR-codes onto the previously prepared EXT and IJP ODFs, thus, likely improving patient safety by enhancing the identification of the dosage form.

Requirements for utilizing printing techniques in hospital pharmacy environment is the use of pharmaceutical grade excipients and printers that fulfill the demands of good manufacturing practice (GMP) [24]. One such aspect is the cleaning of the printer parts that come into contact with the pharmaceutical product. In EXT it is possible to use disposable parts thus avoiding cleaning procedures and validations. The IJP printer used in this study needs to be flushed with a suitable solvent after use in order to ensure that contamination between different drugs and/or formulations do not occur. Separate print heads (IJP) for specific drug solutions might decrease the burden of cleaning in cases where the same printer is used for different formulations or drugs. Moreover, disposable ink cartridges and tubing or alternatively stainless steel parts that may be cleaned would be compulsory in order to be able to transfer the printers from laboratories into hospitals. As for all medicines, the safety of excipients for use in neonates and infants must be taken into consideration as well as the suitability of the formulation for administration through a naso-gastric tube without causing blockage of the tube. The solvents ethanol and PG used in this study are excipients that might cause adverse reactions in children, especially neonates and infants, and the use of such excipients should be based on a risk assessment [62]. In future studies, PG could be replaced with another viscosity modifier and residual amounts of ethanol in the dosage forms could be measured to better evaluate the risk as in this study, the residual solvent was not analytically determined, but instead theoretically calculated to be well below the permitted daily exposure of 50 mg/day for ethanol [63]. Excipient availability from reliable suppliers is also important from GMP and safety point of view as well as for assuring the continuous supply of extemporaneously prepared dosage forms. The transparency sheet, as part of manufacturing equipment, could be replaced by a printing platform made of, e.g., glass, which could be easily removed and cleaned to fulfill GMP requirements.

Investment costs and annual costs for maintenance and qualification are factors that might have an impact when deciding on the choice of printing method to be implemented in a hospital. For on-demand manufacturing purposes, it would be necessary to have duplicates of devices to ensure a continuous supply of printed dosage forms even in case of malfunction. Devices for high-end IJP equipped with a camera needed for analysis of droplets are more expensive than the basic devices used for EXT. The training necessary for pharmacists using the devices and the batch specific premanufacturing tests ensuring the correct function of the devices is probably easier to perform for the EXT than the IJP, at least with the printers utilized in this study. In EXT, one could print test dosages and weigh them prior to printing of patient doses as an excellent correlation between the wet weight and the drug content was shown in this study. For IJP one has to test the functioning of all nozzles before printing, which may be time-consuming, but can be automated. Hence, in the future devices for IJP should have an automatic quality check of the nozzles, excluding nozzles deviating from the set droplet volume range. It is worth noticing that laborsome and time-consuming quality checks (especially manually performed) before manufacturing adds to the total manufacturing time.

Both printing techniques involve some manufacturing steps concerning the formulation that needs to be solved in order for the methods to be suitable for on-demand manufacturing. The printing solution used in both EXT and IJP should be ready-made and kept in stock as the manufacturing of these solutions required stirring overnight. Another option would be to keep the polymer solution in stock and add the API immediately before printing, which could be beneficial as the same drug-free print solution could be used as a base formulation for different APIs. As for the IJP method, the substrates should also be kept in stock enabling on-demand manufacturing. Another time-consuming step in the overall printing process is the drying of the printed drug product, which can be optimized, e.g., by using suitable technical heating and drying solutions. The drying phase should ideally be decreased to much less than an hour in order to make printing a suitable method for manufacturing personalized medicines in hospital pharmacy settings where the time from prescribing to delivery is kept as short as possible. The production of a batch of OPSs takes one hour, at most. Further, studies should be conducted to evaluate suitable drying methods for printed ODFs to decrease the total manufacturing time.

Limitations that are essential for adopting a new manufacturing technique into the hospital pharmacy setting should be resolved before the method transfers from a laboratory environment into hospital pharmacies. In this study, we have discussed the advantages of the printing of dosage forms and showed that the ODFs prepared by means of printing in many aspects were superior to the OPSs currently used at hospitals. However, the present study also underlines the critical aspects that still need to be resolved in order to accept novel printing techniques as manufacturing methods in hospitals. Based on this study, we believe that method and product development, as well as further optimization, should be done in close collaboration between academic research labs, hospitals, and regulatory authorities in order to further excel the innovative printing methods to fit the demands of a hospital pharmacy.

4. Conclusions

Tailored drug doses are of great importance for successful and safe therapies, especially for pediatric patients. This study compared an established manufacturing technique to manufacture OPSs with two novel printing techniques (EXT and IJP) for preparation of ODFs. Dosage forms of various strengths of WS were successfully produced utilizing all of the studied manufacturing methods. The prepared ODFs showed acceptable properties and were found to be superior to the established OPSs regarding uniformity of dosage units, proving that the investigated printing techniques are precise methods that in the future could be implemented in a hospital setting for the preparation of personalized doses. The ODFs prepared by printing may, furthermore, have an advantage in ease of administration for pediatrics and children as they can be administered directly in the mouth of the patient, without the need of water, whereas the OPSs would need to be dissolved or dispersed in a liquid prior to administration. In a hospital setting, both dosage forms can alternatively be administered through a naso-gastric tube in case the patient previously has one in place for, e.g., nutritional purposes or in situations where the patient is unconscious. The stability study revealed no loss in quality for the prepared dosage forms during the studied period, independent of the manufacturing technique used.

The present study successfully implemented QR codes directly on the printed ODFs allowing for numerous possibilities such as additional information and increased patient safety. This study, among other recent studies in the field, have shown the feasibility and potential of using printing techniques for manufacturing of flexible doses, contributing to safer and improved treatments for various patient groups in the future. In order to produce personalized on-demand dosage forms for children in a hospital pharmacy setting, special attention should be paid to the safety of used excipients, implementation of suitable non-destructive and fast quality assurance methods. Furthermore, the possibility to use disposable parts instead of time-consuming cleaning procedures and short turnaround time for the complete manufacturing process including printing solution preparation and drying time of final dosage form should be ensured in order to successfully implement printing methods as a part of the manufacturing techniques used in a hospital pharmacy.

Supplementary Materials: The following are available online at http://www.mdpi.com/1999-4923/11/7/334/s1, Video S1. EXT; Video S2. IJP.

Author Contributions: Conceptualization: H.Ö., E.S., M.R., and N.S.; methodology: H.Ö., E.S., M.R., and N.S.; formal analysis: H.Ö., E.S., M.R., and N.S.; investigation: H.Ö., E.S., M.R., and N.S.; resources: N.S.; data curation: H.Ö., E.S., M.R., and N.S.; writing—original draft preparation: H.Ö. and M.R.; writing—review and editing: H.Ö., E.S., M.R., and N.S.; visualization: H.Ö., and E.S.; supervision: N.S.; project administration: N.S.; funding acquisition: N.S.

Funding: This research was funded by Suomen Kulttuurirahasto (Elli Turusen Rahasto) (personal grant for Heidi Öblom), and the Åbo Akademi University Foundation (personal grant for Erica Sjöholm). The APC was funded by Åbo Akademi University.

Acknowledgments: The authors would like to thank Aino Nenonen, Jiri Vehviläinen, Marjaana Huttunen, and Maria Poukka at HUS Pharmacy for their contribution in the manufacturing of the oral powders in unit dose sachets. We kindly thank Ashland for donating the hydroxypropylcellulose used in the study.

Conflicts of Interest: The authors declare no conflict of interest. The funders had no role in the design of the study; in the collection, analyses, or interpretation of data; in the writing of the manuscript; or in the decision to publish the results.

Appendix A

Table A1. Drug content, content uniformity, uniformity of dosage units (acceptance value, according to Ph.Eur 9th ed.), and dose accuracy compared to target doses for the various batches prepared by different manufacturing techniques. Drug content is expressed as average ± SD, $n = 10$, while AV and UC are calculated based on 10 dosage forms from each batch. Note that the weight of the OPSs are given without a decimal as that is how it is routinely done when manufacturing OPS in the hospital pharmacy. The weight of the ODFs are, however, given with one decimal to show differences between the dosage forms.

Dosage Form; Batch	Weight (mg)	Thickness (mm)	Average Drug Content (mg)	Acceptable 15% Limits (mg)	Largest Individual Deviation (mg)	Maximum Deviation (%)	Amount of Drug (% of Target Dose) min/average/max	Acceptance Value
				0.1 mg				
EXT ODF								
1	1.5 ± 0.0	0.04 ± 0.00	0.14 ± 0.00	0.119–0.161	0.004	+2.9 [a]	132.9/136.8/139.7	41.0 [d]
2	1.3 ± 0.1	0.04 ± 0.00	0.11 ± 0.00	0.094–0.127	0.001	+1.1 [a]	110.0/110.7/111.9	10.9 [c]
3	1.2 ± 0.2	0.04 ± 0.01	0.10 ± 0.02	0.085–0.115	0.030	−30.0 [b,***]	71.6/102.2/116.5	47.1 [d]
IJP ODF								
1	2.1 ± 0.1	0.06 ± 0.00	0.07 ± 0.01	0.060–0.081	0.017	+25.9 [b,***]	52.1/66.3/83.4	55.0 [d]
2	2.3 ± 0.2	0.06 ± 0.00	0.09 ± 0.00	0.077–0.104	0.008	−9.0 [a]	82.3/90.5/95.4	17.6 [d]
3	2.2 ± 0.0	0.06 ± 0.00	0.09 ± 0.01	0.077–0.104	0.020	+21.4 [a,*]	84.5/92.1/111.8	25.4 [d]
OPS								
1	200 ± 0	N/A	0.05 ± 0.01	0.043–0.058	0.010	−22.5 [e,***]	36.9/46.2/54.1	67.8 [d]
2	200 ± 0	N/A	0.09 ± 0.01	0.077–0.104	0.021	−23.3 [a,*]	71.6/93.4/104.5	29.0 [d]
3	200 ± 0	N/A	0.08 ± 0.01	0.068–0.092	0.015	+18.3 [a,*]	69.7/82.1/97.2	37.6 [d]
				0.5 mg				
EXT ODF								
1	6.2 ± 0.1	0.04 ± 0.00	0.59 ± 0.00	0.502–0.679	0.006	+1.2 [a]	116.1/117.2/118.5	17.5 [d]
2	5.2 ± 0.1	0.04 ± 0.00	0.48 ± 0.01	0.408–0.552	0.009	−1.8 [a]	94.5/96.2/97.6	4.9 [c]
3	5.5 ± 0.1	0.05 ± 0.00	0.52 ± 0.01	0.442–0.598	0.012	−2.5 [a]	100.4/103.1/104.7	4.5 [c]
IJP ODF								
1	8.6 ± 0.1	0.06 ± 0.00	0.51 ± 0.04	0.434–0.587	0.070	−13.8 [a]	87.6/101.6/108.8	20.8 [d]
2	9.3 ± 0.2	0.06 ± 0.00	0.51 ± 0.03	0.434–0.587	0.070	−13.7 [a]	88.7/102.8/107.8	16.1 [d]
3	9.5 ± 0.0	0.06 ± 0.00	0.52 ± 0.02	0.442–0.598	0.025	−4.6 [a]	99.9/104.7/108.9	11.6 [c]
OPS								
1	200 ± 0	N/A	0.47 ± 0.05	0.400–0.541	0.120	−18.9 [e,**]	76.0/93.7/106.6	30.4 [d]
2	200 ± 0	N/A	0.54 ± 0.02	0.459–0.621	0.070	+5.7 [a]	102.6/107.9/114.1	15.5 [d]
3	200 ± 0	N/A	0.48 ± 0.06	0.408–0.552	0.145	−26.1 [b,**]	71.1/96.2/119.2	32.5 [d]

Table A1. Cont.

Dosage Form; Batch	Weight (mg)	Thickness (mm)	Average Drug Content (mg)	Acceptable 15% Limits (mg)	Largest Individual Deviation (mg)	Maximum Deviation (%)	Amount of Drug (% of Target Dose) min/average/max	Acceptance Value
1 mg								
EXT ODF								
1	12.2 ± 0.1	0.05 ± 0.00	1.16 ± 0.01	0.986–1.336	0.013	+1.2 [a]	114.5/115.8/117.1	16.6 [d]
2	10.7 ± 0.1	0.04 ± 0.00	1.01 ± 0.05	0.859–1.162	0.149	−14.8 [a]	86.0/100.9/106.7	13.7 [c]
3	11.5 ± 0.1	0.05 ± 0.00	1.09 ± 0.01	0.927–1.254	0.015	+1.3 [a]	107.4/108.8/110.3	9.9 [c]
IJP ODF								
1	17.0 ± 0.6	0.06 ± 0.00	1.09 ± 0.07	0.927–1.254	0.131	−11.1 [a]	96.9/109.0/117.4	23.4 [d]
2	17.2 ± 0.3	0.06 ± 0.00	1.06 ± 0.07	0.901–1.219	0.127	−12.0 [a]	92.9/105.6/111.9	21.3 [d]
3	18.2 ± 0.6	0.06 ± 0.00	1.05 ± 0.03	0.893–1.208	0.043	−4.2 [a]	101.7/104.9/108.1	10.3 [c]
OPS								
1	200 ± 0	N/A	1.01 ± 0.03	0.859–1.162	0.060	−6.0 [a]	95.2/101.2/105.5	6.9 [c]
2	200 ± 0	N/A	1.10 ± 0.06	0.935–1.266	0.089	+8.0 [a]	101.9/110.1/119.0	22.7 [d]
3	200 ± 0	N/A	1.11 ± 0.06	0.944–1.277	0.079	+7.1 [a]	96.9/110.7/118.6	23.5 [d]
2 mg								
EXT ODF								
1	23.0 ± 0.7	0.05 ± 0.00	2.12 ± 0.06	1.802–2.438	0.114	−5.4 [a]	100.5/106.2/109.3	12.5 [c]
2	22.4 ± 0.1	0.05 ± 0.00	2.11 ± 0.01	1.794–2.427	0.031	+1.5 [a]	104.5/105.3/106.9	5.4 [c]
3	22.7 ± 0.2	0.05 ± 0.00	2.13 ± 0.03	1.811–2.450	0.050	−2.4 [a]	103.8/106.3/108.4	8.2 [c]
IJP ODF								
1	34.7 ± 0.2	0.06 ± 0.00	2.06 ± 0.10	1.751–2.369	0.202	−9.8 [a]	93.1/103.2/107.5	14.8 [c]
2	34.9 ± 0.8	0.06 ± 0.00	2.13 ± 0.10	1.811–2.450	0.270	−12.7 [a]	93.1/106.7/109.4	17.6 [d]
3	40.1 ± 1.2	0.06 ± 0.00	2.10 ± 0.02	1.785–2.415	0.032	+1.5 [a]	103.8/105.0/106.6	5.8 [c]
OPS								
1	200 ± 0	N/A	2.17 ± 0.07	1.845–2.496	0.128	+14.9 [a]	100.1/108.4/114.9	15.98 [d]
2	200 ± 0	N/A	2.24 ± 0.03	1.904–2.576	0.062	+2.8 [a]	108.9/112.1/114.1	14.32 [c]
3	200 ± 0	N/A	2.25 ± 0.05	1.913–2.588	0.079	+3.5 [a]	108.4/112.3/116.2	17.14 [d]

Number of individual doses outside ± 15% limits: * = 1 dose, ** = 2 doses, *** = 3 doses. [a] = complies with the requirements for UC, [b] = does not comply with the requirements for UC, [c] = complies with the requirements for AV, [d] = does not comply with the requirements for AV, [e] = an additional 20 units should be tested to reveal if the test passed or failed.

Table A2. Mechanical properties of the ODFs. Results are reported as average ± SD, n = 5, except for the humidity and temperature, which describes the conditions at the beginning of the first measurement. RH = relative humidity, T = temperature, WS = warfarin sodium, P = placebo.

Sample	Time (days)	Thickness (mm [a])	Weight (mg)	Burst Strength (N)	Burst Distance (mm [b])	n/mm [a]	mm [b]/mm [a]	RH (%)	T (°C)
EXT WS ODF	1	0.04 ± 0.00	21.4 ± 1.5	5.6 ± 0.7	1.2 ± 0.1	146.5 ± 27.3	30.8 ± 5.9	18.4	23.1
	7	0.05 ± 0.00	22.2 ± 1.8	3.1 ± 1.4	0.7 ± 0.2	66.8 ± 34.6	16.0 ± 5.3	14.9	21.8
	14	0.04 ± 0.00	22.2 ± 0.1	4.2 ± 1.6	0.9 ± 0.2	96.2 ± 37.9	20.2 ± 5.1	15.9	21.8
	21	0.05 ± 0.01	20.8 ± 0.2	5.6 ± 1.2	1.1 ± 0.2	124.0 ± 28.3	25.1 ± 4.4	18.5	21.6
	28	0.04 ± 0.00	22.2 ± 1.1	5.8 ± 1.1	1.3 ± 0.2	136.2 ± 33.7	29.7 ± 5.4	24.2	22.3
EXT P ODF	1	0.04 ± 0.00	20.8 ± 1.2	6.2 ± 0.9	2.1 ± 0.3	156.4 ± 33.0	52.0 ± 12.0	18.4	23.1
	7	0.04 ± 0.00	20.5 ± 0.3	6.4 ± 0.8	2.0 ± 0.2	160.3 ± 19.4	49.6 ± 5.2	14.9	21.8
	14	0.04 ± 0.00	20.2 ± 0.3	5.3 ± 1.7	1.8 ± 0.5	137.2 ± 34.9	46.2 ± 8.4	15.9	21.8
	21	0.04 ± 0.01	19.7 ± 1.6	6.4 ± 1.4	2.1 ± 0.3	167.4 ± 38.2	56.2 ± 11.3	18.2	22.1
	28	0.04 ± 0.00	20.2 ± 0.3	6.3 ± 0.8	2.3 ± 0.2	149.4 ± 17.3	53.9 ± 4.5	24.2	22.3
IJP WS ODF	1	0.06 ± 0.00	38.4 ± 1.0	4.12 ± 0.60	5.61 ± 0.35	71.77 ± 8.07	98.39 ± 12.15	22.1	21.2
	7	0.06 ± 0.00	34.1 ± 0.9	5.1 ± 0.5	5.4 ± 0.1	88.1 ± 6.5	94.0 ± 6.6	18.0	22.2
	14	0.06 ± 0.00	34.8 ± 0.9	4.9 ± 0.5	5.4 ± 0.4	80.4 ± 10.0	87.5 ± 4.2	23.5	22.3
	21	0.07 ± 0.00	39.1 ± 0.5	6.5 ± 0.2	5.0 ± 0.4	98.9 ± 3.5	76.9 ± 7.1	23.5	21.9
	28	0.07 ± 0.00	40.5 ± 0.8	9.0 ± 0.6	4.2 ± 0.1	126.9 ± 6.4	59.9 ± 2.5	10.8	22.0
IJP P ODF	1	0.05 ± 0.00	31.4 ± 1.9	13.1 ± 1.2	2.6 ± 0.2	276.4 ± 20.8	55.8 ± 6.0	21.1	21.9
	7	0.05 ± 0.00	30.1 ± 0.6	12.1 ± 0.8	2.5 ± 0.2	230.3 ± 26.4	47.0 ± 5.5	18.0	22.2
	14	0.06 ± 0.00	30.8 ± 1.7	11.4 ± 1.2	2.5 ± 0.3	203.7 ± 25.0	44.4 ± 6.4	23.3	22.3
	21	0.06 ± 0.01	33.0 ± 2.8	13.3 ± 1.0	2.7 ± 0.1	215.9 ± 29.4	44.6 ± 9.0	24.1	21.7
	28	0.07 ± 0.00	34.2 ± 0.8	14.5 ± 1.8	2.3 ± 0.2	197.8 ± 28.0	32.1 ± 3.3	10.8	22.1

Table A3. Disintegration time of drug-loaded and placebo ODFs one day after manufacturing. Disintegration times are shown as average ± SD, n = 3. WS = warfarin sodium, P = placebo.

Sample	Target Dose (mg)	Thickness (mm)	Weight (mg)	Disintegration (s)
EXT WS ODF	0.1	0.03 ± 0.00	1.1 ± 0.2	30 ± 8
	0.5	0.04 ± 0.00	5.6 ± 0.2	32 ± 4
	1	0.04 ± 0.00	11.6 ± 0.1	37 ± 1
	2	0.04 ± 0.00	21.4 ± 0.2	39 ± 4
EXT P ODF	0.1	0.04 ± 0.01	1.2 ± 0.2	31 ± 3
	0.5	0.04 ± 0.00	5.7 ± 0.1	37 ± 2
	1	0.04 ± 0.00	10.5 ± 0.2	35 ± 2
	2	0.04 ± 0.00	19.4 ± 2.3	28 ± 9
IJP WS ODF	0.1	0.06 ± 0.00	2.2 ± 0.0	104 ± 1
	0.5	0.05 ± 0.01	9.8 ± 0.2	106 ± 5
	1	0.05 ± 0.00	18.2 ± 0.1	96 ± 1
	2	0.05 ± 0.00	41.0 ± 0.9	123 ± 5
IJP P ODF	0.1	0.05 ± 0.01	1.7 ± 0.1	102 ± 7
	0.5	0.05 ± 0.00	7.8 ± 0.1	84 ± 2
	1	0.06 ± 0.00	16.5 ± 0.8	100 ± 13
	2	0.05 ± 0.00	30.7 ± 0.3	90 ± 1

Table A4. Disintegration of the ODFs at different time-points during the stability study. Results presented as average ± SD, n = 3. WS = warfarin sodium, P = placebo.

Sample	Target Dose (mg)	Time Point (day)	Thickness (mm)	Weight (mg)	Disintegration (s)
EXT WS ODF	2	1	0.04 ± 0.00	21.4 ± 0.2	39 ± 4
	2	7	0.04 ± 0.00	22.0 ± 0.3	41 ± 3
	2	14	0.04 ± 0.00	21.9 ± 0.1	41 ± 2
	2	21	0.04 ± 0.00	21.1 ± 0.1	39 ± 1
	2	28	0.04 ± 0.00	22.6 ± 0.4	44 ± 3
Average		All	0.04 ± 0.00	21.8 ± 0.6	41 ± 2
EXT P ODF	2	1	0.04 ± 0.00	19.4 ± 2.3	28 ± 9
	2	7	0.04 ± 0.00	19.4 ± 0.8	32 ± 2
	2	14	0.04 ± 0.00	19.9 ± 1.2	31 ± 1
	2	21	0.05 ± 0.00	20.5 ± 0.2	36 ± 3
	2	28	0.04 ± 0.00	19.5 ± 0.4	32 ± 3
Average		All	0.04 ± 0.00	19.8 ± 0.5	32 ± 3
IJP WS ODF	2	1	0.05 ± 0.00	41.0 ± 0.9	123 ± 5
	2	7	0.06 ± 0.00	38.1 ± 0.4	119 ± 3
	2	14	0.06 ± 0.00	39.5 ± 0.4	115 ± 1
	2	21	0.06 ± 0.00	39.2 ± 0.4	122 ± 4
	2	28	0.06 ± 0.00	41.3 ± 0.4	137 ± 3
Average		All	0.06 ± 0.00	39.8 ± 1.3	123 ± 8
IJP P ODF	2	1	0.05 ± 0.00	30.7 ± 0.3	90 ± 1
	2	7	0.05 ± 0.00	30.1 ± 0.9	93 ± 8
	2	14	0.05 ± 0.00	30.6 ± 0.7	91 ± 2
	2	21	0.06 ± 0.00	39.2 ± 0.4	122 ± 4
	2	28	0.06 ± 0.00	38.4 ± 0.5	121 ± 2
Average		All	0.05 ± 0.00	33.8 ± 4.6	103 ± 17

Table A5. The drug amount, acceptance value (AV), and uniformity of content of single-dose preparations (test B) (UC) of the manufactured dosage forms during the stability study. Results are presented as average ± SD, $n = 10$. No further testing of an additional 20 dosage forms in case the batch failed to comply with the requirements stated in the Ph. Eur. was carried out, however, the batches that could have been further tested to determine if the batch pass or fail are marked with "*".

Stability	Day	Weight (mg)	Average Drug Amount (mg)	AV	Fulfills UC
EXT ODF	1	22.7 ± 0.2	2.13 ± 0.03	8.2	Yes
	7	23.2 ± 0.5	2.19 ± 0.04	13.5	Yes
	14	22.1 ± 0.2	2.13 ± 0.01	6.9	Yes
	21	21.4 ± 0.3	2.02 ± 0.03	3.4	Yes
	28	22.6 ± 0.3	2.12 ± 0.04	9.9	Yes
IJP ODF	1	40.1 ± 1.2	2.10 ± 0.02	5.8	Yes
	7	33.7 ± 0.8	2.02 ± 0.03	3.5	Yes
	14	34.5 ± 1.1	2.02 ± 0.03	3.6	Yes
	21	39.4 ± 0.5	2.05 ± 0.02	4.1	Yes
	28	40.9 ± 0.9	2.01 ± 0.02	3.0	Yes
OPS	1	200 ± 0	2.25 ± 0.05	17.1*	Yes
	7	200 ± 0	2.23 ± 0.08	20.3*	Yes
	14	200 ± 1	2.23 ± 0.07	18.7*	Yes
	21	200 ± 0	2.26 ± 0.05	17.7*	Yes
	28	200 ± 0	2.24 ± 0.06	17.7*	Yes

References

1. Nunn, A.J. Making medicines that children can take. *Arch. Dis. Child.* **2003**, *88*, 369–371. [CrossRef] [PubMed]
2. Young, G. Anticoagulation therapies in children. *Pediatr. Clin. N. Am.* **2017**, *64*, 1257–1269. [CrossRef] [PubMed]
3. Santos, B.B.; Heineck, I.; Negretto, G.W. Use of warfarin in pediatrics: Clinical and pharmacological characteristics. *Rev. Paul. Pediatr.* **2017**, *35*, 375–382. [CrossRef] [PubMed]
4. Hill, S.; Varker, A.S.; Karlage, K.; Myrdal, P.B. Analysis of drug content and weight uniformity for half-tablets of 6 commonly split medications. *J. Manag. Care Pharm.* **2016**, *15*, 253–261. [CrossRef] [PubMed]
5. Helmy, S.A. Tablet splitting: Is it worthwhile? Analysis of drug content and weight uniformity for half tablets of 16 commonly used medications in the outpatient setting. *J. Manag. Care Spec. Pharm.* **2016**, *21*, 76–88. [CrossRef] [PubMed]
6. Madathilethu, J.; Roberts, M.; Peak, M.; Blair, J.; Prescott, R.; Ford, J.L. Content uniformity of quartered hydrocortisone tablets in comparison with mini-tablets for paediatric dosing. *BMJ Paediatr. Open* **2018**, *2*, e000198. [CrossRef]
7. Watson, C.; Webb, E.A.; Kerr, S.; Davies, J.H.; Stirling, H.; Batchelor, H. How close is the dose? Manipulation of 10 mg hydrocortisone tablets to provide appropriate doses to children. *Int. J. Pharm.* **2018**, *545*, 57–63. [CrossRef]
8. Brion, F.; Nunn, A.; Rieutord, A. Extemporaneous (magistral) preparation of oral medicines for children in European hospitals. *Acta Paediatr.* **2010**, *92*, 486–490. [CrossRef]
9. Visser, J.C.; Woerdenbag, H.J.; Hanff, L.M.; Frijlink, H.W. Personalized medicine in pediatrics: The clinical potential of orodispersible films. *AAPS PharmSciTech* **2017**, *18*, 267–272. [CrossRef]
10. Thabet, Y.; Klingmann, V.; Breitkreutz, J. Drug formulations: standards and novel strategies for drug administration in pediatrics. *J. Clin. Pharmacol.* **2018**, *58*, S26–S35. [CrossRef]
11. Preis, M. Orally disintegrating films and mini-tablets—Innovative dosage forms of choice for pediatric use. *AAPS PharmSciTech* **2015**, *16*, 234–241. [CrossRef]
12. Van Riet-Nales, D.A.; De Neef, B.J.; Schobben, A.F.A.M.; Ferreira, J.A.; Egberts, T.C.G.; Rademaker, C.M.A. Acceptability of different oral formulations in infants and preschool children. *Arch. Dis. Child.* **2013**, *98*, 725–731. [CrossRef]
13. Klingmann, V. Acceptability of mini-tablets in young children: Results from three prospective cross-over studies. *AAPS PharmSciTech* **2016**, *18*, 263–266. [CrossRef] [PubMed]
14. Orlu, M.; Ranmal, S.R.; Sheng, Y.; Tuleu, C.; Seddon, P. Acceptability of orodispersible films for delivery of medicines to infants and preschool children. *Drug Deliv.* **2017**, *24*, 1243–1248. [CrossRef]
15. Scarpa, M.; Paudel, A.; Kloprogge, F.; Hsiao, W.K.; Bresciani, M.; Gaisford, S.; Orlu, M. Key acceptability attributes of orodispersible films. *Eur. J. Pharm. Biopharm.* **2018**, *125*, 131–140. [CrossRef] [PubMed]
16. Janßen, E.M.; Schliephacke, R.; Breitenbach, A.; Breitkreutz, J. Drug-printing by flexographic printing technology—A new manufacturing process for orodispersible films. *Int. J. Pharm.* **2013**, *441*, 818–825. [CrossRef] [PubMed]
17. Bala, R.; Khanna, S.; Pawar, P.; Arora, S. Orally dissolving strips: A new approach to oral drug delivery system. *Int. J. Pharm. Investig.* **2013**, *3*, 67–76. [CrossRef]
18. Borges, A.F.; Silva, C.; Coelho, J.F.J.; Simões, S. Oral films: Current status and future perspectives: I—Galenical development and quality attributes. *J. Control. Release* **2015**, *206*, 1–19. [CrossRef]
19. Preis, M.; Breitkreutz, J.; Sandler, N. Perspective: Concepts of printing technologies for oral film formulations. *Int. J. Pharm.* **2015**, *494*, 578–584. [CrossRef]
20. Scarpa, M.; Stegemann, S.; Hsiao, W.-K.; Pichler, H.; Gaisford, S.; Bresciani, M.; Paudel, A.; Orlu, M. Orodispersible films: Towards drug delivery in special populations. *Int. J. Pharm.* **2017**, *523*, 327–335. [CrossRef]
21. Sandler, N.; Preis, M. Printed drug-delivery systems for improved patient treatment. *Trends Pharmacol. Sci.* **2016**, *37*, 1070–1080. [CrossRef] [PubMed]
22. Preis, M.; Öblom, H. 3D-printed drugs for children—Are we ready yet? *AAPS PharmSciTech* **2017**, *18*, 303–308. [CrossRef] [PubMed]

23. Rahman, Z.; Barakh Ali, S.F.; Ozkan, T.; Charoo, N.A.; Reddy, I.K.; Khan, M.A. Additive manufacturing with 3D printing: Progress from bench to bedside. *AAPS J.* **2018**, *20*, 101. [CrossRef] [PubMed]
24. Trenfield, S.J.; Awad, A.; Goyanes, A.; Gaisford, S.; Basit, A.W. 3D printing pharmaceuticals: Drug development to frontline care. *Trends Pharmacol. Sci.* **2018**, *39*, 440–451. [CrossRef] [PubMed]
25. Awad, A.; Trenfield, S.J.; Gaisford, S.; Basit, A.W. 3D printed medicines: A new branch of digital healthcare. *Int. J. Pharm.* **2018**, *548*, 586–596. [CrossRef]
26. Öblom, H.; Zhang, J.; Pimparade, M.; Speer, I.; Preis, M.; Repka, M.; Sandler, N. 3D-printed isoniazid tablets for the treatment and prevention of tuberculosis—Personalized dosing and drug release. *AAPS PharmSciTech* **2019**, *20*, 52. [CrossRef] [PubMed]
27. Goole, J.; Amighi, K. 3D printing in pharmaceutics: A new tool for designing customized drug delivery systems. *Int. J. Pharm.* **2016**, *499*, 376–394. [CrossRef]
28. El Aita, I.; Breitkreutz, J.; Quodbach, J. On-demand manufacturing of immediate release levetiracetam tablets using pressure-assisted microsyringe printing. *Eur. J. Pharm. Biopharm.* **2019**, *134*, 29–36. [CrossRef]
29. Khaled, S.A.; Alexander, M.R.; Wildman, R.D.; Wallace, M.J.; Sharpe, S.; Yoo, J.; Roberts, C.J. 3D extrusion printing of high drug loading immediate release paracetamol tablets. *Int. J. Pharm.* **2018**, *538*, 223–230. [CrossRef]
30. Jamróz, W.; Szafraniec, J.; Kurek, M.; Jachowicz, R. 3D printing in pharmaceutical and medical—Recent achievements and challenges. *Pharm. Res.* **2018**, *35*, 176. [CrossRef]
31. Tian, P.; Yang, F.; Xu, Y.; Lin, M.-M.; Yu, L.-P.; Lin, W.; Lin, Q.-F.; Lv, Z.-F.; Huang, S.-Y.; Chen, Y.-Z. Oral disintegrating patient-tailored tablets of warfarin sodium produced by 3D printing. *Drug Dev. Ind. Pharm.* **2018**, *44*, 1918–1923. [CrossRef] [PubMed]
32. Vuddanda, P.R.; Alomari, M.; Dodoo, C.C.; Trenfield, S.J.; Velaga, S.; Basit, A.W.; Gaisford, S. Personalisation of warfarin therapy using thermal ink-jet printing. *Eur. J. Pharm. Sci.* **2018**, *117*, 80–87. [CrossRef] [PubMed]
33. Sjöholm, E.; Sandler, N. Additive manufacturing of personalized orodispersible warfarin films. *Int. J. Pharm.* **2019**, *564*, 117–123. [CrossRef] [PubMed]
34. Niese, S.; Quodbach, J. Formulation development of a continuously manufactured orodispersible film containing warfarin sodium for individualized dosing. *Eur. J. Pharm. Biopharm.* **2019**, *136*, 93–101. [CrossRef] [PubMed]
35. Sivén, M.; Kovanen, S.; Siirola, O.; Hepojoki, T.; Isokirmo, S.; Laihanen, N.; Eränen, T.; Pellinen, J.; Juppo, A.M. Challenge of paediatric compounding to solid dosage forms sachets and hard capsules—Finnish perspective. *J. Pharm. Pharmacol.* **2017**, *69*, 593–602. [CrossRef] [PubMed]
36. *Pharmacopoeia Europea (Ph. Eur.), edition 9.0*; European Directorate for the Quality of Medicines & HealthCare (EDQM): Strasbourg, France, 2017.
37. Garsuch, V.; Breitkreutz, J. Comparative investigations on different polymers for the preparation of fast-dissolving oral films. *J. Pharm. Pharmacol.* **2010**, *62*, 539–545. [CrossRef] [PubMed]
38. Liew, K.B.; Tan, Y.T.F.; Peh, K.K. Characterization of oral disintegrating film containing donepezil for alzheimer disease. *AAPS PharmSciTech* **2012**, *13*, 134–142. [CrossRef]
39. Pechová, V.; Gajdziok, J.; Muselík, J.; Vetchý, D. Development of orodispersible films containing benzydamine hydrochloride using a modified solvent casting method. *AAPS PharmSciTech* **2018**, *19*, 2509–2518. [CrossRef]
40. Genina, N.; Janßen, E.M.; Breitenbach, A.; Breitkreutz, J.; Sandler, N. Evaluation of different substrates for inkjet printing of rasagiline mesylate. *Eur. J. Pharm. Biopharm.* **2013**, *85*, 1075–1083. [CrossRef]
41. Edinger, M.; Bar-Shalom, D.; Sandler, N.; Rantanen, J.; Genina, N. QR encoded smart oral dosage forms by inkjet printing. *Int. J. Pharm.* **2018**, *536*, 138–145. [CrossRef]
42. Visser, J.C.; Woerdenbag, H.J.; Crediet, S.; Gerrits, E.; Lesschen, M.A.; Hinrichs, W.L.J.; Breitkreutz, J.; Frijlink, H.W. Orodispersible films in individualized pharmacotherapy: The development of a formulation for pharmacy preparations. *Int. J. Pharm.* **2015**, *478*, 155–163. [CrossRef] [PubMed]
43. Boateng, J.S.; Stevens, H.N.E.; Eccleston, G.M.; Auffret, A.D.; Humphrey, M.J.; Matthews, K.H. Development and mechanical characterization of solvent-cast polymeric films as potential drug delivery systems to mucosal surfaces. *Drug Dev. Ind. Pharm.* **2009**, *35*, 986–996. [CrossRef] [PubMed]
44. Szakonyi, G.; Zelkó, R. The effect of water on the solid state characteristics of pharmaceutical excipients: Molecular mechanisms, measurement techniques, and quality aspects of final dosage form. *Int. J. Pharm. Investig.* **2012**, *2*, 18–25. [CrossRef] [PubMed]

45. Hoffmann, E.M.; Breitenbach, A.; Breitkreutz, J. Advances in orodispersible films for drug delivery. *Expert Opin. Drug Deliv.* **2011**, *8*, 299–316. [CrossRef] [PubMed]
46. Liew, K.B.; Tan, Y.T.F.; Peh, K.K. Effect of polymer, plasticizer and filler on orally disintegrating film. *Drug Dev. Ind. Pharm.* **2014**, *40*, 110–119. [CrossRef] [PubMed]
47. Ashland KlucelTM. Hydroxypropylcellulose—Physical and Chemical Properties for Pharmaceutical Applications. Available online: https://www.ashland.com/file_source/Ashland/Product/Documents/Pharmaceutical/PC_11229_Klucel_HPC.pdf (accessed on 22 August 2018).
48. ElMeshad, A.N.; El Hagrasy, A.S. Characterization and optimization of orodispersible mosapride film formulations. *AAPS PharmSciTech* **2011**, *12*, 1384–1392. [CrossRef] [PubMed]
49. Nair, A.B.; Kumria, R.; Harsha, S.; Attimarad, M.; Al-Dhubiab, B.E.; Alhaider, I.A. In vitro techniques to evaluate buccal films. *J. Control. Release* **2013**, *166*, 10–21. [CrossRef] [PubMed]
50. DFE. Pharma Lactose Some Basic Properties and Characteristics. Available online: https://www.dfepharma.com/-/media/documents/technical-documents/technical-papers/lactose-some-basic-properties.pdf (accessed on 3 April 2019).
51. Thabet, Y.; Lunter, D.; Breitkreutz, J. Continuous manufacturing and analytical characterization of fixed-dose, multilayer orodispersible films. *Eur. J. Pharm. Sci.* **2018**, *117*, 236–244. [CrossRef]
52. Jamróz, W.; Kurek, M.; Łyszczarz, E.; Szafraniec, J.; Knapik-Kowalczuk, J.; Syrek, K.; Paluch, M.; Jachowicz, R. 3D printed orodispersible films with Aripiprazole. *Int. J. Pharm.* **2017**, *533*, 413–420. [CrossRef]
53. Sandler, N.; Määttänen, A.; Ihalainen, P.; Kronberg, L.; Meierjohann, A.; Viitala, T.; Peltonen, J. Inkjet printing of drug substances and use of porous substrates-towards individualized dosing. *J. Pharm. Sci.* **2011**, *100*, 3386–3395. [CrossRef]
54. Genina, N.; Fors, D.; Vakili, H.; Ihalainen, P.; Pohjala, L.; Ehlers, H.; Kassamakov, I.; Haeggström, E.; Vuorela, P.; Peltonen, J.; et al. Tailoring controlled-release oral dosage forms by combining inkjet and flexographic printing techniques. *Eur. J. Pharm. Sci.* **2012**, *47*, 615–623. [CrossRef] [PubMed]
55. Raijada, D.; Genina, N.; Fors, D.; Wisaeus, E.; Peltonen, J.; Rantanen, J.; Sandler, N. A step toward development of printable dosage forms for poorly soluble drugs. *J. Pharm. Sci.* **2013**, *102*, 3694–3704. [CrossRef]
56. Wickström, H.; Palo, M.; Rijckaert, K.; Kolakovic, R.; Nyman, J.O.; Määttänen, A.; Ihalainen, P.; Peltonen, J.; Genina, N.; de Beer, T.; et al. Improvement of dissolution rate of indomethacin by inkjet printing. *Eur. J. Pharm. Sci.* **2015**, *75*, 91–100. [CrossRef] [PubMed]
57. Speer, I.; Preis, M.; Breitkreutz, J. Novel dissolution method for oral film preparations with modified release properties. *AAPS PharmSciTech* **2018**, *20*, 7. [CrossRef] [PubMed]
58. Eguchi, N.; Kawabata, K.; Goto, H. Electrochemical polymerization of 4,4-dimethyl-2,2′-bithiophene in concentrated polymer liquid crystal solution. *J. Mater. Sci. Chem. Eng.* **2017**, *5*, 64–70. [CrossRef]
59. Yang, M.-L.; Song, Y.-M. Synthesis and investigation of water-soluble anticoagulant warfarin/ferulic acid grafted rare earth oxide nanoparticle materials. *RSC Adv.* **2015**, *5*, 17824–17833. [CrossRef]
60. Parfenyuk, E.V.; Dolinina, E.S. Development of novel warfarin-silica composite for controlled drug release. *Pharm. Res.* **2017**, *34*, 825–835. [CrossRef]
61. Reddy, K.S.; Prabhakar, M.N.; Rao, K.M.; Suhasini, D.M.; Subha, M.C.S.; Rao, K.C. Development and characterization of hydroxy propyl cellulose/poly(vinyl alcohol) blends and their physico-chemical studies. *Indian J. Adv. Chem. Sci.* **2013**, *2*, 38–45.
62. World Health Organization. *Development of Pediatric Medicines: Points to Consider in Pharmaceutical Development (Working Document QAS/08.257/Rev.3)*; World Health Organization: Geneva, Switzerland, 2012.
63. European Medicines Agency. *ICH Guideline Q3C (R7) on Impurities: Guideline for Residual Solvents Step 5*; European Medicines Agency: Amsterdam, The Netherlands, 2018.

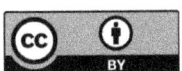

© 2019 by the authors. Licensee MDPI, Basel, Switzerland. This article is an open access article distributed under the terms and conditions of the Creative Commons Attribution (CC BY) license (http://creativecommons.org/licenses/by/4.0/).

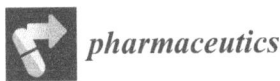

Review

Polymers for Extrusion-Based 3D Printing of Pharmaceuticals: A Holistic Materials–Process Perspective

Mohammad A. Azad [1,*], Deborah Olawuni [1], Georgia Kimbell [1], Abu Zayed Md Badruddoza [2], Md. Shahadat Hossain [3] and Tasnim Sultana [4]

1. Department of Chemical, Biological and Bioengineering, North Carolina A&T State University, Greensboro, NC 27411, USA; doolawuni@aggies.ncat.edu (D.O.); glkimbell@aggies.ncat.edu (G.K.)
2. Department of Chemical and Life Sciences Engineering, Virginia Commonwealth University, Richmond, VA 23284, USA; azmbadruddoza@vcu.edu
3. Department of Engineering Technology, Queensborough Community College, City University of New York (CUNY), Bayside, NY 11364, USA; MSHossain@qcc.cuny.edu
4. Department of Public Health, School of Arts and Sciences, Massachusetts College of Pharmacy and Health Sciences (MCPHS), Boston, MA 02115, USA; m0378698@stu.mcphs.edu
* Correspondence: maazad@ncat.edu; Tel.: +1-336-285-3701

Received: 1 January 2020; Accepted: 30 January 2020; Published: 3 February 2020

Abstract: Three dimensional (3D) printing as an advanced manufacturing technology is progressing to be established in the pharmaceutical industry to overcome the traditional manufacturing regime of 'one size fits for all'. Using 3D printing, it is possible to design and develop complex dosage forms that can be suitable for tuning drug release. Polymers are the key materials that are necessary for 3D printing. Among all 3D printing processes, extrusion-based (both fused deposition modeling (FDM) and pressure-assisted microsyringe (PAM)) 3D printing is well researched for pharmaceutical manufacturing. It is important to understand which polymers are suitable for extrusion-based 3D printing of pharmaceuticals and how their properties, as well as the behavior of polymer–active pharmaceutical ingredient (API) combinations, impact the printing process. Especially, understanding the rheology of the polymer and API–polymer mixtures is necessary for successful 3D printing of dosage forms or printed structures. This review has summarized a holistic materials–process perspective for polymers on extrusion-based 3D printing. The main focus herein will be both FDM and PAM 3D printing processes. It elaborates the discussion on the comparison of 3D printing with the traditional direct compression process, the necessity of rheology, and the characterization techniques required for the printed structure, drug, and excipients. The current technological challenges, regulatory aspects, and the direction toward which the technology is moving, especially for personalized pharmaceuticals and multi-drug printing, are also briefly discussed.

Keywords: polymers; pharmaceuticals; extrusion-based 3D printing; fused deposition modeling (FDM); pressure-assisted microsyringe (PAM); materials; process

1. Introduction

Additive manufacturing, commonly known as three dimensional printing (3D printing), is seeing increased use in several different industries such as aerospace, motor vehicles, industrial machines, consumer products, electronics, military, medical, dental, etc. [1–3]. Prototyping, directly printed functional parts, patient-specific hearing aids, and dental restoration are a few examples where 3D printing contributes significantly [1]. 3D printing has also expanded to the pharmaceutical industry where it is used to manufacture pharmaceuticals (drug products, implants, drug delivery systems, etc.). 3D printing is especially advantageous in the manufacturing of personalized drug products, where current scale-focused industrial pharmaceutical processes fall short [1], which allows on-demand production of the drug product [4]. A drug product is comprised of an active pharmaceutical ingredient (API) and inactive functional excipients, which can be in the form of a solid dosage (pills, film, implantable devices, etc.) or as a liquid [5]. 3D printing has boomed in the pharmaceutical sector since the Food and Drug Administration's (FDA) approval of the first 3D printed medicine, SPRITAM®, a levetiracetam drug manufactured by Aprecia Pharmaceuticals Company (USA) for the treatment of seizures [6].

Healthcare treatment has recently seen a movement toward personalized medicine. Ginsberg et al. define personalized medicine as medicine created from the analysis of an individual's molecular profile. Progress in human genome research is quickly advancing its growth of personalized medicine [7]. This can be seen with the 2015 implementation of the Precision Medicine Initiative, an Obama administration (in the USA) national initiative focused on individualized care [8]. Current pharmaceutical manufacturing practices are not cost-effective for personalized medicine [2]. 3D printing pharmaceuticals are more suitable than current manufacturing practices for tailored solid dosages.

3D printing was established by Sachs et al. in 1992 at Massachusetts Institute of Technology (MIT) [9,10]. Over the years, many different types of printing technologies have been developed [1,5,11]. The first wave of 3D printed pharmaceutical was fabricated using continuous inkjet printing. Wu et al. first used 3D printing in 1996 to make drug delivery devices [12]. Since this work, there have been significant advancements in 3D printing pharmaceuticals using inkjet printing as well as other printing technologies. The technologies used for drug product development are powder-based printing (powder bed and powder jetting) [13–16], extrusion (solid or semi-solid) based printing (fused deposition modelling (FDM), pressure-assisted microsyringes (PAM)) [17–26], stereolithographic (SLA) printing [27–29], selective laser sintering (SLS) printing [30–32], inkjet printing [33–35], digital light processing (DLP) [36,37], etc. Among all these printing processes, extrusion-based printing (FDM, PAM) has shown a growing interest among researchers due to the advantage of low cost, ability to fabricate hollow objects, ability to print using a range of polymers with or without drug, ability to tune drug release by tuning the geometry and polymer, and ability to print at room temperature (using PAM), etc. [38]. Figure 1a summarizes the published literature in the last five years on existing 3D printing technologies for pharmaceutical manufacturing and shows the proportion of research articles published on extrusion-based printing. Figure 1b presents the number of scientific publications over the last five years on extrusion-based 3D printing and shows the growing interest.

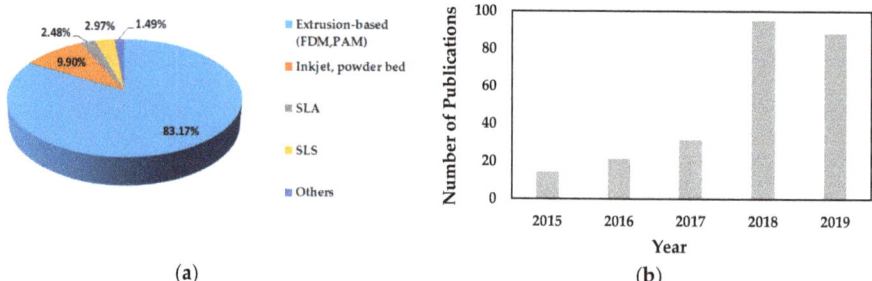

Figure 1. (a) The proportion of research articles published on different types of 3D printing processes in the last five years (2015-2019, total 202 articles); (b) The number of published scientific articles (research and review) in the period from 2015 to 2019 which reported the use of extrusion-based (fused deposition modeling (FDM) or pressure-assisted microsyringe (PAM)) 3D printing (source: Scopus database and PubMed).

Each extrusion-based 3D printing technology requires certain material requirements in order for the successful printing of pharmaceuticals. The requirements are based on the nature of the printing process. To guarantee the successful printing of solid dosage pharmaceuticals, it is necessary to choose the appropriate polymers and other functional excipients besides the drugs [39]. Pharmaceuticals must also have proper criteria in order to meet FDA regulations. The selection of unsuitable polymers will result in unsatisfactory pharmaceuticals. Jones reviewed the different roles that polymers play specifically for solid dosage pharmaceuticals, i.e., tablets and caplets [40]. In tablets and caplets, polymers can be used as binders, disintegrants, compression aids, diluents, or fillers. Polymers can also be used for controlled drug release applications. Hence, polymers are used in the 3D printing of pharmaceuticals for different purposes such as to control the dosage shape, size, drug release, etc. Polymers' multifaceted utilization in solid dosage drug delivery systems solidifies its importance in pharmaceutical 3D printing applications.

There are several review articles published on extrusion-based 3D printing [11,41–51]. However, those published articles focused on different aspects of this technology. For example, Araujo et al. discussed updates on FDM technology, its challenges, and how it can be integrated with the pharmaceutical production process [43]. Tan et al. discussed hot-melt extrusion, FDM 3D printing, and how both can be combined for advanced pharmaceutical applications [44]. Goole and Amighi discussed different 3D printing (including extrusion-based) processes and process parameters that can be controlled [11]. Kjar and Huang et al. discussed different 3D printing processes, then emphasized on micro-sized pharmaceutical applications [45]. Gioumouxouzis et al. discussed different dosage forms and devices that can be printed using a different 3D printing process [46]. Vithani et al. discussed potential opportunities for the 3D printing of soft materials such as lipids [48]. Joo et al. discussed different FDM process and parameters and discussed how FDM 3D printers can be used to control the release, make a novel dosage form, and deliver the customized doses [49]. Long et al. discussed appropriate polymers and key parameters required for FDM 3D printing and its usage in the printing of personalized tablets and drug delivery devices [50]. He et al. discussed FDM 3D printing methodology, suitable polymers, and important parameters that are required to print personalized tablets and drug delivery devices [51]. Konta et al. reviewed several 3D printing technologies and the polymers that are used successfully in those printing methods [52]. Unfortunately, there is no detailed discussion on how polymers should be selected based on materials characteristics, how their rheology impact on the printing process, and the required characterization for the 3D printed pharmaceuticals. The objective of this review is to discuss all these in detail to guide the researchers in selecting the right polymers and extrusion process to 3D print pharmaceuticals. In addition, a comparison between FDM and PAM 3D printing, the current challenges, regulatory aspects, and opportunities for extrusion-based printing are discussed.

2. Extrusion-Based 3D Printing

Extrusion-based 3D printing can be categorized into two main types: Fused deposition modeling (FDM) and pressure-assisted microsyringe (PAM) [11]. Extrusion-based printing is also known as a nozzle-based deposition system [11]. It relies on a computer-controlled manufacturing method that deposit materials layer by layer through a nozzle to create a 3D structure with controlled composition and architecture. FDM also known as fused filament fabrication (FFF) is one of the most commonly used low-cost 3D printing techniques [53]. In FDM, the filament of the thermoplastic materials is melted or softened, then extruded from the printer's head, and layer by layer deposited to form the 3D object (see Figure 2a). For pharmaceutical printing thermoplastic polymers have been used as a drug carrier and thermo-resistant drug molecules are used. Polyvinylpyrrolidone (PVP), polyvinyl alcohol (PVA), and polylactic acid (PLA) are the most commonly used pharmaceutical grade polymers for FDM [54]. The process parameters that must be controlled for FDM are the infill density, printer speed, layer height, and the temperature of the nozzle and build platform [19,20,38,55,56]. Prednisone, theophylline, etc. are examples of drug molecules [52]. The drugs can be loaded into the polymer filament by impregnation (known as FDMi) [11,38,56] or integrated with the polymer and make the filament by hot-melt extrusion (HME). If necessary additional functional excipients (e.g., plasticizer) are added during the filament making by HME [11]. Most recently, Pietrzak et al. showed the integration of HME and FDM in an attempt to increase the range of polymers that can be used to make filament for FDM [20]. Their study also showed that the drug loading can be increased to 50%.

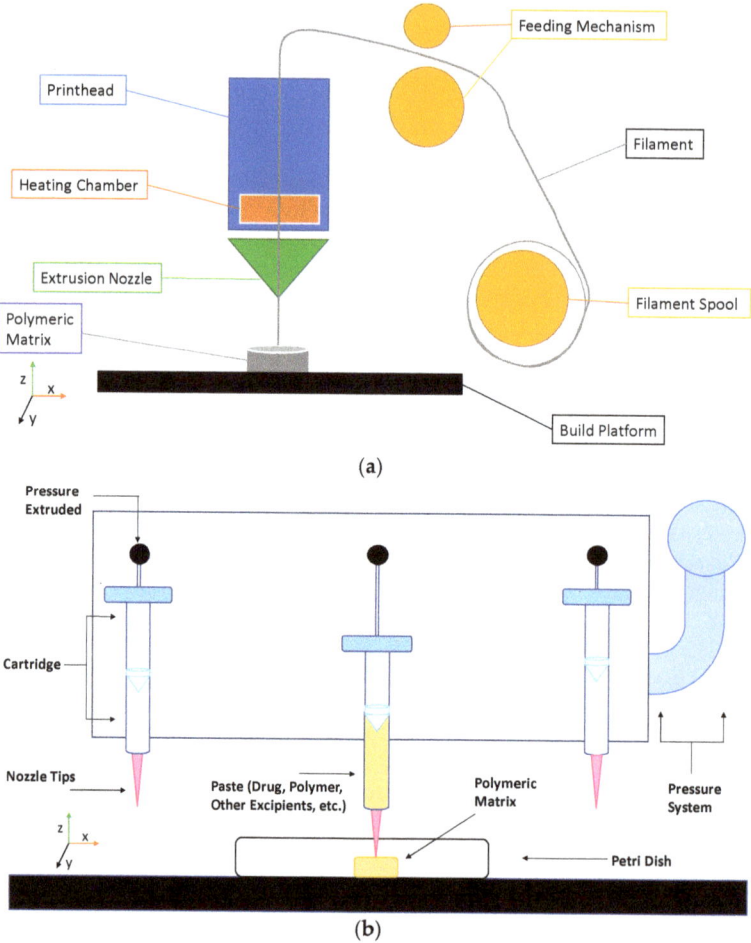

Figure 2. 2-dimensional (2D) schematic of the extrusion-based 3D printing process: (**a**) fused deposition modeling (FDM), (**b**) pressure-assisted microsyringe (PAM).

Pressure assisted microsyringe (PAM) was used extensively in tissue engineering to create soft tissue scaffolds [11]. PAM has recently gained popularity in pharmaceutical applications. Semi-solids (gels or pastes) are extruded continuously layer-by-layer through a syringe based tool-head (Figure 2b). The extrusion is usually based on a pneumatic (pressured-air), mechanical, and solenoid piston, [17,57]. Semi solids contain an optimal mixture of polymer, solvent, and other functional excipients (if needed) having appropriate rheological properties that make it suitable for printing. PAM does not require high temperature whereas, drying as post-print processing is required. However, shrinking or deformation of the product may occur following the drying process. The printed object may also collapse if the deposited layer did not strengthen sufficiently to withstand the weight of the successive layers [53]. Nifedipine, Glipizide, etc. are drug examples that have been used in PAM [52]. It is also noted that for extrusion-based (FDM, PAM) 3D printing infill type, e.g., rectilinear, hexagonal, or honeycomb affect the mechanical strength (i.e., flexural strength) of the printed structure [58,59]. Table 1 provides a comparison between FDM and PAM 3D printing technologies [38,60–63].

Table 1. Comparison of FDM and PAM 3D printing technologies.

Technology	FDM 3D Printing	PAM 3D Printing
Advantages	<ul><li>Low-cost printing technology.</li><li>No post-processing is required.</li><li>Better drug uniformity.</li></ul>	<ul><li>Works at room temperature.</li><li>High drug loading is achieved.</li><li>Suitable for multi-drug pill (polypill) printing.</li></ul>
Limitations	<ul><li>High-temperature processing is required which is not suitable for thermally labile drugs.</li><li>Pre-processing steps of filament making are required.</li><li>Lack of suitable biocompatible/biodegradable thermoplastic polymers.</li><li>Active pharmaceutical ingredient (API) degradation may occur due to the high processing temperature.</li></ul>	<ul><li>Post-processing, drying, is required.</li><li>Polymer rheological properties impact on structure formation and printing process.</li><li>Printing resolution is depended on nozzle size.</li><li>Toxicity and drug instability may occur due to the usage of organic solvents.</li></ul>

Figure 3 shows a workflow diagram or decision matrix that is required to consider from the beginning to the end of the printing process. The overall process starts with the decision making of dosage, types of application intended, then design using Computer-Aided Design (CAD), translating the design to machine language, deciding materials and process parameters, and finally printing the dosage. It is noted that printer resolution can also be a decision parameter when selecting the printer types. Due to the advances in technology standard 3D printing equipment now enable to achieve a print resolution of the order of a few hundred micrometers [64]. However, getting print resolution below a hundred micrometers is yet a major technical challenge [65].

A comparison of processing steps required for traditional pharmaceutical manufacturing direct compressions (DC) vs. 3D printing (FDM and PAM) is shown in Figure 4. DC is considered the simplest manufacturing process for pharmaceutical tablets [66,67]. Both FDM and PAM require the same number of processing steps to manufacture deliverable finished products from raw materials (API and excipients). However, the added advantage for 3D printing is that it requires a smaller footprint, can be remotely controlled, and is not only for use with small batches but also for individual pills to be fabricated within a single batch of materials. These characteristics make 3D printing manufacturing closer to the patient's specifications. The important aspects for 3D printing, similar to DC processing are that stable, reproducible starting materials need to be supplied.

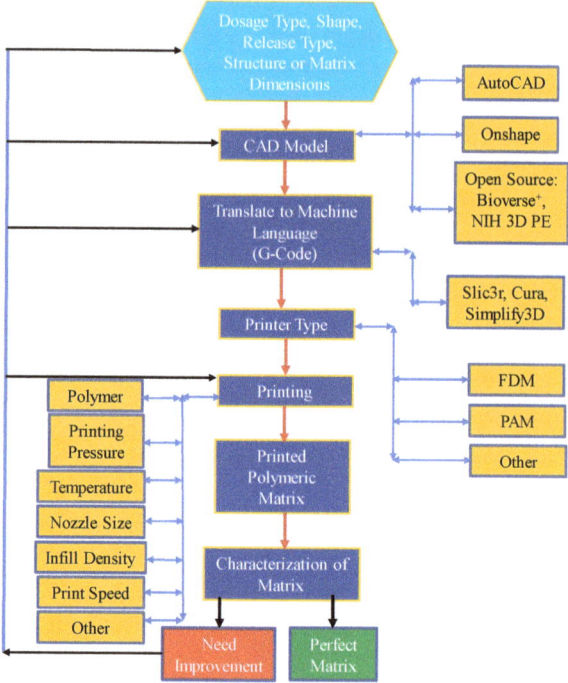

Figure 3. Workflow diagram or decision matrix for a 3D printing process. (CAD: computer-aided design, FDM: fused deposition modeling, PAM: pressure-assisted microsyringe, NIH 3D PE: National Institutes of Health 3D Print Exchange).

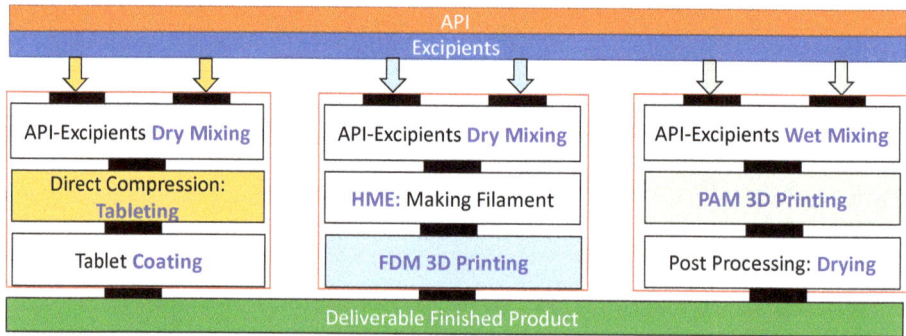

Figure 4. Comparison of different processing steps required for traditional direct compression (DC) tablet manufacturing vs. advanced manufacturing, 3D printing (FDM or PAM).

3. Polymers Role on Extrusion-Based 3D Printing of Pharmaceuticals

Table 2 summarizes the materials (drugs, polymers, and other functional excipients) compositions used in recently published articles that utilized extrusion-based (either FDM or PAM) 3D printing for pharmaceuticals. Typically, in FDM the drug and polymer are mixed and made into filament by using HME (hot melt extrusion) and then extruded through the nozzle whereas, for PAM they are mixed in a solvent to make a paste. The semi-solid paste is then extruded through the nozzle. HME is used primarily for pharmaceutical solid dispersion manufacturing. It is a solvent-free process, employing heat and mechanical shear, and can be coupled with 3D printing [68,69]. Besides polymers, there are other functional excipients (plasticizer, insoluble filler, antioxidants, etc.) that are also used in either FDM or PAM 3D printing [60,69]. However, the polymer contains a large proportion of all ingredients. Hence, the polymer plays a critical role in forming the drug–polymer matrix suitable for dosage, and overall materials processability through process unit. This is applicable for both FDM and PAM. In this review, polymers are analyzed from both materials and process perspective. In the materials perspective (Section 3.1), polymers' physicochemical properties, their suitability for the FDM or PAM printing process, dosage types, and types of drug release from the matrix are discussed. From the process perspective (Section 3.2), how these polymers impact the process operations are discussed.

Table 2. Examples of material compositions used in extrusion-based 3D printing.

Extrusion Method	Materials Composition	Drug Release Type	References
FDM	95% Polyvinyl alcohol (PVA), 5% drug (Paracetamol)	Controlled Release	[55]
	90–100% Hydroxypropyl cellulose (HPC), 2–10% Poly (ethylene glycol) (PEG), 2% drug (acetaminophen)	Pulsatile Release	[70]
	45.5% Hydroxypropyl methylcellulose (HPMC E5) and 19.5% Ethylcellulose (EC) or HPC, 30% drug Acetaminophen (APAP), 5% Kollidon	Controlled Release	[71]
	45% HPC, 50% drug (Theophylline), 5% triaceten	Immediate Release	[72]
	65–90% PVA, 10–35% drug (Ciprofloxacin hydrochloride), 2% dibutyl sebacate	Controlled Release	[73]
	60.35% PVA, drugs = 5% Lisinopril dihydrate, 2.5% Amlodipine besylate, 1.25% indapamide, 5% rosuvastatin calcium. 25.9% sorbitol	Various (Depends on Drug)	[74]
	60% HPMC, 15% Eudragit, 20% drug (Carvedilol), 5% D-α-Tocopheryl polyethylene glycol 1000 succinate (TPGS)	Extended Release	[75]
PAM	2% HPMC, 81% drug (Guaifenesin), 7% Sodium starch glycolate (SSG), 10% Microcrystalline cellulose (MCC)	Controlled Release	[17]
	7.1% HPMC, 3.5% drug (Glipizide), 17.8% PEG, 25% tromethamine, 46.6% lactose	Sustained Release	[76]
	72.1% 2-Hydroxypropyl-β-cyclodextrin (HPβCD), 2.4% HPMC, 24% drug (Carbamazepine)	Immediate Release	[77]
	2% Carbopol, 35% drug (Diclofenac sodium), 20% Lactose, 5% Polyplasdone, 21% Avicel PH101, 14% Avicel PH105	Modified Release	[60]

3.1. Materials Perspective

3.1.1. Carbopol®

Carbopol® homopolymers are high molecular weight, crosslinked polyacrylic acid polymers [78]. Crosslinking is done with allyl sucrose or allyl pentaerythritol. Polymers are synthesized in either ethyl acetate or cosolvent ethyl acetate/cyclohexane mixture. Carbopol® 971P and 974P are suitable for PAM 3D printing. Carbopol® 971P is a lightly crosslinked polymer having a viscosity of 4000–11,000 cP (0.5 wt% suspension), which will result in flow like honey in a semisolid formulation [78,79]. It is suitable for extended/controlled-release tablets, oral liquids and suspension [79]. Carbopol® 974P is a highly crosslinked polymer and produces highly viscous gels [80]. The viscosity of 0.5 wt% suspension of Carbopol® 974P is 29,400–39,400 cP [78]. It is suitable for extended-release tablet formulation.

3.1.2. Ethylcellulose (EC)

Ethylcellulose (EC) is often used as a polymer in pharmaceuticals and has recently found use in 3D printed pharmaceuticals. It is a water-insoluble thermoplastic polymer. These properties associated with EC are taken advantage of its usage in FDM 3D printing in the pharmaceutical industry. As a polymer in drug formulations, it is often used for its sustained release capabilities [81]. EC must undergo some form of sample preparation, such as dissolution in acetone or the addition of a plasticizer before it can be used in FDM printing [82].

3.1.3. Eudragit®

Eudragit® polymers are a set of synthetic polymethacrylate used in pharmaceutical drug formulations. They are non-biodegradable, non-absorbable, nontoxic and amorphous polymer [83]. According to Evonik, all Eudragit polymers have thermoplastic properties, low glass transition temperatures (between 9 °C and > 150 °C), high thermostability, and high miscibility with APIs and other excipients [83,84]. Hence, they are suitable for hot-melt extrusion. Varying the functional group on the polymer dictates the type of drug release it is best suited for. For example, the Eudragit E series is for immediate release drugs. Eudragit® E series is suitable for gastric fluid as it is soluble at lower pH up to pH-5. Eudragit® L and S series show delayed release in drug formulations. The L and S series vary in pH. Eudragit® RL and Eudgrait® RS are used for time-controlled release purposes. These series are insoluble with pH-independent swelling [84]. Eudragit® RL has high permeability while Eudragit® RS has low permeability. Combining the series together enables pharmaceuticals with customized time-controlled release profiles. While it has been used successfully with FDM methods to create immediate-release tablets when used with a plasticizer, the 3D printing process was unreliable and the nozzle was frequently clogged [85].

3.1.4. Hydroxypropyl Cellulose (HPC)

Hydroxypropyl cellulose (HPC) is a flexible, water-soluble polymer. HPC is made up of a monomer that is comprised of a glucose molecule with multiple hydroxypropyl substituents. HPC is available in different viscosity grades, making it suitable for formulating drugs with different release profiles. Overheating and rapid changes in temperature drastically affect the stability of HPC and its viscosity. HPC has a low glass transition temperature in the range of −25 °C to 0 °C as moisture varies from ~10% to 1%approximately [86]. It has high thermostability, making it suitable for processes that require melting and extrusion. The viscosity of HPC decreases as temperature increases, which in turn increases the release rate of the selected API. High molecular weight HPC, compared to its low molecular weight counterparts, exhibits high swellability that is suitable for controlled-release matrices [87].

3.1.5. Hydroxypropyl Methylcellulose (HPMC)

Hydroxypropyl methylcellulose (HPMC) is a swellable, water-soluble polymer that enhances the sustained release capabilities of active ingredients in pharmaceuticals [88]. The high swellability of HPMC has significant effects on the release kinetics of pharmaceuticals [89]. HPMC E5 is used for immediate-release tablets and suitable for the PAM printing method [11]. Under high UV-light exposure, HPMC remains stable [90]. The glass transition temperature (T_g) of HPMC is 170–198 °C [91]. When heated above certain temperatures, an aqueous solution composed of HPMC will gel out of the solution. The thermal gelation may impact drug stability in regards to 3D printing.

3.1.6. Polycaprolactone (PCL)

Polycaprolactone (PCL) is a semi-crystalline, biocompatible polyester with a melting point of 55–60 °C and T_g of −54°C [92,93]. It has a great organic solvent solubility. It is used for long-term implant delivery devices due to its very low in vivo degradation [92,94]. PCL is often blended or co-polymerized with PLLA (poly(L-lactic acid)), PDLLA (a racemic mixture of PLLA and PDLA (poly(D-lactic acid)), PLGA poly(lactic-*co*-glycolic acid), etc. to improve polymer erosion [94]. PCL is considered a good elastic biomaterial due to its low tensile strength (~0.023 GPa) and high elongation at breakage (4700%) [95].

3.1.7. Polylactic Acid (PLA)

Polylactic acid (PLA) is an insoluble, synthetic biodegradable polymer [96,97]. It is the most extensively researched and utilized biodegradable aliphatic polyester. PLA is a thermoplastic, high-strength, and high modulus polymer [93,98]. It is non-toxic because its monomers can be made from the fermentation of sugar. The drug release of PLA encapsulated medicines can be influenced by the manipulation of PLA crystallinity degree and mechanical stability [98]. PLA is a very brittle material with less than 10% elongation at break, which limits its use in the application where plastic deformation is required at higher stress levels [98]. PLA has four forms as it possesses chiral molecules. Among them PLLA and PDLLA are promising for pharmaceutical applications. PLLA has a melting temperature of around 175 °C, a T_g of 60–65 °C, and a mechanical strength of 4.8 GPa; whereas, PDLLA has a slightly lower T_g of 55–60 °C and a mechanical strength of 1.9 GPa [94]. PLA can last up to three hours in acid, which is more suited to drugs that require a delayed release [99].

3.1.8. Polyvinyl Alcohol (PVA)

Polyvinyl alcohol (PVA) is a biocompatible, swellable water-soluble synthetic polymer [100,101]. It is also a thermoplastic polymer [62], exhibiting a T_g of 85 °C, melting point range of 180 (partially hydrolyzed) to 228 °C (fully hydrolyzed), and a partially hydrolyzed viscosity ranging from 3.4 mPa·s to 52 mPa·s [11,52]. It is widely used in FDM [102]. PVA is suitable for immediate release tablets as it dissolves more readily in hydrochloric acid [99]. However, controlled release can be achieved using PVA if the capsule is designed as a series of concentric circles to delay release [103].

3.1.9. Polyvinylpyrrolidone (PVP)

Polyvinylpyrrolidone (PVP) is a water-soluble polymer [53]. It is also capable of solubilizing in other organic solvents. PVP's solubility properties are attributed to its chemical structure, where it displays hydrophilic and hydrophobic components [104]. The chemical structure also yields hydrogen bonding of PVP. The hydrogen bonding causes interactions and the formation of complexes with low molecular weight compounds. The T_g of PVP has a direct relationship with its molecular weight and it reaches a plateau at about 175 °C which corresponds to a molecular weight of 100,000 [104].

3.1.10. Poly(Ethylene Glycol) (PEG)

PEG is a water-soluble, biocompatible, and amphiphilic polymer whose derivatives are used for a variety of applications. PEG is also known as polyethylene oxide (PEO) or polyoxyethylene (POE), depending on its molecular weight [105]. Polymers with Mw <100,000 are usually called PEGs, while higher molecular weight polymers are classified as PEOs [105]. PEGDA (PEG diacrylate) is a polymer that is a derivative of polyethylene glycol (PEG). To create PEGDA, an acrylic group is added to the terminal hydroxyl end group in PEG. The acrylic groups aid in its polymerization process where photopolymerization and other techniques are used [106]. PEGDA has better mechanical strength than PEG due to the formation of cross-link [94].

3.1.11. Soluplus®

Soluplus® is a polymeric solubilizer with an amphiphilic chemical structure. It is a graft copolymer composed of polyethylene glycol, polyvinyl acetate, and polyvinyl caprolactam. BASF designed this copolymer to solubilize APIs that are typically poorly soluble. It is also very suitable for HME because of its T_g of about 70 °C and low hygroscopicity [107].

In summary, all the polymers available are classified based on water solubility and the types of drug release which have been summarized in Figure 5a. Figure 5b shows their suitability to use for either FDM or PAM 3D printing process.

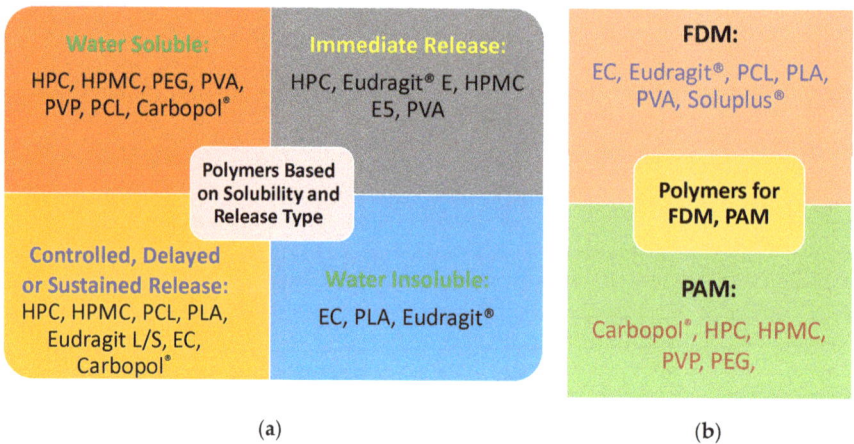

Figure 5. Summary of polymers based on (**a**) water solubility and drug release type, (**b**) their selection for either FDM or PAM 3D printing method.

3.2. Process Perspective

In the FDM 3D printing process, melted materials are used in the creation of products. This printing method requires constructing the material into printable filament and passing the filament through a heated nozzle [52]. In most experiments, filaments are either bought or created using HME. Printable filaments must have adequate rheological properties and mechanical strength to ensure proper processability in FDM 3D printing [52,93]. Goyanes et al. used commercially available PVA filaments impregnated with drugs to 3D printed pharmaceutical tablets. There was no indication that the rheological properties of the commercial PVA filaments changed. Therefore, there were no issues with processing the filaments through the printer [19,38]. In other studies, Goyanes et al. used HME to mix commercial PVA filament with active pharmaceutical ingredients. The mixture of PVA and API is extruded through a single screw extruder with a diameter of 1.75 mm at a screw speed of 15 rpm and a temperature of 170 °C. The filaments were able to be processed through the printer successfully. Goyanes et al. noted that the HME filaments were not significantly different from the commercial PVA filaments relative to the physical appearance, size, and mechanical behavior. The study did not include any rheological testing done on the created filaments [100,108].

The thermoplastic properties of a filament produced from HME may be affected if the filament has a high drug to polymer ratio [11]. If the drug-loading percentages are to be increased, a plasticizer may need to be added in order to soften the filament to suitable flexibility for printing [55]. Aho et al. described that soluble APIs can act as plasticizers when mixed with polymers during HME [109]. This leads to the mixture's melt/glass transition temperature and viscosity decreasing. Yang et al. found a similar result and showed that when ibuprofen is the active ingredient, it acted as a plasticizer for the HME filaments, decreasing the stiffness (resistance to deflection or deformation by an applied force) of the filaments [110]. Yang et al. used a tensile test to determine the stiffness of the Ethyl Cellulose filaments and found a linear relationship between ibuprofen content and stiffness [110].

Stiffness and brittleness (and viscosity) are important properties to determine whether a filament will be suitable for FDM processing. Stiffness is typically defined using the ratio of load and deformation [111].

$$Stiffness = \frac{Load}{Deformation} \quad (1)$$

Zhang et al. used breaking stress as load and breaking distance as deformation [71]. They used the 3-point bending flexural test to measure the stiffness and brittleness. In the study, the filaments were produced solely with EC and the model drug. They have suitable stiffness but are too brittle for FDM. The HPMC filaments created high stiffness and toughness but had low processability because of high melt viscosities and rough surfaces. The HPC LF and the HPC EF filaments are too soft and flexible to be processed by the FDM 3D printer. Soluplus® and Eudragit® L100 melt are unable to form HME extruded filaments at high temperatures, such as 140°C [71]. Okwuosa et al. used HME to create PVA filaments for 3D printing of pharmaceuticals. During the printing process, the PVA filaments exhibited poor flow from the nozzle in the FDM printer and could not form a stable structure. It was necessary to add talc to the filament as a thermostable filler [112]. Filaments composed of different combinations of polymers, created with HME, exhibited better mechanical and rheological properties suitable for FDM 3D printing compared to the individual polymer formulations [71].

Viscosity, an important rheological property, is largely dependent on temperature [109]. In FDM 3D printing, the recommended temperatures for printing are typically too high for printing pharmaceuticals. In a study by Pietrazk et al., a lower printing temperature was used in order to avoid thermal degradation of the API and the polymer [20]. At lower than optimal temperatures, the filament can block the nozzle when attempting to print because of increased viscosity. Similarly, in another study by Yang et al., low printing temperatures had an increase in the viscosity of the EC tablets which caused nozzle blockage and low bond strength between layers [110].

PAM printing eliminates the need for prior formulations of filament that is necessary for FDM. The materials extruded during PAM printing should be in a semi-solid form, also referred to as a paste or gel. These are typically formed by mixing polymer(s), functional excipient(s), and drug with an appropriate solvent(s) at a ratio that results in a paste suitable for printing [53]. Optimal paste should have suitable rheological properties to enable it to process through the printing system. These properties include viscosity, yield stress under shear and compression, and viscoelastic properties [113]. Rattanakit et al. developed an extrusion printer with the purpose of printing a Dexamethasone-21-phosphate disodium salt (Dex21P) tablet encapsulated by PLGA and PVA [114]. In this extrusion system, an air pressure line is connected to dispensing the paste. Paste with varying molecular weights of PVA is used for printing. The viscosities of the different ink solutions are measured and deemed suitable viscosities for printing, with values between 16.4 cP and 861.9 cP. As the molecular weight of PVA in the paste increases, the amount of air pressure for extrusion increases. For the solution with a viscosity of 16.4cP, an air pressure line was not necessary for extrusion. Rheological parameters of the paste must be configured to the needle of the print head for successful extrusion.

Khaled et al. produced various pharmaceuticals using PAM printing. In 2015, Khaled et al. created a three-drug (multi-active) tablet [76]. To ensure that the print head nozzle does not experience blockage, they made the paste smooth and homogeneous. The proper flowability of the paste ensures that the printing process is successful. HPMC was used for the sustained-release compartments of the tablet. To keep the HPMC at an optimal viscosity for printing, hydroalcoholic gel, instead of water, was used as the binder. In another study Khaled et al. created a polypill with five different drug doses, using PAM printing [18]. HPMC and cellulose acetate are chosen as the polymers for the shell and sustained release compartments, respectively. To prevent nozzle blockage, both polymers were mixed with solvents to be made into a smooth and homogeneous paste. Khaled et al. state that if a polymer can be processed into a powder form, it can be printed using PAM printing [17]. A detail on polymer rheology and its impact on structure and process are elaborated in the next section.

4. Polymers Rheology and Its Impact on Structure and Process

Rheological properties of the polymers and polymer–API mixture play a vital role in predicting the processability of FDM and PAM 3D printing and the properties of the final pharmaceutical products (solid dosages) such as drug release. These rheological properties that depend on types of materials, i.e., polymers, excipients and formulation compositions are influenced by the nozzle diameter, pressure drop and feed rate, as well as the thermal properties of the feed, such as specific heat capacity, thermal conductivity, density and glass transition temperature [109,115]. The knowledge and better understanding of how the flow behavior of the feed materials changes as a function of time, shear and/or extensional deformation, and deformation rate, is of great help in tailoring the process conditions and choosing suitable polymer-carriers for melt processing by FDM and paste or gel processing by PAM 3D printing. Moreover, the addition of solid matters such as APIs, plasticizers, non-melting fillers particularly at high content in the polymer melts dramatically influences the flow properties of the pharmaceutical formulations, and therefore adjustment of the processing parameters, e.g., the extrusion temperature or nozzle speed is required [96,115,116]. The rheological properties are also considered as the major parameter that controls the reproducibility of the printed structure. Of particular concern to PAM 3D printing method is the polymer's response to being extruded, how well it is able to adhere to previously printed layers, and its ability to hold the weight of subsequent layers [60]. Hence, the polymer–drug paste should be characterized by suitable apparent viscosity, viscoelastic properties, and yield stress under shearing and compression to be smooth and homogeneous to avoid nozzle blockage [113]. Figure 6 shows important rheological tests are required for the polymer–drug melts or paste to use it for FDM or PAM 3D printing. Aho et al. summarize the various rheological tools and measurement techniques that can be used to evaluate the flow behavior and processability of polymers and APIs with HME or FDM processing [109]. Hence, for extrusion based-3D printing, rheological measurements should be considered as a key part of the basic physicochemical characterization toolbox when selecting suitable polymer candidates, yet it remains underutilized [109].

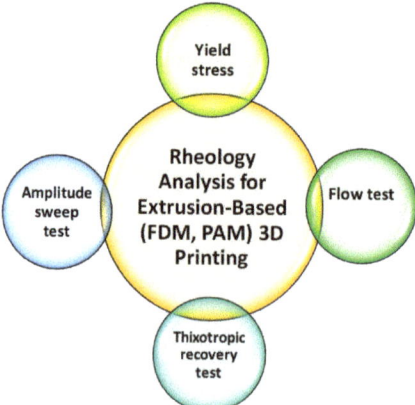

Figure 6. Important rheological tests are required for polymer–drug paste or molten dispersions to ensure their suitability and processability for extrusion-based (FDM, PAM) 3D printing.

The viscosity is the most important rheological parameter that plays a major role in determining optimal processing conditions for FDM and PAM 3D printing. It describes the resistance to flow and is given as a relationship of stress to the deformation rate. In the FDM process, a different force would be applied to the filament as it is pushed down by the drive gear and directs the heated filament toward the nozzle, where they are subjected to different shear rates. The shear rate at the printer liquefier depends on its dimensions and the printing speed, and because of the narrow nozzle diameter, it is typically very high [96]. Both temperature and shear rate affect melt viscosity, flow, and deformation behavior of materials during melt extrusion. The flow behavior index measures the degree of non-Newtonian characteristics for a material. The more the index deviates from 1, the more non-Newtonian its character becomes and the more viscosity is affected by strain. If a fluid has a flow behavior exponent less than 1, it is shear-thinning and exhibits more non-Newtonian characteristics [117]. The changes in viscosity of polymers can be associated with a shear-thinning behavior; whereas the viscosity of polymer can significantly be reduced when a higher shear rate is exerted during the printing process. A fluid that is shear-thinning is favored in PAM or FDM applications as the 'shear-thinning' property influences not only the capability to be pushed through a narrow nozzle at a given temperature but also the ability to regain structure and shape after deposition. Knowing the ideal viscosity range can help in predicting whether the new melt or paste formulation is extrudable. The viscosity has to be much lower than that for melt or paste extrusion for efficient printing and, at the same time, it should not be so low that it flows as liquids or very soft filaments from the printing nozzle. Viscosity data at high shear rates are more representative of the materials' rheological properties during extrusion [118]. However, very few published works are available on the evaluation of the flow behavior by considering the process shear rates and access to the printability window of the FDM or PAM process. Nevertheless, the actual viscosity of the polymers during FDM is unable to be measured; and therefore, to date, no indicator or acceptable viscosity range can be provided to predict the success of the FDM process [119]. A straightforward approach is to compare the viscosity of the new formulation to that of a successfully extruded formulation (e.g., a commercial filament) using a rheometer. A dissimilar viscosity profile may not necessarily equate to an unextrudable melt, provided that they possess comparable viscosity at the operating shear rate; hence the shear rate of interest will need to be identified.

In order to estimate the feed filament viscosity in the 3D printing process, the volume flow rate through the printer nozzle was calculated from the pre-set nozzle speed, i.e., the speed at which molten material is deposited/extruded from the nozzle. The volume flow rate, Q can be calculated using the radius of the nozzle exit, r and the speed of extrusion v (i.e., printing speed):

$$Q = \pi r^2 v \quad (2)$$

The corresponding apparent shear rate at the nozzle wall can be semi-empirically determined using the following equation:

$$\dot{\gamma}_{app} = \frac{4Q}{\pi r^3} \quad (3)$$

For example, a printing speed (v) of 50 mm/s and a printer nozzle radius (r) of 0.1 mm equates to a flow rate of 6.3 mm^3/s and consequently an apparent shear rate ($\dot{\gamma}_{app}$) of ~1000 s^{-1}. Due to the flow instabilities and sample rupture for high-viscosity fluids like polymer melts, measuring steady-state shear viscosity at the range of high shear rate is not possible by rotational rheometers [120], thus capillary rheometers should be used to access a high shear rate regime. Using the small amplitude oscillatory shear (SAOS) measurements and applying the Cox–Merz rule [121] which links together the dynamic and steady-state rheological properties, one can make estimations of the higher shear rate range too, albeit this is also limited to shear rates below 700 s^{-1} [109]. If the Cox–Merz rule is applicable, the complex viscosity from SAOS test and steady shear viscosity can be correlated to each other:

$$\eta(\dot{\gamma}) = |\eta^*(\omega)|, \text{ when } \dot{\gamma} = \omega \quad (4)$$

In other words, if the Cox–Merz rule is valid, one can directly compare the complex viscosity vs. angular frequency results to shear viscosity vs. shear rate. A good overlapping between the results measured in SAOS and steady-state rotation shear (SSRS) was noticed for the green PLA, whilst the Cox–Merz rule failed for the white PLA [122]. The viscoelastic data shows that the typical Maxwellian behavior that is expected for pure polymers (storage modulus, G' ~ ω^2 and loss modulus, G" ~ ω^1 at low frequency) was observed for the green PLA, which behaved similarly to a viscous liquid with negligible elasticity. Storage modulus (G′) and loss modulus (G″) are measure of elastic response and viscous response of a polymer, respectively. The white samples, on the other hand, exhibited a marked elasticity and a much weaker ω-dependence of the moduli. The printing quality of these samples with the FDM technique could be correlated to the viscoelastic properties outside the printing apparatus [122]. Usually, amplitude sweep test or dynamic frequency sweeps or dynamic mechanical analysis is commonly used to measure the viscoelastic properties of polymer melts or paste such as storage modulus (G′), loss modulus (G″), and yield stress (σ).The crossover point (G′ = G″) provides information on the solid- or viscous-like behavior of the materials at various temperatures [118,123]. Its measurement essentially indicates how well the material withstands oscillation stress and how quickly it will break down. The higher the storage modulus, the more rigid the sample, and the more difficult it is to begin flow from the nozzle of a PAM printer [117]. This can lead to the nozzle becoming clogged before printing even begins, though after printing it will be the most rigid structure. Conversely, if this indicator is too low, the polymer will fall apart and not withstand oscillation. If G″ is greater than G′ at all frequency investigated, the polymer solution behaves and flows like a viscous material, and the printed material will generally retain its shape [124]. Yield stress is the point at which storage and loss modulus meet and is indicative of the amount of force required to make a material flowable, or transition from a solid to a liquid-like character. In PAM printing, this corresponds to the moment that the polymer is extruded through the nozzle. Therefore, the polymer should not have so great a storage modulus that it cannot be extruded and becomes clogged, but the loss modulus must not be so low as to allow the material to drain freely from the nozzle or fail to hold its shape. The yield stress of the polymer should be adequate for use on a standard PAM printer at a reasonable printing pressure [60]. A yield stress fluid is also desirable for its structural characteristics [124]. Thixotropic properties of the polymers which relate to the ability of a material to recover after the application of shear, are also important during PAM or FDM extrusion. Ideally, the polymer should be able to recover completely to its original state after a shear force is applied during extrusion, and as quickly as possible [125]. Recovery time is also important so that when the polymer is deposited on the printing platform, it can be given the time it needs to recover before any subsequent layers are added [77].

Controlling the dose of 3D printed tablets is also a challenge in single head FDM 3D printing. Previously commercially available filaments composed of widely used polymers such as polyvinyl alcohol (PVA) [19,56,126,127] in addition to newer ones such as Eudragit® RL, Kollicoat®, IR and Soluplus® [54] have been explored to make drug-loaded tablets by FDM 3D printing. All those studies highlighted several challenges involved in employing the printing techniques for pharmaceutical applications. The use of elevated temperatures (185–220 °C) and limited drug loading (0.063–9.5% w/w) renders it less suitable for many drugs particularly thermo-labile ones. HME has been used to compound high drug-loaded filaments as a feed for FDM 3D printing [61,62,71,128–132]. Tuning drug loading in such filaments, however, would significantly impact the plasticity as well as drug release profiles [82,128]. Although FDM is an extension of HME, the mode of shearing differs between the two technologies, and thus viscoelastic properties suitable for HME may not be suitable for FDM. As the FDM 3D printing process is particularly sensitive to changes in plasticity and rheological properties of the filament, it is therefore of paramount importance to craft compatible filaments so the printer can fabricate structures of a similar release profile from a wide range of doses. Recent studies have linked a filament's 3D printing compatibility with the rheological properties of the backbone polymers used in FDM 3D printing process: polymethacrylate [62,132], PLA [96], polyvinylpyrrolidone-vinyl acetate (PVP-VA) [133], PCL [134], and polyethylene oxide (PEO)-PEG [135]. Pharmaceutical literature presents some examples of how rheology can be used in the FDM 3D printing process to rationalize the effect of melt behavior on printing quality, and Table 3 summarizes the polymers (excipients) and APIs, and the rheological analysis tools reported in the literature for extrusion-based (FDM, PAM) 3D printing.

Table 3. Application of rheological techniques for extrusion-based (FDM, PAM) 3D printing and the used API-excipient combinations; literature examples.

Rheological Techniques; Application	Excipients (Polymers, Plasticizers, Other)	APIs	Reference
FDM 3D Printing			
Oscillatory shear; controlling the dosage forms	Eudragit EPO, Tri-calcium phosphate (TCP), triethyl citrate (TEC)	Enalapril maleate (EM) and hydrochlorothiazide (HCT)	[132]
Oscillatory shear; effect of excipient content on the flow properties and API release	PLA, Hydroxypropyl methylcellulose (Metolose®)	Nitrofurantoin	[96]
Oscillatory shear; evaluation of materials for FDM printability and process modulation	Hydroxypropyl methylcellulose (HPMC) Affinisol HME 15LV, Kollidon SR [a mixture of insoluble poly(vinyl acetate) (PVAc) and soluble povidone (PVP)], Eudragit EPO, hydroxypropyl cellulose (HPC) SSL, Kolliphor TPGS	Carvedilol	[136]
Oscillatory shear; effect of polymer molecular weights on the flow properties and FDM printability	PEO, PEG	Theophylline	[135]
Steady-state (zero-shear) viscosity and Oscillatory shear; API–polymer miscibility, assessment of FDM 3D printability	Poly(ε-caprolactone)	Indomethacin	[134]
Oscillatory shear; drug-polymer, polymer–polymer, and drug–polymer–polymer miscibility, and evaluation of polymers or polymer blends for FDM 3D printability and drug release	Polyvinylpyrrolidone-vinyl acetate copolymer (Kollidon® VA64), polyvinyl alcohol-polyethylene glycol graft copolymer (Kollicoat® IR), Hydroxypropyl Methylcellulose (HPMC), hydroxypropyl methylcellulose acetate succinate (HPMCAS)	Haloperidol	[137]
Steady-state (zero-shear) viscosity and Oscillatory shear; drug-polymer miscibility, effects of particle morphological changes in the drug-polymer mixture on the flow behaviours	Polyethylene oxide (PEO), methacrylate copolymer (Eudragit® E PO)	Paracetamol and ibuprofen	[138]
Oscillatory shear; effect of non-melting filler on FDM 3D printing quality and drug release	Methacrylic polymer (Eudragit EPO), tri-calcium phosphate (TCP)	5-aminosalicylic acid (5-ASA), captopril, theophylline, and prednisolone	[62]
Oscillatory shear; effects of plasticizer on processing parameters of FDM 3D printing	Polycaprolactone, poly-(ethylene glycol) (PEG, M_w = 200, 4000 and 8000 g/mol)	Ciprofloxacin	[116]
PAM 3D Printing			
Creep recovery, cross-over modulus; probe the viscoelastic properties of paste	Carbopol (CP-794), Avicel PH101 and PH105, Polyplasdone, and glycerol	Diclofenac Sodium	[139]
Rheogram (plot of shear stress vs. shear rate); appropriate extrusion of paste and 3D printability	Hydroxypropyl methylcellulose (HPMC 2208 type), Crospovidone (Kollidon CL-F), D-Mannitol, and Polyethylene glycol (PEG) 4000	Naftopidil	[63]

The miscibility between polymers and other materials in the blends can significantly affect the rheological properties of the systems which in turn impacts the processability and the qualities of 3D printed pharmaceuticals and also their performance. Recent studies by Sadia et al. showed that the complex viscosity of Eudragit EPO was ~8750 Pa·s at the FDM 3D printing temperature [132]. Upon compounding into filament via HME, the complex viscosity was dropped to approximately 4000 Pa·s at 1 rad/s angular frequency (with the 0% hydrochlorothiazide (HCT) drug). This drop-in viscosity could be linked to the reduced T_g in these filaments (with the addition of plasticizer) and the decreased polymeric chain interaction. In a previous study, they reported that the introduction of a non-melting filler (tribasic calcium phosphate, TCP) can enhance the viscoelastic behavior in the system [62]. Replacing a non-melting filler (TCP) with an equivalent amount of low miscibility drug, HCT at a wide range of percentages (2.5–50%) resulted in comparable rheological behaviors with a predominantly viscous character with G' < G''. However, when a drug with high miscibility with the polymer is incorporated in the filament, the complex viscosity dropped significantly (~743 Pa·s at 1 rad/s angular frequency). This illustrates the importance of drug miscibility with the polymer on the rheological performance of the filament in FDM 3D printing. Alhijjaj et al. explored the use of polymer blends as a formulation strategy to overcome the processability issues associated with commercially available FDM printers and to provide adjustable drug release rates from the printed dispersions [22]. The solid dispersions of felodipine with Eudragit® and Soluplus® were prepared using FDM printing after blending with plasticizers—PEG, PEO and Tween 80. The results demonstrated that the interplay between the miscibility of the excipients in the blends and the solubility of the polymer in the media can be used to manipulate the drug release rates of the dispersions. Many miscible/ soluble small-molecule APIs act also as plasticizers when mixed with polymers, lowering the molecular friction between the long, entangled polymer chains, which leads to decreasing of the melting/glass transition temperature and viscosity of the drug-polymer systems [109,118,137,138]. The solubility of a drug substance in the polymer matrix can be measured by a rheological method suggested by Suwardie and Yang [118,123]. The curves of the viscosity of a drug-polymer mixture vs. the drug loading generally have a 'V' shape, and the minimal point gives the drug's solubility in the polymeric excipient as shown in Figure 7. If the API does not dissolve into the polymer matrix, it will form a solid dispersion, and the drug particles can be considered to behave the same way as inorganic filler particles in polymers. At high filler content, some particles are believed to form networks whose breaking down requires a certain amount of stress, yield stress, which causes a significant increase in viscosity at low deformation rates [62]. Both the plasticization by the dissolved drug and the presence of solid drug particles have implications on the melt processes such as hot melt extrusion or FDM 3D printing of concentrated mixtures [140]. The plasticization potentially enables the production of dosage forms with a high drug load using a low processing temperature and therefore avoiding thermal degradation of the drug [61,138].

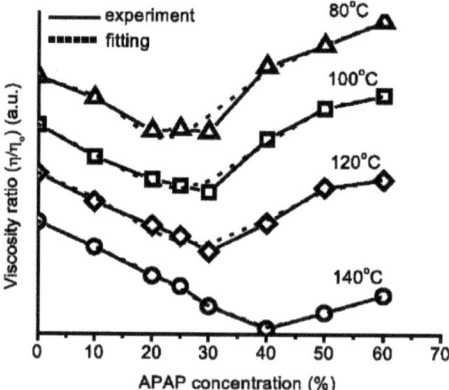

Figure 7. Viscosity ratio (η/η_o) of acetaminophen (APAP) in poly (ethylene oxide) (PEO) at different temperatures to determine the solubility of the drug. Reprinted with permission from M Yang, International Journal of Pharmaceutics, Published by Elsevier, 2011 [123].

The selection of the FDM 3D printing process parameters such as extrusion temperature, shear rate requires the knowledge of the rheological properties of feedstock materials. The extrusion temperature should be set such that the complex viscosity falls within this range. It was reported that certain polymers, such as Affinisol™ 15 LV, can undergo shear-thinning during the extrusion process, which further reduces melt viscosity and facilitates melt extrusion at a lower temperature [141]. Recently Solanki et al. attempted to identify pharmaceutically acceptable polymers for the formulation of 3D printed tablets by FDM that would provide relatively rapid drug release [137]. They studied the rheological properties, i.e., complex viscosity of individual polymers, polymer–polymer binary mixture, drug–polymer binary mixtures, and drug–polymer–polymer ternary mixtures to rationalize their viscosities on FDM 3D printability. K. Ilyés et al. also reported the assessment of the printability window of different filaments based on pharmaceutically relevant polymer blends from the rheo-mechanical properties standpoint [136]. Each component in the blends modifies the rheology of the polymer matrix as shown in Figure 8, improving the shear thinning behavior and positively influencing the FDM processability window. Measuring G′, G″ and the crossover point (G′ = G″) for polymer–drug mixtures at different concentration and temperature also provides an idea to select the processing temperature during FDM 3D printing. In a study by Suwardie et al., the extrusion temperatures for acetaminophen-PEO system were selected between 120 °C and 140 °C as the mixture samples do not show crossover points at 120 °C and 140 °C within the tested frequency, and G″ is always higher than G′ in the temperature range, suggesting the viscous behavior of the mixture [118,123]. The molecular weight (MW) and molecular weight distribution (MWD) of the polymers can affect their printability because of their variable flow behaviour [116]. Increasing polydispersity (broader MWD) broadens the glass transition area and melting endotherm peak (for semi-crystalline polymers) observed in the DSC, as well as the transition area from the Newtonian plateau to the shear-thinning area in the viscosity curve profile [109]. Isreb et al. recently studied the effect of PEO of different molecular weight on the compatibility of HME compounded filaments for FDM 3D printing and their rheological properties to rationalize the effect of melt behaviors on their printability [135]. A lower molecular weight of PEO (100–200 K) yielded mechanically incompatible HME compounded filaments and a larger molecular weight of PEO (900 K) contributed to significantly high complex viscosity and inhibited material flow at a printing temperature of 110 °C and 145 °C. The molecular weight of PEO between 300 K and 600 K was shown to have optimal mechanical and rheological properties for the FDM 3D printing process.

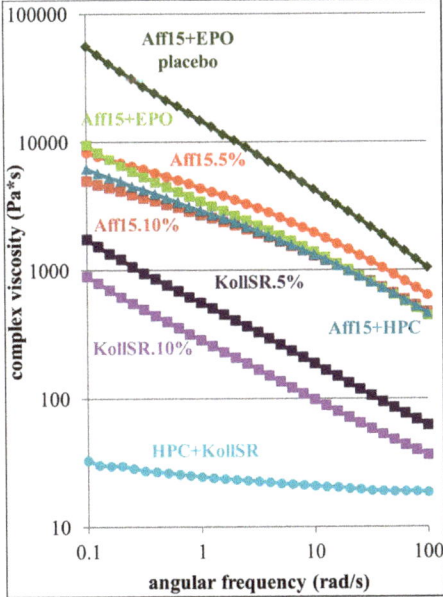

Figure 8. The rheological characterization of the blends of different polymers [Affinisol 15LV (Aff15), Kollidon SR (KollSR), Eudragit EPO (EPO), hydroxypropyl cellulose (HPC)]. Constituent effect visualized with frequency sweep at the maximum processing temperature (200 °C). Reprinted with permission from K Ilyés, European Journal of Pharmaceutical Sciences, Published by Elsevier, 2019 [136].

5. Characterization of the 3D Printed Pharmaceuticals

Table 4 shows different dosage shapes that have been reported in the literature. 3D printing has the advantage of the ability to design and print dosages of different shapes and sizes to control the release profile. However, in the 3D printing of pharmaceuticals, one of the important parameters is the degree of accuracy between the CAD model and the printed structure.

Table 4. Pharmaceutical dosages of different shapes or forms, sizes and complexities that had been 3D printed and reported in the literature.

Dosage Shape, Size, Complexity	References
FDM 3D Printing	

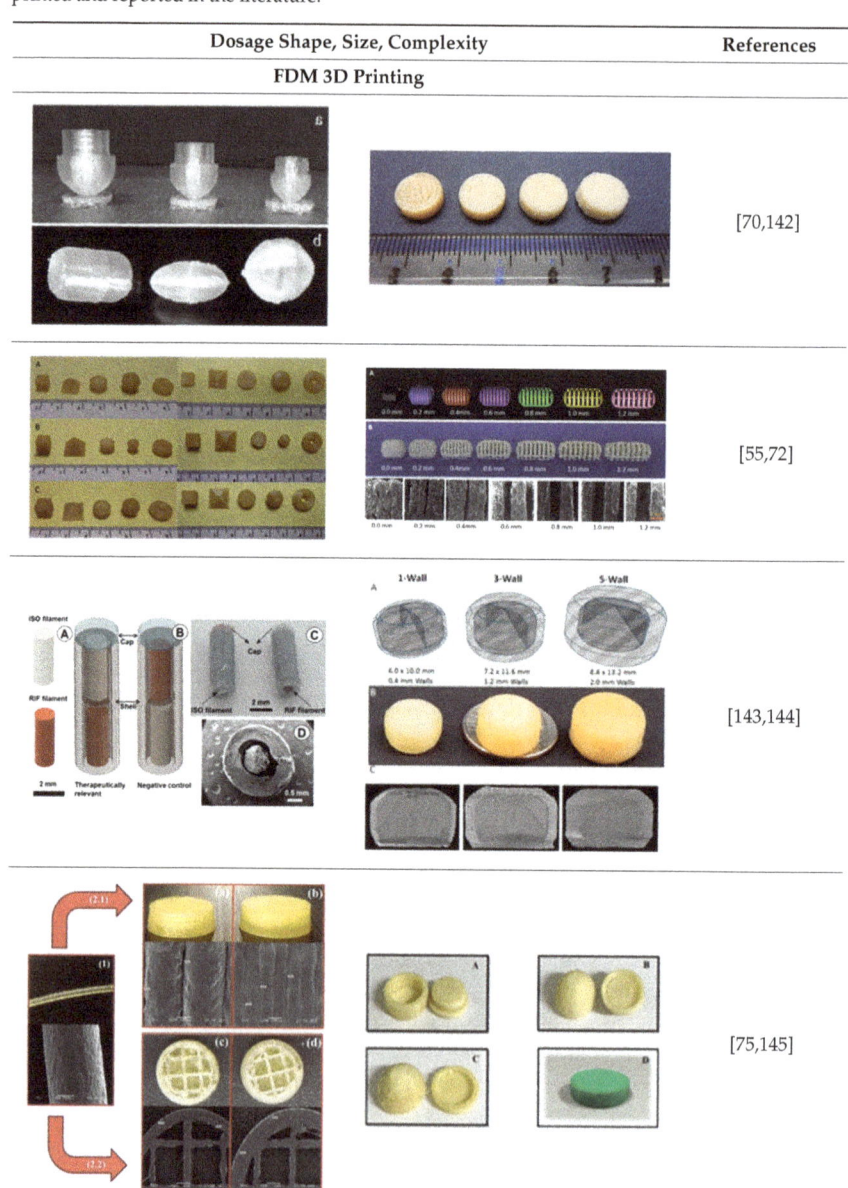

	[70,142]
	[55,72]
	[143,144]
	[75,145]

Table 4. *Cont.*

Dosage Shape, Size, Complexity	References
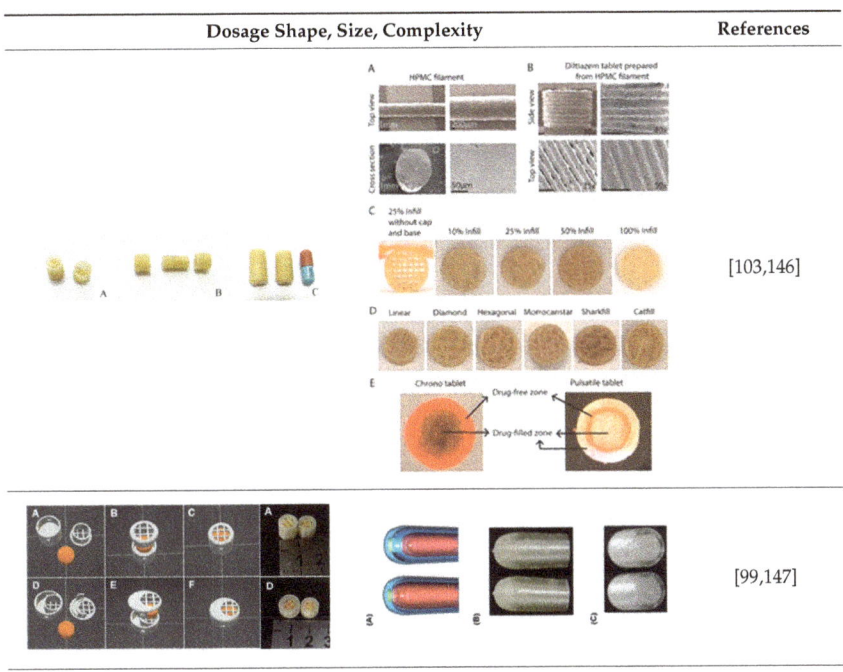	[103,146]
	[99,147]
PAM 3D Printing	
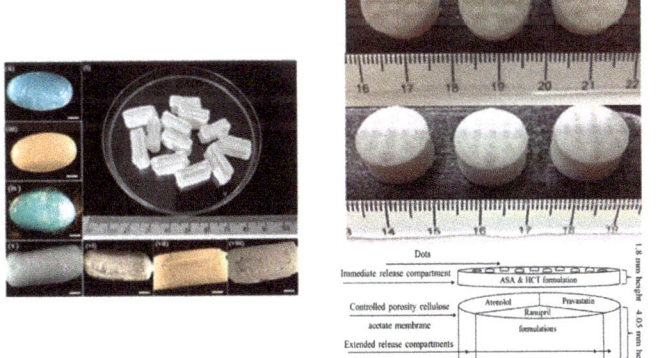	[17,18]

Table 4. *Cont.*

Dosage Shape, Size, Complexity	References
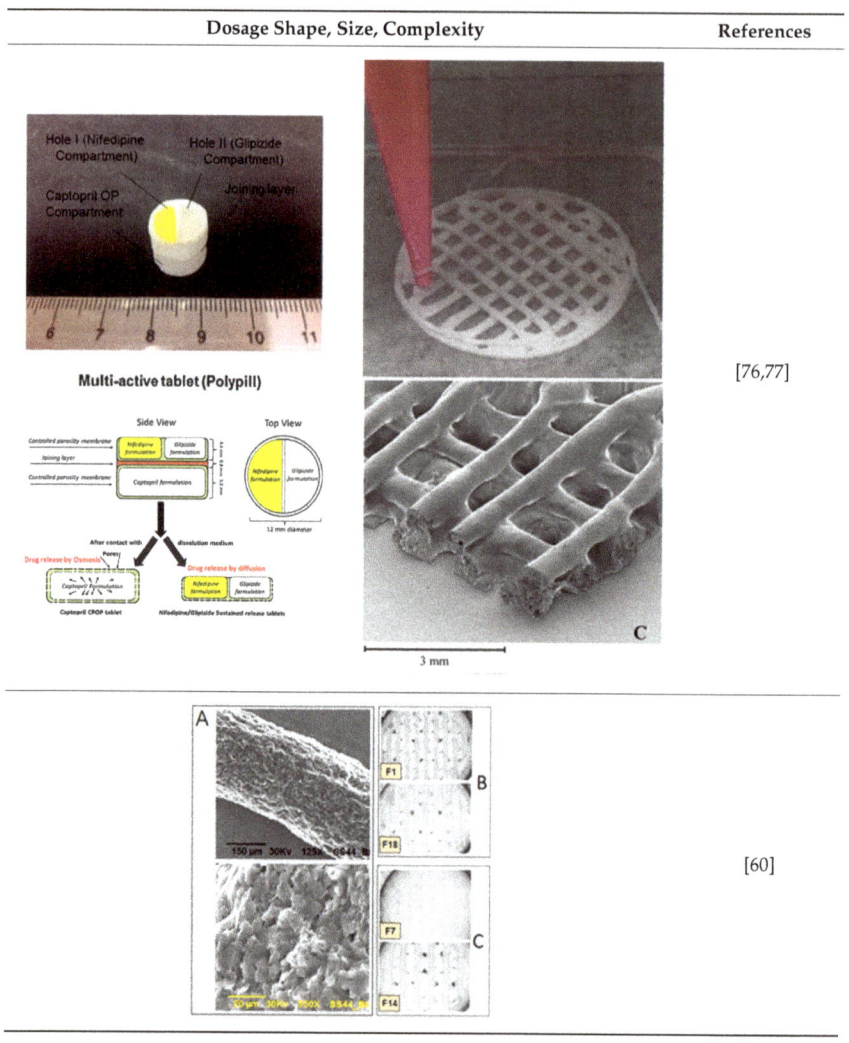	[76,77]
	[60]

FDM and PAM 3D printing technologies rely on the extrusion of polymer melts and semi-solids through the nozzle. The major challenge here is to maintain a reproducible and consistent flow of materials throughout the printing process to make the printed dosage form flawless [53]. Typically, surface imperfections are observed in the printed object. Post-treatment method such as the drying method and duration can also affect the structure and properties of the finished products. Several drying conditions (process types, temperature, and duration) are reported for PAM 3D printing. El Aita et al. investigated the drying process and found only 3 h of drying at 200 mbar in a vacuum dryer was sufficient for the complete drying (loss on drying, LOD, <1%) of their printed structure [148]. Other drying conditions reported as using a vacuum dryer at 40 °C for 24 h [18,76,139], on the heated printing platform at 80 °C for 3 h [149], in an oven at 40 °C for 12 h [150,151], left at 20 °C for 12 h [152], in an incubator containing a silica gel bead cartridge at 40 °C for 24 h [63] etc. Drying effect on structure and properties of the finished products are reported as during the drying process shell formation may occur on the outer surface of the tablet which might cause inefficient drying and result in the mechanical properties (friability, hardness) of the tablet [148], deformation of the structure [63,76,150], formation of pores on the surface [152], paste shrinkage [139], etc. The mechanical strength of 3D printed tablets is also important. Materials choices also impact the tensile strength of the tablets. A thorough characterization is required to ensure that the 3D printed structure or dosage form can reliably deliver the right amount of drug in a consistent manner. Figure 9 shows the characterization methods/techniques required for the 3D printed structure, drug, and excipients to ensure the right surface and mechanical strength of the structure as well as drug and excipients' physical properties and stability maintained.

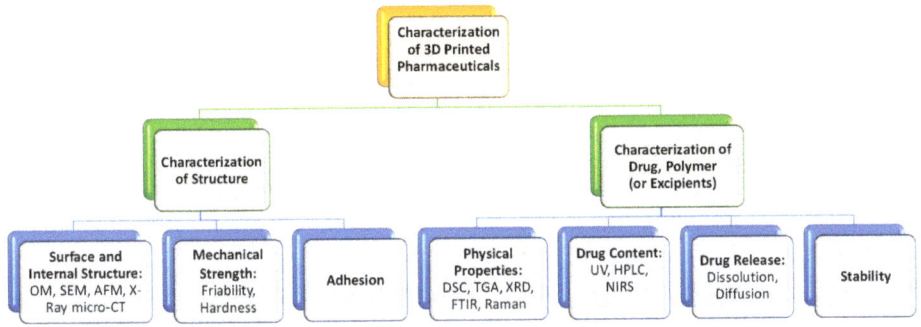

Figure 9. Characterizations required for 3D printed structure, drug, and polymer (or other functional excipients, if necessary).

The surface or cross-section images of the structure can be depicted using optical microscopy (OM), scanning electron microscopy (SEM), and atomic force microscopy (AFM). Images can provide more detailed information about the nature of the surface of the material, such as the presence of pores, cracks, or other inconsistencies [100]. To visualize the internal structure, density, and porosity of the 3D printed structure X-ray Micro Computed Tomography (Micro-CT) can be used [131]. Mechanical tests such as friability and hardness test the strength of a tablet. Ideally, a tablet should be able to remain intact through transportation and storage without breaking or losing material [150]. Adhesion is the interatomic and intermolecular interaction at the interface of two surfaces. Whether the two surfaces adhere well to each other depends on the characteristics of both surfaces at the interface. Interfacial adhesion refers to adhesion between two layers of different compositions. If adhesion is poor between two different polymers, it can lead to brittleness in the final product [153]. Interfacial adhesion is improved when the two different layers have similar properties, such as hydrophilicity [154]. Adhesion can also be achieved by polar functional groups [155]. Adhesion is important when different types of polymers are used in the same structure. Adhesion can be measured by shear tension and torsion tests [156]. Some other tests include a delamination resistance test which measures the force required to separate two layers. A qualitative tape test can be performed, in which an adhesive is attached to one layer and then removed so that the percentage of the layer that becomes detached can be measured [153]. Fourier-transform infrared spectroscopy (FTIR) can be used to examine whether two polymers have chemically bonded to each other, by observing whether certain bonds are present or not. Adhesion can be also be analyzed visually at the interface surface, with a microscope [157].

Tests such as X-ray diffraction (XRD), differential scanning calorimetry (DSC), and FTIR, etc. are used to determine a variety of physical properties. XRD for crystalline, semi-crystalline, and amorphous materials show sharp peaks, a combination of sharp peaks and amorphous halo, and only amorphous halo, respectively. The thermal analysis of the drug or excipient can be done using DSC. Thermogravimetric analysis (TGA) data helps to detect drug degradation [158]. Goyanes et al. determined the degradation of salicylic acid by comparing the weight of the sample with the starting weight at different temperatures [93]. Salicylic acid weight percentage is greatly reduced at temperatures above 140 °C, whereas it completely degrades at about 200 °C [93]. Typically drug content is measured by UV spectrophotometer or high-performance liquid chromatography (HPLC) [60,93]. However, in both methods, the structure needs to be dissolved in a suitable solvent. Vakili et al. have used near infra-red (NIR) hyperspectral imaging technique as a tool to quantify the drug content in 3D printed dosage forms of each printed layer [159]. The tool is currently heavily used in the agricultural and food industries for quality and safety assessments. With future research, NIR hyperspectral imaging can be used as a reliable, rapid and non-destructive method to validate the dosage of printed pharmaceuticals and ensure that the pharmaceuticals are meeting quality standards [159]. Kyobula et al. used Raman spectroscopy to understand the drug distribution on the printed structure [33]. Boetker et al. reported Raman spectroscopy can be considered as a potential PAT (process analytical tool) for the robust production of different 3D printed structures [96]. Dissolution and diffusion tests simulate how the drug would break down in the human body. They are used to determine release profiles and time the drug spends in the body. A drug diffusion test is conducted in vertical glass Franz cells [93] whereas, the dissolution test is done in dissolution tester [18]. The long-term stability can be eliminated by on-demand printing of dosage using 3D printing. However, the dosage should have some short period of stability at least for one or two weeks. Tablet properties such as assay, tensile strength, and dissolution after a short period of stability need to be checked to ensure that the drug does not degrade [67].

6. Challenges and Opportunities

6.1. Quality and Sterility Aspects

3D printing is well taken in many applications of pharmaceuticals but there still needs improvement of quality and safety aspects of the 3D printed drug products. Several issues such as variation in product qualities (shrinkage, warping, residuals, etc.), mechanical instability, high friability, low drug loading, high post-processing cycles, and an unidentified suitable combination of API and excipient materials need improvement to obtain a quality product in a reproducible manner [5].

Pharmaceutical manufacturing is a regulated and complex process. To meet the requirements of current good manufacturing practice (cGMP), sterilization of manufacturing equipments is essential. Sterility is needed to ensure that the product is contamination free. It should be noted that there is not much mention of sterility in regards to 3D printing of pharmaceuticals. Alomari et al. summarized different methods of the printer cartridge and printer nozzle in inkjet printing of pharmaceuticals [160]. Cheah et al. reported that the parts in SLS printing to be sterile by nature because of the high processing temperature and inert nitrogen-filled fabrication environment [161]. The print head for PAM printing is designed to use disposable tubes that hold the feed material, paste [162]. Several other techniques can be adopted to consider sterility of printings such as the use of removable head, print on surfaces treated with ethanol, print under UV light, etc. [160,163]. More research must be done to get a complete idea of sterilization aspects in FDM and PAM printing of pharmaceuticals.

6.2. Regulatory Aspects

The future of 3D printed pharmaceuticals appears to be geared towards the ability of patients to 3D print their necessary pharmaceuticals at home. Printing at home creates a new issue of how to regulate that process. Regulatory issues arise when considering how to ensure that what a patient is printing at home is safe and of adequate quality. In the future, the FDA will have to tackle the problem of how to regulate drug algorithms or drug recipes that individuals could have easy access to at home [164].

The FDA has already approved the 3D printed drug, Spritam® (levetiracetam), in August 2015 for commercial use. There are still numerous issues such as variation in product qualities, mechanical instability, etc. [5] mentioned above that must be improved to completely regulate the 3D printed pharmaceuticals. Alhnan et al. noted that it is likely that the FDA will have to overhaul its traditional regulations in order to adapt to the regulatory needs of 3D printing [53]. The FDA is currently doing its own research on 3D printing and the development of a clear and complete regulatory pathway may take some time [53].

6.3. Commercial Manufacturing

Mass manufacturing commercially is always a factor considered when a new technology is developed. However, it is noted that traditional mass manufacturing cannot be replaced by 3D printing, at least in the short term, and it is unlikely to be used for mass production [160]. The use of 3D printing in the fabrication of pharmaceuticals offers major advantages in commercial manufacturing. Combining HME with 3D printing eliminates the need for downstream processing that is present in current pharmaceutical manufacturing practices [165]. FDM printing is known for its use of relatively cheap printers and having minimal to no post-operating processing [62]. The current manufacturing process has limitations related to drug release rates. Drug release rates produced by current manufacturing techniques decrease as a function of time. Ideally, constant release rates are desired, especially for personalized pharmaceuticals. 3D printing enables us to create different polymer matrices that determine tunable release profiles [12]. Using conventional production techniques, such as powder compaction, it is difficult to manufacture the dosage of complex shapes. With 3D printing methods, like FDM or PAM, complex shapes like the torus shape can be created. The torus shape provides increased surface area as well as offers a relatively constant surface area during dissolution [166].

There are some significant challenges in replacing the current commercial manufacturing with 3D printing technology. Compared to current manufacturing processes for drug delivery systems, 3D printing has a low throughput as a result of low processing speeds [167]. Another problem for commercial 3D printing is that all pharmaceuticals manufactured in the United States have to follow the cGMP regulations enforced by the FDA [168]. Melocchi et al. set up a pilot plant that industrialized the FDM 3D printing process. To create the necessary filaments, hot-melt extrusion was carried out using a micro-extrusion manufacturing system. The team paid close attention to the operating temperature and pressure in order to ensure the maintenance of the chemical properties of the starting materials. The group considered non-traditional cooling options because of the water solubility of the polymer. They also designed a prototype FDM 3D printing to follow the cGMP [169].

A few companies are dipping their toes into the 3D printing pharmaceutical industry. Aprecia Pharmaceuticals have already filed a patent application and commercialized Zipdose®, a 3D printing system that produces Spritam, a printed medicine. FabRx, a small startup company, is developing and commercializing technology that uses 3D printing to produce personalized pharmaceuticals on-site in pharmacies or clinical trial units. GlaxoSmithKline (GSK) is also looking into the 3D printing of drugs, dedicating a research and development project towards the technology [170].

6.4. Personalized Pharmaceuticals

Typically, oral solid dosages are manufactured in pre-defined strength which is determined during early clinical trials based on therapeutic effects observed in the greatest portion of the population [160]. Current approaches to personalized pharmaceuticals involve manually splitting tablets or measuring out specific amounts of liquid dosages. Both of these methods can lead to errors and lack the necessary precision needed for exact personalization [160]. Having the ability to control the dose via 3D printing is a vital tool in the goal to create personalized medicines. Pharmaceuticals can be individualized for each patient by controlling the dose.

Skowyra et al. investigated how the FDM 3D printing process can be used to control the dose of the active ingredient by changing the printed volume using computer software [56]. Skowyra et al. compared the theoretical doses determined by tablet mass with HPLC measured doses of prednisolone, a model pharmaceutical drug, to establish a linear correlation between the parameters. This linear relationship is used to determine an equation that calculates the required dimension needed to achieve the target dosage. Results show (Figure 10) a strong correlation between the target dose and the measured dose proving the possibility of controlling the dose using FDM 3D printing via volume manipulation and make it suitable for personalized pharmaceuticals development [56].

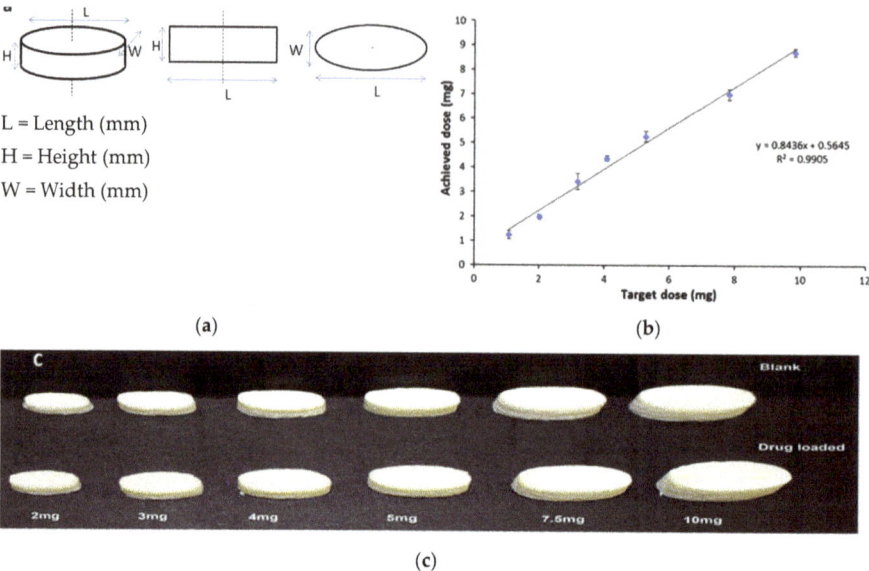

Figure 10. (a) Design of tablets, (b) the relationship between the target and achieved prednisolone dose, and (c) PVA based FDM 3D printed tablets having different dose strengths [56].

Target or theoretical dose D (mg) = M.S/100

The mass of the printed tablet M (mg) = 1.0322 V + 24.898

The volume of the design V (mm^3) = L × W × H = 0.04 × π × L^3 (Consider ellipse shape and W = H = 0.4L)

The filament loading percentage S = 100× (Mass of drug/Total mass of filament)

The required dimension (L) to achieve a target dose (D) from the filament with loading percentage (S) can be calculated as

$$L = \sqrt[3]{25\frac{\left(\frac{1000}{S}\right) - 24.898}{1.0322}} \tag{5}$$

6.5. Medication Adherence and Multi-Drug Printing

Medication adherence, or taking drugs correctly, is usually defined as the extent to which patients take drugs as prescribed by the doctor [171]. A drug that is not taken or taken at the wrong intervals, in under-dose or over-dose defeats its intended efficacy to patient's disease treatment [172]. The difficulty of tracking with multiple drugs, complex dosing regimen, and swallowing difficulties commonly causes poor adherence [173]. Poor adherence can interfere with the proper treatment of diseases and aggravate the complications. One of the approaches to improve poor adherence is by incorporating multiple drugs in the same matrix and tuning their release profile in a controlled manner. This is also known as poly-pharmacy or polypill [174].

To the extent of the authors' knowledge, there is only one commercially available multidrug pill named Polycap^{TM}, manufactured by Cadila Pharmaceuticals Ltd. India [175,176]. It is a five-drug capsule that is used to treat cardiovascular disease and stroke. Current manufacturing practices provide limitations to the successful creation of multi-drug pills [18]. Traditional direct compression manufacturing processes is unable to make multi-drug pills due to challenges of drug processing without functional excipients, limited capacity to compress multiple bulk materials having different drugs, and eventually control the pill size to make it swallowable. In current practices, manufacturers are only able to control release profiles by using a different material or polymer during fabrication [165]. With the advent of 3D printing, drug makers have the ability to formulate pharmaceuticals that have a complex design and fabricate multi-drug pills. 3D printing has made it possible by the creation of different infill densities and patterns that would be an advantage in multi-drug printing. Varying the infills provides a method to control the release profiles [146].

Recently, there have been several publications that reported multi-drug printing using 3D printing [18,74,76,177–181]. In 2015, Khaled et al. used PAM printing to create a multi-drug pill with five drugs and two different release profiles [18]. Melocchi et al. designed a hollow multidrug capsule that is made up of two separate compartments connected by a joint [169]. Goyanes et al. used FDM 3D printing to construct a multilayer pill with alternating layers of two different drugs [108]. With these attempts, researchers are seeking solutions to different problems related to the fabrication of multi-drug pills. Goyanes et al. observed that the layers of the fabricated multi-drug pill are difficult to separate because they adhere independently of the type of layers during the printing process. This addresses a current problem in current bilayer technology where insufficient layer bonding and bilayer hardness damage the products of the technology [182]. One problem that still needs to be addressed is the size of the multi-drug pills. Incidentally, a multi-drug pill with multiple release capabilities often requires large amounts of excipients which can make the pill too large for swallowing [11]. There is still room for improvement to decrease the size of the multi-drug pill for easy swallowing, control drug release, tune the dose strength, etc.

7. Conclusions and Outlook

3D printing of pharmaceuticals is an emerging technique that is especially advantageous for personalized medicine, offers design flexibility, high complexity, on-demand, and cost-effective production. With an exceptionally high degree of control and flexibility, 3D printing technology opens up the possibility of producing any types of pharmaceutical formulations, dosages and tailor-made drug delivery systems. Despite the last decade has seen massive achievements in other manufacturing industries, such as aerospace and automobile, 3D printing of pharmaceuticals is still at its infancy and its potential yet to be fully explored. Various technical and regulatory challenges need to be overcome to fulfill its real potential in the pharmaceutical industry. Though a large scale production of pharmaceuticals using 3D printing might be a long way from now, personalized medicine is possible in-house for immediate use. Future work to enable drug product manufacture using FDM and PAM 3D printing technologies should include the suitability and characterization of polymers and other excipients amenable to processing. Polymer materials and their properties, specifically their rheology should be investigated to allow a wider formulation and 3D printing design space. A better understanding of the rheological properties of API–polymer mixtures and their measurement is necessary for the successful 3D printing of pharmaceuticals. This review provides a holistic materials–processing perspective for the extrusion-based 3D printing technologies which provides a guideline in selecting suitable polymers for FDM and PAM 3D printing processes, and also the proper characterization techniques for printed structures, drugs, and excipients. The authors hope that the insights of this review will provide a useful stimulus to encourage future research into the optimization of the pharmaceutical extrusion-based 3D printing process.

Author Contributions: M.A.A. conceived the concept of the review article and prepared the content outline. M.A.A., D.O., G.K., A.Z.M.B., M.S.H., and T.S. contributed to the review writing for different sections. M.A.A. supervised the writing of this review paper and guided the major review and editing of the manuscript. All authors have read and agreed to the published version of the manuscript.

Funding: This work is supported by the startup fund provided by North Carolina A&T State University (NCAT) College of Engineering.

Conflicts of Interest: The authors declare no conflict of interest.

References

1. Ligon, S.C.; Liska, R.; Stampfl, J.; Gurr, M.; Mülhaupt, R. Polymers for 3D printing and customized additive manufacturing. *Chem. Rev.* **2017**, *117*, 10212–10290. [CrossRef] [PubMed]
2. Hofmann, M. 3D printing gets a boost and opportunities with polymer materials. *ACS Macro Lett.* **2014**, *3*, 382–386. [CrossRef]
3. Vikram Singh, A.; Hasan Dad Ansari, M.; Wang, S.; Laux, P.; Luch, A.; Kumar, A.; Patil, R.; Nussberger, S. The Adoption of Three-Dimensional Additive Manufacturing from Biomedical Material Design to 3D Organ Printing. *Appl. Sci.* **2019**, *9*, 811. [CrossRef]
4. Norman, J.; Madurawe, R.D.; Moore, C.M.; Khan, M.A.; Khairuzzaman, A. A new chapter in pharmaceutical manufacturing: 3D-printed drug products. *Adv. Drug Deliv. Rev.* **2017**, *108*, 39–50. [CrossRef]
5. Liaw, C.-Y.; Guvendiren, M. Current and emerging applications of 3D printing in medicine. *Biofabrication* **2017**, *9*, 024102. [CrossRef]
6. Yoo, J.; Bradbury, T.J.; Bebb, T.J.; Iskra, J.; Surprenant, H.L.; West, T.G. Three-Dimensional Printing System and Equipment Assembly. U.S. Patent US8888480B2, 18 November 2014.
7. Ginsburg, G.S.; McCarthy, J.J. Personalized medicine: Revolutionizing drug discovery and patient care. *Trends Biotechnol.* **2001**, *19*, 491–496. [CrossRef]
8. Schork, N.J. Personalized medicine: Time for one-person trials. *Nature* **2015**, *520*, 609–611. [CrossRef]
9. Yu, D.G.; Zhu, L.-M.; Branford-White, C.J.; Yang, X.L. Three-Dimensional Printing in Pharmaceutics: Promises and Problems. *J. Pharm. Sci.* **2008**, *97*, 3666–3690. [CrossRef]
10. Sachs, E.; Cima, M.; Williams, P.; Brancazio, D.; Cornie, J. Three dimensional printing: Rapid tooling and prototypes directly from a CAD model. *J. Manuf. Sci. Eng.* **1992**, *114*, 481–488. [CrossRef]
11. Goole, J.; Amighi, K. 3D printing in pharmaceutics: A new tool for designing customized drug delivery systems. *Int. J. Pharm.* **2016**, *499*, 376–394. [CrossRef]
12. Wu, B.M.; Borland, S.W.; Giordano, R.A.; Cima, L.G.; Sachs, E.M.; Cima, M.J. Solid free-form fabrication of drug delivery devices. *J. Control. Release* **1996**, *40*, 77–87. [CrossRef]
13. Rowe, C.; Katstra, W.; Palazzolo, R.; Giritlioglu, B.; Teung, P.; Cima, M. Multimechanism oral dosage forms fabricated by three dimensional printing™. *J. Control. Release* **2000**, *66*, 11–17. [CrossRef]
14. Wang, C.-C.; Tejwani, M.R.; Roach, W.J.; Kay, J.L.; Yoo, J.; Surprenant, H.L.; Monkhouse, D.C.; Pryor, T.J. Development of near zero-order release dosage forms using three-dimensional printing (3-DP™) technology. *Drug Dev. Ind. Pharm.* **2006**, *32*, 367–376. [CrossRef] [PubMed]
15. Yu, D.G.; Yang, X.L.; Huang, W.D.; Liu, J.; Wang, Y.G.; Xu, H. Tablets with material gradients fabricated by three-dimensional printing. *J. Pharm. Sci.* **2007**, *96*, 2446–2456. [CrossRef]
16. Infanger, S.; Haemmerli, A.; Iliev, S.; Baier, A.; Stoyanov, E.; Quodbach, J. Powder bed 3D-printing of highly loaded drug delivery devices with hydroxypropyl cellulose as solid binder. *Int. J. Pharm.* **2019**, *555*, 198–206. [CrossRef]
17. Khaled, S.A.; Burley, J.C.; Alexander, M.R.; Roberts, C.J. Desktop 3D printing of controlled release pharmaceutical bilayer tablets. *Int. J. Pharm.* **2014**, *461*, 105–111. [CrossRef]
18. Khaled, S.A.; Burley, J.C.; Alexander, M.R.; Yang, J.; Roberts, C.J. 3D printing of five-in-one dose combination polypill with defined immediate and sustained release profiles. *J. Control. Release* **2015**, *217*, 308–314. [CrossRef]
19. Goyanes, A.; Buanz, A.B.; Hatton, G.B.; Gaisford, S.; Basit, A.W. 3D printing of modified-release aminosalicylate (4-ASA and 5-ASA) tablets. *Eur. J. Pharm. Biopharm.* **2015**, *89*, 157–162. [CrossRef]
20. Pietrzak, K.; Isreb, A.; Alhnan, M.A. A flexible-dose dispenser for immediate and extended release 3D printed tablets. *Eur. J. Pharm. Biopharm.* **2015**, *96*, 380–387. [CrossRef]
21. Chen, D.; Xu, X.-Y.; Li, R.; Zang, G.-A.; Zhang, Y.; Wang, M.-R.; Xiong, M.-F.; Xu, J.-R.; Wang, T.; Fu, H.; et al. Preparation and In vitro Evaluation of FDM 3D-Printed Ellipsoid-Shaped Gastric Floating Tablets with Low Infill Percentages. *AAPS PharmSciTech* **2020**, *21*, 6. [CrossRef]
22. Alhijjaj, M.; Nasereddin, J.; Belton, P.; Qi, S. Impact of Processing Parameters on the Quality of Pharmaceutical Solid Dosage Forms Produced by Fused Deposition Modeling (FDM). *Pharmaceutics* **2019**, *11*, 633. [CrossRef] [PubMed]

23. Eleftheriadis, G.K.; Ritzoulis, C.; Bouropoulos, N.; Tzetzis, D.; Andreadis, D.A.; Boetker, J.; Rantanen, J.; Fatouros, D.G. Unidirectional drug release from 3D printed mucoadhesive buccal films using FDM technology: In vitro and ex vivo evaluation. *Eur. J. Pharm. Biopharm.* **2019**, *144*, 180–192. [CrossRef] [PubMed]
24. Viidik, L.; Seera, D.; Antikainen, O.; Kogermann, K.; Heinämäki, J.; Laidmäe, I. 3D-printability of aqueous poly(ethylene oxide) gels. *Eur. Polym. J.* **2019**, *120*, 109206. [CrossRef]
25. Feuerbach, T.; Callau-Mendoza, S.; Thommes, M. Development of filaments for fused deposition modeling 3D printing with medical grade poly(lactic-co-glycolic acid) copolymers. *Pharm. Dev. Technol.* **2018**, *24*, 487–493. [CrossRef]
26. Nukala, P.K.; Palekar, S.; Patki, M.; Patel, K. Abuse Deterrent Immediate Release Egg-Shaped Tablet (Egglets) Using 3D Printing Technology: Quality by Design to Optimize Drug Release and Extraction. *AAPS PharmSciTech* **2019**, *20*, 80. [CrossRef]
27. Healy, A.V.; Fuenmayor, E.; Doran, P.; Geever, L.M.; Higginbotham, C.L.; Lyons, J.G. Additive Manufacturing of Personalized Pharmaceutical Dosage Forms via Stereolithography. *Pharmaceutics* **2019**, *11*, 645. [CrossRef]
28. Martinez, P.R.; Goyanes, A.; Basit, A.W.; Gaisford, S. Influence of Geometry on the Drug Release Profiles of Stereolithographic (SLA) 3D-Printed Tablets. *AAPS PharmSciTech* **2018**, *19*, 3355–3361. [CrossRef]
29. Wang, J.; Goyanes, A.; Gaisford, S.; Basit, A.W. Stereolithographic (SLA) 3D printing of oral modified-release dosage forms. *Int. J. Pharm.* **2016**, *503*, 207–212. [CrossRef]
30. Awad, A.; Fina, F.; Trenfield, S.J.; Patel, P.; Goyanes, A.; Gaisford, S.; Basit, A.W. 3D Printed Pellets (Miniprintlets): A Novel, Multi-Drug, Controlled Release Platform Technology. *Pharmaceutics* **2019**, *11*, 148. [CrossRef]
31. Fina, F.; Madla, C.M.; Goyanes, A.; Zhang, J.; Gaisford, S.; Basit, A.W. Fabricating 3D printed orally disintegrating printlets using selective laser sintering. *Int. J. Pharm.* **2018**, *541*, 101–107. [CrossRef]
32. Fina, F.; Goyanes, A.; Gaisford, S.; Basit, A.W. Selective laser sintering (SLS) 3D printing of medicines. *Int. J. Pharm.* **2017**, *529*, 285–293. [CrossRef] [PubMed]
33. Kyobula, M.; Adedeji, A.; Alexander, M.R.; Saleh, E.; Wildman, R.; Ashcroft, I.; Gellert, P.R.; Roberts, C.J. 3D inkjet printing of tablets exploiting bespoke complex geometries for controlled and tuneable drug release. *J. Control. Release* **2017**, *261*, 207–215. [CrossRef] [PubMed]
34. Clark, E.A.; Alexander, M.R.; Irvine, D.J.; Roberts, C.J.; Wallace, M.J.; Sharpe, S.; Yoo, J.; Hague, R.J.M.; Tuck, C.J.; Wildman, R.D. 3D printing of tablets using inkjet with UV photoinitiation. *Int. J. Pharm.* **2017**, *529*, 523–530. [CrossRef] [PubMed]
35. Cader, H.K.; Rance, G.A.; Alexander, M.R.; Gonçalves, A.D.; Roberts, C.J.; Tuck, C.J.; Wildman, R.D. Water-based 3D inkjet printing of an oral pharmaceutical dosage form. *Int. J. Pharm.* **2019**, *564*, 359–368. [CrossRef]
36. Kadry, H.; Wadnap, S.; Xu, C.; Ahsan, F. Digital light processing (DLP) 3D-printing technology and photoreactive polymers in fabrication of modified-release tablets. *Eur. J. Pharm. Sci.* **2019**, *135*, 60–67. [CrossRef]
37. Krkobabić, M.; Medarević, D.; Cvijić, S.; Grujić, B.; Ibrić, S. Hydrophilic excipients in digital light processing (DLP) printing of sustained release tablets: Impact on internal structure and drug dissolution rate. *Int. J. Pharm.* **2019**, *572*, 118790. [CrossRef]
38. Goyanes, A.; Buanz, A.B.; Basit, A.W.; Gaisford, S. Fused-filament 3D printing (3DP) for fabrication of tablets. *Int. J. Pharm.* **2014**, *476*, 88–92. [CrossRef]
39. Godwin, A.; Bolina, K.; Clochard, M.; Dinand, E.; Rankin, S.; Simic, S.; Brocchini, S. New strategies for polymer development in pharmaceutical science—A short review. *J. Pharm. Pharmacol.* **2001**, *53*, 1175–1184. [CrossRef]
40. Jones, D.S. *Pharmaceutical Applications of Polymers for Drug Delivery*; Rapra Technology Ltd.: Shawbury, UK, 2004.
41. Park, B.J.; Choi, H.J.; Moon, S.J.; Kim, S.J.; Bajracharya, R.; Min, J.Y.; Han, H.-K. Pharmaceutical applications of 3D printing technology: Current understanding and future perspectives. *J. Pharm. Investig.* **2019**, *49*, 575–585. [CrossRef]
42. Souto, E.B.; Campos, J.C.; Filho, S.C.; Teixeira, M.C.; Martins-Gomes, C.; Zielinska, A.; Carbone, C.; Silva, A.M. 3D printing in the design of pharmaceutical dosage forms. *Pharm. Dev. Technol.* **2019**, *24*, 1044–1053. [CrossRef]

43. Araújo, M.R.P.; Sa-Barreto, L.L.; Gratieri, T.; Gelfuso, G.M.; Cunha-Filho, M. The Digital Pharmacies Era: How 3D Printing Technology Using Fused Deposition Modeling Can Become a Reality. *Pharmaceutics* **2019**, *11*, 128. [CrossRef] [PubMed]
44. Deck Khong, T.; Mohammed, M.; Ali, N. Advanced Pharmaceutical Applications of Hot-Melt Extrusion Coupled with Fused Deposition Modelling (FDM) 3D Printing for Personalised Drug Delivery. *Pharmaceutics* **2018**, *10*, 203.
45. Kjar, A.; Huang, Y. Application of Micro-Scale 3D Printing in Pharmaceutics. *Pharmaceutics* **2019**, *11*, 390. [CrossRef] [PubMed]
46. Gioumouxouzis, C.I.; Karavasili, C.; Fatouros, D.G. Recent advances in pharmaceutical dosage forms and devices using additive manufacturing technologies. *Drug Discov. Today* **2019**, *24*, 636–643. [CrossRef]
47. Aimar, A.; Palermo, A.; Innocenti, B. The Role of 3D Printing in Medical Applications: A State of the Art. *J. Health Eng.* **2019**, *2019*, 5340616. [CrossRef]
48. Vithani, K.; Goyanes, A.; Jannin, V.; Basit, A.W.; Gaisford, S.; Boyd, B.J. An Overview of 3D Printing Technologies for Soft Materials and Potential Opportunities for Lipid-based Drug Delivery Systems. *Pharm. Res.* **2019**, *36*, 4. [CrossRef]
49. Joo, Y.; Shin, I.; Ham, G.; Abuzar, S.M.; Hyun, S.-M.; Hwang, S.-J. The advent of a novel manufacturing technology in pharmaceutics: Superiority of fused deposition modeling 3D printer. *J. Pharm. Investig.* **2019**, 1–15. [CrossRef]
50. Long, J.; Gholizadeh, H.; Lu, J.; Bunt, C.; Seyfoddin, A. Application of fused deposition modelling (FDM) method of 3D printing in drug delivery. *Cur. Pharm. Des.* **2017**, *23*, 433–439. [CrossRef]
51. He, D.; Han, F.; Wang, Z.; Liu, Q. A review of 3D printing via fused deposition modeling in pharmaceutics. *Acta Pharm. Sin.* **2016**, *51*, 1659–1665.
52. Konta, A.A.; García-Piña, M.; Serrano, D.R. Personalised 3D printed medicines: Which techniques and polymers are more successful? *Bioengineering* **2017**, *4*, 79. [CrossRef]
53. Alhnan, M.A.; Okwuosa, T.C.; Sadia, M.; Wan, K.-W.; Ahmed, W.; Arafat, B. Emergence of 3D printed dosage forms: Opportunities and challenges. *Pharm. Res.* **2016**, *33*, 1817–1832. [CrossRef] [PubMed]
54. Melocchi, A.; Parietti, F.; Maroni, A.; Foppoli, A.; Gazzaniga, A.; Zema, L. Hot-melt extruded filaments based on pharmaceutical grade polymers for 3D printing by fused deposition modeling. *Int. J. Pharm.* **2016**, *509*, 255–263. [CrossRef] [PubMed]
55. Goyanes, A.; Martinez, P.R.; Buanz, A.; Basit, A.W.; Gaisford, S. Effect of geometry on drug release from 3D printed tablets. *Int. J. Pharm.* **2015**, *494*, 657–663. [CrossRef] [PubMed]
56. Skowyra, J.; Pietrzak, K.; Alhnan, M.A. Fabrication of extended-release patient-tailored prednisolone tablets via fused deposition modelling (FDM) 3D printing. *Eur. J. Pharm. Sci.* **2015**, *68*, 11–17. [CrossRef] [PubMed]
57. Firth, J.; Basit, A.W.; Gaisford, S. The role of semi-solid extrusion printing in clinical practice. In *3D Printing of Pharmaceuticals*; Springer: Cham, Switzerland, 2018; pp. 133–151.
58. Jamróz, W.; Szafraniec, J.; Kurek, M.; Jachowicz, R. 3D Printing in Pharmaceutical and Medical Applications—Recent Achievements and Challenges. *Pharm. Res.* **2018**, *35*, 1–22. [CrossRef] [PubMed]
59. Ehtezazi, T.; Algellay, M.; Islam, Y.; Roberts, M.; Dempster, N.M.; Sarker, S.D. The Application of 3D Printing in the Formulation of Multilayered Fast Dissolving Oral Films. *J. Pharm. Sci.* **2018**, *107*, 1076–1085. [CrossRef]
60. Zidan, A.; Alayoubi, A.; Coburn, J.; Asfari, S.; Ghammraoui, B.; Cruz, C.N.; Ashraf, M. Extrudability analysis of drug loaded pastes for 3D printing of modified release tablets. *Int. J. Pharm.* **2019**, *554*, 292–301. [CrossRef]
61. Kollamaram, G.; Croker, D.M.; Walker, G.M.; Goyanes, A.; Basit, A.W.; Gaisford, S. Low temperature fused deposition modeling (FDM) 3D printing of thermolabile drugs. *Int. J. Pharm.* **2018**, *545*, 144–152. [CrossRef]
62. Sadia, M.; Sośnicka, A.; Arafat, B.; Isreb, A.; Ahmed, W.; Kelarakis, A.; Alhnan, M.A. Adaptation of pharmaceutical excipients to FDM 3D printing for the fabrication of patient-tailored immediate release tablets. *Int. J. Pharm.* **2016**, *513*, 659–668. [CrossRef]
63. Tagami, T.; Ando, M.; Nagata, N.; Goto, E.; Yoshimura, N.; Takeuchi, T.; Noda, T.; Ozeki, T.J.J. Fabrication of Naftopidil-Loaded Tablets Using a Semisolid Extrusion-Type 3D Printer and the Characteristics of the Printed Hydrogel and Resulting Tablets. *J. Pharm. Sci.* **2019**, *108*, 907–913. [CrossRef]
64. Capel, A.J.; Rimington, R.P.; Lewis, M.P.; Christie, S.D. 3D printing for chemical, pharmaceutical and biological applications. *Nat. Rev. Chem.* **2018**, *2*, 422–436. [CrossRef]

65. Okwuosa, T.C.; Pereira, B.C.; Arafat, B.; Cieszynska, M.; Isreb, A.; Alhnan, M.A. Fabricating a Shell-Core Delayed Release Tablet Using Dual FDM 3D Printing for Patient-Centred Therapy. *Pharm. Res.* **2017**, *34*, 427–437. [CrossRef] [PubMed]
66. Azad, M.A.; Osorio, J.G.; Brancazio, D.; Hammersmith, G.; Klee, D.M.; Rapp, K.; Myerson, A. A compact, portable, re-configurable, and automated system for on-demand pharmaceutical tablet manufacturing. *Int. J. Pharm.* **2018**, *539*, 157–164. [CrossRef] [PubMed]
67. Azad, M.A.; Osorio, J.G.; Wang, A.; Klee, D.M.; Eccles, M.E.; Grela, E.; Sloan, R.; Hammersmith, G.; Rapp, K.; Brancazio, D.; et al. On-Demand Manufacturing of Direct Compressible Tablets: Can Formulation Be Simplified? *Pharm. Res.* **2019**, *36*, 167. [CrossRef]
68. Maniruzzaman, M. Pharmaceutical Applications of Hot-Melt Extrusion: Continuous Manufacturing, Twin-Screw Granulations, and 3D Printing. *Pharmaceutics* **2019**, *11*, 218. [CrossRef]
69. Kempin, W.; Domsta, V.; Grathoff, G.; Brecht, I.; Semmling, B.; Tillmann, S.; Weitschies, W.; Seidlitz, A. Immediate release 3D-printed tablets produced via fused deposition modeling of a thermo-sensitive drug. *Pharm. Res.* **2018**, *35*, 124. [CrossRef]
70. Melocchi, A.; Parietti, F.; Loreti, G.; Maroni, A.; Gazzaniga, A.; Zema, L. 3D printing by fused deposition modeling (FDM) of a swellable/erodible capsular device for oral pulsatile release of drugs. *J. Drug Deliv. Sci. Technol.* **2015**, *30*, 360–367. [CrossRef]
71. Zhang, J.; Feng, X.; Patil, H.; Tiwari, R.V.; Repka, M.A. Coupling 3D printing with hot-melt extrusion to produce controlled-release tablets. *Int. J. Pharm.* **2017**, *519*, 186–197. [CrossRef]
72. Arafat, B.; Wojsz, M.; Isreb, A.; Forbes, R.T.; Isreb, M.; Ahmed, W.; Arafat, T.; Alhnan, M.A. Tablet fragmentation without a disintegrant: A novel design approach for accelerating disintegration and drug release from 3D printed cellulosic tablets. *Eur. J. Pharm. Sci.* **2018**, *118*, 191–199. [CrossRef]
73. Saviano, M.; Aquino, R.P.; Del Gaudio, P.; Sansone, F.; Russo, P. Poly (vinyl alcohol) 3D printed tablets: The effect of polymer particle size on drug loading and process efficiency. *Int. J. Pharm.* **2019**, *561*, 1–8. [CrossRef]
74. Pereira, B.C.; Isreb, A.; Forbes, R.T.; Dores, F.; Habashy, R.; Petit, J.-B.; Alhnan, M.A.; Oga, E.F. 'Temporary Plasticiser': A novel solution to fabricate 3D printed patient-centred cardiovascular 'Polypill' architectures. *Eur. J. Pharm. Biopharm.* **2019**, *135*, 94–103. [CrossRef] [PubMed]
75. Ilyés, K.; Balogh, A.; Casian, T.; Igricz, T.; Borbás, E.; Démuth, B.; Vass, P.; Menyhárt, L.; Kovács, N.K.; Marosi, G. 3D Floating tablets: Appropriate 3d design from the perspective of different in vitro dissolution testing methodologies. *Int. J. Pharm.* **2019**, *567*, 118433. [CrossRef] [PubMed]
76. Khaled, S.A.; Burley, J.C.; Alexander, M.R.; Yang, J.; Roberts, C.J. 3D printing of tablets containing multiple drugs with defined release profiles. *In. J. Pharm.* **2015**, *494*, 643–650. [CrossRef] [PubMed]
77. Conceição, J.; Farto-Vaamonde, X.; Goyanes, A.; Adeoye, O.; Concheiro, A.; Cabral-Marques, H.; Sousa Lobo, J.M.; Alvarez-Lorenzo, C. Hydroxypropyl-β-cyclodextrin-based fast dissolving carbamazepine printlets prepared by semisolid extrusion 3D printing. *Carbohydr. Polym.* **2019**, *221*, 55–62. [CrossRef]
78. Corporation, T.L. Carbopol®Polymer Products. Available online: https://www.lubrizol.com/Life-Sciences/Products/Carbopol-Polymer-Products (accessed on 29 December 2019).
79. Corporation, T.L. Carbopol®971P NF Polymer. Available online: https://www.lubrizol.com/en/Life-Sciences/Products/Carbopol-Polymer-Products/Carbopol-971P-NF-Polymer (accessed on 29 December 2019).
80. Corporation, T.L. Carbopol®974P NF Polymer. Available online: https://www.lubrizol.com/Life-Sciences/Products/Carbopol-Polymer-Products/Carbopol-974P-NF-Polymer (accessed on 29 December 2019).
81. Cellulosics, D. *ETHOCEL™: Ethylcellulose Polymers Technical Handbook*; TDC Company: Fairfield, NJ, USA, 2005; p. 28.
82. Kempin, W.; Franz, C.; Koster, L.-C.; Schneider, F.; Bogdahn, M.; Weitschies, W.; Seidlitz, A. Assessment of different polymers and drug loads for fused deposition modeling of drug loaded implants. *Eur. J. Pharm. Biopharm.* **2017**, *115*, 84–93. [CrossRef]
83. Thakral, S.; Thakral, N.K.; Majumdar, D.K. Eudragit®: A technology evaluation. *Exp. Opin. Drug Deliv.* **2013**, *10*, 131–149. [CrossRef]
84. Evonik. Eudragit®Setting Benchmarks in Oral Solid Dosage Forms Since 1954. Available online: https://healthcare.evonik.com/sites/lists/NC/DocumentsHC/Evonik-Eudragit_brochure.pdf (accessed on 22 December 2019).
85. Prasad, L.K.; Smyth, H. 3D Printing technologies for drug delivery: A review. *Drug Dev. Ind. Pharm.* **2016**, *42*, 1019–1031. [CrossRef]

86. Picker-Freyer, K.M.; Dürig, T. Physical mechanical and tablet formation properties of hydroxypropylcellulose: In pure form and in mixtures. *AAPS PharmSciTech* **2007**, *8*, 82. [CrossRef]
87. Ashland Inc. Klucel™ Hydroxypropylcellulose—Physical and Chemical Properties. Available online: https://www.ashland.com/file_source/Ashland/Product/Documents/Pharmaceutical/PC_11229_Klucel_HPC.pdf (accessed on 22 December 2019).
88. Li, C.L.; Martini, L.G.; Ford, J.L.; Roberts, M. The use of hypromellose in oral drug delivery. *J. Pharm. Pharmacol.* **2005**, *57*, 533–546. [CrossRef]
89. Siepmann, J.; Peppas, N. Modeling of drug release from delivery systems based on hydroxypropyl methylcellulose (HPMC). *Adv. Drug Deliv. Rev.* **2012**, *64*, 163–174. [CrossRef]
90. Ethers, M.C. *Technical Handbook*; Dow Chemical Company: Midland, MI, USA, 1997.
91. Gómez-Carracedo, A.; Alvarez-Lorenzo, C.; Gómez-Amoza, J.; Concheiro, A. Chemical structure and glass transition temperature of non-ionic cellulose ethers. *J. Therm. Anal. Calorim.* **2003**, *73*, 587–596. [CrossRef]
92. Patlolla, A.; Collins, G.; Arinzeh, T.L. Solvent-dependent properties of electrospun fibrous composites for bone tissue regeneration. *Acta Biomater.* **2010**, *6*, 90–101. [CrossRef] [PubMed]
93. Goyanes, A.; Det-Amornrat, U.; Wang, J.; Basit, A.W.; Gaisford, S. 3D scanning and 3D printing as innovative technologies for fabricating personalized topical drug delivery systems. *J. Control. Release* **2016**, *234*, 41–48. [CrossRef] [PubMed]
94. Ulery, B.D.; Nair, L.S.; Laurencin, C.T. Biomedical applications of biodegradable polymers. *J. Polym. Sci. Part B* **2011**, *49*, 832–864. [CrossRef]
95. Gunatillake, P.; Mayadunne, R.; Adhikari, R. Recent developments in biodegradable synthetic polymers. *Biotechnol. Annu. Rev.* **2006**, *12*, 301–347.
96. Boetker, J.; Water, J.J.; Aho, J.; Arnfast, L.; Bohr, A.; Rantanen, J. Modifying release characteristics from 3D printed drug-eluting products. *Eur. J. Pharm. Sci.* **2016**, *90*, 47–52. [CrossRef]
97. Dwivedi, C.; Pandey, H.; Pandey, A.C.; Patil, S.; Ramteke, P.W.; Laux, P.; Luch, A.; Singh, A.V. In vivo biocompatibility of electrospun biodegradable dual carrier (antibiotic+ growth factor) in a mouse model—Implications for rapid wound healing. *Pharmaceutics* **2019**, *11*, 180. [CrossRef]
98. Farah, S.; Anderson, D.G.; Langer, R. Physical and mechanical properties of PLA, and their functions in widespread applications—A comprehensive review. *Adv. Drug Deliv. Rev.* **2016**, *107*, 367–392. [CrossRef]
99. Fu, J.; Yin, H.; Yu, X.; Xie, C.; Jiang, H.; Jin, Y.; Sheng, F. Combination of 3D printing technologies and compressed tablets for preparation of riboflavin floating tablet-in-device (TiD) systems. *Int. J. Pharm.* **2018**, *549*, 370–379. [CrossRef]
100. Goyanes, A.; Kobayashi, M.; Martínez-Pacheco, R.; Gaisford, S.; Basit, A.W. Fused-filament 3D printing of drug products: Microstructure analysis and drug release characteristics of PVA-based caplets. *Int. J. Pharm.* **2016**, *514*, 290–295. [CrossRef]
101. Morita, R.; Honda, R.; Takahashi, Y. Development of oral controlled release preparations, a PVA swelling controlled release system (SCRS): I. Design of SCRS and its release controlling factor. *J. Control. Release* **2000**, *63*, 297–304. [CrossRef]
102. Gupta, S.; Webster, T.J.; Sinha, A. Evolution of PVA gels prepared without crosslinking agents as a cell adhesive surface. *J. Mater. Sci. Mater. Med.* **2011**, *22*, 1763–1772. [CrossRef] [PubMed]
103. Matijašić, G.; Gretić, M.; Vinčić, J.; Poropat, A.; Cuculić, L.; Rahelić, T. Design and 3D printing of multi-compartmental PVA capsules for drug delivery. *J. Drug Deliv. Sci.* **2019**, *52*, 677–686. [CrossRef]
104. Haaf, F.; Sanner, A.; Straub, F. Polymers of N-vinylpyrrolidone: Synthesis, characterization and uses. *Polym. J.* **1985**, *17*, 143. [CrossRef]
105. Sigma, M. Poly(ethylene glycol) and Poly(ethylene oxide). Available online: https://www.sigmaaldrich.com/materials-science/material-science-products.html?TablePage=20204110 (accessed on 20 December 2019).
106. Pelras, T.; Glass, S.; Scherzer, T.; Elsner, C.; Schulze, A.; Abel, B. Transparent low molecular weight poly (ethylene glycol) diacrylate-based hydrogels as film media for photoswitchable drugs. *Polymers* **2017**, *9*, 639. [CrossRef]
107. Hardung, H.; Djuric, D.; Ali, S. Combining HME & solubilization: Soluplus®—The solid solution. *Drug Deliv. Technol.* **2010**, *10*, 20–27.
108. Goyanes, A.; Chang, H.; Sedough, D.; Hatton, G.B.; Wang, J.; Buanz, A.; Gaisford, S.; Basit, A.W. Fabrication of controlled-release budesonide tablets via desktop (FDM) 3D printing. *Int. J. Pharm.* **2015**, *496*, 414–420. [CrossRef]

109. Aho, J.; Boetker, J.P.; Baldursdottir, S.; Rantanen, J. Rheology as a tool for evaluation of melt processability of innovative dosage forms. *Int. J. Pharm.* **2015**, *494*, 623–642. [CrossRef]
110. Yang, Y.; Wang, H.; Li, H.; Ou, Z.; Yang, G. 3D printed tablets with internal scaffold structure using ethyl cellulose to achieve sustained ibuprofen release. *Eur. J. Pharm. Sci.* **2018**, *115*, 11–18. [CrossRef]
111. Baumgart, F. Stiffness-an unknown world of mechanical science? *Injury* **2000**, *31*, 14–23.
112. Okwuosa, T.C.; Stefaniak, D.; Arafat, B.; Isreb, A.; Wan, K.-W.; Alhnan, M.A. A lower temperature FDM 3D printing for the manufacture of patient-specific immediate release tablets. *Pharm. Res.* **2016**, *33*, 2704–2712. [CrossRef] [PubMed]
113. Lewis, J.A.; Gratson, G.M. Direct writing in three dimensions. *Mater. Today* **2004**, *7*, 32–39. [CrossRef]
114. Rattanakit, P.; Moulton, S.E.; Santiago, K.S.; Liawruangrath, S.; Wallace, G.G. Extrusion printed polymer structures: A facile and versatile approach to tailored drug delivery platforms. *Int. J. Pharm.* **2012**, *422*, 254–263. [CrossRef]
115. Solanki, N.G.; Gumaste, S.G.; Shah, A.V.; Serajuddin, A.T. Effects of Surfactants on Itraconazole-Hydroxypropyl Methylcellulose Acetate Succinate Solid Dispersion Prepared by Hot Melt Extrusion. II: Rheological Analysis and Extrudability Testing. *J. Pharm. Sci.* **2019**, *108*, 3063–3073. [CrossRef]
116. Elbadawi, M. Rheological and Mechanical Investigation into the Effect of Different Molecular Weight Poly (ethylene glycol) s on Polycaprolactone-Ciprofloxacin Filaments. *ACS Omega* **2019**, *4*, 5412–5423. [CrossRef] [PubMed]
117. Polamaplly, P.; Cheng, Y.; Shi, X.; Manikandan, K.; Zhang, X.; Kremer, G.E.; Qin, H. 3D printing and characterization of hydroxypropyl methylcellulose and methylcellulose for biodegradable support structures. *Polymer* **2019**, *173*, 119–126. [CrossRef]
118. Suwardie, H.; Wang, P.; Todd, D.B.; Panchal, V.; Yang, M.; Gogos, C.G. Rheological study of the mixture of acetaminophen and polyethylene oxide for hot-melt extrusion application. *Eur. J. Pharm.* **2011**, *78*, 506–512. [CrossRef] [PubMed]
119. Rahim, T.N.A.T.; Abdullah, A.M.; Md Akil, H. Recent Developments in Fused Deposition Modeling-Based 3D Printing of Polymers and Their Composites. *Polym. Rev.* **2019**, *59*, 589–624. [CrossRef]
120. Tanner, R.; Keentok, M. Shear fracture in cone-plate rheometry. *J. Rheol.* **1983**, *27*, 47–57. [CrossRef]
121. Cox, W.; Merz, E. Correlation of dynamic and steady flow viscosities. *J. Polym. Sci.* **1958**, *28*, 619–622. [CrossRef]
122. Cicala, G.; Giordano, D.; Tosto, C.; Filippone, G.; Recca, A.; Blanco, I. Polylactide (PLA) filaments a biobased solution for additive manufacturing: Correlating rheology and thermomechanical properties with printing quality. *Materials* **2018**, *11*, 1191. [CrossRef] [PubMed]
123. Yang, M.; Wang, P.; Suwardie, H.; Gogos, C. Determination of acetaminophen's solubility in poly (ethylene oxide) by rheological, thermal and microscopic methods. *Int. J. Pharm.* **2011**, *403*, 83–89. [CrossRef] [PubMed]
124. Hu, Y.; Wang, J.; Li, X.; Hu, X.; Zhou, W.; Dong, X.; Wang, C.; Yang, Z.; Binks, B.P. Facile preparation of bioactive nanoparticle/poly(ε-caprolactone) hierarchical porous scaffolds via 3D printing of high internal phase Pickering emulsions. *J. Colloid Interface Sci.* **2019**, *545*, 104–115. [CrossRef] [PubMed]
125. Kim, M.H.; Lee, Y.W.; Jung, W.-K.; Oh, J.; Nam, S.Y. Enhanced rheological behaviors of alginate hydrogels with carrageenan for extrusion-based bioprinting. *J. Mech. Behav. Biomed. Mater.* **2019**, *98*, 187–194. [CrossRef]
126. Ibrahim, M.; Barnes, M.; McMillin, R.; Cook, D.W.; Smith, S.; Halquist, M.; Wijesinghe, D.; Roper, T.D. 3D Printing of Metformin HCl PVA Tablets by Fused Deposition Modeling: Drug Loading, Tablet Design, and Dissolution Studies. *AAPS PharmSciTech* **2019**, *20*, 195. [CrossRef]
127. Tagami, T.; Fukushige, K.; Ogawa, E.; Hayashi, N.; Ozeki, T. 3D printing factors important for the fabrication of polyvinylalcohol filament-based tablets. *Biol. Pharm. Bull.* **2017**, *40*, 357–364. [CrossRef]
128. Prasad, E.; Islam, M.T.; Goodwin, D.J.; Megarry, A.J.; Halbert, G.W.; Florence, A.J.; Robertson, J. Development of a hot-melt extrusion (HME) process to produce drug loaded Affinisol™ 15LV filaments for fused filament fabrication (FFF) 3D printing. *Addit. Manuf.* **2019**, *29*, 100776. [CrossRef]
129. Öblom, H.; Zhang, J.; Pimparade, M.; Speer, I.; Preis, M.; Repka, M.; Sandler, N. 3D-Printed Isoniazid Tablets for the Treatment and Prevention of Tuberculosis—Personalized Dosing and Drug Release. *AAPS PharmSciTech* **2019**, *20*, 52. [CrossRef]
130. Verstraete, G.; Samaro, A.; Grymonpré, W.; Vanhoorne, V.; Van Snick, B.; Boone, M.; Hellemans, T.; Van Hoorebeke, L.; Remon, J.P.; Vervaet, C. 3D printing of high drug loaded dosage forms using thermoplastic polyurethanes. *Int. J. Pharm.* **2018**, *536*, 318–325. [CrossRef]

131. Goyanes, A.; Fina, F.; Martorana, A.; Sedough, D.; Gaisford, S.; Basit, A.W. Development of modified release 3D printed tablets (printlets) with pharmaceutical excipients using additive manufacturing. *Int. J. Pharm.* **2017**, *527*, 21–30. [CrossRef] [PubMed]

132. Sadia, M.; Isreb, A.; Abbadi, I.; Isreb, M.; Aziz, D.; Selo, A.; Timmins, P.; Alhnan, M.A. From 'fixed dose combinations' to 'a dynamic dose combiner': 3D printed bi-layer antihypertensive tablets. *Eur. J. Pharm. Sci.* **2018**, *123*, 484–494. [CrossRef] [PubMed]

133. Fuenmayor, E.; Forde, M.; Healy, A.; Devine, D.; Lyons, J.; McConville, C.; Major, I. Material considerations for fused-filament fabrication of solid dosage forms. *Pharmaceutics* **2018**, *10*, 44. [CrossRef]

134. Aho, J.; Genina, N.; Edinger, M.; Botker, J.P.; Baldursdottir, S.; Rantanen, J. Drug-loaded poly (ε-caprolactone) for 3D printing of personalized medicine: A rheological study. In Proceedings of the 25th Nordic Rheology Conference, Helsinki, Finland, 30 May–1 June 2016; pp. 97–100.

135. Isreb, A.; Baj, K.; Wojsz, M.; Isreb, M.; Peak, M.; Alhnan, M.A. 3D printed oral theophylline doses with innovative 'radiator-like'design: Impact of polyethylene oxide (PEO) molecular weight. *Int. J. Pharm.* **2019**, *564*, 98–105. [CrossRef] [PubMed]

136. Ilyés, K.; Kovács, N.K.; Balogh, A.; Borbás, E.; Farkas, B.; Casian, T.; Marosi, G.; Tomuță, I.; Nagy, Z.K. The applicability of pharmaceutical polymeric blends for the fused deposition modelling (FDM) 3D technique: Material considerations–printability–process modulation, with consecutive effects on in vitro release, stability and degradation. *Eur. J. Pharm. Sci.* **2019**, *129*, 110–123. [CrossRef] [PubMed]

137. Solanki, N.G.; Tahsin, M.; Shah, A.V.; Serajuddin, A.T. Formulation of 3D printed tablet for rapid drug release by fused deposition modeling: Screening polymers for drug release, drug-polymer miscibility and printability. *J. Pharm. Sci.* **2018**, *107*, 390–401. [CrossRef] [PubMed]

138. Aho, J.; Van Renterghem, J.; Arnfast, L.; De Beer, T.; Rantanen, J. The flow properties and presence of crystals in drug-polymer mixtures: Rheological investigation combined with light microscopy. *Int. J. Pharm.* **2017**, *528*, 383–394. [CrossRef] [PubMed]

139. Zidan, A.; Alayoubi, A.; Asfari, S.; Coburn, J.; Ghammraoui, B.; Aqueel, S.; Cruz, C.N.; Ashraf, M. Development of mechanistic models to identify critical formulation and process variables of pastes for 3D printing of modified release tablets. *Int. J. Pharm.* **2019**, *555*, 109–123. [CrossRef]

140. Van Renterghem, J.; Vervaet, C.; De Beer, T. Rheological characterization of molten polymer-drug dispersions as a predictive tool for pharmaceutical hot-melt extrusion processability. *Pharm. Res.* **2017**, *34*, 2312–2321. [CrossRef]

141. Gupta, S.S.; Solanki, N.; Serajuddin, A.T. Investigation of thermal and viscoelastic properties of polymers relevant to hot melt extrusion, IV: Affinisol™ HPMC HME polymers. *AAPS PharmSciTech* **2016**, *17*, 148–157. [CrossRef]

142. Goyanes, A.; Allahham, N.; Trenfield, S.J.; Stoyanov, E.; Gaisford, S.; Basit, A.W. Direct powder extrusion 3D printing: Fabrication of drug products using a novel single-step process. *Int. J. Pharm.* **2019**, *567*, 118471. [CrossRef]

143. Genina, N.; Boetker, J.P.; Colombo, S.; Harmankaya, N.; Rantanen, J.; Bohr, A. Anti-tuberculosis drug combination for controlled oral delivery using 3D printed compartmental dosage forms: From drug product design to in vivo testing. *J. Control. Release* **2017**, *268*, 40–48. [CrossRef] [PubMed]

144. Smith, D.; Kapoor, Y.; Hermans, A.; Nofsinger, R.; Kesisoglou, F.; Gustafson, T.P.; Procopio, A. 3D printed capsules for quantitative regional absorption studies in the GI tract. *Int. J. Pharm.* **2018**, *550*, 418–428. [CrossRef] [PubMed]

145. Huanbutta, K.; Sangnim, T. Design and development of zero-order drug release gastroretentive floating tablets fabricated by 3D printing technology. *J. Drug Deliv. Sci. Technol.* **2019**, *52*, 831–837. [CrossRef]

146. Kadry, H.; Al-Hilal, T.A.; Keshavarz, A.; Alam, F.; Xu, C.; Joy, A.; Ahsan, F. Multi-purposable filaments of HPMC for 3D printing of medications with tailored drug release and timed-absorption. *Int. J. Pharm.* **2018**, *544*, 285–296. [CrossRef]

147. Tagami, T.; Hayashi, N.; Sakai, N.; Ozeki, T. 3D printing of unique water-soluble polymer-based suppository shell for controlled drug release. *Int. J. Pharm.* **2019**, *568*, 118494. [CrossRef]

148. El Aita, I.; Breitkreutz, J.; Quodbach, J. On-demand manufacturing of immediate release levetiracetam tablets using pressure-assisted microsyringe printing. *Eur. J. Pharm. Biopharm.* **2019**, *134*, 29–36. [CrossRef]

149. Khaled, S.A.; Alexander, M.R.; Wildman, R.D.; Wallace, M.J.; Sharpe, S.; Yoo, J.; Roberts, C.J. 3D extrusion printing of high drug loading immediate release paracetamol tablets. *Int. J. Pharm.* **2018**, *538*, 223–230. [CrossRef]
150. Li, Q.; Guan, X.; Cui, M.; Zhu, Z.; Chen, K.; Wen, H.; Jia, D.; Hou, J.; Xu, W.; Yang, X.; et al. Preparation and investigation of novel gastro-floating tablets with 3D extrusion-based printing. *Int. J. Pharm.* **2018**, *535*, 325–332. [CrossRef]
151. Li, P.; Zhang, S.; Sun, W.; Cui, M.; Wen, H.; Li, Q.; Pan, W.; Yang, X. Flexibility of 3D Extruded Printing for a Novel Controlled-Release Puerarin Gastric Floating Tablet: Design of Internal Structure. *AAPS PharmSciTech* **2019**, *20*, 1–13. [CrossRef]
152. Siyawamwaya, M.; du Toit, L.C.; Kumar, P.; Choonara, Y.E.; Kondiah, P.; Pillay, V. 3D printed, controlled release, tritherapeutic tablet matrix for advanced anti-HIV-1 drug delivery. *Eur. J. Pharm. Biopharm.* **2019**, *138*, 99–110. [CrossRef]
153. Heidemann, H.M.; Laurindo, J.B.; Carciofi, B.A.M.; Costa, C.; Dotto, M.E.R. Cold plasma treatment to improve the adhesion of cassava starch films onto PCL and PLA surface. *Colloids Surfaces A* **2019**, *580*, 123739. [CrossRef]
154. Azman Mohammad Taib, M.N.; Julkapli, N.M. 4-Dimensional stability of natural fiber-based and hybrid composites. In *Mechanical and Physical Testing of Biocomposites, Fibre-Reinforced Composites and Hybrid Composites*; Jawaid, M., Thariq, M., Saba, N., Eds.; Woodhead Publishing: Cambridge, UK, 2019; pp. 61–79.
155. Awaja, F.; Gilbert, M.; Kelly, G.; Fox, B.; Pigram, P.J. Adhesion of polymers. *Prog. Polym. Sci.* **2009**, *34*, 948–968. [CrossRef]
156. Messimer, S.L.; Patterson, A.E.; Muna, N.; Deshpande, A.P.; Rocha Pereira, T. Characterization and Processing Behavior of Heated Aluminum-Polycarbonate Composite Build Plates for the FDM Additive Manufacturing Process. *J. Manuf. Mater. Process.* **2018**, *2*, 12. [CrossRef]
157. Ortega-Toro, R.; Santagata, G.; Gomez d'Ayala, G.; Cerruti, P.; Talens Oliag, P.; Chiralt Boix, M.A.; Malinconico, M. Enhancement of interfacial adhesion between starch and grafted poly(ε-caprolactone). *Carbohydr. Polym.* **2016**, *147*, 16–27. [CrossRef]
158. Gioumouxouzis, C.I.; Baklavaridis, A.; Katsamenis, O.L.; Markopoulou, C.K.; Bouropoulos, N.; Tzetzis, D.; Fatouros, D.G. A 3D printed bilayer oral solid dosage form combining metformin for prolonged and glimepiride for immediate drug delivery. *Eur. J. Pharm. Sci.* **2018**, *120*, 40–52. [CrossRef] [PubMed]
159. Vakili, H.; Kolakovic, R.; Genina, N.; Marmion, M.; Salo, H.; Ihalainen, P.; Peltonen, J.; Sandler, N. Hyperspectral imaging in quality control of inkjet printed personalised dosage forms. *Int. J. Pharm.* **2015**, *483*, 244–249. [CrossRef]
160. Alomari, M.; Mohamed, F.H.; Basit, A.W.; Gaisford, S. Personalised dosing: Printing a dose of one's own medicine. *Int. J. Pharm.* **2015**, *494*, 568–577. [CrossRef]
161. Cheah, C.; Leong, K.; Chua, C.; Low, K.; Quek, H. Characterization of microfeatures in selective laser sintered drug delivery devices. *Proc. Inst. Mech. Eng. Part H J. Eng. Med.* **2002**, *216*, 369–383. [CrossRef]
162. Amza, C.; Zapciu, A.; Popescu, D. Paste Extruder—Hardware Add-On for Desktop 3D Printers. *Technologies* **2017**, *5*, 50. [CrossRef]
163. Neches, R.Y.; Flynn, K.J.; Zaman, L.; Tung, E.; Pudlo, N. On the intrinsic sterility of 3D printing. *PeerJ* **2016**, *4*, e2661. [CrossRef]
164. Campbell, R. Pharma to table: 3-D printing and the regulatory future of home remedies. *Conn. L. Rev. CONNtemplations* **2017**, *49*, 1.
165. Zhang, J.; Yang, W.; Vo, A.Q.; Feng, X.; Ye, X.; Kim, D.W.; Repka, M.A. Hydroxypropyl methylcellulose-based controlled release dosage by melt extrusion and 3D printing: Structure and drug release correlation. *Carbohydr. Polym.* **2017**, *177*, 49–57. [CrossRef] [PubMed]
166. Cheng, K.; Zhu, J.; Song, X.; Sun, L.; Zhang, J. Studies of Hydroxypropyl Methylcellulose Donut-Shaped Tablets. *Drug Dev. Ind. Pharm.* **1999**, *25*, 1067. [CrossRef] [PubMed]
167. Lim, S.H.; Kathuria, H.; Tan, J.J.Y.; Kang, L. (2018). 3D printed drug delivery and testing systems—A passing fad or the future. *Adv. Drug Delivery Rev.* **2018**, *132*, 139–168. [CrossRef]
168. Food, U.; Administration, D. Facts about the Current Good Manufacturing Practices (CGMPs). Available online: https://www.fda.gov/drugs/pharmaceutical-quality-resources/facts-about-current-good-manufacturing-practices-cgmps (accessed on 15 December 2019).

169. Melocchi, A.; Parietti, F.; Maccagnan, S.; Ortenzi, M.A.; Antenucci, S.; Briatico-Vangosa, F.; Maroni, A.; Gazzaniga, A.; Zema, L. Industrial Development of a 3D-Printed Nutraceutical Delivery Platform in the Form of a Multicompartment HPC Capsule. *AAPS PharmSciTech* **2018**, *19*, 3343–3354. [CrossRef]
170. Sanderson, K. 3D printing: The future of manufacturing medicine. *Pharm. J.* **2015**, *294*, 598–600.
171. FDA. Are You Taking Medication as Prescribed? Available online: https://www.fda.gov/consumers/consumer-updates/are-you-taking-medication-prescribed (accessed on 16 December 2019).
172. Florence, A.T.; Lee, V.H. Personalised medicines: More tailored drugs, more tailored delivery. *Int. J. Pharm.* **2011**, *415*, 29–33. [CrossRef]
173. Schiele, J.T.; Quinzler, R.; Klimm, H.-D.; Pruszydlo, M.G.; Haefeli, W.E. Difficulties swallowing solid oral dosage forms in a general practice population: Prevalence, causes, and relationship to dosage forms. *Eur. J. Clinical Pharmacol.* **2013**, *69*, 937–948. [CrossRef]
174. Spence, J.D. Polypill: For Pollyanna. *Int. J. Stroke* **2008**, *3*, 92–97. [CrossRef]
175. Pharmaceuticals, C. About PolycapTM. Available online: http://www.polycap.org/ (accessed on 16 December 2019).
176. Urquhart, J. The indian polycap study (TIPS). *Lancet* **2009**, *374*, 781–782. [CrossRef]
177. Wu, W.; Zheng, Q.; Guo, X.; Sun, J.; Liu, Y. A programmed release multi-drug implant fabricated by three-dimensional printing technology for bone tuberculosis therapy. *Biomed. Mater.* **2009**, *4*, 065005. [CrossRef] [PubMed]
178. Acosta-Vélez, G.; Linsley, C.; Zhu, T.; Wu, W.; Wu, B. Photocurable Bioinks for the 3D Pharming of Combination Therapies. *Polymers* **2018**, *10*, 1372. [CrossRef] [PubMed]
179. Haring, A.P.; Tong, Y.; Halper, J.; Johnson, B.N. Programming of multicomponent temporal release profiles in 3D printed polypills via core–shell, multilayer, and gradient concentration profiles. *Adv. Healthc. Mater.* **2018**, *7*, 1800213. [CrossRef] [PubMed]
180. Fastø, M.M.; Genina, N.; Kaae, S.; Sporrong, S.K. Perceptions, preferences and acceptability of patient designed 3D printed medicine by polypharmacy patients: A pilot study. *Int. J. Clin. Pharm.* **2019**, *41*, 1290–1298. [CrossRef] [PubMed]
181. Robles-Martinez, P.; Xu, X.; Trenfield, S.J.; Awad, A.; Goyanes, A.; Telford, R.; Basit, A.W.; Gaisford, S. 3D Printing of a Multi-Layered Polypill Containing Six Drugs Using a Novel Stereolithographic Method. *Pharmaceutics* **2019**, *11*, 274. [CrossRef]
182. Goyanes, A.; Wang, J.; Buanz, A.; Martínez-Pacheco, R.; Telford, R.; Gaisford, S.; Basit, A.W. 3D Printing of Medicines: Engineering Novel Oral Devices with Unique Design and Drug Release Characteristics. *Mol. Pharm.* **2015**, *12*, 4077–4084. [CrossRef]

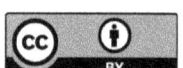

© 2020 by the authors. Licensee MDPI, Basel, Switzerland. This article is an open access article distributed under the terms and conditions of the Creative Commons Attribution (CC BY) license (http://creativecommons.org/licenses/by/4.0/).

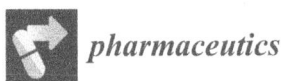

Review

Application of Micro-Scale 3D Printing in Pharmaceutics

Andrew Kjar and Yu Huang *

Department of Biological Engineering, Utah State University, Logan, UT 84322, USA
* Correspondence: yu.huang@usu.edu

Received: 30 June 2019; Accepted: 1 August 2019; Published: 3 August 2019

Abstract: 3D printing, as one of the most rapidly-evolving fabrication technologies, has released a cascade of innovation in the last two decades. In the pharmaceutical field, the integration of 3D printing technology has offered unique advantages, especially at the micro-scale. When printed at a micro-scale, materials and devices can provide nuanced solutions to controlled release, minimally invasive delivery, high-precision targeting, biomimetic models for drug discovery and development, and future opportunities for personalized medicine. This review aims to cover the recent advances in this area. First, the 3D printing techniques are introduced with respect to the technical parameters and features that are uniquely related to each stage of pharmaceutical development. Then specific micro-sized pharmaceutical applications of 3D printing are summarized and grouped according to the provided benefits. Both advantages and challenges are discussed for each application. We believe that these technologies provide compelling future solutions for modern medicine, while challenges remain for scale-up and regulatory approval.

Keywords: additive manufacturing; 3D printing; drug delivery; micromedicine; drug development; micro-swimmer; micro-implant; oral dosages; microneedle; high-precision targeting; controlled release; geometry; resolution; feature size; personalized medicine; release profile; vascularization

1. Introduction

Pharmaceutical development is commonly considered to proceed in three main stages: drug discovery, drug development, and drug delivery [1]. In drug discovery, a suitable target is first identified. Afterwards, a library of compounds is screened for activity with the biological target, from which an active compound is selected. In drug development, the active compound is then tested in various settings, including in vitro models, in vivo animal studies, and clinical trials. During these regulatory phases of intense development and testing, the exact dosing and delivery methods are optimized. Drug delivery is comprised of precise delivery of the active pharmaceutical compound and encompasses possibilities from oral dosages to drug-eluting micro-implants.

There are challenges which currently face each phase of pharmaceutical development. Drug development is a long, costly process. Typically, a new pharmaceutical entity will take over a decade to enter the market, requiring upwards of one billion dollars [2]. However, many drugs fail in later stages of clinical trials [3], as in vitro and animal models fail to fully predict drug reaction in humans. Animal models often produce data that are limited in their ability to translate to humans [4]. To this end, a heavy focus of drug development research seeks more realistic and effective in vitro models.

Manufacturing better models for drug development proves to be challenging because the in vivo response is highly nuanced [5]. A key feature of human biological systems is exquisite spatial patterning and organization, down to the micron range It has long been known that cell response, morphology, chemotaxis, messaging, and differentiation depend on the micro-scale environmental conditions. Thus, in vitro models seek to faithfully recapitulate critical features of in vivo as closely as possible [6].

The goal of pharmaceutical drug delivery is similarly complex: the ideal drug should be highly specific in reaching and affecting its intended target, while minimizing side effects [7]. Many compounds display inhibitory or therapeutic effects at some minimum concentration, but increase in toxicity and side effects with increased dose, having some functional therapeutic window. Some drugs may have narrow therapeutic windows [8], need to be tissue-specific [9], or are specific to certain patients' genetics. Individual biological systems are incredibly sensitive to location, dose, and timing of medication. Because these effects are sophisticated, medicine tailored to an individual is an attractive target for the industry [9].

However, today's market has a limited possibility to produce personalized medicines [10]. For example, in the case of oral delivery, conventional batch methods cannot feasibly make every dose size. Splitting doses to overcome this is associated with dose variation, and it compromises dose coatings [11]. Additionally, current manufacturing cannot make different shaped tablets [10]. Inflexible dosage regimes highlight a need in the pharmaceutical industry that cannot be met through current manufacturing methods. Thus, innovative solutions are necessary.

This review aims to cover recent advances in additive manufacturing with regards to micro-sized biomedical applications, and the potential solutions they provide to these stated challenges in drug delivery and development. The purpose of this article is to show that the integration of 3D printing technology has unique advantages. At a micro-scale, 3D-printed materials can provide nuanced solutions to controlled release, minimally invasive delivery, high-precision targeting, biomimetic models for drug discovery and development, and future opportunities for personalized medicine. Specific micro-sized pharmaceutical applications of 3D printing are summarized and grouped according to the provided benefits.

2. Additive Manufacturing: Methods and Resolution

3D printing, more formally known as additive manufacturing, is rapidly becoming one of the most well-known and innovative technologies of the 21st century. Additive manufacturing is a number of manufacturing techniques in which material is selectively placed in a layer-by-layer fashion (Figure 1), including material extrusion, material jetting, binder jetting, selective laser sintering, and vat polymerization. Each of these techniques is currently applied in the pharmaceutical field, and thus are presented here [12–35].

2.1. Material Extrusion

Material extrusion is the least costly and most common type of 3D printing [36]. There are two major categories: fused deposition modeling and semisolid extrusion [37]. In both approaches, the preprinting material is extruded in a continuous stream through a nozzle. The nozzle or the platform (or a combination of the two) is moved in the x, y, and z directions to produce the final desired geometry.

Fused deposition modeling utilizes a heated extrusion nozzle. Filaments are fed through the heated nozzle and then deposited onto the print bed containing the emerging part. As the filament cools, the layers fuse together. Heat-based printer nozzles are essentially limited to thermoplastics, as the material must decrease in solidity and viscosity as the temperature is increased, and then harden and bond on the print bed [38]. For pharmaceutical applications, filaments are usually prepared by incorporating active compounds via hot melt extrusion; however, recent advances include direct powder extrusion, which circumvents this process, and may enable a larger number of printable materials [39].

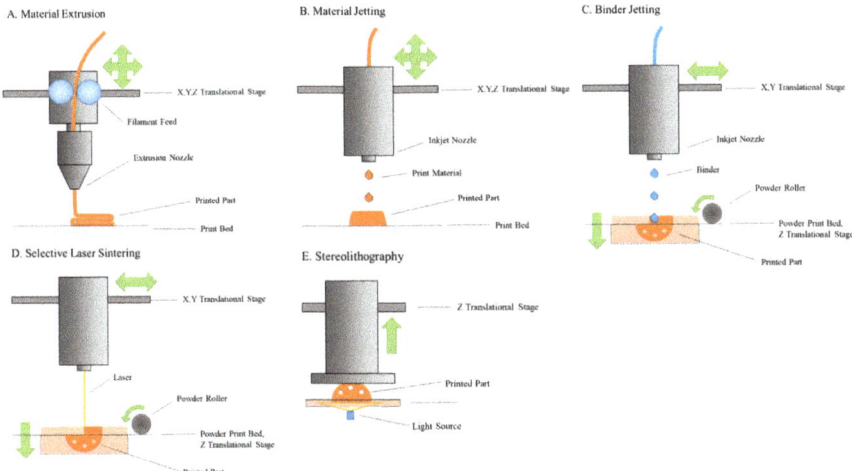

Figure 1. Typical additive manufacturing mechanisms. Additive manufacturing techniques are classified by their deposition of material in a layer-by-layer fashion. Material extrusion (**A**) traditionally deposits thermoplastic materials, but also includes pneumatic and mechanical deposition of semisolid materials. Both material jetting (**B**) and binder jetting (**C**) rely on familiar inkjet heads; in material jetting the entire print material passes through the nozzle, while in binder jetting, only a binder is deposited. An advantage of binder jetting is the support of the powder bed, negating the need for support structures or sacrificial material. This mechanism is also seen in selective laser sintering (**D**), where the powder bed is selectively fused by a laser. Finally, stereolithography (**E**) selectively polymerizes a liquid resin vat, thereby producing the desired part.

Semisolid extrusion techniques extend extrusion printing to a wider range of temperatures and materials, including living material (termed "bioprinting") [40]. Instead of relying solely on heat, semisolid extrusion printers can print a variety of materials using pneumatic or mechanical extrusion forces. In these systems, the rheological properties of the fluid to be printed and the method of solidification must be carefully considered. For steady extrusion, fluids must have the correct viscosity. Non-Newtonian fluid behavior, such as shear rate dependence, is often a factor that must be taken into account [41]. After extrusion, solidification can occur through physical or chemical processes. For example, printers fitted with UV lamps can cross-link newly printed layers of photolinked hydrogels. Alternatively, the crosslinking agent may be printed at the same time as the print material [42]. These gelation processes are a key consideration in the design of materials to be used in semisolid extrusion prints.

The motions in the x–y plane and z-axis are typically actuated with extreme precision—down to 1 micron. In terms of feature resolution, fused deposition modeling is essentially limited by the size of the extrusion nozzle. Typical sizes of fused deposition nozzles are in the range of 400 microns [43–46]. Semisolid extrusion usually has relatively poor feature resolution, as lower-viscosity substances spread upon printing [37].

Hybrid techniques can push the feature resolution of extrusion printing to the range of ten microns [47]. In these printers, the extruded filament is subjected to an electric force, producing a much smaller filament stream. These "electrospinning" hybrids are commercially available and represent the highest resolution extrusion-based methods currently available [48,49].

2.2. Material Jetting

The mechanism of material jetting is similar to that of familiar inkjet printers. For 3D materials, the print head and platform are actuated to move in the x-, y-, and z-axis. For successful printing, the material must be cross-linkable upon delivery. As with semisolid extrusion, cross-linking processes include photo, thermal, ionic, and pH-dependent effects [41]. One of the greatest advantages of this technique is that it may be used to print multiple materials simultaneously, even materials with different properties [50]. Material jetting is used for both small molecules and bioprinting [40,41].

The final feature resolution of material-jetted prints depends on the droplet size. Print feature resolution is also highly dependent upon the rheological properties of the fluid and print speed, which must be carefully parametrized. Upon arrival onto the print, droplets tend to spread before they are fully cross-linked, which limits inkjet resolution. Additionally, the most defined features tend to be printed in parallel to the inkjet direction [36]. Inkjet manufacturers advertise feature resolution in the range of 20 to 100 microns [51].

2.3. Binder Jetting

While material extrusion and material jetting may be printed onto a variety of surfaces, binder jetting requires the use of a powder which may be selectively bound by the addition of a liquid binder. For the creation of each layer of the part, a layer of powder is spread across a printing surface [36]. An inkjet head then deposits binder in the desired geometry. The powder bed is then lowered, the new powder is spread, and another layer is selectively bound. This technique can require high volumes of powder, but has no need for sacrificial materials, as the powder bed can support the emerging part [52].

Advantages of this technique include the possibility of multimaterial printing, as multiple binding agents may be used [36]. Additionally, this manufacturing process can often occur at room temperature, and it easily makes porous structures [36]. Metals and ceramics are commonly used, but polymers may also be printed [36]. Materials printed in this way require postprocessing, such as chemical treatment, for better mechanical properties. Many printers have a feature resolution of two millimeters [36], but better printers can produce up to 50-micron feature resolution [12], dependent on powder particle size [36].

2.4. Selective Laser Sintering

Selective laser sintering occurs in a similar fashion to binder jetting, but instead of using a binder to fuse powder particles, a laser is used to sinter them together. Because of this mechanism, only materials that can be fused by laser are utilized. Metals and ceramics are common, although the use of thermoplastics is increasingly prevalent, especially in biomedical applications [13,53–55]. For all materials, careful calibration of the powder to be used is important, as particle size will affect feature print resolution, workability of particle spreading, and final print mechanical properties [56,57].

The feature resolution of selective laser sintering depends highly on the material. While some report feature resolutions in the range of 100 microns [12], selective laser sintering can be a high-resolution technique, producing features as small as 30 microns [58]. As with binder jetting, parts are usually porous and need postprocessing for smooth surfaces and mechanical strength. Additionally, selective laser sintering is usually fast and economical, requiring no support materials. When printing metals or ceramics, sterilization via an autoclave is a viable option.

2.5. Stereolithography

The oldest form of additive manufacturing, stereolithography, relies on the same techniques as its predecessor, photolithography. Stereolithography is based on the reaction of light with photopolymer resins. First, a large vat is filled with resin and subjected to a radiation source from the top or the bottom, in a desired geometric pattern. The bottom-up method, which features lower resin volumes, places the light source under the resin tank with a transparent base (as pictured in Figure 1) [37].

The light-cured layer polymerizes, and the build platform moves upwards, peeling the cured layer off the bottom surface. Another layer is then polymerized in a similar fashion. Alternatively, in top-down stereolithography, the actuator platform is lowered for each layer, requiring larger volumes of material for the part to remain fully immersed [59]. Continuous liquid interface processing (CLIP) and digital light processing (DLP) are other techniques related to stereolithography [37]. Stereolithographic techniques can offer relatively high resolution, by reaching the diffraction limit of light simply using conventional radiation sources. Some print quality can suffer from nonspecific photopolymerization due to light leakage [60]; however, the highest feature resolution is often reported as 20–30 microns in commercially available printers [61–63].

The printing process often requires post-curing, postprocessing, and sacrificial support structures. There is also a limited number of materials that may be used, but these include, prominently, photocurable polymers [37]. Some metals and ceramics may be printed in specialized machines and processes [64]. Recent studies have demonstrated the incorporation of active pharmaceuticals in the resin to be effective [65,66].

With increased cost, increased feature resolution is possible with two-photon polymerization, a specialized form of stereolithography. In two-photon polymerization, resins are polymerized using two laser beams. These machines can exceed the diffraction limit and produce feature resolution of 120 nm [67,68].

2.6. Resolution

The preceding feature resolutions are given as a range based on manufacturer specifications and literature (Figure 2 and Table 1). However, the reporting of resolution is non-standard across the industry. Manufacturers report any of the following specifications; x–y resolution, layer thickness, part accuracy, and nozzle size [43,69].

Typically, the layer thickness is the most straightforward specification to find, and values range as low as 5 microns, depending on the type of printing being used [12]. This same value may, however, be inaccurately reported as x–y resolution. Print x–y resolution is often a function of the material printing method: material extrusion rarely can provide structures finer than the nozzle, powder methods are limited by the powder size, and inkjet printers are limited by droplet size [12].

The smallest feature resolution, which is dependent on geometry, print speed, temperature, and material, is of the uppermost relevance to the biomedical designer. However, the smallest feature resolutions are not standardly reported. For example, material extrusion manufacturers commonly report accuracy to 100 microns using a 400-micron nozzle, indicating a difference between accuracy and smallest feature size [43,46]. Literature has attempted to address this [70,71], but more research in the area would be invaluable.

Continued innovation will push the boundaries of the current resolution limits, but standard printing techniques are within the range of critical biological entities [72]. All printer types can print in the micro-scale, which is defined as printing of features smaller than 1000 microns. Additive manufacturing brings unique capability to this field. While topography on a micro-scale can be created relying solely on material properties, additive manufacturing allows engineering design of specific micro geometries. As discussed in the following sections, printing on a micro-scale—within the range of single cells and microvasculature—can produce unique solutions for drug discovery, development, and delivery.

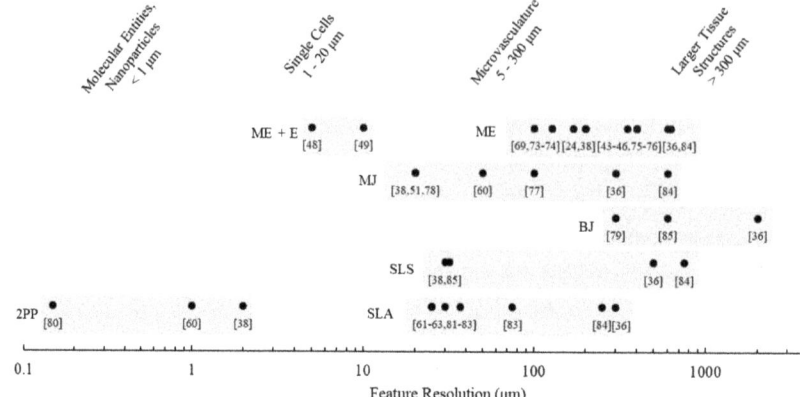

Figure 2. Maximum feature resolution of various 3D printing techniques, as compared to typical biological entities. Most techniques can print in the range of microvasculature; expensive, specialized methods, such as two-photon polymerization (2PP) and electrospinning hybrid extrusion (ME + E) are required for printing sizes comparable to single cells. Material extrusion (ME) feature resolution is essentially limited by nozzle size, while material jetting (MJ) and binder jetting (BJ) feature resolution is limited to droplet size. Binder jetting and selective laser sintering (SLS) feature resolution both depend on particle powder size, while stereolithography (SLA) has superior feature resolution based on the light source. However, for all print types, feature resolution depends highly on the designed geometry and print orientation. Data was compiled from manufacturer technical specification sheets [43–46,48,49,51,61–63,69,73–83] and literature [24,36,38,60,84,85]. Material extrusion values extracted from specification sheets are based on nozzle diameter.

Table 1. Representative commercial printers with their associated feature resolutions and applications in the literature. Feature resolution data is taken from manufacturer technical specification sheets. Material extrusion values extracted from specification sheets are based on nozzle diameter. However, the smallest feature size is dependent on geometry, print speed, temperature, and material, and is not standardly reported. High-resolution printing techniques find applications in the printing of oral dosages, microneedles, micro-swimmers, and micro-implants. Material extrusion is a popular technique in the printing of oral dosages, whereas the feature resolution of stereolithography and two-photon polymerization are necessary for use in microneedles and micro-swimmers.

3D-Printing Type	Printer	Resolution (μm)	Applications
Electrospinning Hybrid Extrusion	RegenHU Benchtop 3D Discovery Evolution	5 [48]	Oral Dosages [25,26]
	GeSiM Bioscaffolder 3.2/4.2	10 [49]	Micro-implants [29]
Material Extrusion	LulzBot TAZ 5	350 [75]	Microneedles [24]
	MakerBot Replicator 2, ZMorph 2.0 SX	400 [43–45]	Oral Dosages [30–35,86]
	Solidoodle 2 Base	400 [46]	Micro-implants [21]
Material Jetting	3D Systems Phenix PXM	20 [51]	Micro-implants [14,15]
Binder Jetting	Z Corporation Spectrum Z510	300 [79]	Micro-implants [16]
Two-Photon Polymerization	NanoScribe Photonic Professional	0.15 [80]	Microneedles [22] Micro-swimmers [19,20]
Stereolithography	Envisiontec Perfactory DSP III Standard SXGA+, Kudo 3D Titan 1, Carbon M2	25–75 [61,63,83]	Microneedles [17,27,28]
	3D Systems ProJet 6000	25 [62]	Micro-swimmers [23]

3. Controlled Release

Additive manufacturing is gaining traction for use in drug delivery, having applications in drug delivery methods and devices [87–89]. Oral drug delivery devices, tablets, are one such application of additive manufacturing in the medical field, Spritam® being the first FDA approved 3D-printed medicine. The incorporation of micro-geometry has unique advantages in terms of controlled release. Additive manufacturing can produce geometries that are impossible or impractical via typical pharmaceutical manufacturing processes (Figure 3).

One of the most straightforward geometric modifications—infill percentage—relies on the intrinsic material extrusion methods. Parts to be printed via material extrusion are commonly printed by first depositing an outer shell and subsequently filling this shell with preset infill geometry; 0% infill would leave the part fully hollow, while 100% infill creates a solid part. For use in oral drug delivery, Verstraete et al. demonstrated that lower infill percentages have faster release profiles [90]. Immediate release profiles are often desirable, as in pain relievers. Verstraete's release profile results are due to the increase of surface area to volume ratio for the prints. Importantly, Kyobula et al. likewise demonstrated that this process is also dependent on wettability [91]. Spaces and cavities under the size of 600 microns were less wettable, producing longer release times than counterparts with >600-micron cavities. Other literature reports the correlation between infill, micro-geometry creation, and release profile [92,93]. Similarly, Li et al. showed that varied infill percentage could be tailored to create gastro-flotation tablets [94]. Prolonged retention enhances the bioavailability, and lower infill percentages produce floating without sacrificing mechanical properties such as friability.

Conventional tablet release profiles are dominated by various physical forces, of which surface area to volume ratio plays a significant part. In these systems, drug release is often dominated by diffusion patterns. One method for creating more complex release profiles is the incorporation of outer layers, to produce, for example, enteric coatings which delay the release until the intestinal tract. These controlled release tablets are achievable through additive manufacturing, as demonstrated by Okwuosa et al., who showed that an outer coating of ≥520 microns was necessary to produce the intended release profile [95]. The feature resolution of the printer was also shown to affect the release profile, where low-resolution printing resulted in coating layers thicker than the nominal dimension.

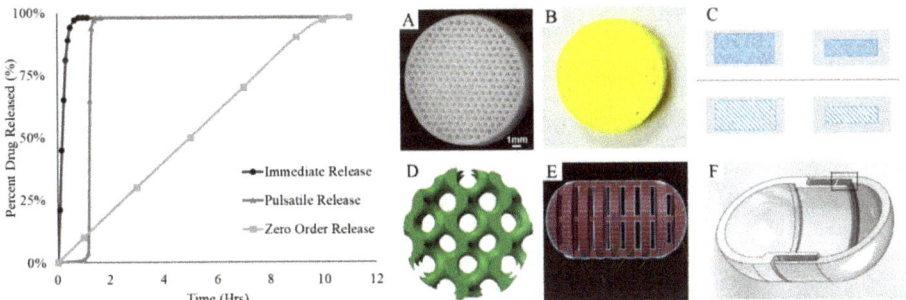

Figure 3. Idealized release profiles (left) and micro-geometry incorporation in oral dosages produced by additive manufacturing techniques (A–F). Immediate release is desirable for quick action drugs, such as pain relievers. Immediate release profiles are correlated to infill percentage (A) [91], and other factors such as wettability. Infill percentage may also be exploited for gastro-floating devices (B) [94]. If combined with a shell of variable thickness (C) [96], infill variation can also achieve tunable zero-order release. More complicated geometries offer release profiles that are dependent on erosion, providing immediate release profiles (D,E) [34,55]. Additionally, pulsatile release is possible with the fabrication of an outer shell of tunable thickness, here designed to be 600 microns (F) [33]. Reproduced with permission from Elsevier (A–F).

For multilayer tablets, Zhang et al. demonstrated that release mechanisms are dependent on several parameters, including both infill percentage and shell thickness [96]. By varying these parameters, release profiles could be dominated by diffusion or swelling (or a combination), and the authors were capable of tuning until a zero-order release was achieved. Other literature similarly reports zero-order (or constant sustained) release [97,98]. These applications demonstrate the importance of small features in CAD designs for drug delivery. Micro-geometry and feature resolution have also been shown to be important in orodispersible, thin-layer films [99,100].

Other, less familiar shapes are also possible with additive manufacturing [35,101]. Whereas varied infill produces pores that are initially separated from the aqueous media, several groups have made channels and holes that cross the entire tablet. These channels were demonstrated by both Sadia et al. and Arafat et al. to produce much faster release profiles, putting them within the pharmacopeial regulations for immediate release [30,34]. These release profiles were a function of geometry; features in the range of 1000 microns seem optimal. Erosion becomes a dominant force in the dissolution of these tablets, as the tablet breaks into pieces as time progresses. Likewise, Fina et al. found faster dissolution for their gyroid structures, which could be paired with nonporous regions for complex release profiles [55].

Many of the presented examples rely on specific pairings of active pharmaceutical and polymer, which are then extruded through hot-melt extrusion [30,33,35,86,90,96,102]. The properties (rheology for material jetting, thermoplasticity for material extrusion, and particle size for binder jetting) must be carefully tuned and parameterized for each drug. Typically, active pharmaceutical is incorporated into filament at a rate of 4–8% w/w [31,35,55,91,94]. Some attempts have been made to create fully flexible systems. For example, Melocchi et al. have demonstrated a pulsatile release profile based on material extrusion of a shell (thickness 600 microns) which could be used for any number of active pharmaceuticals [33].

4. Minimally Invasive Delivery

Hypodermal needles are common for drug delivery in which oral ingestion is inappropriate; the method, however, is invasive. Additive manufacturing provides alternative solutions for minimally invasive delivery through the design of microneedle arrays.

The first transdermal drug delivery system was introduced in 1979, and since these systems have become more sophisticated with the addition of microneedle arrays [103]. Microneedle arrays, as compared to hypodermal needles, improve patient compliance, decrease pain and tissue damage, decrease the need for skilled healthcare professionals for administration, and inhibit microbial entrance [104,105]. Additionally, transdermally delivered drugs can elicit a higher immunogenic response and increased bioavailability.

The efficacy of such systems is highly dependent on geometric properties. As Johnson et al. note, key parameters in the design of microneedle arrays include microneedle shape (height and diameter) aspect ratio, composition, strength, sharpness, spacing, and quantity [28]. For example, a decrease in aspect ratio corresponds to an increase in microneedle mechanical strength [106], whereas material composition and toughness facilitate penetration deepness [28]. Needle spacing is directly related to how much force is necessary for penetration [107]. Dimensions are variable, depending on the application. As Lu et al. note, various microneedle heights ranging from 150 to 2000 microns have been reported [103]. The microneedle array must at least penetrate the stratum corneum layer, the outermost layer of the skin, which is in the range of 10 to 20 microns [108]. To draw blood, the microneedle height must be at least 900 microns [109]. Optimal tip size is a function of material—robust materials have improved penetration at small tip sizes, while polymers at the same dimensions easily fracture [106]. The possibility of creating these structures via additive manufacturing is, therefore, limited by the feature resolution of the technology. Stereolithography (including two-photon polymerization) is the additive manufacturing technique most widely used for this purpose [22,27,28,104,109–115].

Different shapes are possible, each tailored for various applications (Figure 4). Pere et al. demonstrated that between cones and pyramids, cones took less force to penetrate, perhaps due to the decrease in microneedle-to-skin contact area [104]. Solid microneedles such as these are coated with active pharmaceutical ingredients, which are then deposited upon application. These systems must be carefully tuned for full biocompatibility and resistance to fracture. Another approach is to puncture the skin using solid microneedle arrays, and then apply drug topically, improving topical access via the punctures. Daraiswamy and Gittard developed various hollow microneedles with complex hollow geometry [111,115]. After puncture, an active pharmaceutical may be added, facilitating delivery. Alternatively, active pharmaceuticals may be incorporated with the needles and applied simultaneously. Needles are removed after application.

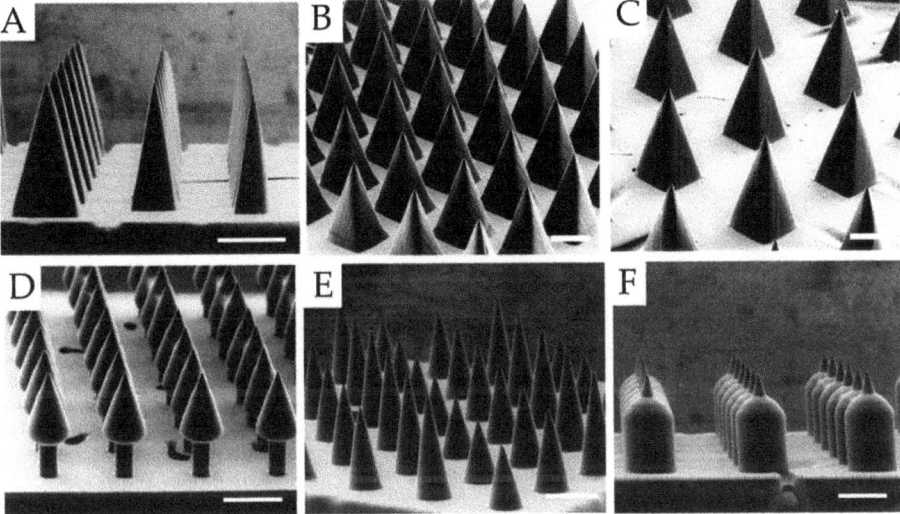

Figure 4. Microneedle providing minimally invasive delivery. Additive manufacturing brings enhanced flexibility, as shown in arbitrarily shaped microneedle arrays (**A–F**) [28]. Scale bars: 500 µm (**A–F**). Reproduced with permission from PLOS.

Fully dissolvable microneedle arrays are a viable strategy for prolonged release. These arrays are typically made through polymer molding, which is not an additive manufacturing technique [116]. Limited print material capability in stereolithography and resolution limits in other methods challenge additive manufacturing for needles of this kind. As innovative materials are developed for stereolithography, and high-resolution versions of other printing types become available, this strategy may be realized. Currently, inkjet printing for coatings of microneedle arrays has received attention as a high-resolution, highly flexible method [104,105,116–120].

Luzuriaga et al. showed an innovative approach to the fabrication of microneedles, extending the technology to material extrusion [24]. However, as expected, the feature resolution of the printer resulted in the impossibility of creating sharp peaks. The smallest producible tip diameter was more than twice the optimal size, so postprocessing in basic solution was necessary to produce viable microneedles. This speaks to why stereolithographic techniques dominate these applications. It should be noted, however, that standard resolution stereolithographic printing reports distortion in final print features, compared to the CAD model [27]. Despite challenges, additive manufacturing of microneedle arrays can streamline prototyping and enable the fabrication of complex geometries [28].

5. High-Precision Targeting

Some drug delivery applications require high-precision targeting, as do cancer treatments [7]. Highly specific delivery aims to provide a higher dose to a localized area while simultaneously reducing systemic toxicity. This delivery is often intended for parts of the body that are hard-to-reach and confined, thus making them difficult to approach through conventional methods. Thus, two lines of innovation—micro-swimmer devices and micro-implants—are fabricated to provide solutions (Figure 5).

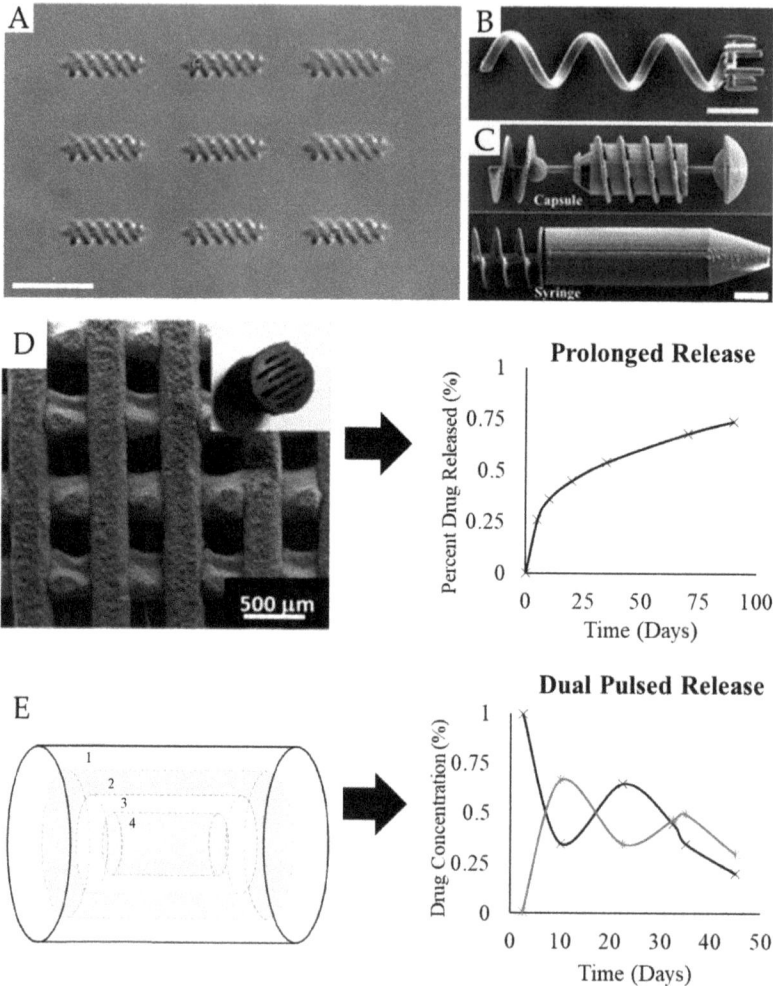

Figure 5. Examples of high-precision targeting in drug delivery. Micro-swimmer double helices (**A**) [121] are guided by a magnetic field to their target, being loaded during fabrication, while other micro-swimmers mechanically pick up the cargo (**B**) [122]. With high-resolution printing, complex micromachine structures can be fabricated, including capsules and syringes (**C**) [18]. Micro-implants can offer long term release profiles, based on drug incorporation within the scaffold in material extrusion (**D**) [123]. The dual-pulsed release is also possible, via geometric patterning in binder jetting (**E**) [124]. Scale bars: 20 μm (**A,C**) and 10 μm (**B**). (**A**) Reproduced with permission from American Chemical Society (**A**), Wiley (**B,C**), and Elsevier (**D**).

5.1. Micro-Swimmer Devices

Micro-swimmers are motile delivery devices currently under developmental research. These devices are reviewed elsewhere [125,126]; the basic principles are summarized here to highlight the incorporation of additive manufacturing into the field. Micro-swimmer devices function on a variety of mechanisms, but all have essentially three stages: loading, transportation, and release. Micro-scale geometry can contribute significantly to each stage.

Loading can be achieved through passive adsorption [19,127], surface chemistry, incorporation of pharmaceuticals in the print material [23], or mechanical trapping within arms or syringes [18,122]. In the case of arms, the micro-swimmer needs to be maneuvered carefully to entrap the particle in a ring of extending rods (Figure 5B) [122]. In the case of syringes, Huang et al. designed micro-swimmers with Archimedean screw pumps, which were magnetically actuated (Figure 5C) [18]. By alternating the magnetic field, the pump could be selectively turned one way or another, producing fluid vortices sufficient for particle trapping. These latter approaches are complex and not fully efficient—incorporation of the desired particles within the object material may prove to be the superior method. These latter means are, however, fully dependent on geometry.

Transportation mechanisms are then engineering for motion to the target tissue. Actuation methods may be based on magnetic, thermal, chemical, electrostatic, or mechanical stimuli [18]. Upon excitation by one of these stimuli, micro-swimmers will move in the desired direction, depending on their shape, working their way through in vivo vascular systems. Of these methods, magnetic actuation is prominent, as magnetic fields are noninvasive and body tissue may be considered essentially nonmagnetic. Micro-swimmer devices using this mechanism are either plated with magnetic material [18,127] or have magnetic material incorporated [23,121], so the devices will respond to a magnetic gradient or a rotating magnetic field. A rotating magnetic field is preferable for its increased strength [23].

At the micro-scale, viscous forces dominate inertial forces, especially for small devices in body fluid, a non-Newtonian fluid [128]. Thus, the geometry must be carefully constructed for motion on this scale. Natural solutions to this problem include flagella and cilia, and these solutions have inspired many of the current micro-swimmer devices [20]. A typical shape is a cylinder encased by a helix or double helix. Ceylan et al. remark that double helices are more stable than a single helix, and carefully parameterized their helix to produce optimal swimming velocity [20]. Size is also important, as micro-swimmers are meant to maneuver easily within the target tissue. However, as Hunter et al. demonstrate, there is a trade-off between smaller size and higher possible velocity [23]. Typical helical structures have a length of 20 microns with a diameter of 5 microns. Other approaches to transport are not dependent on helical geometry, but instead on the incorporation of motile sperm cells [19]. Because these devices are currently in research development, testing of motion in vivo is limited. Similarly, testing in low-Reynolds regime fluids that accurately model body fluids is not consistent in all literature, a challenge which will need to be addressed for the application of these devices in pharmaceutical administration.

Release mechanisms vary and may be dependent on simple diffusion [23], light [121], magnetic fields [18], or mechanical stimuli [19]. Even structurally similar systems can be highly variable. One hydrogel system demonstrated enzymatic degradation to release the payload [20], whereas another used light as a trigger for tunable release [121]. Akin to oral dosages, release profiles are affected by erosion and swelling processes for hydrogel micro-swimmers or diffusion for non-hydrogel systems.

For these applications, high feature resolution is necessary. Thus two-photon polymerization is almost exclusively used. Two-photon polymerization is a cutting-edge technique for prototyping these devices: no other manufacturing methods parallel in shear flexibility. However, two-photon polymerization is essentially limited to photopolymers. Incorporation of particles (such as pharmaceuticals or magnets) in the resin is one strategy to achieve a wider variety of functional materials. Micromolding from 3D-printed molds has also been demonstrated [23], boasting a wider variety of possible materials.

5.2. Micro-Implants

Non-mobile drug delivery devices can also provide high-precision targeting and release. These drug delivery methods, termed micro-implants, can provide long-lasting release profiles, regenerative tissue effects, and restoration of tissue function. Implants are a long-standing part of conventional medicine; the use of additive manufacturing in implants is similarly well established [129]. Design considerations are important for both drug-eluting and inert implants. As shown here, additive manufacturing can enable solutions for both.

Microstructure is a key feature of implanted materials as it governs interactions with resident cells [130]. Optimal pore size, for example, is dependent on tissue type. Bone implants are made with pores in the range of 200 to 400 microns [131–133]. Pore size plays a role in differentiation, cell perfusion, and nutrient exchange, and stands as an example of important micro-geometry.

Additive manufacturing has the unique capability of fabricating macrostructure and micro-geometry simultaneously. Most additive manufacturing techniques have been applied to making implant materials and tissue scaffolds, including material extrusion (both fused deposition modeling [21] and semisolid extrusion [29,134]), binder jetting [131,135], and selective laser sintering [14]. Because the microstructured design for many scaffolds is above 200 microns, the design of biomimetic pores is within the resolution range of most printers.

Ideal bone implant materials should be biodegradable, osteoconductive, osteoinductive, angiogenic, and resistant to bacteria [132]. The incorporation and controlled release of compounds into the scaffold can help create these properties. Research has shown the incorporation of growth factors (esp. recombinant human bone morphogenetic proteins (rhBMP) or vascular endothelial growth factor (VGEF)) to enhance proliferation and bone response [29,134,136]. Antibiotics may also be feasibly incorporated [16,135].

Besides merely augmenting the properties of the scaffold, controlled release can provide pharmaceutical solutions (Figure 5). For example, in tuberculosis treatment, Zhu et al. and Wu et al. have demonstrated the incorporation of multiple drugs to provide programmed release [123,124]. While Zhu et al. showed prolonged release from a scaffold printing via material extrusion, Wu et al. designed dual-pulsed release by incorporating multiple layers of different drugs, manufacturing via binder jetting. In cancer treatment, Maher et al. showed biphasic release from their implant material [14]. This release is highly specific—providing stronger therapeutic effects and, importantly, lower systemic toxicity. While micro-swimmers must be guided to the target tissue, micro-implants are surgically placed in the area needing the most pharmaceutical treatment.

In these systems, the spatial distribution of the drug layers is a determining factor in the release profile, as was seen in oral dosages. For example, Martinez-Vazquez et al. showed first order kinetics due to their design [137]. Often, however, drug release profiles from scaffolds are biphasic: a quick release burst followed by prolonged release [14,131,134]. Prolonged release may be as long as 80 days [123]. Thus, there are clear benefits to the incorporation of additive manufacturing and pharmaceuticals into implants.

6. Biomimetic Models for Drug Discovery and Development

Whereas the preceding examples have all dealt with drug delivery, additive manufacturing can also be employed in the drug discovery and drug development phases. Perhaps the most viable application of additive manufacturing in drug development is the creation of organ models.

In manufacturing organ models, numerous techniques are currently employed. Monolayer cultures are an industry standard, due to their ease and reproducibility, despite the fact that the response of cells in such cultures is often different than in three-dimensional counterparts [138]. No methods have been able to produce fully biomimetic structures with the resolution and three-dimensional architecture found in vivo. However, fully functional organ models have the potential to provide better translational data towards clinical trials [6]. They also have a capacity to limit the cost later in the drug development process, excluding compounds earlier and increasing the accuracy of testing. This provides a strong impetus for development in this industry.

Additive manufacturing for use in drug development has been extensively reviewed elsewhere [139]. Thus, we focus on demonstrating how micro-scale geometry is a key consideration in the design of organ models and functional tissue (Figure 6).

Vascularization in vivo is a prime example of the importance of micro-scale geometry. Microvasculature is composed of arterioles, capillaries, and venules, which form a complex network [140]. In this network, lumen diameters range between 5 and 200 µm for capillaries and arterioles, respectively [140]. Without vascularization, the nutrient exchange is weak, and necrosis occurs. Much research, therefore, has sought to create vascularization, the realization of which would provide more fully biomimetic structures [141]. For pharmaceutical development, the incorporation of vasculature helps promote realistic cell viability and drug response [142,143].

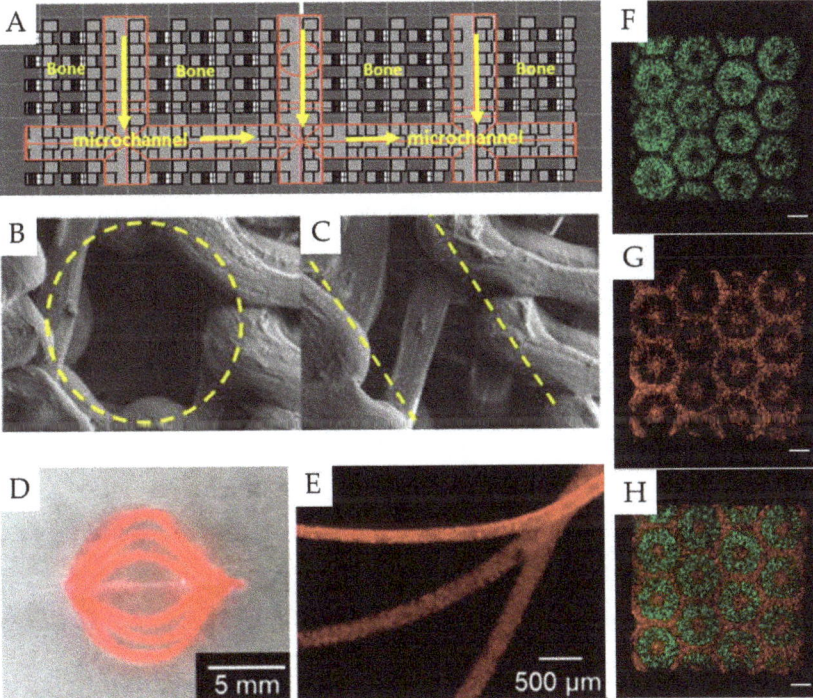

Figure 6. Examples of microstructured tissue constructs made via additive manufacturing techniques. Vascularization is a major component of functional tissue, and may be printed by leaving micron size spaces in the CAD file; 500-micron spaces are designed in this model (**A–C**) [15]. Another approach involves the printing of sacrificial material (**D,E**) [143]. Finally, tissues function depends on desired arrangement of cells, which may be achieved by direct bioprinting (**F–H**) [144]. Hepatic progenitor cells are marked in green, whereas support cells are marked in red. Scale bar: 500 µm. Vascularized, functional tissue provides better data for drug development. Reproduced with permission from Wiley (**A–C**), AIP (**D,E**), and PNAS (**F–H**).

Various strategies exist in the creation of microvasculature; additive manufacturing brings unique approaches. Printing methods include the incorporation of sacrificial materials, designed spaces, or even direct printing of endothelial cells (Figure 6A–E) [140]. Scaffolds printed with sacrificial materials or designed spaces are typically seeded after printing and postprocessing, while bioprinting is capable of placing cells throughout the scaffold. The defining feature of these systems is a need for simultaneous design of macro and micro features, which additive manufacturing is uniquely suited to create. However, capillary-sized features are beyond the current printer feature resolution for the majority of extrusion printing, the most common type of bioprinting [139]. Advances in the feature resolution for additive manufacturing are of importance for this aim.

Various tissues are the focus for bioprinting, including skin, liver, bone, cartilage, cardiac, and adipose tissue [6]. Of these, the liver is most important to pharmaceutical drug development, as many drugs fail clinical trials due to the detection of toxicity to the liver. Liver function depends on its microenvironment [5]. In vivo, functional liver tissue is made of both hepatocytes and supporting endodermal and mesodermal cells [144,145]. With this in mind, Ma et al. designed a bioprinted organ slice, which depends on the micron resolution placement of hepatic and supporting cells (Figure 6F–H) [144]. As in the case of vasculature, designs of this complexity are made possible through high-resolution additive manufacturing techniques. Multimaterial printing methods bring an increased spatial control unseen with other manufacturing methods [142].

Other cells that might be used in drug discovery display responses to micro-scale geometry: cardiomyocytes display alignment based on feature widths [146], and have been patterned in a filamentous matrix for drug discovery based on these effects [147]. As discussed previously, pore size plays a role in cell differentiation for bone cells and adipose-derived mesenchymal stem cells [148]. Thus, cell response to the engineered environment should be carefully tailored to produce the intended cell morphology and differentiation. Micro-scale, cell-size features are a key design parameter. The goal of these engineering systems is to provide the optimal cell response for use in drug development, allowing for data with better translational and predictive qualities. Besides the use of bioprinted scaffolds for application in drug discovery and organ-on-a-chip and microfluidic devices are also emerging as alternatives that may be created via additive manufacturing [149].

7. Future Challenges and Opportunities

The future is bright for the use of additive manufacturing in the pharmaceutical field; however, this future is not without obstacles. Traditional methods are more suited for mass-production than is additive manufacturing. Whereas injection molding becomes more cost-effective as the production rate rises, additive manufacturing of prints remains constant in cost per part [150]. While additive manufacturing significantly reduces prototyping time, it takes more time per part than traditional methods such as injection molding [52]. Increasing print speed is challenging, as there is generally a trade-off between feature resolution and print speed [60]. Higher feature resolution printing methods, such as stereolithography, selective laser sintering, or electrospinning hybrid extrusion have increased the cost for materials and a higher amount of energy necessary for processing [52]. Thus, additive manufacturing is historically well suited for rapid prototyping and design of devices, but not mass production. However, the features discussed previously are dependent on geometry only possible with additive manufacturing. Therefore, the development of additive manufacturing for mass-production is of great interest to the pharmaceutical industry.

Material science will continue to be a key field for additive manufacturing development. While the selection of materials for printing has grown exponentially in the last decade [41,151], materials specifications will continue to limit and inform the feasibility of additive manufacturing processes for specific applications. In consideration of materials, bioprinting of extracellular matrix material is poised for high impact in the field of 3D bioprinted scaffolds [152]. Improvements in material possibilities and printing methods may facilitate larger-scale solutions.

While this article has mainly focused on resolution, other important material properties include printability, mechanical properties, and drug loading capacity [41,153]. For example, bone implants should mimic in vivo bone stiffness, and research on micro-implants characterizes mechanical properties such as Young's modulus [21], compressive strength [29], and yield stress [15]. These properties are dependent on printing method, geometry, and drug loading content. Mechanical properties are also important in oral dosages; as previously stated, microstructured oral dosages can be carefully designed for zero friability [30]. High-resolution printing is complex and requires geometric design, material selection, and printing parametrization to achieve biomedical solutions.

These technologies are making personalized medicine more feasible, as the customizability of additive manufacturing remains the most apparent benefit. The time necessary to print to identical shapes is comparable to the time necessary to print to customized shapes. Additive manufacturing already has a widespread application in the dental industry, where patient-specific parts are necessary [154]. In a similar way, patient-specific therapy remains a promising application of additive manufacturing in the pharmaceutical industry. Point-of-care fabrication of tailored medications is becoming increasingly possible [155]. Orphan medications, which cannot profitably be manufactured at a large scale, could be produced on an individual, small-batch level to reach the needs of patients [156]. Additive manufacturing is uniquely suited for this application.

In the case of oral drug delivery, various authors have addressed the printing of tablets with fully customizable release profiles [157]. As presented, these release profiles are tuned by infill percentage or geometric structure. For example, dose combination or "polypills" are an emerging possibility afforded by additive manufacturing [86]. Maroni et al. demonstrated a shelled capsule capable of dual-pulse controlled release [32]. Their design took advantage of wall thickness and polymer selection for the timing of release. Khaled et al. showed both a three-in-one combination and a five-in-one combination based on spatial separation of active ingredients [25,26]. For each of the preceding cases, the microstructure is a key feature enabled by additive manufacturing.

Larger features are also personalized. Lim et al. designed a finger splint which could be 3D-printed in tandem with microneedles for drug delivery [27]. The design hoped to optimize skin-to-microneedle contact, thereby increasing efficiency, being made specifically for the user's hand. Drug releasing implants made via additive manufacturing also show macrostructure easily tailored to each patient [123]. Printed pediatric stints have already been shown to be effective personalized medical implants in hospital settings [158]. High-resolution printing, therefore, augments current efforts towards personalized medicine. These tablets could be designed, fabricated, and distributed on a case-by-case basis, the entire process occurring at the local clinic.

Regulation of these applications will likely prove to be one of the most challenging hurdles before the wide-spread application of this technology [159]. However, the implementation of microstructured devices made via additive manufacturing promises to shift the paradigm of the industry and enable solutions to the challenging and nuanced problems currently faced.

Funding: Research reported in this publication was supported by the National Institute of General Medical Sciences of the National Institutes of Health under award number R15GM132877.

Acknowledgments: We thank Utah State University's Honors Program and the College of Engineering Undergraduate Research Program (EURP) for supporting Andrew Kjar.

Conflicts of Interest: The authors declare no conflicts of interest.

References

1. Prashansa, A. A Perspective on Drug Discovery, Development, and Delivery. *J. Drug Discov. Dev. Deliv.* **2014**, *1*, 1–3.
2. Suresh, P.; Basu, P.K. Improving Pharmaceutical Product Development and Manufacturing: Impact on Cost of Drug Development and Cost of Goods Sold of Pharmaceuticals. *J. Pharm. Innov.* **2008**, *3*, 175–187. [CrossRef]
3. Sertkaya, A.; Birkenbach, A.; Berlind, A.; Eyraud, J. *Examination of Clinical Trial Costs and Barriers for Drug Development|ASPE*; U.S. Department of Health and Human Services: Washington, DC, USA, 2014.
4. Mak, I.W.; Evaniew, N.; Ghert, M. Lost in translation: Animal models and clinical trials in cancer treatment. *Am. J. Transl. Res.* **2014**, *6*, 114. [PubMed]

5. Nguyen, D.G.; Funk, J.; Robbins, J.B.; Crogan-Grundy, C.; Presnell, S.C.; Singer, T.; Roth, A.B. Bioprinted 3D Primary Liver Tissues Allow Assessment of Organ-Level Response to Clinical Drug Induced Toxicity In Vitro. *PLoS ONE* **2016**, *11*, e0158674. [CrossRef] [PubMed]
6. Pati, F.; Gantelius, J.; Svahn, H.A. 3D Bioprinting of Tissue/Organ Models. *Angew. Chem. Int. Ed.* **2016**, *55*, 4650–4665. [CrossRef] [PubMed]
7. Hofmann, F.; Editorial Board Beavo, M.J.; Busch, W.A.; Ganten, B.D.; J-A Karlsson, B.; Michel, S.M.; Page, A.C.; Rosenthal, L.W. *Handbook of Experimental Pharmacology*; Springer-Verlag: Berlin/Heidelberg, Germany, 2010.
8. Sjöholm, E.; Sandler, N. Additive manufacturing of personalized orodispersible warfarin films. *Int. J. Pharm.* **2019**, *564*, 117–123. [CrossRef] [PubMed]
9. Jain, K.K. Basic Aspects. In *Textbook of Personalized Medicine*; Springer: New York, NY, USA, 2015; pp. 1–33.
10. Genina, N.; Fors, D.; Vakili, H.; Ihalainen, P.; Pohjala, L.; Ehlers, H.; Kassamakov, I.; Haeggström, E.; Vuorela, P.; Peltonen, J.; et al. Tailoring controlled-release oral dosage forms by combining inkjet and flexographic printing techniques. *Eur. J. Pharm. Sci.* **2012**, *47*, 615–623. [CrossRef] [PubMed]
11. Peek, B.T.; Al-Achi, A.; Coombs, S.J. Accuracy of tablet splitting by elderly patients. *JAMA* **2002**, *288*, 451–452. [CrossRef]
12. George, E.; Liacouras, P.; Rybicki, F.J.; Mitsouras, D. Measuring and Establishing the Accuracy and Reproducibility of 3D Printed Medical Models. *RadioGraphics* **2017**, *37*, 1424–1450. [CrossRef]
13. Shirazi, S.F.S.; Gharehkhani, S.; Mehrali, M.; Yarmand, H.; Metselaar, H.S.C.; Adib Kadri, N.; Osman, N.A.A. A review on powder-based additive manufacturing for tissue engineering: Selective laser sintering and inkjet 3D printing. *Sci. Technol. Adv. Mater.* **2015**, *16*, 033502. [CrossRef]
14. Maher, S.; Kaur, G.; Lima-Marques, L.; Evdokiou, A.; Losic, D. Engineering of Micro- to Nanostructured 3D-Printed Drug-Releasing Titanium Implants for Enhanced Osseointegration and Localized Delivery of Anticancer Drugs. *ACS Appl. Mater. Interfaces* **2017**, *9*, 29562–29570. [CrossRef] [PubMed]
15. Cui, H.; Zhu, W.; Holmes, B.; Zhang, L.G. Biologically Inspired Smart Release System Based on 3D Bioprinted Perfused Scaffold for Vascularized Tissue Regeneration. *Adv. Sci.* **2016**, *3*, 1600058. [CrossRef] [PubMed]
16. Vorndran, E.; Klammert, U.; Ewald, A.; Barralet, J.E.; Gbureck, U. Simultaneous Immobilization of Bioactives During 3D Powder Printing of Bioceramic Drug-Release Matrices. *Adv. Funct. Mater.* **2010**, *20*, 1585–1591. [CrossRef]
17. Gittard, S.D.; Miller, P.R.; Jin, C.; Martin, T.N.; Boehm, R.D.; Chisholm, B.J.; Stafslien, S.J.; Daniels, J.W.; Cilz, N.; Monteiro-Riviere, N.A.; et al. Deposition of antimicrobial coatings on microstereolithography-fabricated microneedles. *JOM* **2011**, *63*, 59–68. [CrossRef]
18. Huang, T.-Y.; Sakar, M.S.; Mao, A.; Petruska, A.J.; Qiu, F.; Chen, X.-B.; Kennedy, S.; Mooney, D.; Nelson, B.J. 3D Printed Microtransporters: Compound Micromachines for Spatiotemporally Controlled Delivery of Therapeutic Agents. *Adv. Mater.* **2015**, *27*, 6644–6650. [CrossRef] [PubMed]
19. Xu, H.; Medina-Sánchez, M.; Magdanz, V.; Schwarz, L.; Hebenstreit, F.; Schmidt, O.G. Sperm-Hybrid Micromotor for Targeted Drug Delivery. *ACS Nano* **2018**, *12*, 327–337. [CrossRef]
20. Ceylan, H.; Ceren Yasa, I.; Yaşa, Ö.; Tabak, A.F. 3D-Printed Biodegradable Microswimmer for Drug Delivery and Targeted Cell Labeling. *BioRxiv* **2018**, 379024. [CrossRef]
21. Holmes, B.; Bulusu, K.; Plesniak, M.; Zhang, L.G. A synergistic approach to the design, fabrication and evaluation of 3D printed micro and nano featured scaffolds for vascularized bone tissue repair. *Nanotechnology* **2016**, *27*, 064001. [CrossRef]
22. Kavaldzhiev, M.; Perez, J.E.; Ivanov, Y.; Bertoncini, A.; Liberale, C.; Kosel, J. Biocompatible 3D printed magnetic micro needles. *Biomed. Phys. Eng. Express* **2017**, *3*, 025005. [CrossRef]
23. Hunter, E.E.; Brink, E.W.; Steager, E.B.; Kumar, V. Toward Soft Micro Bio Robots for Cellular and Chemical Delivery. *IEEE Robot. Autom. Lett.* **2018**, *3*, 1592–1599. [CrossRef]
24. Luzuriaga, M.A.; Berry, D.R.; Reagan, J.C.; Smaldone, R.A.; Gassensmith, J.J. Biodegradable 3D printed polymer microneedles for transdermal drug delivery. *Lab Chip* **2018**, *18*, 1223–1230. [CrossRef]
25. Khaled, S.A.; Burley, J.C.; Alexander, M.R.; Yang, J.; Roberts, C.J. 3D printing of tablets containing multiple drugs with defined release profiles. *Int. J. Pharm.* **2015**, *494*, 643–650. [CrossRef]
26. Khaled, S.A.; Burley, J.C.; Alexander, M.R.; Yang, J.; Roberts, C.J. 3D printing of five-in-one dose combination polypill with defined immediate and sustained release profiles. *J. Control. Release* **2015**, *217*, 308–314. [CrossRef]

27. Lim, S.H.; Ng, J.Y.; Kang, L. Three-dimensional printing of a microneedle array on personalized curved surfaces for dual-pronged treatment of trigger finger. *Biofabrication* **2017**, *9*, 015010. [CrossRef]
28. Johnson, A.R.; Caudill, C.L.; Tumbleston, J.R.; Bloomquist, C.J.; Moga, K.A.; Ermoshkin, A.; Shirvanyants, D.; Mecham, S.J.; Luft, J.C.; DeSimone, J.M. Single-Step Fabrication of Computationally Designed Microneedles by Continuous Liquid Interface Production. *PLoS ONE* **2016**, *11*, e0162518. [CrossRef]
29. Ahlfeld, T.; Akkineni, A.R.; Förster, Y.; Köhler, T.; Knaack, S.; Gelinsky, M.; Lode, A. Design and Fabrication of Complex Scaffolds for Bone Defect Healing: Combined 3D Plotting of a Calcium Phosphate Cement and a Growth Factor-Loaded Hydrogel. *Ann. Biomed. Eng.* **2017**, *45*, 224–236. [CrossRef]
30. Sadia, M.; Arafat, B.; Ahmed, W.; Forbes, R.T.; Alhnan, M.A. Channelled tablets: An innovative approach to accelerating drug release from 3D printed tablets. *J. Control. Release* **2018**, *269*, 355–363. [CrossRef]
31. Goyanes, A.; Wang, J.; Buanz, A.; Martínez-Pacheco, R.; Telford, R.; Gaisford, S.; Basit, A.W. 3D Printing of Medicines: Engineering Novel Oral Devices with Unique Design and Drug Release Characteristics. *Mol. Pharm.* **2015**, *12*, 4077–4084. [CrossRef]
32. Maroni, A.; Melocchi, A.; Parietti, F.; Foppoli, A.; Zema, L.; Gazzaniga, A. 3D printed multi-compartment capsular devices for two-pulse oral drug delivery. *J. Control. Release* **2017**, *268*, 10–18. [CrossRef]
33. Melocchi, A.; Parietti, F.; Loreti, G.; Maroni, A.; Gazzaniga, A.; Zema, L. 3D printing by fused deposition modeling (FDM) of a swellable/erodible capsular device for oral pulsatile release of drugs. *J. Drug Deliv. Sci. Technol.* **2015**, *30*, 360–367. [CrossRef]
34. Arafat, B.; Wojsz, M.; Isreb, A.; Forbes, R.T.; Isreb, M.; Ahmed, W.; Arafat, T.; Alhnan, M.A. Tablet fragmentation without a disintegrant: A novel design approach for accelerating disintegration and drug release from 3D printed cellulosic tablets. *Eur. J. Pharm. Sci.* **2018**, *118*, 191–199. [CrossRef]
35. Goyanes, A.; Martinez, P.R.; Basit, A.W. Effect of geometry on drug release from 3D printed tablets. *Int. J. Pharm.* **2015**, *494*, 657–663. [CrossRef]
36. Bhushan, B.; Caspers, M. An overview of additive manufacturing (3D printing) for microfabrication. *Microsyst. Technol.* **2017**, *23*, 1117–1124. [CrossRef]
37. Vithani, K.; Goyanes, A.; Jannin, V.; Basit, A.W.; Gaisford, S.; Boyd, B.J. An Overview of 3D Printing Technologies for Soft Materials and Potential Opportunities for Lipid-based Drug Delivery Systems. *Pharm. Res.* **2019**, *36*, 4. [CrossRef]
38. Vaezi, M.; Seitz, H.; Yang, S. A review on 3D micro-additive manufacturing technologies. *Int. J. Adv. Manuf. Technol.* **2013**, *67*, 1721–1754. [CrossRef]
39. Goyanes, A.; Allahham, N.; Trenfield, S.J.; Stoyanov, E.; Gaisford, S.; Basit, A.W. Direct powder extrusion 3D printing: Fabrication of drug products using a novel single-step process. *Int. J. Pharm.* **2019**, *567*, 118471. [CrossRef]
40. Murphy, S.V.; Atala, A. 3D bioprinting of tissues and organs. *Nat. Biotechnol.* **2014**, *32*, 773–785. [CrossRef]
41. Hospodiuk, M.; Dey, M.; Sosnoski, D.; Ozbolat, I.T. The bioink: A comprehensive review on bioprintable materials. *Biotechnol. Adv.* **2017**, *35*, 217–239. [CrossRef]
42. Ahn, S.H.; Lee, H.J.; Lee, J.-S.; Yoon, H.; Chun, W.; Kim, G.H. A novel cell-printing method and its application to hepatogenic differentiation of human adipose stem cell-embedded mesh structures. *Sci. Rep.* **2015**, *5*, 13427. [CrossRef]
43. MakerBot. MakerBot Replicator 2 Brochure. Available online: http://downloads.makerbot.com/replicator2/MakerBot_Replicator2_brochure.pdf (accessed on 21 June 2019).
44. ZMorph. ZMorph 2.0 SX. 2018. Available online: https://zmorph3d.com/products/zmorph-2-0-sx (accessed on 21 June 2019).
45. Dynamism. Ultimaker 3 Extended. 2018. Available online: https://www.dynamism.com/3d-printers/ultimaker-3-extended.shtml?gclid=EAIaIQobChMIhJafktfu4QIVEdtkCh2_DQA3EAQYASABEgIp_vD_BwE (accessed on 21 June 2019).
46. Treatstock. Solidoodle 2 Base. 2019. Available online: https://www.treatstock.com/machines/item/64-solidoodle-2-base (accessed on 21 June 2019).
47. Zhang, B.; Seong, B.; Nguyen, V.; Byun, D. 3D printing of high-resolution PLA-based structures by hybrid electrohydrodynamic and fused deposition modeling techniques. *J. Micromech. Microeng.* **2016**, *26*, 025015. [CrossRef]
48. Aniwaa Pte. Ltd. 3DDiscovery Regenhu. 2019. Available online: https://www.aniwaa.com/product/3d-printers/regenhu-3ddiscovery/ (accessed on 21 June 2019).

49. GeSiM. BioScaffolder 3.2/4.2 BS32-42. 2019. Available online: https://gesim-bioinstruments-microfluidics.com/wp-content/uploads/2019/04/GeSiM_BS32-42_2019_web.pdf (accessed on 21 June 2019).
50. Bhattacharjee, N.; Urrios, A.; Kang, S.; Folch, A. The upcoming 3D-printing revolution in microfluidics. *Lab Chip* **2016**, *16*, 1720–1742. [CrossRef]
51. Aniwaa Pte. Ltd. Phenix PXM 3D Systems. 2019. Available online: https://www.aniwaa.com/product/3d-printers/3d-systems-phenix-pxm/ (accessed on 21 June 2019).
52. Ngo, T.D.; Kashani, A.; Imbalzano, G.; Nguyen, K.T.Q.; Hui, D. Additive manufacturing (3D printing): A review of materials, methods, applications and challenges. *Compos. Part B Eng.* **2018**, *143*, 172–196. [CrossRef]
53. Mazzoli, A. Selective laser sintering in biomedical engineering. *Med. Biol. Eng. Comput.* **2013**, *51*, 245–256. [CrossRef]
54. Fina, F.; Madla, C.M.; Goyanes, A.; Zhang, J.; Gaisford, S.; Basit, A.W. Fabricating 3D printed orally disintegrating printlets using selective laser sintering. *Int. J. Pharm.* **2018**, *541*, 101–107. [CrossRef]
55. Fina, F.; Goyanes, A.; Madia, C.M.; Awad, A.; Trenfield, S.J.; Kuek, J.M.; Patel, P.; Gaisford, S.; Basit, A.W. 3D printing of drug-loaded gyroid lattices using selective laser sintering. *Int. J. Pharm.* **2018**, *547*, 44–52. [CrossRef]
56. Olakanmi, E.O. Selective laser sintering/melting (SLS/SLM) of pure Al, Al–Mg, and Al–Si powders: Effect of processing conditions and powder properties. *J. Mater. Process. Technol.* **2013**, *213*, 1387–1405. [CrossRef]
57. Dadbakhsh, S.; Verbelen, L.; Vandeputte, T.; Strobbe, D.; van Puyvelde, P.; Kruth, J.-P. Effect of Powder Size and Shape on the SLS Processability and Mechanical Properties of a TPU Elastomer. *Phys. Procedia* **2016**, *83*, 971–980. [CrossRef]
58. Regenfuss, P.; Streek, A.; Hartwig, L.; Klötzer, S.; Brabant, T.; Horn, M.; Ebert, R.; Exner, H. Principles of laser micro sintering. *Rapid Prototyp. J.* **2007**, *13*, 204–212. [CrossRef]
59. Manapat, J.Z.; Chen, Q.; Ye, P.; Advincula, R.C. 3D Printing of Polymer Nanocomposites via Stereolithography. *Macromol. Mater. Eng.* **2017**, *302*, 1600553. [CrossRef]
60. Hwang, H.H.; Zhu, W.; Victorine, G.; Lawrence, N.; Chen, S. 3D-Printing of Functional Biomedical Microdevices via Light- and Extrusion-Based Approaches. *Small Methods* **2018**, *2*, 1700277. [CrossRef]
61. Exapro. Envisiontec Perfactory DSP III Standard SXGA+. 2019. Available online: https://www.exapro.com/envisiontec-perfactory-dsp-iii-standard-sxga-p70626007/ (accessed on 21 June 2019).
62. 3D Systems. 3D Stereolithography Printers. 2018. Available online: https://www.3dsystems.com/sites/default/files/2018-11/3d-systems-sla-tech-specs-a4-us-2018-11-01-web_0.pdf (accessed on 21 June 2019).
63. Kudo3D Inc. Kudo 3D Titan 1 Specifications. 2017. Available online: https://www.kudo3d.com/titan1/ (accessed on 21 June 2019).
64. Halloran, J.W.; Griffith, M.; Chu, T.M. Stereolithography resin for rapid prototyping of ceramics and metals. U.S. Patent 6,117,612, 8 October 1997.
65. Bloomquist, C.J.; Mecham, M.B.; Paradzinsky, M.D.; Janusziewicz, R.; Warner, S.B.; Luft, J.C.; Mecham, S.J.; Wang, A.Z.; DeSimone, J.M. Controlling release from 3D printed medical devices using CLIP and drug-loaded liquid resins. *J. Control. Release* **2018**, *278*, 9–23. [CrossRef]
66. Martinez, P.R.; Goyanes, A.; Basit, A.W.; Gaisford, S. Fabrication of drug-loaded hydrogels with stereolithographic 3D printing. *Int. J. Pharm.* **2017**, *532*, 313–317. [CrossRef]
67. Kawata, S.; Sun, H.-B.; Tanaka, T.; Takada, K. Finer features for functional microdevices. *Nature* **2001**, *412*, 697–698. [CrossRef]
68. Maruo, S.; Nakamura, O.; Kawata, S. Three-dimensional microfabrication with two-photon-absorbed photopolymerization. *Opt. Lett.* **1997**, *22*, 132–134. [CrossRef]
69. Stratasys. F900 3D Printer Series Spec Sheet. 2018. Available online: https://www.stratasys.com/3d-printers/stratasys-f900 (accessed on 21 June 2019).
70. Guo, T.; Holzberg, T.R.; Lim, C.G.; Gao, F.; Gargava, A.; Trachtenberg, J.E.; Mikos, A.G.; Fisher, J.P. 3D printing PLGA: A quantitative examination of the effects of polymer composition and printing parameters on print resolution. *Biofabrication* **2017**, *9*, 024101. [CrossRef]
71. Rebaioli, L.; Fassi, I. A review on benchmark artifacts for evaluating the geometrical performance of additive manufacturing processes. *Int. J. Adv. Manuf. Technol.* **2017**, *93*, 2571–2598. [CrossRef]
72. Mao, M.; He, J.; Li, X.; Zhang, B.; Lei, Q.; Liu, Y.; Li, D.; Mao, M.; He, J.; Li, X.; et al. The Emerging Frontiers and Applications of High-Resolution 3D Printing. *Micromachines* **2017**, *8*, 113. [CrossRef]

73. Aniwaa Pte. Ltd. Biobots Full Specs. 2019. Available online: https://www.aniwaa.com/product/3d-printers/biobots-biobots/ (accessed on 21 June 2019).
74. Stratasys. Fortus 380mc and 450mc. 2018. Available online: https://www.stratasys.com/3d-printers/fortus-380mc-450mc (accessed on 21 June 2019).
75. Lulzbot. Lulzbot TAZ 5. 2019. Available online: https://www.lulzbot.com/store/printers/lulzbot-taz-5 (accessed on 21 June 2019).
76. Wanhao 3D Printer. Catalogue Duplicator 4S. 2012. Available online: http://www.wanhao3dprinter.com/xiazai/D4S.pdf (accessed on 21 June 2019).
77. Stratasys. Objet 260 Connex 3. 2019. Available online: https://www.stratasys.com/3d-printers/objet260-connex3 (accessed on 21 June 2019).
78. Stratasys. PolyJet 3D Printers Systems and Materials. 2018. Available online: https://www.stratasys.com/3d-printers/objet30-pro (accessed on 21 June 2019).
79. Corporation, Z. Spectrum Z510 Technical Specs. Available online: https://www.3dcreationlab.co.uk/pdfs/spectrum-z510-v3.pdf (accessed on 21 June 2019).
80. Nanoscribe. Data Sheet Photonic Professional. 2016. Available online: http://www.nanoscribe.de/files/4414/7393/1095/DataSheet_PP_V05_2016_Web.pdf (accessed on 21 June 2019).
81. Formlabs. Form 3. Available online: https://formlabs.com/3d-printers/form-3/ (accessed on 21 June 2019).
82. Gesswein. EnvisionTEC Micro Plus. Available online: https://www.gesswein.com/p-11761-envisiontec-micro-plus.aspx?gclid=EAIaIQobChMIpdKQsKvx4QIVC8NkCh3Y0gjeEAYYASABEgJ0L_D_BwE (accessed on 21 June 2019).
83. Snider, J. 2019 Carbon M2 3D Printer—Review the Specs and Price. 2018. Available online: https://all3dp.com/1/carbon-m2-review-specs/ (accessed on 21 June 2019).
84. Lifton, V.A.; Lifton, G.; Simon, S. Options for additive rapid prototyping methods (3D printing) in MEMS technology. *Rapid Prototyp. J.* **2014**, *20*, 403–412. [CrossRef]
85. Miyanaji, H.; Zhang, S.; Lassell, A.; Zandinejad, A.; Yang, L. Process Development of Porcelain Ceramic Material with Binder Jetting Process for Dental Applications. *JOM* **2016**, *68*, 831–841. [CrossRef]
86. Sadia, M.; Isreb, A.; Abbadi, I.; Isreb, M.; Aziz, D.; Selo, A.; Timmins, P.; Alhnan, M.A. From 'fixed dose combinations' to 'a dynamic dose combiner': 3D printed bi-layer antihypertensive tablets. *Eur. J. Pharm. Sci.* **2018**, *123*, 484–494. [CrossRef]
87. Prasad, L.K.; Smyth, H. 3D Printing technologies for drug delivery: A review. *Drug Dev. Ind. Pharm.* **2016**, *42*, 1019–1031. [CrossRef]
88. Awad, A.; Trenfield, S.J.; Gaisford, S.; Basit, A.W. 3D printed medicines: A new branch of digital healthcare. *Int. J. Pharm.* **2018**, *548*, 586–596. [CrossRef]
89. Norman, J.; Madurawe, R.D.; Moore, C.M.V.; Khan, M.A.; Khairuzzaman, A. A new chapter in pharmaceutical manufacturing: 3D-printed drug products. *Adv. Drug Deliv. Rev.* **2017**, *108*, 39–50. [CrossRef]
90. Verstraete, G.; Samaro, A.; Grymonpré, W.; Vanhoorne, V.; Van Snick, B.; Boone, M.N.; Hellemans, T.; Van Hoorebeke, L.; Remon, J.P.; Vervaet, C. 3D printing of high drug loaded dosage forms using thermoplastic polyurethanes. *Int. J. Pharm.* **2018**, *536*, 318–325. [CrossRef]
91. Kyobula, M.; Adedeji, A.; Alexander, M.R.; Saleh, E.; Wildman, R.; Ashcroft, I.; Gellert, P.R.; Roberts, C.J. 3D inkjet printing of tablets exploiting bespoke complex geometries for controlled and tuneable drug release. *J. Control. Release* **2017**, *261*, 207–215. [CrossRef]
92. Goyanes, A.; Fina, F.; Martorana, A.; Sedough, D.; Gaisford, S.; Basit, A.W. Development of modified release 3D printed tablets (printlets) with pharmaceutical excipients using additive manufacturing. *Int. J. Pharm.* **2017**, *527*, 21–30. [CrossRef]
93. Goyanes, A.; Buanz, A.B.M.; Hatton, G.B.; Gaisford, S.; Basit, A.W. 3D printing of modified-release aminosalicylate (4-ASA and 5-ASA) tablets. *Eur. J. Pharm. Biopharm.* **2015**, *89*, 157–162. [CrossRef]
94. Li, Q.; Guan, X.; Cui, M.; Zhu, Z.; Chen, K.; Wen, H.; Jia, D.; Hou, J.; Xu, W.; Yang, X.; et al. Preparation and investigation of novel gastro-floating tablets with 3D extrusion-based printing. *Int. J. Pharm.* **2018**, *535*, 325–332. [CrossRef]
95. Okwuosa, T.C.; Pereira, B.C.; Arafat, B.; Cieszynska, M.; Isreb, A.; Alhnan, M.A. Fabricating a Shell-Core Delayed Release Tablet Using Dual FDM 3D Printing for Patient-Centred Therapy. *Pharm. Res.* **2017**, *34*, 427–437. [CrossRef]

96. Zhang, J.; Yang, W.; Vo, A.Q.; Feng, X.; Ye, X.; Kim, D.W.; Repka, M.A. Hydroxypropyl methylcellulose-based controlled release dosage by melt extrusion and 3D printing: Structure and drug release correlation. *Carbohydr. Polym.* **2017**, *177*, 49–57. [CrossRef]
97. Huanbutta, K.; Sangnim, T. Design and development of zero-order drug release gastroretentive floating tablets fabricated by 3D printing technology. *J. Drug Deliv. Sci. Technol.* **2019**, *52*, 831–837. [CrossRef]
98. Tagami, T.; Nagata, N.; Hayashi, N.; Ogawa, E.; Fukushige, K.; Sakai, N.; Ozeki, T. Defined drug release from 3D-printed composite tablets consisting of drug-loaded polyvinylalcohol and a water-soluble or water-insoluble polymer filler. *Int. J. Pharm.* **2018**, *543*, 361–367. [CrossRef]
99. Jamróz, W.; Kurek, M.; Czech, A.; Szafraniec, J.; Gawlak, K.; Jachowicz, R. 3D printing of tablets containing amorphous aripiprazole by filaments co-extrusion. *Eur. J. Pharm. Biopharm.* **2018**, *131*, 44–47. [CrossRef]
100. Ehtezazi, T.; Algellay, M.; Islam, Y.; Roberts, M.; Dempster, N.M.; Sarker, S.D. The Application of 3D Printing in the Formulation of Multilayered Fast Dissolving Oral Films. *J. Pharm. Sci.* **2018**, *107*, 1076–1085. [CrossRef]
101. Martinez, P.R.; Goyanes, A.; Basit, A.W.; Gaisford, S. Influence of Geometry on the Drug Release Profiles of Stereolithographic (SLA) 3D-Printed Tablets. *AAPS PharmSciTech* **2018**, *19*, 3355–3361. [CrossRef]
102. Jamróz, W.; Kurek, M.; Łyszczarz, E.; Szafraniec, J.; Knapik-Kowalczuk, J.; Syrek, K.; Paluch, M.; Jachowicz, R. 3D printed orodispersible films with Aripiprazole. *Int. J. Pharm.* **2017**, *533*, 413–420. [CrossRef]
103. Lu, Y.; Mantha, S.N.; Crowder, D.C.; Chinchilla, S.; Shah, K.N.; Yun, Y.H.; Wicker, R.B.; Choi, J.-W. Microstereolithography and characterization of poly (propylene fumarate)-based drug-loaded microneedle arrays. *Biofabrication* **2015**, *7*, 045001. [CrossRef]
104. Pere, C.P.P.; Economidou, S.N.; Lall, G.; Ziraud, C.; Boateng, J.S.; Alexander, B.D.; Lamprou, D.A.; Douroumis, D. 3D printed microneedles for insulin skin delivery. *Int. J. Pharm.* **2018**, *544*, 425–432. [CrossRef]
105. O'Mahony, C.; Hilliard, L.; Kosch, T.; Bocchino, A.; Sulas, E.; Kenthao, A.; O'Callaghan, S.; Clover, A.J.P.; Demarchi, D.; Bared, G. Accuracy and feasibility of piezoelectric inkjet coating technology for applications in microneedle-based transdermal delivery. *Microelectron. Eng.* **2017**, *172*, 19–25. [CrossRef]
106. Gittard, S.D.; Chen, B.; Xu, H.; Ovsianikov, A.; Chichkov, B.N.; Monteiro-Riviere, N.A.; Narayan, R.J. The effects of geometry on skin penetration and failure of polymer microneedles. *J. Adhes. Sci. Technol.* **2013**, *27*, 227–243. [CrossRef]
107. Kochhar, J.S.; Quek, T.C.; Soon, W.J.; Choi, J.; Zou, S.; Kang, L. Effect of Microneedle Geometry and Supporting Substrate on Microneedle Array Penetration into Skin. *J. Pharm. Sci.* **2013**, *102*, 4100–4108. [CrossRef]
108. Holbrook, K.A.; Odland, G.F. Regional differences in the thickness (cell layers) of the human stratum corneum: An ultrastructural analysis. *J. Investig. Dermatol.* **1974**, *62*, 415–422. [CrossRef]
109. Ovsianikov, A.; Chichkov, B.; Mente, P.; Monteiro-Riviere, N.A.; Doraiswamy, A.; Narayan, R.J. Two Photon Polymerization of Polymer-Ceramic Hybrid Materials for Transdermal Drug Delivery. *Int. J. Appl. Ceram. Technol.* **2007**, *4*, 22–29. [CrossRef]
110. Ali, Z.; Türeyen, E.B.; Karpat, Y.; Çakmakcı, M. Fabrication of Polymer Micro Needles for Transdermal Drug Delivery System Using DLP Based Projection Stereo-lithography. *Procedia CIRP* **2016**, *42*, 87–90. [CrossRef]
111. Gittard, S.D.; Miller, P.R.; Boehm, R.D.; Ovsianikov, A.; Chichkov, B.N.; Heiser, J.; Gordon, J.; Monteiro-Riviere, N.A.; Narayan, R.J. Multiphoton microscopy of transdermal quantum dot delivery using two photon polymerization-fabricated polymer microneedles. *Faraday Discuss.* **2011**, *149*, 171–185. [CrossRef]
112. Gittard, S.D.; Ovsianikov, A.; Chichkov, B.N.; Doraiswamy, A.; Narayan, R.J. Two-photon polymerization of microneedles for transdermal drug delivery. *Expert Opin. Drug Deliv.* **2010**, *7*, 513–533. [CrossRef]
113. Gittard, S.D.; Ovsianikov, A.; Monteiro-Riviere, N.A.; Lusk, J.; Morel, P.; Minghetti, P.; Lenardi, C.; Chichkov, B.N.; Narayan, R.J. Fabrication of Polymer Microneedles Using a Two-Photon Polymerization and Micromolding Process. *J. Diabetes Sci. Technol.* **2009**, *3*, 304–311. [CrossRef]
114. Gittard, S.D.; Ovsianikov, A.; Akar, H.; Chichkov, B.; Monteiro-Riviere, N.A.; Stafslien, S.; Chisholm, B.; Shin, C.-C.; Shih, C.-M.; Lin, S.-J.; et al. Two Photon Polymerization-Micromolding of Polyethylene Glycol-Gentamicin Sulfate Microneedles. *Adv. Eng. Mater.* **2010**, *12*, B77–B82. [CrossRef]
115. Doraiswamy, A.; Ovsianikov, A.; Gittard, S.D.; Monteiro-Riviere, N.A.; Crombez, R.; Montalvo, E.; Shen, W.; Chichkov, B.N.; Narayan, R.J. Fabrication of microneedles using two photon polymerization for transdermal delivery of nanomaterials. *J. Nanosci. Nanotechnol.* **2010**, *10*, 6305–6312. [CrossRef]
116. Boehm, R.D.; Jaipan, P.; Skoog, S.A.; Stafslien, S.; VanderWal, L.; Narayan, R.J. Inkjet deposition of itraconazole onto poly (glycolic acid) microneedle arrays. *Biointerphases* **2016**, *11*, 011008. [CrossRef]

117. Allen, E.A.; O'Mahony, C.; Cronin, M.; O'Mahony, T.; Moore, A.C.; Crean, A.M. Dissolvable microneedle fabrication using piezoelectric dispensing technology. *Int. J. Pharm.* **2016**, *500*, 1–10. [CrossRef]
118. Uddin, M.J.; Scoutaris, N.; Klepetsanis, P.; Chowdhry, B.; Prausnitz, M.R.; Douroumis, D. Inkjet printing of transdermal microneedles for the delivery of anticancer agents. *Int. J. Pharm.* **2015**, *494*, 593–602. [CrossRef]
119. Boehm, R.D.; Daniels, J.; Stafslien, S.; Nasir, A.; Lefebvre, J.; Narayan, R.J. Polyglycolic acid microneedles modified with inkjet-deposited antifungal coatings. *Cit. Biointerphases* **2015**, *10*, 11004. [CrossRef]
120. Boehm, R.D.; Miller, P.R.; Hayes, S.L.; Monteiro-Riviere, N.A.; Narayan, R.J. Modification of microneedles using inkjet printing. *AIP Adv.* **2011**, *1*, 022139. [CrossRef]
121. Bozuyuk, U.; Yasa, O.; Yasa, I.C.; Ceylan, H.; Kizilel, S.; Sitti, M. Light-Triggered Drug Release from 3D-Printed Magnetic Chitosan Microswimmers. *ACS Nano* **2018**, *12*, 9617–9625. [CrossRef]
122. Tottori, S.; Zhang, L.; Qiu, F.; Krawczyk, K.K.; Franco-Obregón, A.; Nelson, B.J. Magnetic Helical Micromachines: Fabrication, Controlled Swimming, and Cargo Transport. *Adv. Mater.* **2012**, *24*, 811–816. [CrossRef]
123. Zhu, M.; Li, K.; Zhu, Y.; Zhang, J.; Ye, X. 3D-printed hierarchical scaffold for localized isoniazid/rifampin drug delivery and osteoarticular tuberculosis therapy. *Acta Biomater.* **2015**, *16*, 145–155. [CrossRef]
124. Wu, W.; Zheng, Q.; Guo, X.; Sun, J.; Liu, Y. A programmed release multi-drug implant fabricated by three-dimensional printing technology for bone tuberculosis therapy. *Biomed. Mater.* **2009**, *4*, 065005. [CrossRef]
125. Erkoc, P.; Yasa, I.C.; Ceylan, H.; Yasa, O.; Alapan, Y.; Sitti, M. Mobile Microrobots for Active Therapeutic Delivery. *Adv. Ther.* **2019**, *2*, 1800064. [CrossRef]
126. Li, J.; de Ávila, B.E.; Gao, W.; Zhang, L.; Wang, J. Micro/nanorobots for biomedicine: Delivery, surgery, sensing, and detoxification. *Sci. Robot.* **2017**, *2*, 1–9. [CrossRef]
127. Mhanna, R.; Qiu, F.; Zhang, L.; Ding, Y.; Sugihara, K.; Zenobi-Wong, M.; Nelson, B.J. Artificial Bacterial Flagella for Remote-Controlled Targeted Single-Cell Drug Delivery. *Small* **2014**, *10*, 1953–1957. [CrossRef]
128. Qiu, T.; Lee, T.-C.; Mark, A.G.; Morozov, K.I.; Münster, R.; Mierka, O.; Turek, S.; Leshansky, A.M.; Fischer, P. Swimming by reciprocal motion at low Reynolds number. *Nat. Commun.* **2014**, *5*, 5119. [CrossRef]
129. Ventola, C.L. Medical Applications for 3D Printing: Current and Projected Uses. *Pharm. Ther.* **2014**, *39*, 704–711.
130. Sanz-Herrera, J.A.; Doblaré, M.; García-Aznar, J.M. Scaffold microarchitecture determines internal bone directional growth structure: A numerical study. *J. Biomech.* **2010**, *43*, 2480–2486. [CrossRef]
131. Huang, W.; Zheng, Q.; Sun, W.; Xu, H.; Yang, X. Levofloxacin implants with predefined microstructure fabricated by three-dimensional printing technique. *Int. J. Pharm.* **2007**, *339*, 33–38. [CrossRef]
132. Lai, Y.; Li, Y.; Cao, H.; Long, J.; Wang, X.; Li, L.; Li, C.; Jia, Q.; Teng, B.; Tang, T.; et al. Osteogenic magnesium incorporated into PLGA/TCP porous scaffold by 3D printing for repairing challenging bone defect. *Biomaterials* **2019**, *197*, 207–219. [CrossRef]
133. Flautre, B.; Descamps, M.; Delecourt, C.; Blary, M.C.; Hardouin, P. Porous HA ceramic for bone replacement: Role of the pores and interconnections—Experimental study in the rabbit. *J. Mater. Sci. Mater. Med.* **2001**, *12*, 679–682. [CrossRef]
134. Wang, H.; Wu, G.; Zhang, J.; Zhou, K.; Yin, B.; Su, X.; Qiu, G.; Yang, G.; Zhang, X.; Zhou, G.; et al. Osteogenic effect of controlled released rhBMP-2 in 3D printed porous hydroxyapatite scaffold. *Colloids Surf. B Biointerfaces* **2016**, *141*, 491–498. [CrossRef]
135. Inzana, J.A.; Trombetta, R.P.; Schwarz, E.M.; Kates, S.L.; Awad, H.A. 3D printed bioceramics for dual antibiotic delivery to treat implant-associated bone infection. *Eur. Cell. Mater.* **2015**, *30*, 232–247. [CrossRef]
136. Shim, J.-H.; Yoon, M.-C.; Jeong, C.-M.; Jang, J.; Jeong, S.-I.; Cho, D.-W.; Huh, J.-B. Efficacy of rhBMP-2 loaded PCL/PLGA/ β-TCP guided bone regeneration membrane fabricated by 3D printing technology for reconstruction of calvaria defects in rabbit. *Biomed. Mater.* **2014**, *9*, 065006. [CrossRef]
137. Martínez-Vázquez, F.J.; Cabañas, M.V.; Paris, J.L.; Lozano, D.; Vallet-Regí, M. Fabrication of novel Si-doped hydroxyapatite/gelatine scaffolds by rapid prototyping for drug delivery and bone regeneration. *Acta Biomater.* **2015**, *15*, 200–209. [CrossRef] [PubMed]
138. Edmondson, R.; Broglie, J.J.; Adcock, A.F.; Yang, L. Three-Dimensional Cell Culture Systems and Their Applications in Drug Discovery and Cell-Based Biosensors. *Assay Drug Dev. Technol.* **2014**, *12*, 207–218. [CrossRef]
139. Ma, X.; Liu, J.; Zhu, W.; Tang, M.; Lawrence, N.; Yu, C.; Gou, M.; Chen, S. 3D bioprinting of functional tissue models for personalized drug screening and in vitro disease modeling. *Adv. Drug Deliv. Rev.* **2018**, *132*, 235–251. [CrossRef] [PubMed]

140. Datta, P.; Ayan, B.; Ozbolat, I.T. Bioprinting for vascular and vascularized tissue biofabrication. *Acta Biomater.* **2017**, *51*, 1–20. [CrossRef] [PubMed]
141. Sasmal, P.; Datta, P.; Wu, Y.; Ozbolat, I.T. 3D bioprinting for modelling vasculature. *Microphysiol. Syst.* **2018**, *2*. [CrossRef] [PubMed]
142. Kang, H.-W.; Lee, S.J.; Ko, I.K.; Kengla, C.; Yoo, J.J.; Atala, A. A 3D bioprinting system to produce human-scale tissue constructs with structural integrity. *Nat. Biotechnol.* **2016**, *34*, 312–319. [CrossRef] [PubMed]
143. Massa, S.; Sakr, M.A.; Seo, J.; Bandaru, P.; Arneri, A.; Bersini, S.; Zare-Eelanjegh, E.; Jalilian, E.; Cha, B.-H.; Antona, S.; et al. Bioprinted 3D vascularized tissue model for drug toxicity analysis. *Biomicrofluid.* **2017**, *11*, 044109. [CrossRef]
144. Ma, X.; Qu, X.; Zhu, W.; Li, Y.-S.; Yuan, S.; Zhang, H.; Liu, J.; Wang, P.; Lai, C.S.E.; Zanella, F.; et al. Deterministically patterned biomimetic human iPSC-derived hepatic model via rapid 3D bioprinting. *Proc. Natl. Acad. Sci. USA* **2016**, *113*, 2206–2211. [CrossRef]
145. Chang, R.; Emami, K.; Wu, H.; Sun, W. Biofabrication of a three-dimensional liver micro-organ as an in vitro drug metabolism model. *Biofabrication* **2010**, *2*, 045004. [CrossRef]
146. Salick, M.R.; Napiwocki, B.N.; Sha, J.; Knight, G.T.; Chindhy, S.A.; Kamp, T.J.; Ashton, R.S.; Crone, W.C. Micropattern width dependent sarcomere development in human ESC-derived cardiomyocytes. *Biomaterials* **2014**, *35*, 4454–4464. [CrossRef]
147. Ma, Z.; Koo, S.; Finnegan, M.A.; Loskill, P.; Huebsch, N.; Marks, N.C.; Conklin, B.R.; Grigoropoulos, C.P.; Healy, K.E. Three-dimensional filamentous human diseased cardiac tissue model. *Biomaterials* **2014**, *35*, 1367–1377. [CrossRef]
148. Theodoridis, K.; Aggelidou, E.; Vavilis, T.; Manthou, M.E.; Tsimponis, A.; Demiri, E.C.; Boukla, A.; Salpistis, C.; Bakopoulou, A.; Mihailidis, A.; et al. Hyaline cartilage next generation implants from Adipose Tissue Derived Mesenchymal Stem Cells: Comparative study on 3D-Printed Polycaprolactone scaffold patterns. *J. Tissue Eng. Regen. Med.* **2019**, *13*, 342–355. [CrossRef]
149. Yi, H.-G.; Lee, H.; Cho, D.-W. 3D Printing of Organs-On-Chips. *Bioengineering* **2017**, *4*, 10. [CrossRef]
150. Awad, A.; Trenfield, S.J.; Goyanes, A.; Gaisford, S.; Basit, A.W. Reshaping drug development using 3D printing. *Drug Discov. Today* **2018**, *23*, 1547–1555. [CrossRef]
151. Lee, J.-Y.; An, J.; Chua, C.K. Fundamentals and applications of 3D printing for novel materials. *Appl. Mater. Today* **2017**, *7*, 120–133. [CrossRef]
152. Hinderer, S.; Layland, S.L.; Schenke-Layland, K. ECM and ECM-like materials—Biomaterials for applications in regenerative medicine and cancer therapy. *Adv. Drug Deliv. Rev.* **2016**, *97*, 260–269. [CrossRef]
153. Hölzl, K.; Lin, S.; Tytgat, L.; van Vlierberghe, S.; Gu, L.; Ovsianikov, A. Bioink properties before, during and after 3D bioprinting. *Biofabrication* **2016**, *8*, 032002. [CrossRef]
154. Bhargav, A.; Sanjairaj, V.; Rosa, V.; Feng, L.W.; Fuh, Y.H.J. Applications of additive manufacturing in dentistry: A review. *J. Biomed. Mater. Res. Part B Appl. Biomater.* **2018**, *106*, 2058–2064. [CrossRef]
155. Trenfield, S.J.; Awad, A.; Goyanes, A.; Gaisford, S.; Basit, A.W. 3D Printing Pharmaceuticals: Drug Development to Frontline Care. *Trends Pharmacol. Sci.* **2018**, *39*, 440–451. [CrossRef]
156. Araújo, M.R.P.; Sa-Barreto, L.L.; Gratieri, T.; Gelfuso, G.M.; Cunha-Filho, M. The digital pharmacies era: How 3D printing technology using fused deposition modeling can become a reality. *Pharmaceutics* **2019**, *11*, 128. [CrossRef]
157. Sun, Y.; Soh, S. Printing Tablets with Fully Customizable Release Profiles for Personalized Medicine. *Adv. Mater.* **2015**, *27*, 7847–7853. [CrossRef]
158. Morrison, R.J.; Hollister, S.J.; Niedner, M.F.; Mahani, M.G.; Park, A.H.; Mehta, D.K.; Ohye, R.G.; Green, G.E. Mitigation of tracheobronchomalacia with 3D-printed personalized medical devices in pediatric patients. *Sci. Transl. Med.* **2015**, *7*, 285ra64. [CrossRef]
159. Alhnan, M.A.; Okwuosa, T.C.; Sadia, M.; Wan, K.-W.; Ahmed, W.; Arafat, B. Emergence of 3D Printed Dosage Forms: Opportunities and Challenges. *Pharm. Res.* **2016**, *33*, 1817–1832. [CrossRef]

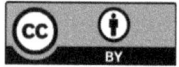

© 2019 by the authors. Licensee MDPI, Basel, Switzerland. This article is an open access article distributed under the terms and conditions of the Creative Commons Attribution (CC BY) license (http://creativecommons.org/licenses/by/4.0/).

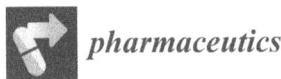

Review

The Digital Pharmacies Era: How 3D Printing Technology Using Fused Deposition Modeling Can Become a Reality

Maisa R. P. Araújo, Livia L. Sa-Barreto, Tais Gratieri, Guilherme M. Gelfuso and Marcilio Cunha-Filho *

Laboratory of Food, Drugs and Cosmetics (LTMAC), University of Brasília (UnB), Brasília 70910-900, Brazil; maisaraposo@gmail.com (M.R.P.A.); liviabarreto@unb.br (L.L.S.-B.); tgratieri@gmail.com (T.G.); gmgelfuso@unb.br (G.M.G.)
* Correspondence: marciliocunha@unb.br; Tel.: +55-61-31071990

Received: 24 February 2019; Accepted: 14 March 2019; Published: 19 March 2019

Abstract: The pharmaceutical industry is set to join the fourth industrial revolution with the 3D printing of medicines. The application of 3D printers in compounding pharmacies will turn them into digital pharmacies, wrapping up the telemedicine care cycle and definitively modifying the pharmacotherapeutic treatment of patients. Fused deposition modeling 3D printing technology melts extruded drug-loaded filaments into any dosage form; and allows the obtainment of flexible dosages with different shapes, multiple active pharmaceutical ingredients and modulated drug release kinetics—in other words, offering customized medicine. This work aimed to present an update on this technology, discussing its challenges. The co-participation of the pharmaceutical industry and compounding pharmacies seems to be the best way to turn this technology into reality. The pharmaceutical industry can produce drug-loaded filaments on a large scale with the necessary quality and safety guarantees; while digital pharmacies can transform the filaments into personalized medicine according to specific prescriptions. For this to occur, adaptations in commercial 3D printers will need to meet health requirements for drug products preparation, and it will be necessary to make advances in regulatory gaps and discussions on patent protection. Thus, despite the conservatism of the sector, 3D drug printing has the potential to become the biggest technological leap ever seen in the pharmaceutical segment, and according to the most optimistic prognostics, it will soon be within reach.

Keywords: digital pharmacy; fused deposition modeling 3D printing; modified drug release; personalized medicines; telemedicine

1. Introduction

The industrial revolution in its beginning transformed drug therapy with large-scale production in assembly line, symbolized by the production of tablets in 1834. Thenceforward, despite the modernization of industrial facilities and advances in quality issues, the bases of the pharmaceutical production process were not modified. 3D printing has revolutionized various sectors of human activity over the last few decades, being one of the pillars of the fourth industrial revolution. In recent years, the use of this technology in medicine preparation has demonstrated such potential. This is why experts around the world point out that the pharmaceutical field has finally been given, after two centuries, the opportunity to make a significant technological jump [1].

3D technology offers unique benefits to drug products manufacturing, when compared to traditional methods—notably, the capacity of designing personalized pharmaceutical forms with flexible dosage [2–5], different shapes [3,6,7], multiple active pharmaceutical ingredients (even incompatible ones) [8,9], and modulated release kinetics [10–13]. Moreover, the most diversified and sophisticated drug delivery devices for oral, dermal, and implantable administration can be produced with high accuracy using 3D printers [14].

Nonetheless, competing against the mass production of pharmaceutical manufacturing is not a simple task. The FDM 3D printer may not be an optimal solution for largescale production. For instance, a tablet machine can be 60 times faster than a printer [15]. 3D printers cannot match the velocity of industrial tablet machines, but they certainly serve to address an existing therapeutic gap with regard to the need for individualization of drug therapy, acting in a complementary or alternative manner to the conventional drug product production [16,17].

On the other hand, in a small scale at compounding pharmacies, the speed difference between manually encapsulating powders and using a printer may not be so discrepant. The printer can also be adapted with multiple heads, making it possible to print several units at the same time, accelerating the process. The artisanal processes employed today at compounding pharmacies to meet patient's individuals needs are similar to those used in apothecaries hundreds of years ago. For instance, they are not capable of elaborating controlled-release dosage forms and are not sufficiently equipped to guarantee the quality specifications required by the pharmacopoeia, risking patient safety [18]. The automation of the 3D printing process and particularly the high accuracy achieved by FDM technology makes the printing of drug products potentially safer. It could also prevent low-quality issues and meet the necessary requirements to take drug personalization to another level [14,15,19–21].

Fused deposition modeling (FDM), a type of 3D printing technology, is the most quoted when dealing with production of drug delivery devices, because of the low cost of printers; printing precision, fundamental to guaranteeing medicine quality parameters; and hot-melt extrusion, a technological process incorporated in the pharmaceutical field a decade ago [22,23] The FDM 3D printer uses heat to melt a polymeric filament and deposit it layer by layer in the x, y and z-axes, creating a three-dimensional product [24,25]. The filament used to feed the printer is produced by hot-melt extrusion using active pharmaceutical ingredients and pharmaceutical grade polymers [26].

The co-participation of both pharmaceutical industry and compounding pharmacy seems to be the best way to cross the barrier of research and reach the market. The FDM 3D printer is portable and relatively simple to operate, making it eligible for implementation in compounding pharmacies. On the other hand, the hot-melt extruded drug loaded filaments can be produced by the industry on a large scale as an intermediate product. These filaments can be transformed into personalized medicines for medical prescriptions at local pharmacies [27].

Moreover, personalized 3D printed medicines appear as the missing piece in the care cycle of trendy telemedicine (Figure 1). Launched as the future of medicine, telemedicine has the capacity to expand access to health, making it possible to contact patients from the neediest regions of the globe with the most qualified physicians on the planet employing the latest technological resources that allow remote consultations and accurate diagnoses. 3D printed medicines offer pharmacotherapeutic treatment as a response to a virtual prescription, paving the way for digital pharmacy [28], which completes the care cycle that can definitively mark the 21st century (Figure 1).

Despite the fast development of 3D printing in the pharmaceutical field and the market release of the first 3D printed drug product, Spritam® (levetiracetam), there are technical and regulatory issues that need to be addressed [29]. This work aimed to update the theme of FDM 3D printing used for elaborate drug delivery devices, discussing the challenges and possible solutions that could allow this technology to enter the market.

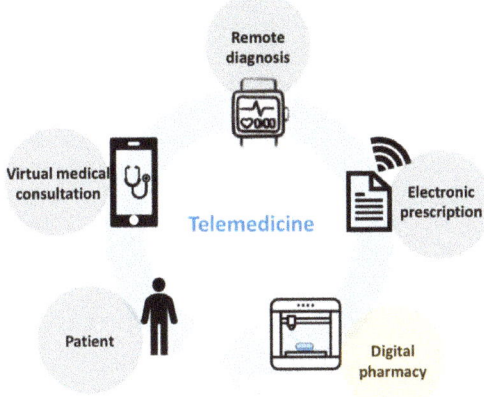

Figure 1. Telemedicine care cycle with insertion of digital pharmacy.

2. The Versatility of FDM 3D Printing for Drug-Delivery Devices

FDM 3D printers can produce a wide range of different drug delivery devices, as evidenced by recently published scientific reports on the subject. A search of the combined terms, "3D printing", "FDM" and "drug" in SciFinder® for 2014 to 2018 resulted in 54 papers on the subject. These works give a glimpse of the technology's potential (Figure 2).

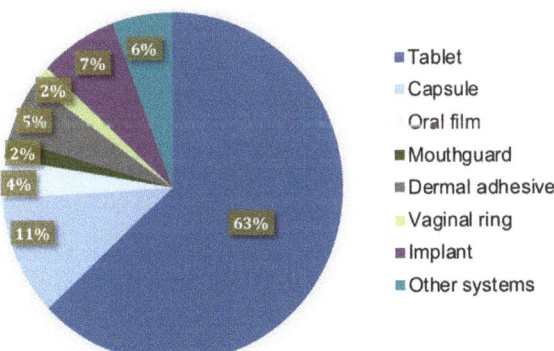

Figure 2. The share of drug-delivery devices (n = 54) that could be printed using fused deposition modeling 3D printing, as published in research papers between years 2014 and 2018 (SciFinder®).

As expected, the majority of studies explored the development of oral dosage forms, with tablets accounting for the largest share of the pie (63%), followed by capsules (11%). Oral pharmaceutical presentations represent more than 40% of the drug products in the market [30]. Simple control of printing variables can offer interesting therapeutic advantages to 3D printed drug products. Precision in dosage personalization is undoubtedly one of the great benefits of FDM 3D printing technology, as opportunely explored in the case of warfarin tablets. This active pharmaceutical ingredient was printed in tailored doses safely administered to rats, eliminating the need to split and facilitate the progression and regression of doses, as is usually employed in treatments with this drug [31].

Another distinguished approach was the printing of domperidone disks with low infill, increasing the drug time in the stomach through flotation, thus decreasing the frequency of tablet intake [32]. Moreover, several drugs can be easily associated with the same pharmaceutical unit, such as in the case of a "polypill" printed with intercalated layers of paracetamol and caffeine, leading to simultaneous release of both drugs [33]. FDM 3D printing could also produce immediate release tablets using distinct pharmaceutical grade polymers [34] or by adding gaps to the tablet design, called "gaplets", which increase the porosity of the tablets [35].

Innovative geometries to increase patient compliance could also be created. Tests performed in vivo have revealed that patients are open to experimenting with new geometries, such as in donut form (torus) [6]. Pediatric dosage forms imitating candy may improve children's acceptance of oral forms and the extrusion and printing processes using polymers may help mask the bitterness of active pharmaceutical ingredients [36]. Control of tablet shapes can also help modulate drug-release rates, which are dependent on surface area/volume of the tablet [7]. Figure 3 shows different shapes of FDM printed tablets and capsules.

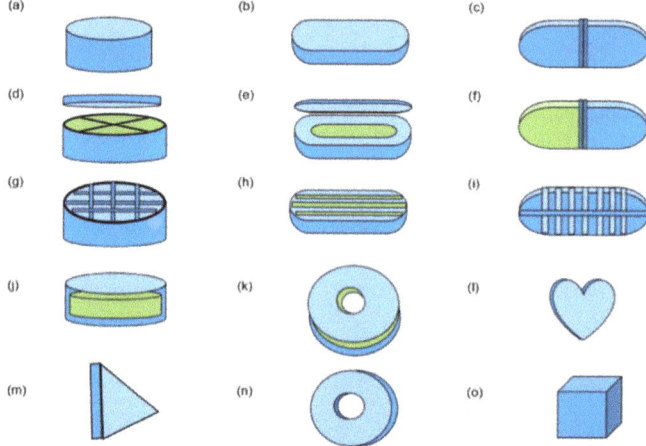

Figure 3. Different shapes of oral drug-delivery devices produced using fused deposition modeling 3D printing (blue = API 1, green = API 2). (**a**) [32], (**b**) [31], (**c**) [38], (**d**) [39], (**e**) [40], (**f**) [37], (**g**) [34], (**h**) [33], (**i**) [35], (**j**) [10], (**k**) [41], (**l**) [36], (**m**) [33], (**n**) [6], (**o**) [6].

In addition, 3D printing of capsules has advantageous performances. Studies have revealed that a capsule combining two different polymer compartments can produce a two-pulse release kinetic [37] and dual release for caffeine [38]. Hollow printed capsules containing complex compartments filled with liquid metformin, where the liquid formulation is not exposed to heating, lead to controlled drug release by capsule dissolution rate [39]. Printed capsules may also create different release rates of drug solutions by changing the shell thickness and core volume [40], whereas for printed cores, the infill and polymeric matrix even helps achieve a zero-order release rate [10]. Zero-order release was also reached in a three-part donut shaped tablet composed of polymeric water insoluble outside layers and a soluble polymeric drug loaded center [41].

Other oral forms printed using FDM are oral films and medicinal mouthguards, for example, aripiprazole oral films printed by 3D FDM that have improved drug dissolution rate using a porous polymeric matrix [42]; and the new personalized drug delivery device, shaped as a mouthguard, which contains clobetasol propionate to treat mouth inflammation [2].

Dermal adhesives for cutaneous drug delivery have also been produced using the same technique. Printed polylactic acid microneedles devices have been shown to be able to pierce porcine skin and deliver a model drug [43]. Vaginal rings and drug implants represented 2% and 7%, respectively, of studies on printed drug delivery devices (Figure 2). Printed progesterone vaginal rings in different shapes have distinct dissolution rates based on surface area/volume and release the drug over a period of one week [3]. A polylactic acid sub cutaneous implant for sustained release of disulfiram [44] and even ethylene vinyl acetate intrauterine devices loaded with indomethacin [45] have also been printed using 3D FDM.

Other complex delivery systems correspond to 6% of the devices described in Figure 2. For example, 'tablet-in-devices', which were developed to keep the riboflavin tablet floating in stomach acid for a longer period, enhances drug absorption and ensures a sustained release [46]. 'Dual-compartmental dosage unit' can combine two incompatible drugs (rifampicin and isoniazid) used in tuberculosis treatment, using polylactic acid to separate the drug filaments and generate distinct dissolution patterns [47].

3D printing technology has proven, therefore, to be capable of producing very complex anatomical shapes, with multiple active pharmaceutical ingredients and different release kinetics. However, despite this research, this topic is not exhaustive, and new pharmaceutical devices could be produced in future to deliver drugs to specific body requirements. Drug-loaded contact lens to treat eye disorders, pharmaceutical polymeric nails to treat fungal infections, and drug delivery head caps to treat baldness are obvious alternatives that have not been tested yet.

3. Adaptations of FDM 3D Printer for Pharmaceutical Production

As mentioned above, FDM printing is the most researched technique for 3D-printed drug delivery devices today, when compared to other 3D printing techniques such as selective laser sintering and powder bed. The equipment is affordable, easy to operate, and shows high print accuracy and reproducibility [22]. MakerBot® (USA), Multirap M420® (Germany) and Prusa i3® (Czech Republic) are printer brands used in several studies; and their process variables, such as temperature, speed and infill, have been correlated with pharmaceutical production variables [22,48].

Despite this, no commercial model is available for pharmaceutical use. Moreover, recent studies point out that numerous adaptations of commercial machines are needed to meet pharmaceutical production requirements [49]. Figure 4 shows the main FDM printer parts that require adjustments.

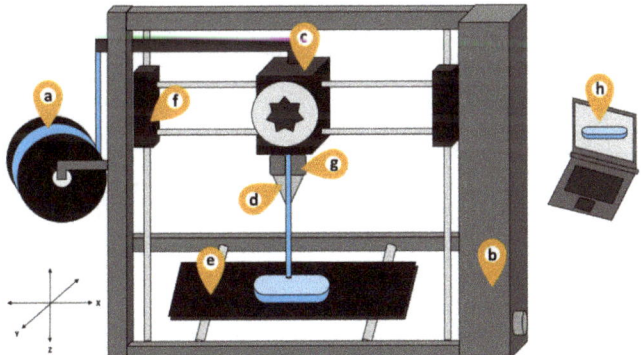

Figure 4. Schematic representation of a pharmaceutical fused deposition modeling 3D printer with indications of the specific points in which adaptations will be required for pharmaceutical production. (a) Spool, (b) printer enclosure, (c) extruder head, (d) nozzle, (e) build platform, (f) motor, (g) heater, (h) 3D design software.

The spool containing the extruded drug loaded filament (Figure 4a) is attached to the printer through a tube, from where it reaches the equipment nozzle through a gear system [50]. In several printers, the filament coil in the spool is not protected from particles or humidity during the printing process. This exposure could lead to cross-contamination of filament spools, which could ideally be reused. To solve this problem, a closed compartment could be connected to the printer, covering the spool attachment. Store boxes for filaments are now available; they can be coupled with the 3D printer to protect the filaments from moisture, dust contamination; and keep them heated for a better printing result (eBox®, eSUN, China). The printer enclosure (Figure 4b) should also be sealed against contaminants, as in MakerBot Replicator 2x® (USA), protecting the printed drug delivery device and eliminating the need for a laminar airflow or strict particle control of the production area [38].

In order to meet Good Manufacturing Practices, all the printer parts, such as extruder head, nozzle and build platform (Figure 4c–e), which are in direct contact with the drug-loaded filament should be made of an inert material that can be easily cleaned—accordingly, stainless steel is the most recommended. Similar to what happens in hot-melt extruders, the use of cleaning polymers may be more efficient in removing residues from the machine than the use of solvent and chemical products, such as water and soap. In addition, the mechanical parts of the FDM printer, such as the motors (Figure 4f), need to be completely closed, preventing lubricant oil from spilling over the product [38].

The thermal processing of the formulation involved in FDM 3D printing and its risks to drug stability cannot be ignored. In fact, stability issues for thermosensitive drugs have already been noted by initial application of this technology [51]. The problem has been addressed by using polymers with low glass transition temperature or by using plasticizers, which can reduce the polymers glass transition and consequently the nozzle temperature [34,52]. Taking this into consideration, an important point for pharmaceutical use concerns the need of a more precise and sensitive control of the heater's temperature (Figure 4g). Overheating could lead to modifications of the polymer viscoelasticity compromising drug control release and, eventually, stability of the drug.

Another operational problem with some FDM 3D printers is the lack of flexibility in the size of the nozzle (Figure 4d), since commercial filaments have a standard 1.75 mm diameter. However, for pharmaceutical use, a wide range of polymeric materials is extruded generating diameter oscillations due to their viscoelastic characteristics. In that case, it is necessary to choose a printer with adjustable nozzles [53]. Furthermore, an optimized FDM printer with multiple nozzles could improve the printing time of a batch or even produce devices with multiple APIs without the need to change filaments during the process [33]. Currently there are certain commercial models that comply with those needs, such as Stacker S4® (Stacker Corp., USA), an industrial multi nozzle 3D printer capable of printing four objects at the same time, and RoVa3D® (ORD Solutions Inc., Canada), which possesses 0.2 mm, 0.35 mm, 0.5 mm, 0.7 mm, 1.0 mm diameter nozzles and can print up to five filaments simultaneously.

In order to extend the possibilities of FDM 3D printing and to increase the automation of the process, it would be desirable to fill scaffolds printed with a liquid or semisolid containing the drug using a piston or syringe coupled to the printer [40,54]. For instance, the use of thermogelling materials such as poloxamers may be of particular utility in modulating drug release [55]. The HYREL 3D company (USA) developed an interesting solution for the same—a set of different printer heads compatible with their machines. The modular heads are assembled to the printers to allow the introduction of different materials in the 3D device, such as hot flow heads for FDM filaments, cold and warm flow heads for pastes and resins, and cold flow syringe heads for liquids and gels.

The software used to control the printer (Figure 4h) should be designed to receive electronic prescriptions from the physician's office and to suggest the most recommended conditions of printing. The more complex information, such as nozzle and platform temperature, speed, layer height and infill, would be supplied by pharmacy technicians, based on filament manufacturer information. After training, the professional should be qualified to operate the machine. The 3D design of devices would be preferably pre-selected from a database, thus saving time when defining device shape [56,57].

4. Integrated Production Process

Diversified drug delivery devices using 3D FDM technology are being developed at a fast pace by dozens of researches groups in different parts of the globe [58]. Nevertheless, another step has to be taken to allow the commercial viability of this technology. In the light of previous works and considering the extrusion process already used by the pharmaceutical industry, a partnership between pharmaceutical industries and compounding pharmacies in a complementary production chain appears as the most viable alternative to create a new pathway to the market (Figure 5).

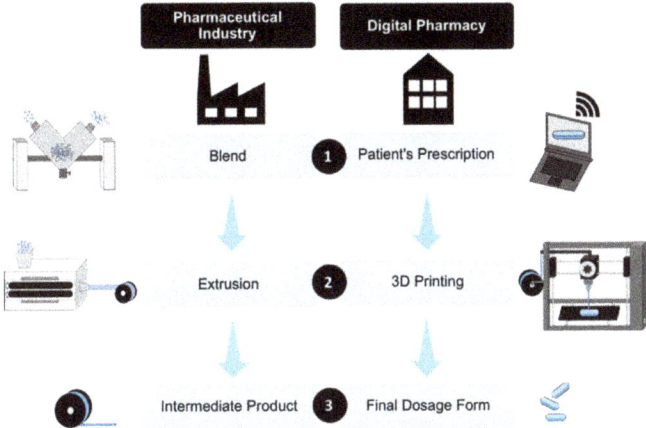

Figure 5. Schematic steps required for the industrial production of filaments and the elaboration of personalized drug delivery device in digital pharmacies.

4.1. Pharmaceutical Industry: Filament Production by Hot-Melt Extrusion

The production of drug-loaded filaments used to feed FDM 3D printers consists of a known process with industrial production profiles. The routine of filament production follows three major steps (Figure 5): First, the components of the batch are mixed, for example in an industrial V-blender. Next, the hot-melt extruder, fed with the component's mixture, produces the drug-loaded filaments by shear and heating. Finally, filament bulk is packed in smaller spools. This intermediate pharmaceutical product should be hermetically packed to prevent product deterioration until it reaches compounding pharmacies.

In the initial phase, the industry dedicated to producing the filaments should conduct research and development for each product, based on the selected drug and desired drug release profile. In this stage, formulation composition, as well as extrusion process, should be defined by following quality-by-design planning [59].

Hot-melt extrusion is an already stablished industrial production process for drugs, but the finer nuances of fabrication of printable filaments needs to be studied further. Thermal and rheological studies should be performed to determine the compatibility between the components and their suitability for the extrusion processing and for the 3D FDM printing. Then, stability studies should be conducted to determine product shelf-life. Different modified drug release profiles can be achieved with the manufacturing of filaments from polymers with delimited solubilization characteristics (fast, slow, pH dependent, etc.).

Filament diameter is crucial for the printing process; improper size can cause the extrudate to clog or lead to a lower feeding rate [60]. Some hygroscopic polymers can cause diameter enlargement, compromising passage of the filament through the printer mechanism [41]. In addition, the heating process could cause diameter deformities, which is why an external pulley with a cooling system should be attached to the extruder dye end in some cases [53].

Routine quality control tests may include organoleptic characteristics, dimensions, rheological properties, tensile strength, thermal behavior, and drug content. In addition, drug release should be evaluated using dissolution apparatus or Franz diffusion cells [61,62].

4.2. Digital Pharmacy: 3D FDM Printing of Personalized Drug Products

Current compounding pharmacies have the necessary infrastructure to produce 3D printed drug delivery devices. In fact, their usual layout is appropriate for FDM pharmaceutical printer installation without requiring major adaptations or masonry work [30]. In a compounding pharmacy, the equipment could be set over existing benches in the solid and liquid preparation rooms, requiring only a power source to operate [63].

The printers could be networked by one or more computers equipped with the necessary interfaces in a central control room. The prescriptions arrive from the doctor's offices remotely, and after authorization of the pharmacy administration and revision by the pharmacist they are sent for impression to one of the available printers. Thus, with investment in the purchase of printers, software, and personnel training, it is possible to transform a regular compounding pharmacy into a digital one. Figure 6 shows the layout of a hypothetical compounding pharmacy with FDM 3D printers.

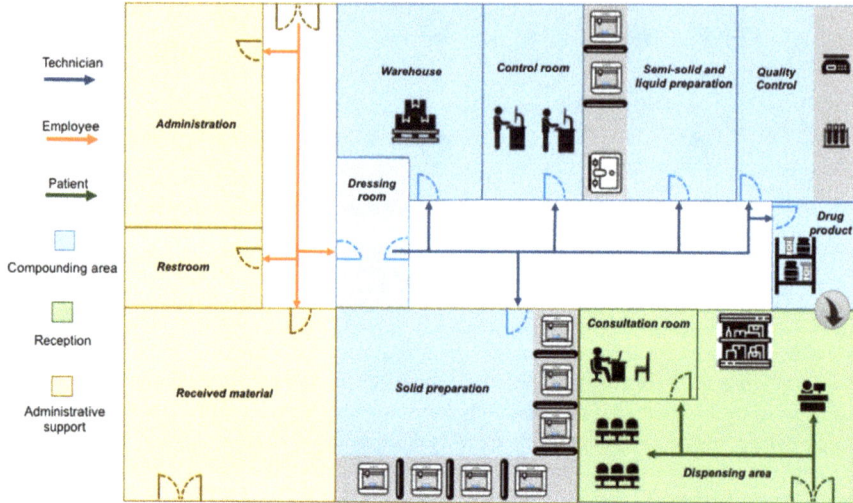

Figure 6. Digital pharmacy layout equipped with FDM 3D printers.

The drug delivery production process should depend on three major steps (Figure 5). First, trained technicians with access to the compounding area should set printer parameters, such as infill, velocity, resolution, temperature, and others, using the pharmaceutical printer software [64]. The information provided by the filament manufacturer and the prescription should serve as guidance. In addition, an adequate design (shape) for the drug delivery device needs to be selected from the database [7]. It is important that the FDM printer is compatible with the filament manufacturer's specifications, so that the intermediate product can be safely used and validated to guarantee process specifications [49].

The second step should include printer preparation and spool attachment. To avoid wastage and exposure of the entire spool to the printing process, the needed amount of filament for the desired batch should be cut and transferred to a smaller spool. The rest of the filament should be hermetically restored using a vacuum device. A FDM-adapted pharmaceutical printer with the modifications discussed before should produce the desired drug tailored for a specific patient. After printing, the product batch should be removed, and the technician could proceed to step three. In this stage, the produced drug delivery device is packed and labeled according to current legislation and dispensed to the patient in the reception room [65]. Before the printer is used again with a different filament, it must be cleaned following a validated method [66].

Besides the use of polymers with characteristics that modulate the drug release from the printed medicine, drug release kinetics can also be directed by adjusting printing parameters such as infill percentage, infill pattern or print speed. In the case of drug combinations in the same dosage form, it is possible to alternate the filaments that are feeding the printer in order to build the desired structure. An innovative approach to do this can be performed with the aid of the Palette 2 device (Mosaic Manufacturing Ltd., Canada), in which different filaments are combined into one that will feed the 3D printer. This filament produced from the merger of numerous fragments of several filaments has its composition defined according to the 3D structure to be built in the printer.

The quality control required for the finished drug products should be the same as those currently required for common solid preparations in compounding pharmacies, which includes average weight and organoleptic characteristics. However, due to the high automation of the 3D printing process and the small number of production steps, there is a lower risk of human error, and consequently a noticeable gain in the safety of printed drug products. Extra tests to determine drug delivery device characteristics, such as hardness, friability, drug content, and drug release could be applied to pilot batches or by sampling in accordance with each country's regulatory demands [37,38,67].

Several studies have shown innumerable cases of intoxication related to the use of medicines produced in compounding pharmacies, resulting, for example, from errors in weighing [18]. This scenario may be overcome by the introduction of 3D printing of drug products. Moreover, new analytical alternatives have been probed for quality control of the 3D printed structures. One is the use of tools with viability for batch-to-batch analysis; such as near infrared spectroscopy, which can perform drug content determinations with a sensitivity comparable to that of chromatographic methods [1]; and terahertz pulsed imaging, which allows acquisition of single-depth scans in a few milliseconds, providing information on the microstructure of the printed devices [54]. These new analytical approaches can make a significant contribution to the safety of printed pharmaceutical preparations.

5. Patent and Regulatory Limitations

In the few last years, 3D printing of medical devices has gained worldwide attention; in particular, products such as cranial implants, artificial knees, and spine prosthesis, which are personalized for each patient. Such products are marketed under current FDA regulations following their similarities with already existing medical devices [68]. In 2017, the FDA released guidelines for the manufacturing of medical devices and implants; however, there are currently no regulatory guidelines on the 3D printing of other products [69,70].

In 2015, the FDA released the first 3D printed drug product, Spritam® (levetiracetam) [71]. This great technological step led to the increase of research on 3D printing technology to produce drug delivery devices. However, despite the fast development in the field, there are legal and regulatory issues that need to be addressed [72].

Spritam® is an oral, fast disintegrating tablet, approved by existing legislation for largescale industrial production. The 3D printing process improved upon a disintegrating process, given that the drug contained a known active pharmaceutical ingredient (levetiracetam), in a permitted dosage (up to 1000 mg) to treat a stablished condition (epilepsy) [20,73]. 3D printing in an industrial scale presents benefits, as the design of complex geometries, when compared to other technologies, such as tableting, is not as competitive. Tailored formulations, 'polypills' and orphan medications produced in small batches can reach places the pharmaceutical industry cannot envision [17].

Many 3D printing technologies have lost their patents over the last decade, which was a decisive factor in making these machines more accessible to the public and to the pharmaceutical industry [56]. The patentability process, especially with regard to intellectual property rights involving 3D printed drug products, should be granted to innovative processes or products. The patent owner has exclusivity on the product or process until the concession expires; in the meantime, other manufactures may not produce, use, or sell without the owner's authorization [74].

Despite this patent right, extemporaneous formulations produced at compounding pharmacies prescribed by professionals to a specific patient are exempted and do not configure patent violation, according to the intellectual property law of several countries, such as UK and Brazil [74]. Unlike in the US and Europe, where compounding pharmacies represent a small share of the market, in Brazil there are about 16,000 compounding pharmacies, which handle more than 60 million prescriptions per year [75]. If the market for compounding pharmacies is not a threat to large pharmaceutical corporations, this technological leap by digital pharmacies can change the global market scenario. However, this could provoke major legal disputes. Other drug delivery technologies already patented and vastly researched on could be rapidly brought back, not because of any drawback of the new technology, but for economic reasons, e.g., microneedles, active drug delivery patches using iontophoresis or sonophoresis [76]. The pharmaceutical industry is known to manage risk by broadening the use of old technologies, instead of accepting novel products. However, the difference here is in the demand chain—not from the industry, which carries the burden of educating and promoting the product; but by patients or healthcare personnel who place demands on small compounding pharmacies; and ultimately on the industry for supply of raw material. Hence, with growing research and small investments by compounding pharmacy owners, the industry might be forced to respond to such demands. The risk then would be consequently diminished, showcasing optimistic prognostics.

6. Conclusions

FDM 3D printing is a versatile technology widely studied for the production of multiple drug delivery devices. Research groups over the world are currently working to identify the nuances of the production process, and despite the great progress made so far, palpable planning to bring these products to life is necessary. The potential of 3D printing for the development of personalized drug products is undeniable; however, machine adaptations are fundamental for proper pharmaceutical use. In addition, a viable production process needs the co-participation of the pharmaceutical industry (to extrude filaments on a large scale), and digital pharmacies (to print drugs according to patient-specific prescriptions). Finally, regulatory and patent agencies should work together with companies to carve a solid path into the market.

Author Contributions: Conceptualization, M.R.P.A., L.L.S.-B. and M.C.-F.; Funding acquisition, L.L.S.-B. and M.C.-F.; Data curation, M.R.P.A., T.G. and M.C.-F.; Supervision, M.C.-F.; Writing—original draft, M.R.P.A., G.M.G. and M.C.-F.; Writing—review & editing, T.G. and G.M.G.

Funding: This research was funded by FAPDF, grant number 193.001741/2017, and CAPES.

Conflicts of Interest: The authors declare no conflict of interest.

References

1. Trenfield, S.J.; Goyanes, A.; Telford, R.; Wilsdon, D.; Rowland, M.; Gaisford, S.; Basit, A.W. 3D printed drug products: Non-destructive dose verification using a rapid point-and-shoot approach. *Int. J. Pharm.* **2018**, *549*, 283–292. [CrossRef] [PubMed]
2. Liang, K.; Carmone, S.; Brambilla, D.; Leroux, J.C. 3D printing of a wearable personalized oral delivery device: A first-in-human study. *Sci. Adv.* **2018**, *4*, eaat2544. [CrossRef]
3. Fu, J.; Yu, X.; Jin, Y. 3D printing of vaginal rings with personalized shapes for controlled release of progesterone. *Int. J. Pharm.* **2018**, *539*, 75–82. [CrossRef]
4. Muwaffak, Z.; Goyanes, A.; Clark, V.; Basit, A.W.; Hilton, S.T.; Gaisford, S. Patient-specific 3D scanned and 3D printed antimicrobial polycaprolactone wound dressings. *Int. J. Pharm.* **2017**, *527*, 161–170. [CrossRef] [PubMed]
5. Goyanes, A.; Det-Amornrat, U.; Wang, J.; Basit, A.W.; Gaisford, S. 3D scanning and 3D printing as innovative technologies for fabricating personalized topical drug delivery systems. *J. Control. Release* **2016**, *234*, 41–48. [CrossRef] [PubMed]
6. Goyanes, A.; Scarpa, M.; Kamlow, M.; Gaisford, S.; Basit, A.; Orlu, M. Patient acceptability of 3D printed medicines. *Int. J. Pharm.* **2017**, *530*, 71–78. [CrossRef] [PubMed]
7. Goyanes, A.; Robles Martinez, P.; Buanz, A.; Basit, A.W.; Gaisford, S. Effect of geometry on drug release from 3D printed tablets. *Int. J. Pharm.* **2015**, *494*, 657–663. [CrossRef]
8. Okwuosa, T.C.; Pereira, B.C.; Arafat, B.; Cieszynska, M.; Isreb, A.; Alhnan, M.A. Fabricating a shell-core delayed release tablet using dual FDM 3D printing for patient-centred therapy. *Pharm. Res.* **2017**, *34*, 427–437. [CrossRef]

9. Gioumouxouzis, C.I.; Baklavaridis, A.; Katsamenis, O.L.; Markopoulou, C.K.; Bouropoulos, N.; Tzetzis, D.; Fatouros, D.G. A 3D printed bilayer oral solid dosage form combining metformin for prolonged and glimepiride for immediate drug delivery. *Eur. J. Pharm. Sci.* **2018**, *120*, 40–52. [CrossRef] [PubMed]
10. Zhang, J.; Yang, W.; Vo, A.Q.; Feng, X.; Ye, X.; Kim, D.W.; Repka, M.A. Hydroxypropyl methylcellulose-based controlled release dosage by melt extrusion and 3D printing: Structure and drug release correlation. *Carbohydr. Polym.* **2017**, *177*, 49–57. [CrossRef] [PubMed]
11. Goyanes, A.; Fina, F.; Martorana, A.; Sedough, D.; Gaisford, S.; Basit, A.W. Development of modified release 3D printed tablets (printlets) with pharmaceutical excipients using additive manufacturing. *Int. J. Pharm.* **2017**, *527*, 21–30. [CrossRef]
12. Goyanes, A.; Buanz, A.B.; Basit, A.W.; Gaisford, S. Fused-filament 3D printing (3DP) for fabrication of tablets. *Int. J. Pharm.* **2014**, *476*, 88–92. [CrossRef]
13. Bloomquist, C.J.; Mecham, M.B.; Paradzinsky, M.D.; Janusziewicz, R.; Warner, S.B.; Luft, J.C.; Mecham, S.J.; Wang, A.Z.; DeSimone, J.M. Controlling release from 3D printed medical devices using CLIP and drug-loaded liquid resins. *J. Control. Release* **2018**, *278*, 9–23. [CrossRef]
14. Ventola, C.L. Medical applications for 3D printing: Current and projected uses. *Pharm. Ther.* **2014**, *39*, 704.
15. Norman, J.; Madurawe, R.D.; Moore, C.M.V.; Khan, M.A.; Khairuzzaman, A. A new chapter in pharmaceutical manufacturing: 3D-printed drug products. *Adv. Drug Deliv. Rev.* **2017**, *108*, 39–50. [CrossRef]
16. Hsiao, W.K.; Lorber, B.; Reitsamer, H.; Khinast, J. 3D printing of oral drugs: A new reality or hype? *Expert Opin. Drug Deliv.* **2018**, *15*, 1–4. [CrossRef]
17. Awad, A.; Trenfield, S.J.; Goyanes, A.; Gaisford, S.; Basit, A.W. Reshaping drug development using 3D printing. *Drug Discov. Today* **2018**, *23*, 1547–1555. [CrossRef]
18. James, K.L.; Barlow, D.; McArtney, R.; Hiom, S.; Roberts, D.; Whittlesea, C. Incidence, type and causes of dispensing errors: A review of the literature. *Int. J. Pharm. Pract.* **2009**, *17*, 9–30. [CrossRef]
19. Palo, M.; Holländer, J.; Suominen, J.; Yliruusi, J.; Sandler, N. 3D printed drug delivery devices: Perspectives and technical challenges. *Expert Rev. Med. Devices* **2017**, *14*, 685–696. [CrossRef]
20. Lim, S.H.; Kathuria, H.; Tan, J.J.Y.; Kang, L. 3D printed drug delivery and testing systems—A passing fad or the future? *Adv. Drug Deliv. Rev.* **2018**, *132*, 139–168. [CrossRef]
21. Trenfield, S.J.; Awad, A.; Goyanes, A.; Gaisford, S.; Basit, A.W. 3D Printing Pharmaceuticals: Drug Development to Frontline Care. *Trends Pharmacol. Sci.* **2018**, *39*, 440–451. [CrossRef] [PubMed]
22. Cunha-Filho, M.; Araújo, M.R.P.; Gelfuso, G.M.; Gratieri, T. FDM 3D printing of modified drug-delivery systems using hot melt extrusion: A new approach for individualized therapy. *Ther. Deliv.* **2017**, *8*, 957–966. [CrossRef] [PubMed]
23. Tan, D.K.; Maniruzzaman, M.; Nokhodchi, A. Advanced Pharmaceutical Applications of Hot-Melt Extrusion Coupled with Fused Deposition Modelling (FDM) 3D Printing for Personalised Drug Delivery. *Pharmaceutics* **2018**, *10*, 203. [CrossRef] [PubMed]
24. Long, J.; Gholizadeh, H.; Lu, J.; Bunt, C.; Seyfoddin, A. Application of fused deposition modelling (FDM) method of 3D printing in drug delivery. *Curr. Pharm. Des.* **2017**, *23*, 433–439. [CrossRef] [PubMed]
25. Prasad, L.K.; Smyth, H. 3D Printing technologies for drug delivery: A review. *Drug. Dev. Ind. Pharm.* **2016**, *42*, 1019–1031. [CrossRef] [PubMed]
26. Moulton, S.E.; Wallace, G.G. 3-dimensional (3D) fabricated polymer based drug-delivery systems. *J. Control. Rel.* **2014**, *193*, 27–34. [CrossRef]
27. Jamróz, W.; Szafraniec, J.; Kurek, M.; Jachowicz, R. 3D Printing in Pharmaceutical and Medical Applications—Recent Achievements and Challenges. *Pharm. Res.* **2018**, *35*, 176. [CrossRef]
28. Trenfield, S.J.; Madla, C.M.; Basit, A.W.; Gaisford, S. The Shape of Things to Come: Emerging Applications of 3D Printing in Healthcare. In *3D Printing of Pharmaceuticals*, 1st ed.; Basit, A., Gaisford, S., Eds.; Springer: London, UK, 2018; Volume 31, pp. 1–19.
29. Pravin, S.; Sudhir, A. Integration of 3D printing with dosage forms: A new perspective for modern healthcare. *Biomed. Pharmacother.* **2018**, *107*, 146–154. [CrossRef]
30. Sadia, M.; Sósnicka, A.; Arafat, B.; Isreb, A.; Ahmed, W.; Kelarakis, A.; Alhnan, M.A. Adaptation of pharmaceutical excipients to FDM 3D printing for the fabrication of patient-tailored immediate release tablets. *Int. J. Pharm.* **2016**, *513*, 659–668. [CrossRef]

31. Arafat, B.; Qinna, N.; Cieszynska, M.; Forbes, R.T.; Alhnan, M.A. Tailored on demand anti-coagulant dosing: An in vitro and in vivo evaluation of 3D printed purpose-designed oral dosage forms. *Eur. J. Pharm. Biopharm.* **2018**, *128*, 282–289. [CrossRef]
32. Chai, X.; Chai, H.; Wang, X.; Yang, J.; Li, J.; Zhao, Y.; Cai, W.; Tao, T.; Xiang, X. Fused Deposition Modeling (FDM) 3D Printed Tablets for Intragastric Floating Delivery of Domperidone. *Sci. Rep.* **2017**, *7*, 2829. [CrossRef] [PubMed]
33. Goyanes, A.; Wang, J.; Buanz, A.; Martínez-Pacheco, R.; Telford, R.; Gaisford, S.; Basit, A.W. 3D printing of medicines: Engineering novel oral devices with unique design and drug release characteristics. *Mol. Pharm.* **2015**, *12*, 4077–4084. [CrossRef]
34. Kempin, W.; Domsta, V.; Grathoff, G.; Brecht, I.; Semmling, B.; Tillmann, S.; Weitschies, W.; Seidlitz, A. Immediate Release 3D-Printed Tablets Produced Via Fused Deposition Modeling of a Thermo-Sensitive Drug. *Pharm. Res.* **2018**, *35*, 124. [CrossRef] [PubMed]
35. Arafat, B.; Wojsz, M.; Isreb, A.; Forbes, R.T.; Isreb, M.; Ahmed, W.; Arafat, T.; Alhnan, M.A. Tablet fragmentation without a disintegrant: A novel design approach for accelerating disintegration and drug release from 3D printed cellulosic tablets. *Eur. J. Pharm. Sci.* **2018**, *118*, 191–199. [CrossRef]
36. Scoutaris, N.; Ross, S.A.; Douroumis, D. 3D Printed "Starmix" Drug Loaded Dosage Forms for Paediatric Applications. *Pharm. Res.* **2018**, *35*, 34. [CrossRef]
37. Maroni, A.; Melocchi, A.; Parietti, F.; Foppoli, A.; Zema, L.; Gazzaniga, A. 3D printed multi-compartment capsular devices for two-pulse oral drug delivery. *J. Control. Release* **2017**, *268*, 10–18. [CrossRef]
38. Melocchi, A.; Parietti, F.; Maccagnan, S.; Ortenzi, M.A.; Antenucci, S.; Briatico-Vangosa, F.; Maroni, A.; Gazzaniga, A.; Zema, L. Industrial Development of a 3D-Printed Nutraceutical Delivery Platform in the Form of a Multicompartment HPC Capsule. *AAPS. PharmSciTech* **2018**, *19*, 3343–3354. [CrossRef]
39. Smith, D.M.; Kapoor, Y.; Klinzing, G.R.; Procopio, A.T. Pharmaceutical 3D printing: Design and qualification of a single step print and fill capsule. *Int. J. Pharm.* **2018**, *544*, 21–30. [CrossRef] [PubMed]
40. Okwuosa, T.C.; Soares, C.; Gollwitzer, V.; Habashy, R.; Timmins, P.; Alhnan, M.A. On demand manufacturing of patient-specific liquid capsules via co-ordinated 3D printing and liquid dispensing. *Eur. J. Pharm. Sci.* **2018**, *118*, 134–143. [CrossRef]
41. Gioumouxouzis, C.I.; Katsamenis, O.L.; Bouropoulos, N.; Fatouros, D.G. 3D printed oral solid dosage forms containing hydrochlorothiazide for controlled drug delivery. *J. Drug. Deliv. Sci. Technol.* **2017**, *40*, 164–171. [CrossRef]
42. Jamróz, W.; Kurek, M.; Łyszczarz, E.; Szafraniec, J.; Knapik-Kowalczuk, J.; Syrek, K.; Paluch, M.; Jachwicz, R. 3D printed orodispersible films with Aripiprazole. *Int. J. Pharm.* **2017**, *533*, 413–420. [CrossRef]
43. Luzuriaga, M.A.; Berry, D.R.; Reagan, J.C.; Smaldone, R.A.; Gassensmith, J.J. Biodegradable 3D printed polymer microneedles for transdermal drug delivery. *Lab. Chip* **2018**, *18*, 1223–1230. [CrossRef]
44. Davies, M.J.; Costley, E.; Ren, J.; Gibbons, P.; Kondor, A.; Naderi, M. On drug base incompatibilities during extrudate manufacture and fused deposition 3D printing. *J. 3D Print. Med.* **2017**, *1*, 31–47. [CrossRef]
45. Genina, N.; Hollander, J.; Jukarainen, H.; Makila, E.; Salonen, J.; Sandler, N. Ethylene vinyl acetate (EVA) as a new drug carrier for 3D printed medical drug delivery devices. *Eur. J. Pharm. Sci.* **2016**, *90*, 53–63. [CrossRef]
46. Fu, J.; Yin, H.; Yu, X.; Xie, C.; Jiang, H.; Jin, Y.; Sheng, F. Combination of 3D printing technologies and compressed tablets for preparation of riboflavin floating tablet-in-device (TiD) systems. *Int. J. Pharm.* **2018**, *549*, 370–379. [CrossRef] [PubMed]
47. Genina, N.; Boetker, J.P.; Colombo, S.; Harmankaya, N.; Rantanen, J.; Bohr, A. Anti-tuberculosis drug combination for controlled oral delivery using 3D printed compartmental dosage forms: From drug product design to in vivo testing. *J. Control. Release* **2017**, *268*, 40–48. [CrossRef] [PubMed]
48. Goyanes, A.; Fernández-Ferreiro, A.; Majeed, A.; Gomez-Lado, N.; Awad, A.; Luaces-Rodríguez, A.; Gaisford, S.; Aguiar, P.; Basit, A.W. PET/CT imaging of 3D printed devices in the gastrointestinal tract of rodents. *Int. J. Pharm.* **2018**, *536*, 158–164. [CrossRef]
49. Feuerbach, T.; Kock, S.; Thommes, M. Characterisation of fused deposition modeling 3D printers for pharmaceutical and medical applications. *Pharm. Dev. Technol.* **2018**, *23*, 1136–1145. [CrossRef]
50. Alhijjaj, M.; Belton, P.; Qi, S. An investigation into the use of polymer blends to improve the printability of and regulate drug release from pharmaceutical solid dispersions prepared via fused deposition modeling (FDM) 3D printing. *Eur. J. Pharm. Biopharm.* **2016**, *108*, 111–125. [CrossRef]

51. Goyanes, A.; Buanz, A.B.; Hatton, G.B.; Gaisford, S.; Basit, A.W. 3D printing of modified-release aminosalicylate (4-ASA and 5-ASA) tablets. *Eur. J. Pharm. Biopharm.* **2015**, *89*, 157–162. [CrossRef] [PubMed]
52. Kollamaram, G.; Croker, D.M.; Walker, G.M.; Goyanes, A.; Basit, A.W.; Gaisford, S. Low temperature fused deposition modeling (FDM) 3D printing of thermolabile drugs. *Int. J. Pharm.* **2018**, *545*, 144–152. [CrossRef]
53. Melocchi, A.; Parietti, F.; Loreti, G.; Maroni, A.; Gazzaniga, A.; Zema, L. 3D printing by fused deposition modeling (FDM) of a swellable/erodible capsular device for oral pulsatile release of drugs. *J. Drug. Deliv. Sci. Technol.* **2015**, *30*, 360–367. [CrossRef]
54. Markl, D.; Zeitler, J.A.; Rasch, C.; Michaelsen, M.H.; Müllertz, A.; Rantanen, J.; Rades, T.; Bøtker, J. Analysis of 3D Prints by X-ray Computed Microtomography and Terahertz Pulsed Imaging. *Pharm. Res.* **2017**, *34*, 1037–1052. [CrossRef]
55. Cunha-Filho, M.S.; Alvarez-Lorenzo, C.; Martínez-Pacheco, R.; Landin, M. Temperature-sensitive gels for intratumoral delivery of β-lapachone: Effect of cyclodextrins and ethanol. *Sci. World J.* **2012**, *2012*, 126723. [CrossRef]
56. Awad, A.; Trenfield, S.J.; Gaisford, S.; Basit, A.W. 3D printed medicines: A new branch of digital healthcare. *Int. J. Pharm.* **2018**, *548*, 586–596. [CrossRef]
57. Skowyra, J.; Pietrzak, K.; Alhnan, M.A. Fabrication of extended-release patient-tailored prednisolone tablets via fused deposition modelling (FDM) 3D printing. *Eur. J. Pharm. Sci.* **2015**, *68*, 11–17. [CrossRef]
58. Trivedi, M.; Jee, J.; Silva, S.; Blomgren, C.; Pontinha, V.M.; Dixon, D.L.; Van Tassel, B.; Bortner, M.J.; Williams, C.; Gilmer, E.; et al. Additive manufacturing of pharmaceuticals for precision medicine applications: A review of the promises and perils in implementation. *Addit. Manuf.* **2018**, *23*, 319–328. [CrossRef]
59. Do Carmo, A.C.M.; Cunha-Filho, M.; Gelfuso, G.M.; Gratieri, T. Evolution of quality on pharmaceutical design: Regulatory requirement? *Accred. Qual. Assur.* **2017**, *22*, 199–205. [CrossRef]
60. Korte, C.; Quodbach, J. Formulation development and process analysis of drug-loaded filaments manufactured via hot-melt extrusion for 3D-printing of medicines. *Pharm. Dev. Technol.* **2018**, *23*, 1117–1127. [CrossRef]
61. Verstraete, G.; Samaro, A.; Grymonpré, W.; Vanhoorne, V.; Van Snick, B.; Boone, M.N.; Hellemans, T.; Van Hoorebeke, L.; Remon, J.P.; Vervaet, C. 3D printing of high drug loaded dosage forms using thermoplastic polyurethanes. *Int. J. Pharm.* **2018**, *536*, 318–325. [CrossRef]
62. Sadia, M.; Arafat, B.; Ahmed, W.; Forbes, R.T.; Alhnan, M.A. Channelled tablets: An innovative approach to accelerating drug release from 3D printed tablets. *J. Control. Release* **2018**, *269*, 355–363. [CrossRef] [PubMed]
63. Weisman, J.A.; Nicholson, J.C.; Tappa, K.; Jammalamadaka, U.; Wilson, C.G.; Mills, D.K. Antibiotic and chemotherapeutic enhanced three-dimensional printer filaments and constructs for biomedical applications. *Int. J. Nanomed.* **2015**, *10*, 357–370.
64. Pietrzak, K.; Isreb, A.; Alhnan, M.A. A flexible-dose dispenser for immediate and extended release 3D printed tablets. *Eur. J. Pharm. Biopharm.* **2015**, *96*, 380–387. [CrossRef] [PubMed]
65. Goyanes, A.; Kobayashi, M.; Martinez-Pacheco, R.; Gaisford, S.; Basit, A.W. Fused-filament 3D printing of drug products: Microstructure analysis and drug release characteristics of PVA-based caplets. *Int. J. Pharm.* **2016**, *514*, 290–295. [CrossRef]
66. Melocchi, A.; Parietti, F.; Maroni, A.; Foppoli, A.; Gazzaniga, A.; Zema, L. Hot-melt extruded filaments based on pharmaceutical grade polymers for 3D printing by fused deposition modeling. *Int. J. Pharm.* **2016**, *509*, 255–263. [CrossRef] [PubMed]
67. Okwuosa, T.C.; Stefaniak, D.; Arafat, B.; Isreb, A.; Wan, K.W.; Alhnan, M.A. A lower temperature FDM 3D printing for the manufacture of patient-specific immediate release tablets. *Pharm. Res.* **2016**, *33*, 2704–2712. [CrossRef] [PubMed]
68. Di Prima, M.; Coburn, J.; Hwang, D.; Kelly, J.; Khairuzzaman, A.; Ricles, L. Additively manufactured medical products—The FDA perspective. *3D Print Med.* **2016**, *2*, 1. [CrossRef]
69. Madla, C.M.; Trenfield, S.J.; Goyanes, A.; Gaisford, S.; Basit, A.W. 3D printing technologies, implementation and regulation: An overview. In *3D Printing of Pharmaceuticals*, 1st ed.; Basit, A., Gaisford, S., Eds.; Springer: London, UK, 2018; Volume 31, pp. 21–40.
70. Economidou, S.N.; Lamprou, D.A.; Douroumis, D. 3D printing applications for transdermal drug delivery. *Int. J. Pharm.* **2018**, *544*, 415–424. [CrossRef]

71. Alhnan, M.A.; Okwuosa, T.C.; Sadia, M.; Wan, K.W.; Ahmed, W.; Arafat, B. Emergence of 3D printed dosage forms: Opportunities and challenges. *Pharm. Res.* **2016**, *33*, 1817–1832. [CrossRef]
72. Jose, P.A. 3D printing of pharmaceuticals—A potential technology in developing personalized medicine. *Asian J. Pharm. Dev.* **2018**, *6*, 46–54. [CrossRef]
73. Zema, L.; Melocchi, A.; Maroni, A.; Gazzaniga, A. Three-Dimensional Printing of Medicinal Products and the Challenge of Personalized Therapy. *J Pharm Sci.* **2017**, *106*, 1697–1705. [CrossRef] [PubMed]
74. Stones, J.A.; Jewell, C.M. 3D printing of pharmaceuticals: Patent and regulatory challenges. *Pharm. Pat. Anal.* **2017**, *6*, 145–149. [CrossRef] [PubMed]
75. Souza, R.P.; Guedes, H. The Compounding Pharmacy in Brazil: A Pharmacist's Perspective. *Int. J. Pharm. Compd.* **2009**, *13*, 87. [PubMed]
76. Karpiński, T.M. Selected Medicines Used in Iontophoresis. *Pharmaceutics* **2018**, *10*, 204. [CrossRef] [PubMed]

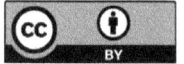

© 2019 by the authors. Licensee MDPI, Basel, Switzerland. This article is an open access article distributed under the terms and conditions of the Creative Commons Attribution (CC BY) license (http://creativecommons.org/licenses/by/4.0/).

MDPI
St. Alban-Anlage 66
4052 Basel
Switzerland
Tel. +41 61 683 77 34
Fax +41 61 302 89 18
www.mdpi.com

Pharmaceutics Editorial Office
E-mail: pharmaceutics@mdpi.com
www.mdpi.com/journal/pharmaceutics

www.ingramcontent.com/pod-product-compliance
Lightning Source LLC
LaVergne TN
LVHW070124100526
838202LV00016B/2228